Cancer prevention and screening

D1333824

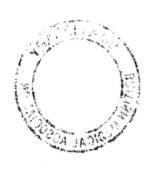

Cancer prevention and screening

Concepts, principles and controversies

EDITED BY

Rosalind A. Eeles, MA (Cantab), PhD, FRCP, FRCR, FMedSci

Professor of Oncogenetics and Team Leader in Oncogenetics,
The Institute of Cancer Research,
Honorary Consultant in Cancer Genetics and Clinical Oncology,
The Royal Marsden NHS Foundation Trust, London, UK

Christine D. Berg, MD

Special Advisor to the Director,
Division of Cancer Epidemiology and Genetics,
National Cancer Institute,
National Institutes of Health, Maryland, USA

Jeffrey S. Tobias, MA (Cantab), MD, FRCP, FRCR

Professor of Cancer Medicine,
Department of Oncology,
University College London,
Honorary Consultant,
University College Hospital Foundation Trust,
London, UK

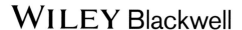

WILEY Blackwell

Registered Office(s)
John Wiley & Sons, Inc., 111 River Street, Hoboken, NJ 07030, USA
John Wiley & Sons Ltd, The Atrium, Southern Gate, Chichester, West Sussex, PO19 8SQ, UK

Editorial Office
9600 Garsington Road, Oxford, OX4 2DQ, UK

For details of our global editorial offices, customer services, and more information about Wiley products visit us at www.wiley.com.

Wiley also publishes its books in a variety of electronic formats and by print-on-demand. Some content that appears in standard print versions of this book may not be available in other formats.

Library of Congress Cataloging-in-Publication Data

Names: Eeles, Rosalind A., 1959– editor. | Berg, Christine D., editor. | Tobias, Jeffrey S., editor.
Title: Cancer prevention and screening : concepts, principles and controversies /
   edited by Rosalind A. Eeles, Christine D. Berg, Jeffrey S. Tobias.
Description: Hoboken, NJ : Wiley, 2018. | Includes bibliographical references and index. |
Identifiers: LCCN 2018007656 (print) | LCCN 2018009190 (ebook) | ISBN 9781118991022 (pdf) |
   ISBN 9781118991060 (epub) | ISBN 9781118990872 (paperback : alk. paper)
Subjects: | MESH: Neoplasms–prevention & control | Mass Screening–methods | Global Health |
   Patient Education as Topic
Classification: LCC RC268 (ebook) | LCC RC268 (print) | NLM QZ 250 | DDC 616.99/4052–dc23
LC record available at https://lccn.loc.gov/2018007656

Cover design: Wiley
Cover image: Mesh Figures gouache on paper, 2004 © Michael Peckham

Set in 9/12pt Meridien by SPi Global, Pondicherry, India

Printed in Singapore by C.O.S. Printers Pte Ltd

10 9 8 7 6 5 4 3 2 1

Contents

List of contributors

Christine D. Berg
Special Advisor to the Director, Division of Cancer Epidemiology and Genetics, National Cancer Institute, National Institutes of Health, Maryland, USA

Otis W. Brawley
Chief Medical Officer, American Cancer Society, Georgia, USA

Richard J. Bryant
Cancer Research UK, Royal College of Surgeons of England Clinician Scientist Fellow, Nuffield Department of Surgical Sciences, Oxford Cancer Research Centre, University of Oxford;
Honorary Consultant Urological Surgeon, Department of Urology, Oxford University Hospitals NHS Foundation Trust, Oxford, UK

John Burn
Professor, Institute of Genetic Medicine, International Centre for Life, Newcastle University, UK

Hilary Burton
Director, PHG Foundation, Cambridge, UK

Pankaj Chaturvedi
Professor, Head & Neck Surgery, Tata Memorial Hospital, Mumbai, India

Susmita Chowdhury
Project Manager and Research Associate, West Suffolk NHS Foundation Trust; PHG Foundation, Cambridge, UK

Jessica S. Donington
Associate Professor, Department of Cardiothoracic Surgery, NYU School of Medicine, New York, USA

Louise S. Donnelly
Research Fellow, Genesis Breast Cancer Prevention Centre, University Hospital of South Manchester NHS Trust, Wythenshawe, UK

Rosalind A. Eeles
Professor of Oncogenetics and Team Leader in Oncogenetics, The Institute of Cancer Research, Honorary Consultant in Cancer Genetics and Clinical Oncology, The Royal Marsden NHS Foundation Trust, London, UK

Mark Elwood
Professor of Cancer Epidemiology, School of Population Health, University of Auckland, New Zealand

D. Gareth Evans
Professor of Medical Genetics, Genesis Breast Cancer Prevention Centre, University Hospital of South Manchester NHS Trust, Wythenshawe, UK; The Christie NHS Foundation Trust & Institute of Cancer Sciences; Manchester Centre for Genomic Medicine, St Mary's Hospital, Manchester Academic Health Sciences Centre (MAHSC), Institute of Human Development, University of Manchester, UK

Kwun M. Fong
Director, University of Queensland Thoracic Research Centre, and Department of Thoracic Medicine, The Prince Charles Hospital, Brisbane, Australia

Apurva Garg
Senior Research Fellow, Head & Neck Surgery, Tata Memorial Hospital, Mumbai, India

Aleksandra Gentry-Maharaj
Trial Coordinator, Gynaecological Cancer
Research Centre, UCL, London, UK

Fiona J. Gilbert
Professor of Radiology, University of
Cambridge, School of Clinical Medicine;
Honorary Consultant Radiologist,
University Hospitals NHS Foundation Trust,
Addenbrooke's Hospital, Cambridge, UK

Michelle Griffin
Honorary Clinical Fellow, Gynaecological
Cancer Research Centre, UCL, London, UK

Andrew E. Grulich
Professor and Head, HIV Epidemiology and
Prevention Program, Kirby Institute,
University of New South Wales, Sydney,
Australia

Alison Hall
Head of Humanities, PHG Foundation,
Cambridge, UK

Freddie C. Hamdy
Professor, Nuffield Department of Surgical
Sciences, Oxford Cancer Research Centre,
University of Oxford; Department of Urology,
Oxford University Hospitals NHS Foundation
Trust, Oxford, UK

Michelle N. Harvie
Research Dietitian, Genesis Breast Cancer
Prevention Centre, University Hospital of
South Manchester NHS Trust, Wythenshawe,
UK

Richard J. Hillman
Associate Professor, HIV, Immunology and
Infectious Diseases, St Vincent's Hospital,
Sydney, Australia

Jonah Himelfarb
Internal Medicine Resident, Division
of Hematology/Oncology, Genetics and
Genome Biology Program, The Hospital for
Sick Children; Department of Pediatrics,
University of Toronto, Ontario, Canada

Margaret G. House
Nurse Consultant, National Cancer Institute,
Rockville, MD, USA

Anthony Howell
Professor in Breast Oncology, Genesis Breast
Cancer Prevention Centre, University
Hospital of South Manchester NHS Trust,
Wythenshawe; The Christie NHS Foundation
Trust & Institute of Cancer Sciences,
University of Manchester, UK

Sacha J. Howell
Senior Clinical Lecturer, Genesis Breast
Cancer Prevention Centre, University
Hospital of South Manchester NHS Trust,
Wythenshawe; The Christie NHS Foundation
Trust & Institute of Cancer Sciences,
University of Manchester, UK

Robert A. Huddart
Professor of Urological Cancer, The Institute
of Cancer Research, London, UK

Ashfaq Khan
Consultant and Head of Colposcopy Service,
Whittington Hospital, and Senior Clinical
Lecturer, UCL Medical School, London, UK

Fleur Kilburn-Toppin
Consultant Radiologist, University of
Cambridge, School of Clinical Medicine;
University Hospitals NHS Foundation Trust,
Addenbrooke's Hospital, Cambridge, UK

Jessica Kirby
Senior Health Information Manager, Cancer
Research UK, London, UK

Eric A. Klein
Chairman, Glickman Urological and
Kidney Institute, Cleveland Clinic,
Cleveland, OH, USA

Harry J de Koning
Professor of Evaluation of Screening,
Department of Public Health, Erasmus
Medical Centre, Rotterdam, The Netherlands

Evan Kovac
Urologic Oncology Fellow, Glickman
Urological and Kidney Institute, Cleveland
Clinic, Cleveland, OH, USA

Kevin Litchfield
Division of Genetics and Epidemiology, The
Institute of Cancer Research; MRC Skills
Development Fellow (Bioinformatics),
Translational Cancer Therapeutics
Laboratory, The Francis Crick Institute,
London, UK

David Malkin
Director, Cancer Genetics Program, Staff
Oncologist, Senior Scientist, Genetics &
Genome Biology Program, The Hospital for
Sick Children, Department of Pediatrics,
University of Toronto, Ontario, Canada

Laura A.V. Marlow
Research Associate, Cancer Research
UK Health Behaviour Research Centre,
Department of Epidemiology & Public
Health, UCL, London, UK

Aileen Marshall
Consultant in Hepatology, The Royal Free
Sheila Sherlock Liver Centre, and UCL
Institute of Liver and Digestive Health,
Royal Free Hospital, London, UK

Henry M. Marshall
Clinical Academic Fellow, University of
Queensland Thoracic Research Centre,
and Department of Thoracic Medicine,
The Prince Charles Hospital, Brisbane,
Australia

Usha Menon
Research Group Lead, Gynaecological Cancer
Research Centre, UCL, London, UK

Tim Meyer
Professor, Department of Oncology, UCL
Medical School, and UCL Cancer Institute,
London, UK

Sabina Musovic
Research Data Coordinator, Department
of Cardiothoracic Surgery, NYU School of
Medicine, New York, USA

Donald Maxwell Parkin
Honorary Senior Research Fellow, Nuffield
Department of Public Health, University of
Oxford, UK

Howard L. Parnes
Chief, National Cancer Institute, Rockville,
MD, USA

Harvey I. Pass
Stephen E. Banner Professor of Thoracic
Oncology, Department of Cardiothoracic
Surgery, NYU School of Medicine, New York,
USA

Julietta Patnick
Visiting Professor, Cancer Screening,
University of Oxford, UK

Paul Pharoah
Professor of Cancer Epidemiology, Centre for
Cancer Genetic Epidemiology, University of
Cambridge, Cambridge, UK

Isobel M. Poynten
Senior Lecturer, HIV Epidemiology and
Prevention Program, Kirby Institute,
University of New South Wales, Sydney,
Australia

Linda Rabeneck
Vice President, Institute for Clinical
Evaluative Sciences; Cancer Care Ontario;
Department of Medicine, Institute of Health
Policy, Management and Evaluation,
and Dalla Lana School of Public Health,
University of Toronto, Toronto, Canada

David F. Ransohoff
Professor of Medicine, Division of
Gastroenterology and Hepatology,
Department of Medicine; Clinical
Professor of Epidemiology, Department of
Epidemiology, University of North Carolina,
Chapel Hill, NC, USA

Andrew G. Renehan
Professor of Cancer Studies and Surgery,
Division of Cancer Sciences, School of
Medical Sciences, University of Manchester;
Manchester Cancer Research Centre and
NIHR Manchester Biomedical Research
Centre; Colorectal and Peritoneal Oncology
Centre, The Christie NHS Foundation Trust,
Manchester, UK

Monique J. Roobol
Professor in Decision making in Urology,
Erasmus University Medical Center,
Rotterdam, Netherlands

Arlinda Ruco
Health Services Researcher, Institute of
Health Policy, Management and Evaluation,
University of Toronto; Department of
Surgery, St. Michael's Hospital, Canada

Jonathan M. Samet
Dean and Professor, Colorado School of
Public Health, Aurora, USA

Valérie D.V. Sankatsing
Department of Public Health, Erasmus
Medical Center, Rotterdam, The Netherlands

Rajiv Sarin
Professor, Radiation Oncology & Cancer
Genetics, Tata Memorial Hospital,
Mumbai, India

Peter David Sasieni
Director of King's Clinical Trials Unit, School
of Cancer and Pharmaceutical Sciences,
King's College London, UK

Joanna Sesti
Thoracic and Cardiac Surgeon, Department
of Cardiothoracic Surgery, NYU School of
Medicine, New York, USA

Harsh Sheth
Research Associate, Institute of Genetic
Medicine, International Centre for Life,
Newcastle University, UK

Albert Singer
Emeritus Professor of Gynaecological
Research, Institute for Women's Health,
UCL, London, UK

Terry Slevin
Director, Education and Research, Cancer
Council of Western Australia, Perth,
Australia

Andrew J. Stephenson
Director, Glickman Urological and Kidney
Institute, Cleveland Clinic, Cleveland, OH,
USA

Jeffrey S. Tobias
Professor of Cancer Medicine, Department
of Oncology, University College London;
Honorary Consultant, University College
Hospital Foundation Trust, London, UK

Clare Turnbull
Professor of Genomic Medicine, William
Harvey Research Institute, Queen Mary
University; Senior Researcher, Division of
Genetics and Epidemiology, The Institute
of Cancer Research; Honorary Consultant
in Clinical Genetics, Department of Clinical
Genetics, Guy's and St Thomas' NHS
Foundation Trust, London, UK

Timothy J. Underwood
Associate Professor in Surgery, Cancer
Sciences Unit, Faculty of Medicine,
University of Southampton, UK

Jane Wardle
(now deceased) Formerly:
Professor, Cancer Research UK Health
Behaviour Research Centre, Department of
Epidemiology & Public Health, UCL,
London, UK

Sarah Woolnough
Executive Director of Policy and
Information, Cancer Research UK,
London, UK

Foreword

Saving lives, saving money, and reducing the huge physical and emotional toll of cancer – the potential gains that can be made through successful cancer prevention and screening should not be underestimated. In the UK, 4 in 10 cancer cases could be prevented, mostly through modifying aspects of our lifestyles which we have the ability to change. Thousands of lives each year are saved through the existing cancer screening programmes. However, there is much scope for improvement, as set out in the chapters in this book.

New screening modalities and refinements to existing screening technologies are in development, which could help save even more lives if the evidence becomes strong enough to support their implementation. More sophisticated risk stratification could lead to tailored screening approaches for individuals or groups, maximizing their efficacy. While these developments hold much promise, research continues to highlight the unintended consequences of screening, and the need for new approaches to minimize harms, as well as clear communication to enable informed decision-making. Public perceptions of screening are extremely positive, but these strong views should not sway a carefully considered and evidence-based approach to screening policy-making.

Legislative changes such as the standardized packaging of cigarettes, and major developments like human papilloma virus vaccination, offer much hope for cancer prevention. But still there are many untapped opportunities. Political discourse on obesity remains predominantly focused on individual choice. We need also to address our obesogenic environment and the influence of industry, while waistlines continue to grow rapidly. The question is, can lessons from tobacco control be transferred to addressing the more complex challenge of obesity?

Our understanding of how and when to deliver health messages for greatest impact is growing, so continued research into successful behaviour change interventions, and making the most of 'teachable moments', should prove fruitful. And as we gain more insight into individual risk prediction, this information can increasingly be used to help target prevention – whether lifestyle or medical – to those who will benefit the most. Successful cancer prevention requires upfront investment, but the large pay-off in savings on cancer care and treatment makes investment in prevention a prudent long-term approach.

Globally, cancer is becoming an extremely important health problem, including in countries where it has historically not been considered a priority. Increases in longevity, together with high tobacco use and the growing prevalence of obesity, have all contributed to rapidly rising cancer rates in many low-income countries with scarce resources for treatment. Prevention, therefore, is essential.

Cancer prevention and screening are central to Cancer Research UK's work. Our empowering, accessible, and engaging public information helps raise awareness of the links between lifestyle choices and cancer risk, and our community-based Roadshow takes nurses into the heart of deprived communities to deliver life-saving messages with impact. We work with general practitioners and a wide range of health professionals to train, inform, and raise confidence in talking about cancer prevention and screening with patients. We successfully influence for policy changes and government activity to support healthy lifestyles and world-class, evidence-based screening programmes.

But effective action on prevention and screening requires many actors working together. From the health professional with a patient, to the marketing we are all exposed to in daily life, nobody can prevent cancer alone. My hope is that increased understanding of the issues surrounding cancer prevention and screening can lead to more effective collaboration and action on these essential issues, and many more lives saved. The potential gains, nationally and globally, are immeasurable.

Sir Harpal S. Kumar
Chief Executive, Cancer Research UK

Prologue

The multitude of different diseases which are generally known by the single word 'cancer' continue to plague humankind. As causes of early mortality such as infectious diseases and malnutrition are increasingly brought further under control even in the developing world, life expectancies are beginning to increase globally and in all probability this trend will continue. So we can realistically expect that the incidence of cancer, for the most part closely associated with increasing age, will continue to grow.

By contrast, however, now that we are developing effective preventive strategies such as tobacco cessation and vaccination against oncogenic viruses, coupled with increasingly successful effective screening methods for many malignancies, there are encouraging signs that many of the major cancers are now capable of being prevented, or at least detected earlier, with an increased cure rate as a result. As editors, we felt it would be timely to produce a book which would address these exciting advances in greater detail, in these critically important fields of prevention and screening. One of our key objectives was to provide a truly global perspective, as in our interconnected world the patients we see are from many highly disparate backgrounds, and the medical and scientific communities worldwide can of course learn so much from each other.

We realize that this is a rapidly evolving field. We have chosen internationally recognized experts who present here their insights and opinions in their particular area of focus. As with any book in an area such as this, advances may possibly outpace the accumulation and subsequent publishing of the chapters. Nonetheless, we have great confidence that our chosen chapter authors are well aware of this inevitability and of the current trends well in advance of them becoming common knowledge. We thank all of them most sincerely for their time and expertise and also for their patience in putting up with the revisions which are – invariably – an intrinsic part of any such endeavour. We hope that this book will be of great interest to professionals in many fields of care, from primary care to policymakers. We are also immensely grateful to Sir Harpal Kumar, Chief Executive Officer of the UK's largest charity, Cancer Research UK, who graciously agreed to write a foreword for us, and to Prof. Sir Michael Peckham, who after a distinguished and varied career as an oncologist and senior academic has now become an acclaimed artist, and kindly allowed us to use one of his striking images for our book cover.

During the gestation of the book our esteemed colleague Prof. Jane Wardle passed away; her contribution to the field of cancer awareness was internationally recognized and we are very privileged that she worked with us as part of this project.

Finally, we would like to thank Dr Michael Sandberg, General Practitioner, London, UK for helpful comments and the editorial and production staff at Wiley-Blackwell for their dedication, assistance, and foresight in helping us along at every stage of what proved to be a very large project.

We hope you will enjoy reading the book and will learn from it as much as we have done while assembling it.

Rosalind A. Eeles
Christine D. Berg
Jeffrey S. Tobias

CHAPTER 1

Global perspectives surrounding cancer prevention and screening

Peter David Sasieni[1] and Donald Maxwell Parkin[2]

[1] School of Cancer and Pharmaceutical Sciences, King's College London, UK
[2] Nuffield Department of Public Health, University of Oxford, UK

SUMMARY BOX

- The primary approach to cancer control will always be the provision of basic treatment and care. It is inconceivable that this would not be the case because of the immediacy of caring for a sick patient. Without treatment, increased awareness, early diagnosis, and screening are pointless.

- Globally, the biggest challenges and greatest successes come from tobacco control and vaccination (against hepatitis B virus and human papilloma virus).

- Although not currently associated with any concerted global action, obesity and alcohol control are the next most important challenges for cancer prevention.

- Cervical screening is the exemplar of a simple test with the potential to prevent the majority of a particular cancer. Even so, cervical cancer remains a major health problem in most low-income countries.

- Most other forms of cancer screening rely on early detection of invasive cancer and their widespread introduction has been restricted to countries with facilities for diagnosis and treatment.

- Screening for early cancers relies on expensive technologies; attempts to use cheap and simple tests have not been successful at a national population level.

- Undoubtedly, early diagnosis of cancer has a large impact on morbidity and survival (and subsequent mortality). There is evidence from developed countries that stage distribution has improved over time (more early-stage disease with a subsequent decline in late stage at presentation). Today, stage distribution in low- and middle-income countries lags behind that of high-income countries.

- Stage at diagnosis can be improved by awareness campaigns, but only when care is available, accessible, and affordable.

Cancer Prevention and Screening: Concepts, Principles and Controversies, First Edition.
Edited by Rosalind A. Eeles, Christine D. Berg, and Jeffrey S. Tobias.
© 2019 John Wiley & Sons, Inc. Published 2019 by John Wiley & Sons, Inc.

Principles of cancer control strategy

Noncommunicable diseases, including cancer, are a current challenge to health services, and one which will increase with the ageing of the world population and changes in lifestyles [1]. The World Health Organization (WHO) strategy is to promote National Cancer Control Programmes (NCCPs) as the most effective approach for reducing the morbidity and mortality from cancer [2]. The development of an NCCP requires adequate information in order to evaluate the nature and magnitude of the cancer burden (and the availability of health-care infrastructure), as well as the potential impact of the various possible strategies in prevention, early diagnosis/screening, treatment, and palliative care.

Prevention of cancer has to be set within the context of prevention of other noncommunicable diseases, because they have many (but not all) risk factors in common, notably those that are lifestyle related, such as smoking, alcohol, diet, overweight/obesity, and lack of physical exercise. We do not, in this chapter, discuss biomedical approaches to prevention (medication, surgery), because globally they have no role at present.

Early diagnosis is a public and health professional awareness activity, to encourage people to recognize early signs of the cancer and to seek prompt medical attention. Screening involves encouraging asymptomatic individuals to undergo tests to detect early cancer, or precancerous states. Both early diagnosis and screening have to be set within an existing health infrastructure that provides adequate resources for the management of detected cancers (without which such programmes would be ineffective). Because of the considerable resources involved, population screening programmes should be undertaken only when the prevalence of the disease to be detected is high enough to justify the effort and costs of screening, and where resources (personnel, equipment, etc.) are sufficient to cover diagnosis, treatment, and follow-up of those with abnormal results.

Magnitude of the problem: Proportion of cancer globally attributable to preventable causes

Noncommunicable diseases accounted for about two-thirds of deaths occurring in the world in 2008 [1]. Considering cancer as a single group, the estimated 7.9 million deaths in that year constituted the leading cause of death (Figure 1.1). In 2012, the most commonly diagnosed cancers were lung cancer (13% of all cancers), breast cancer (11.9%), and colorectal cancer (9.7%); the most common causes of cancer death were lung cancer (19.4% of cancer deaths), liver cancer (9.1%), and stomach cancer (8.8%) [3]. Figure 1.2 shows the numbers of cases and deaths for the most common cancers for males and females.

According to Danaei et al. [4], the major environmental causes of cancer death (in 2001) were tobacco, alcohol, and low consumption of fruit and vegetables.

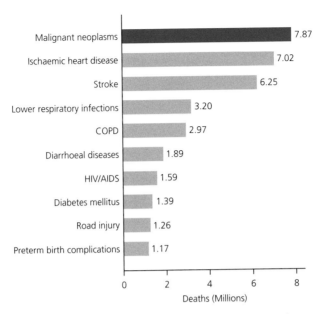

Figure 1.1 The estimated 7.9 million deaths attributed to cancer in comparison to other causes of death. COPD, chronic obstructive pulmonary disease. Source: Global Health Observatory Data Repository.

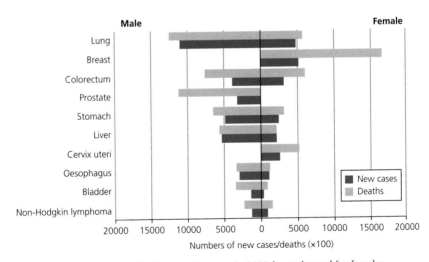

Figure 1.2 The most commonly diagnosed cancers in 2012 for males and for females.

Tobacco smoking is undoubtedly the most important preventable cause of cancer. As estimated by the WHO [5], tobacco was responsible for 22% of the deaths from cancer in 2004 (32% in men, 22% in women), with the major contribution (58% of cancer deaths) coming from lung cancer.

Second in importance in terms of preventable causes of cancer is infection. In 2008, it was estimated that about 16% of the global cancer burden (around 2 million cancers per year) was attributable to infectious agents [6]. The fraction is much larger in low-income than in high-income countries. Each of the three principal infectious agents – *Helicobacter pylori* (stomach cancer), human papilloma virus (HPV; ano-genital, especially cervical, and oropharyngeal cancer), and the hepatitis viruses HBV and HCV (liver cancer) – is responsible for approximately 5% of the global cancer burden. Much smaller fractions are due to Epstein-Barr virus (nasopharynx cancers and some lymphomas) and human herpes virus 8 (Kaposi sarcoma), as well as to parasites such as Schistosoma haematobium (liver cancer) and liver flukes (cholangiocarcinoma).

The International Agency for Research on Cancer (IARC) [7] considers that there is *sufficient evidence* that alcohol consumption causes cancers of the oral cavity, pharynx, larynx, oesophagus, colorectum, liver (hepatocellular carcinoma), and female breast, and also that an association has been observed between alcohol consumption and cancer of the pancreas. The IARC estimated that alcohol was responsible for some 337 400 cancer deaths in 2010, 4.2% of all cancer deaths, with the largest contributions from cancers of the liver and oesophagus (about 23% of such deaths), breast, oral cavity, and colorectum (about 12% each) [7].

Approximately 2.8% of deaths worldwide are attributable to low fruit and vegetable consumption [8]; adequate consumption of fruit and vegetables reduces the risk for cancers of the oral cavity, oesophagus, stomach, and colorectum [9].

Dietary contaminants are a significant problem in some regions; for example aflatoxins, produced by moulds that contaminate cereals and nuts, cause liver cancer, especially in individuals infected with HBV. Aflatoxin has been estimated to have a causative role in 5–28% of all hepatocellular cancers [10].

In 2002, the IARC concluded that overweight and obesity are related to cancers of the colon, endometrium, kidney, and oesophagus (adenocarcinoma), as well as postmenopausal breast cancer. In addition, the report by the World Cancer Research Fund [11] considered that there was convincing evidence for an association with cancers of the pancreas and rectum, and a probable association with cancers of the gall bladder. Overweight and obesity are generally evaluated in terms of body mass index (BMI), with, in 'western' countries, a BMI of 25–29.9 kg/m^2 being considered overweight, and over 30 kg/m^2 obese. Using this definition, Renehan et al. [12] estimated that 5.7% of cancers in Europe in 2008 (3.2% of those in men, 8.6% in women) were caused by overweight/obesity, a figure which is considerably in excess of the 3% estimate (for 2004) for high-income countries by Danaei et al. [4].

Air pollution is known to increase the risk of respiratory (including lung cancer) and heart diseases. In recent years exposure levels have increased significantly in some parts of the world, particularly in rapidly industrializing countries with large populations. The most recent data indicate that in 2010, 223 000 deaths from lung cancer worldwide resulted from air pollution [13];

exposure to outdoor air pollution is also associated with an increased risk of bladder cancer [14].

The IARC has evaluated indoor emissions from household combustion of coal as carcinogenic to humans [7]. In their earlier assessment, Danaei et al. [4] estimated that 1% of lung cancers worldwide could be ascribed to this cause, but it would be a much larger fraction in China, where most such cases occur [15].

The IARC has classified 32 chemical or physical agents and 11 occupations and industries (for which the responsible agent is not specified) as associated with an increased risk of cancer. The most important are asbestos, diesel engine fumes, silica, solar radiation, and second-hand tobacco smoke. It is difficult to arrive at global estimates of cancers attributable to occupation, not least because the numbers of exposed persons in a given country may be totally unknown. Driscoll et al. [16] estimated that there were 102 000 deaths from lung cancer, 43 000 from mesothelioma, and 7000 from leukemia due to occupational carcinogens in 2000 (2.4% of cancer deaths). The total of all occupationally induced cancers would clearly be much greater – estimates for developed countries are in the range of 4–8% [7].

Primary prevention strategies globally

Population attributable fractions give an idea of the numbers (and percentages) of cancers that are, at least in theory, preventable. Almost all of those we have discussed have been the object of preventive efforts, ranging from public education and exhortation, to environmental modification and legislative action at a national or more local level. Globally, there are several well-defined strategies for reducing the burden of cancer.

Tobacco smoking
When the dangers of tobacco smoking became clear, and widely publicized, it was supposed that there would be a reduction in smoking among the public. However, it was soon realized that this was optimistic, and more complex approaches were needed to reduce smoking initiation and promote cessation. Tobacco control programmes are part of national health policy in many countries. Internationally, the WHO initiated a 'framework convention on tobacco control' (FCTC), which became a treaty, signed by member states, in 2003 [17]. By June 2013 there were 176 signatories to its legally binding provisions. These include the following:

Demand reduction
- Article 6. Price and tax measures to reduce the demand for tobacco.
- Article 8. Protection from exposure to tobacco smoke.
- Article 9. Regulation of the contents of tobacco products.
- Article 10. Regulation of tobacco product disclosures.
- Article 11. Packaging and labelling of tobacco products.

- Article 12. Education, communication, training, and public awareness.
- Article 13. Tobacco advertising, promotion, and sponsorship.
- Article 14. Reduction measures concerning tobacco dependence and cessation.

Supply reduction
- Article 15. Illicit trade in tobacco products.
- Article 16. Sales to and by minors.
- Article 17. Provision of support for economically viable alternative activities.

The WHO FCTC also contains provisions for protecting public health policies from commercial and other vested interests in the tobacco industry.

Implementation of the FCTC is monitored by a regular review by the signatories, allowing them to share best practice and present a united, cohesive front against the tobacco industry.

Vaccination
Vaccines are available for two of the important cancer-causing infections: hepatitis B and Human Papilloma Virus (HPV).

Hepatitis B virus (HBV)
HBV is transmitted by percutaneous and permucosal exposure to infected body fluids. The surface antigen of HBV (HBsAg) may be detected in serum 30–60 days following infection and may persist for widely variable periods of time, with some individuals becoming chronic carriers. The prevalence of HBsAg in the general population globally varies considerably: HBsAg prevalences of more than 8% are typical of highly endemic areas, prevalences of 2–7% are found in areas of intermediate endemicity, whereas in areas with low endemicity under 2% of the population is HBsAg positive. Effective vaccines against HBV have been available since the mid-1980s and immunization beginning at birth has been introduced into vaccination schedules in many countries (Figure 1.3). Vaccination results in a dramatic reduction of HBV transmission. This will result in a reduction of HBV-related chronic hepatitis, liver cirrhosis, and hepatocellular carcinoma (HCC). In Taiwan, where infant vaccination was introduced in 1984, there has been a marked reduction in the incidence of HCC in individuals born since that date, compared with preceding birth cohorts [19].

Human papilloma virus (HPV)
Randomized trials have shown the efficacy of two HPV vaccines in preventing infection with virus types 16 and 18 (responsible for about 70% of cervical cancer cases globally) and, more importantly, in preventing cervical intraepithelial neoplasia (CIN) 2 and 3 in females aged 15–25 years [8]. Current vaccines are purely prophylactic; they do not clear existing HPV infection or treat HPV-related disease. They have been approved and are in use in many countries. The primary target group is young adolescent girls (before the onset of sexual activity); current WHO recommendations [20] are for a two-dose schedule if vaccination is initiated

Global Immunization 1989–2016, 3rd dose of Hepatitis B (HepB3) coverage in infants global coverage at 84% in 2016

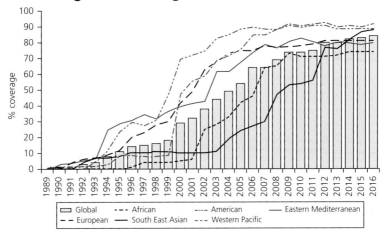

Source: WHO/UNICEF coverage estimates 2016 revision, July 2017.
Immunization Vaccines and Biologicals, (IVB), World Health Organization.
194 WHO Member States. Date of slide: 26 July 2017.

WHO

Immunization coverage with HepB3 in infants, 2016

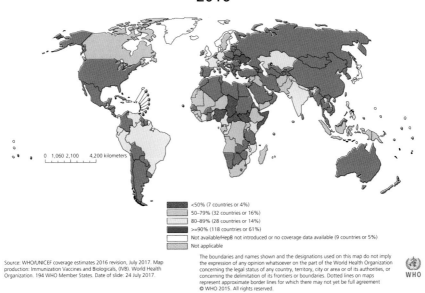

Source: WHO/UNICEF coverage estimates 2016 revision, July 2017. Map production: Immunization Vaccines and Biologicals, (IVB). World Health Organization. 194 WHO Member States. Date of slide: 24 July 2017.

The boundaries and names shown and the designations used on this map do not imply the expression of any opinion whatsoever on the part of the World Health Organization concerning the legal status of any country, territory, city or area or of its authorities, or concerning the delimitation of its frontiers or boundaries. Dotted lines on maps represent approximate border lines for which there may not yet be full agreement
© WHO 2015. All rights reserved.

Figure 1.3 Prevalence of chronic hepatitis B virus infection among adults. Source: Ott 2012 [18]. Reproduced with permission of Elsevier. Note: This map shows the prevalence of chronic HBV infection among adults (aged 19–49 years) globally in 2005; because this analysis grouped countries together regionally, individual country prevalence may be higher or lower than reflected on the map.

prior to age 15 years and a three-dose schedule if immunization is initiated later, but many countries still recommend three doses for all ages.

Routine HPV vaccination has been introduced in many high-income countries (e.g. most of the European Union (EU) [21] and North America [22]), although coverage rates are lower than expected where vaccination is not school based. However, in low- and middle-income countries (where 86% of cervical cancer cases occur), vaccination has often been implemented, if at all, on a limited scale, frequently as demonstration and pilot projects, funded and operated by nongovernmental organizations (NGOs). Certainly, the challenges are greater and include, in addition to financial constraints, problems in reaching girls for two or three doses in settings where school attendance is low and/or irregular [23].

Other prevention programmes

Preventive strategies to reduce cancer incidence are present in many NCCPs, with the emphasis on the exposures most relevant locally. They may include programmes that aim to reduce overweight and obesity (e.g. through reducing consumption of refined sugars), promote exercise and a healthy diet, reduce alcohol consumption (especially by fiscal measures, or reducing access), and salt intake (voluntary or legislative action on the salt content of foods; the World Cancer Research Fund concluded that 'salt is a probable cause of stomach cancer' [24]). None has been the subject of international action like that taken for tobacco and infection.

One area where there is a strong international framework for action is in occupational health. The constituents of the International Labour Organization [25] draw up conventions which are legally binding treaties that may be ratified by member states. Ratifying countries commit to applying the convention in national law and reporting on its application at regular intervals. The conventions most relevant to cancer prevention are as follows:

- The Radiation Protection Convention, 1960 (No. 115), setting out basic requirements with a view to protecting workers against the risks associated with exposure to ionizing radiations.
- The Occupational Cancer Convention, 1974 (No. 139), which provides for the creation of policy to prevent the risks of occupational cancer caused by exposure to chemical and physical agents of various types present in the workplace.
- The Working Environment (Air Pollution, Noise and Vibration) Convention, 1977 (No. 148).
- The Asbestos Convention, 1986 (No. 162), indicating reasonable methods of reducing occupational exposure to asbestos to a minimum.
- The Chemicals Convention, 1990 (No. 170), providing for the adoption and implementation of a coherent policy on safety in the use of chemicals at work (their production, handling, storage, transport, and disposal).

Medication (tamoxifen or aromatase inhibitors for breast; aspirin for bowel) and prophylactic surgery (oophorectomy and/or mastectomy for *BRCA* carriers) as approaches to cancer prevention are not discussed here because of their limited scope globally.

Screening

On a global scale, of all the approaches to cancer control, screening is the least effective. The reasons for this are primarily organizational and monetary. Although screening by NGOs is widespread, there is minimal evidence regarding the effectiveness of these well-meaning interventions, and globally their impact has been minimal.

General principles

Medical screening is an approach to systematically identifying unrecognized disease. In cancer, screening can either be with the intention of identifying cancer early when it has a better chance of being cured, or with the intention of identifying precursor disease that can be treated, thereby preventing it from progressing to cancer.

There is no universally accepted definition of medical screening, but all definitions are based around offering a test to individuals who have not sought medical attention, to identify those who might benefit from further intervention [26]. By definition, testing individuals who consult because of symptoms (no matter how vague) is not screening and will be discussed in the section on early diagnosis.

In 1968, the WHO published the 'Wilson and Jungner criteria' for introducing medical screening [27]:

1 The condition should be an important health problem.
2 There should be a treatment for the condition.
3 Facilities for diagnosis and treatment should be available.
4 There should be a latent stage of the disease.
5 There should be a test or examination for the condition.
6 The test should be acceptable to the population.
7 The natural history of the disease should be adequately understood.
8 There should be an agreed policy on whom to treat.
9 The total cost of finding a case should be economically balanced in relation to medical expenditure as a whole.
10 Case-finding should be a continuous process, not just a 'once and for all' project.

Although the criteria have been debated and modified, they are still widely accepted as sensible. For screening aiming at early diagnosis, it is essential that early-stage disease should have much lower case fatality than late-stage. When screening for cancer precursors, one requires that an affordable, acceptable, and effective treatment of the precursor exists.

When most people think about screening they focus on the screening test, but the existence of an accurate test is just one requirement of a successful screening programme. One needs to consider the whole process, from identifying and contacting the target population, through the screening contact (e.g. obtaining a sample or an image), processing that material (e.g. laboratory testing), communicating the result, arranging triage of those who screen positive, and treatment for those with disease. For many screening modalities, a single screen provides only limited protection and it is necessary to arrange for individuals to be rescreened after a suitable interval (e.g. every three years). All these activities need to be quality assured. The history of screening is plagued by stories such as cervical smears being collected using a finger rather than a spatula; slides being looked at by an inexperienced nonspecialist in a poorly lit room; results not being communicated to the individual screened (or worse, the wrong result being communicated); lack of failsafe measures to ensure that those in need of treatment receive it; and inadequate treatment that causes more harm than good. It should be clear from this discussion that screening is a multidisciplinary activity that should involve a variety of healthcare professionals. All these activities need to be coordinated and that requires considerable infrastructure. Without such an infrastructure, even the best screening test will have little or no impact in reducing morbidity or mortality.

As with all medical interventions, the most robust evidence for the efficacy of screening comes from randomized controlled trials in which it is demonstrated that those offered screening have a lower incidence of or mortality from a particular type of cancer. Nevertheless, it will usually be necessary first to show an impact on surrogate end-points. Occasionally the evidence in favour of screening from nonrandomized trials will be so great that there will no longer be equipoise between screening and no screening.

One surrogate that is often discussed in the context of cancer screening is 'stage shift'. Although a shift in stage is not proof that screening is effective, it is highly unlikely that screening will lead to a reduction in mortality if it does not cause a shift in stage. When claiming a stage shift, many studies simply show that the proportion of cancers diagnosed at early stage has increased. While this is a necessary first step, it is much less powerful than showing that the absolute number of advanced-stage cancers has been decreased. Almost inevitably, early diagnosis through screening will lead to an (initial) increase in early cancers. However, in order for screening to reduce mortality, it must lead to a reduction in advanced cancers.

Another surrogate end-point is survival. If screening for occult cancer does not lead to an improvement in survival post diagnosis, it cannot possibly have an impact on mortality. However, a survival benefit alone is not enough, because screening will create a *lead-time bias* and screen-detected cancers will also have a *length bias* in their survival.

Most cancer screening is offered periodically. The interval between screens should depend on the natural history of the cancer, but will largely come down to cost and what a society is willing to spend for a given improvement in life expectancy or health (often measured in quality-adjusted life years or QALYs). Typically the costs of all screens are very similar, but the benefit from a second screen will be less than that of the first. The first time individuals are screened there will be a lot of occult disease (whether that be precancer or cancer) in the population. The next day, the only undiagnosed disease will be disease that was missed by screening. With time, and no further screening, there will be more incident occult disease. Eventually the prevalence of occult disease will be the same as in an unscreened population. At that point, the benefit of repeat screening should be equal to that of initial screening. The situation may be more complicated, however, because the benefit of screening (with a given test and treatment) depends not only on the prevalence of occult disease, but also on its progressive potential and the likelihood of early intervention being of benefit.

Another cost-effectiveness issue is how long one must wait before benefiting from screening. If screening detects (and then treats) precancer that would on average take 15 years to become invasive and a further 5 years to become fatal, then there is little point in screening someone whose residual life expectancy is only 10 years.

Existing screening options

Specific screening tests will be considered in subsequent chapters. Here, we emphasize the difference between low-tech tests that may require frequent use and high-tech tests that are often expensive and require considerable infrastructure, but can be used infrequently. There are two reasons why low-tech tests often need to be used frequently in order to have a substantial impact. The first is that they may lack sensitivity. That is, on a given test, a theoretically screen-detectable neoplasia may be missed. The second is that the low-tech test may often only be able to detect disease fairly late in its occult natural history. By contrast, one would hope that a high-tech test would be sensitive to very early changes.

The standard method for breast cancer screening is mammography. It is also the only method that has been shown to reduce mortality in randomized controlled trials. Although mammographic screening is standard in many developed countries, other screening modalities which do not require X-ray or other imaging continue to be studied in low- and middle-income countries. Where the infrastructure for mammography is lacking, there is much interest in breast examination performed by a trained health worker. Studies of self-examination have all been negative [28, 29], but many organizations campaign for women to be 'breast aware', which aims at early diagnosis rather than formal self-screening (see the next section). Trials of clinical breast examination are under way in India [30], but whereas such screening can certainly lead to the early diagnosis of breast cancer, it has not yet been demonstrated that it can have an impact on mortality. The Canadian Breast Screening Trials found that physical examination could lead to cancers being screen detected, but also showed that many mammographically detected breast cancers were not palpable. Since, however, they found no mortality benefit of mammography compared to clinical examination, the researchers concluded that the nonpalpable cancers detected by mammography were overdiagnosed. That is, those cancers were indolent and would not have been fatal even in the absence of treatment. A large cluster randomized trial of clinical breast examination (CBE) in the Philippines concluded:

> Although CBE undertaken by health workers seems to offer a cost-effective approach to reducing mortality, the sensitivity of the screening program in the real context was low. Moreover, in this relatively well-educated population, cultural and logistic barriers to seeking diagnosis and treatment persist and need to be addressed before any screening program is introduced. [31]

Cervical screening has seen an explosion of available tests, after many years in which screening was synonymous with the Pap smear. Molecular testing for HPV DNA has become the norm in several developed countries, and visual inspection after application of acetic acid (VIA) is widespread in several low-income countries. Whereas cervical cytology (Pap smear) is subjective and requires repeat screening at relatively short intervals because of poor sensitivity, HPV testing is objective and highly sensitive. Additionally, because HPV infection is the first step in cervical carcinogenesis, a process that typically takes many years, it is sufficient to screen at extended intervals. The downside of HPV testing is that it is less specific (than cytology) for high-grade CIN (the precursor lesion that is treated if found). The majority of women with a cervical HPV would never develop cervical cancer even with no intervention. A drawback of both cytology and HPV testing is that the results are not instant – the collected samples are analysed later in a laboratory. VIA is offered as a simple alternative where facilities are limited and the ability to provide an instant result is considered important. Although a trained nurse can carry out VIA with a couch, a speculum, a simple light source, some acetic acid, and a pair of examination gloves, the results can be very variable. Several studies have shown good sensitivity and specificity for VIA, but it is difficult to quality assure and there has been concern regarding the lack of an independent gold standard to assess sensitivity in some studies. Nevertheless, it is unclear which would be more cost-effective, twice-in-a-lifetime HPV testing (at ages 30 and 45, say) or three-yearly VIA from ages 25 to 60.

The US Preventive Services Task Force recommends colorectal cancer screening for men and women aged 50–75 using high-sensitivity annual fecal occult blood testing (FOBT), five-yearly flexible sigmoidoscopy (with three-yearly FOBT), or ten-yearly colonoscopy. By contrast, the UK National Health Service (NHS) Bowel Cancer Screening Programme offers two-yearly FOBT to men and women aged 60–74 and is piloting the offer of flexible sigmoidoscopy at age 55. Colonoscopy is not offered for general population screening in the UK. The reason that the screening interval (once in a lifetime in the UK) with endoscopy is much longer than with FOBT is because FOBT works primarily by detecting cancer early, whereas during endoscopy all visible polyps are removed, thereby reducing the risk of developing cancer over the next decade. Since flexible sigmoidoscopy only examines the distal bowel, it is often combined with FOBT in order to provide protection against mortality from proximal tumors. Colonoscopy is a much more invasive and expensive procedure compared to sigmoidoscopy, which is why it is only justified in an individual at high risk, either because of a strong family history or a positive result on a simpler screening test. Nevertheless, colonoscopy is still used for bowel screening in some high-income countries.

Screening for other cancer sites is practised in various countries, but is not universally accepted as being effective or cost-effective. Oral screening is mostly by visual inspection of the oral cavity. It has been studied in India [32, 33] and Cuba [34]. The Indian study did not find a reduction in mortality from oral cancer overall, but widely reported a reduction in smokers and drinkers. Undoubtedly, quality assurance is an issue with simple visual inspection. In developed countries there is interest in enhancing visual inspection though use of stains such as acetic acid and devices such as the VELscope Vx, which relies on differential fluorescence of precancerous lesions.

Although incidence rates are declining, gastric cancer remains common in many parts of the world (especially East and Central Asia and South America), and the prognosis when clinically diagnosed is relatively poor. Screening for early disease has been introduced in Japan (barium contrast imaging) and Korea (barium swallow or endoscopy every two years to individuals aged 40 years and older). However, with increasing evidence that treatment of established *H. pylori* infection (by a combination of antibiotics and proton pump inhibitor drugs) can reduce the risk of the disease, there is more interest in programmes of screening for, and treatment of, such infection. At least in relatively affluent countries, these programmes may be cost effective. Currently it is suggested that implementing such programmes should be based on 'local considerations of disease burden, other health priorities, and cost-effectiveness analyses' [35].

Early studies of lung screening using X-rays resulted in downstaging of lung cancer and improved survival, but had no impact on mortality [36]. More recent studies using spiral computed tomography (CT) scanning have shown that this form of screening in individuals at high risk of lung cancer can be effective in reducing lung cancer mortality [37]. Lung screening is still not widely used anywhere and it seems unlikely that it will have a role in cancer control in low- and middle-income countries due to the lack of infrastructure.

Prostate cancer screening remains perhaps the most controversial of screening programmes. While prostate-specific antigen (PSA) testing undoubtedly leads to the diagnosis of occult prostate cancer, many of those cancers are indolent, and many men with screen-detected prostate cancer would have died from other causes before their prostate cancer became symptomatic. Nevertheless, the European Randomized Study of Screening for Prostate Cancer (ERSPC) has shown that screening using PSA testing results in a reduction in mortality from prostate cancer [38]. Of course, it is not the overdiagnosis per se that is so bad, but the side effects of the treatment offered to men with screen-detected cancers.

The harms of screening

Like all medical interventions, screening has the potential to do harm, and it is important to ensure that the benefits exceed the harms before offering screening. The imperative to consider this balance is perhaps even greater for screening than it is for treatment of a medical problem for which the patient has sought help.

The most obvious harm of screening can come from the test itself, but this is very rare, because screening tests with a substantial risk of harm are not used. Harms are more often associated with the work-up of screen-positive individuals. False-positive screening test results are almost always associated with a small amount of harm coming both from anxiety (which will typically resolve after a negative work-up) and the invasive nature of the work-up. In the low-dose CT arm of the National Lung Screening Trial, only 3.8% of individuals with a positive screening had lung cancer; however, the majority of those with a positive screen did not have a biopsy, and of those with a biopsy 53% had cancer [39]. It is also possible that a false-negative test can have a negative impact by providing false reassurance for an individual who subsequently develops symptoms. Such a negative impact can be minimized by providing appropriate information regarding screening with messages such as 'low risk not no risk'.

Targeted screening

From a public health perspective, the greatest gain comes from offering screening to the population at large, but the cost-effectiveness of screening may be improved by offering it only to high-risk groups. Such targeted screening may be offered to groups identified by occupational exposure or to individuals with a strong family history of a particular cancer. Studying the effectiveness of screening in a group already identified as being at very high risk presents a challenge. Globally such targeted screening is of limited importance.

The biggest hurdles to cancer prevention and early diagnosis in low- and middle-income countries relate to social norms and lack of infrastructure rather than the lack of a screening test. As the Breast Health Global Initiative concluded:

> The biggest challenges identified for low-income countries were little community awareness that breast cancer is treatable, inadequate advanced pathology services for diagnosis and staging, and fragmented treatment options, especially for the administration of radiotherapy and the full range of systemic treatments. The biggest challenges identified for middle-resource countries were the establishment and maintenance of data registries, the coordination of multidisciplinary centers of excellence with broad outreach programs to provide community access to cancer diagnosis and treatment, and the resource-appropriate prioritization of breast cancer control programs within the framework of existing, functional health-care systems. [40]

Early diagnosis

Historical importance: Reasons for late presentation

The rationale for early diagnosis is simple: earlier diagnosis improves outcome. Late diagnosis of cancer is thought to relate to inadequate public awareness of cancer signs and symptoms, and barriers (perceived or real) to presentation and diagnosis in the health system.

Many studies have investigated factors related to delayed presentation of cancer patients. Typically, these include demographic factors (age, socio-economic status) as well as disease-related factors (symptoms/signs) [41], and more difficult to define psychological and personality factors [42].

Research in the UK found that (in 2012) the public fear cancer and are largely unwilling to enter a conversation about early diagnosis or vigilance for potential cancer symptoms, and that this is because they feel that there is little to be gained by doing so. Many people see cancer wholly negatively: cure is believed to be unlikely and treatment perceived to be as bad as the disease itself. Individuals likely to present late were characterized as follows:

- Live for Todays
- Unconfident Fatalists
- Balanced Compensators
- Health Conscious Realists
- Hedonistic Immortals.

Approaches to promote early presentation generally aim to increase awareness of the significance of cancer symptoms. A well-known example is the use of the American Cancer Society's seven warning signs (**C**hange in bowel or bladder habits; **A** sore that does not heal; **U**nusual bleeding or discharge; **T**hickening or lump in the breast, testicles, or elsewhere; **I**ndigestion or difficulty swallowing; **O**bvious change in the size, colour, shape, or thickness of a wart, mole, or mouth sore; and **N**agging cough or hoarseness).

Public awareness of the symptoms of cancer is not enough. Early diagnosis requires prompt progression along a pathway from recognition of symptoms through presentation to primary care and general practitioner (GP) referral, to secondary care and prompt diagnosis. The role of primary care delays in late diagnosis globally is unknown, but undoubtedly GPs face a difficult challenge in differentiating between individuals whose vague symptoms are caused by an undiagnosed cancer and the vast majority of their patients. Simple triage tests that can be offered in primary care are desperately needed.

Targeted screening based on nonspecific symptoms

The use of a 'screening test' in those with minor symptoms with the aim of diagnosing cancer while it is treatable by surgery alone (or surgery plus basic radiotherapy) is not screening, because the approach targets symptomatic individuals. The idea is to take a cheap and simple test and to use it in individuals whose risk of having an undiagnosed cancer is low but not negligible. Such an approach has much to offer globally. Currently the only example of such an approach that we know of is the use of PSA testing in men with urinary symptoms. The potential does however exist for offering mammography to women with breast lumps, change in appearance, or discharge from the breast; cervical cytology for women with irregular bleeding or vaginal discharge; and FOBT for middle-aged and elderly adults with persistent change in bowel habits. Such testing should be used to rule in further investigations, not to rule out cancer.

Conclusion

The proportion of cancers attributable to environmental carcinogens (including those in cigarette smoke) and modifiable behaviour globally is substantial, and without concerted efforts in many countries would be even higher. Tobacco control and vaccination are essential components of cancer prevention globally. Increasingly obesity and alcohol control also require coordinated action.

Screening, whether for the identification of precursor disease or the early diagnosis of occult cancer, will most likely always play a relatively minor role in cancer prevention globally, even though it has had substantial impact on specific cancers in many high-income countries. Screening inherently requires a quality-managed system and needs to be continuously monitored to ensure that it remains effective with minimal harms.

The use of drugs such as aspirin and tamoxifen to reduce cancer incidence in high-risk individuals is not discussed in this chapter. Additionally, the use of prophylactic surgery in those at very high risk of a particular cancer is not considered as it is felt to be of little importance globally.

References

1 Alwan, A. and World Health Organization (2011). Global Status Report on Noncommunicable Diseases 2010. Geneva: WHO.

2 World Health Organization (2002). National Cancer Control Programmes: Policies and Managerial Guidelines. Geneva: WHO.

3 Ferlay, J., Soerjomataram, I., Dikshit, R. et al. (2014) Cancer incidence and mortality worldwide: Sources, methods and major patterns in GLOBOCAN 2012. *Int. J. Cancer* 136 (5): E359–E386.

4 Danaei, G., Vander Hoorn, S., Lopez, A.D. et al. (2005) Causes of cancer in the world: Comparative risk assessment of nine behavioural and environmental risk factors. *Lancet* 366 (9499): 1784–1793.

5 World Health Organization (2012). WHO Global Report on Mortality Attributable to Tobacco. Geneva: WHO.

6 de Martel, C., Ferlay, J., Franceschi, S. et al. (2012) Global burden of cancers attributable to infections in 2008: A review and synthetic analysis. *Lancet Oncol.* 13 (6): 607–615.

7 B.W. Stewart and C.W. Wild ed. (2014). World Cancer Report 2014. Lyon: International Agency for Research on Cancer.

8 World Health Organization (2009). Global Health Risks: Mortality and Burden of Disease Attributable to Selected Major Risks. Geneva: WHO.

9 World Health Organization (2003). *Diet, Nutrition and the Prevention of Chronic Diseases: Report of a Joint WHO/FAO Expert Consultation*. New Delhi: Diamond Pocket Books.

10 Pitt, J., Wild, C., Gelderblom, W.C. et al. (2012). Improving public health through mycotoxin control. *World Health* 2012(158): 162.

11 World Cancer Research Fund (2007). Food, Nutrition and the Prevention of Cancer: A Global Perspective. Arlington, VA: American Institute for Cancer Research.

12 Renehan, A.G., Soerjomataram, I., Tyson, M. et al. (2010). Incident cancer burden attributable to excess body mass index in 30 European countries. *Int. J. Cancer* 126 (3): 692–702.

13 Straif, K. and Samet, J. ed. (2014). Air Pollution and Cancer. Lyon: International Agency for Research on Cancer.

14 Loomis, D., Grosse, Y., Lauby-Secretan, B. et al. (2013). The carcinogenicity of outdoor air pollution. *Lancet Oncol.* 14 (13): 1262–1263.

15 Hosgood, H.D., Wei, H., Sapkota, A. et al. (2011). Household coal use and lung cancer: Systematic review and meta-analysis of case-control studies, with an emphasis on geographic variation. *Int. J. Epidemiol.* 40 (3): 719–728.

16 Driscoll, T., Nelson, D.I., Steenland, K. et al. (2005). The global burden of disease due to occupational carcinogens. *Am. J. Ind. Med.* 48 (6): 419–431.

17 World Health Organization (2013). Research for International Tobacco Control: WHO Report on the Global Tobacco Epidemic. Geneva: WHO.

18 Ott, J.J., Stevens, G.A., Groeger, J., and Wiersma, S.T. (2012). Global epidemiology of hepatitis B virus infection: New estimates of age-specific seroprevalence and endemicity. *Vaccine* 30 (12): 2212–2219.

19 Chang, M.H., You, S.L., Chen, C.J. et al. (2009). Decreased incidence of hepatocellular carcinoma in hepatitis B vaccinees: A 20-year follow-up study. *J. Natl Cancer Inst.* 101 (19): 1348–1355.

20 Strategic Advisory Group (2014). Meeting of the Strategic Advisory Group of Experts on Immunization, April 2014 – conclusions and recommendations. *Wkly Epidemiol. Rec.* 89 (21): 221–236.

21 European Centre for Disease Prevention and Control (2012). Introduction of HPV Vaccines in EU Countries – an Update. Stockholm: ECDC. http://ecdc.europa.eu/en/publications/Publications/20120905_GUI_HPV_vaccine_update.pdf (accessed 30 December 2017).

22 Saraiya, M., Steben, M., Watson, M., and Markowitz, L. (2013). Evolution of cervical cancer screening and prevention in United States and Canada: Implications for public health practitioners and clinicians. *Prev. Med.* 57 (5): 426–433.

23 Wigle, J., Coast, E., and Watson-Jones, D. (2013). Human papillomavirus (HPV) vaccine implementation in low and middle-income countries (LMICs): Health system experiences and prospects. *Vaccine* 31 (37): 3811–3817.

24 World Cancer Research Fund/American Institute for Cancer Research (2007). Food, Nutrition, Physical Activity, and the Prevention of Cancer: A Global Perspective. Washington, DC: AICR.

25 International Labour Organization (2014). Conventions and Recommendations. http://ilo.org/global/standards/introduction-to-international-labour-standards/conventions-and-recommendations/lang--en/index.htm (accessed 30 December 2017).

26 Wald, N.J. (2008). Guidance on terminology. *J. Med. Screen.* 15 (1): 50.

27 Wilson, J., and Jungner, G. (1968). Principles and practice of screening for disease. Public Health Papers 34. Geneva: World Health Organization.

28 Thomas, D.B., Gao, D.L., Ray, R.M. et al. (2002). Randomized trial of breast self-examination in Shanghai: Final results. *J. Natl Cancer Inst.* 94 (19): 1445–1457.

29 Semiglazov, V.F., Moiseyenko, V.M., Bavli, J.L. et al. (1992). The role of breast self-examination in early breast cancer detection (results of the 5-years USSR/WHO randomized study in Leningrad). *Eur. J. Epidemiol.* 8 (4): 498–502.

30 Mittra, I., Mishra, G.A., Singh, S. et al. (2010). A cluster randomized, controlled trial of breast and cervix cancer screening in Mumbai, India: Methodology and interim results after three rounds of screening. *Int. J. Cancer* 126 (4): 976–984.

31 Pisani, P., Parkin, D.M., Ngelangel, C. et al. (2006). Outcome of screening by clinical examination of the breast in a trial in the Philippines. *Int. J. Cancer* 118 (1): 149–154.

32 Sankaranarayanan, R., Mathew, B., Jacob, B.J. et al. (2000). Early findings from a community-based, cluster-randomized, controlled oral cancer screening trial in Kerala, India. The Trivandrum Oral Cancer Screening Study Group. *Cancer* 88 (3): 664–673.

33 Sankaranarayanan, R., Ramadas, K., Thara, S. et al. (2013). Long term effect of visual screening on oral cancer incidence and mortality in a randomized trial in Kerala, India. *Oral Oncol.* 49 (4): 314–321.

34 Garrote, L.F., Sankaranarayanan, R., Anta, J.J.L. et al. (1995). An evaluation of the oral cancer control program in Cuba. *Epidemiology* 6 (4): 428–431.

35 IARC *Helicobacter pylori* Working Group (2014). *Helicobacter pylori* Eradication as a Strategy for Preventing Gastric Cancer. Lyon: International Agency for Research on Cancer. http://www.iarc.fr/en/publications/pdfs-online/wrk/wrk8/index.php (accessed 30 December 2017).

36 Parkin, D.M., and Moss, S. (1989). Lung cancer screening: Improved survival but no reduction in deaths. The role of 'overdiagnosis'. *Cancer* 89 (11 Suppl.): 2369–2376.

37 Aberle, D.R., Adams, A.M., Berg, C.D. et al. (2011). Reduced lung-cancer mortality with low-dose computed tomographic screening. *N. Engl. J. Med.* 365 (5): 395–409.

38 Schroder, F.H., Hugosson, J., Roobol, M.J. et al. (2012). Prostate-cancer mortality at 11 years of follow-up. *N. Engl. J. Med.* 366 (11): 981–990.

39 Menon, U., Gentry-Maharaj, A., Hallett, R. et al. (2009). Sensitivity and specificity of multimodal and ultrasound screening for ovarian cancer, and stage distribution of detected cancers: Results of the prevalence screen of the UK Collaborative Trial of Ovarian Cancer Screening (UKCTOCS). *Lancet Oncol.* 10 (4): 327–340.

40 Anderson, B.O., Cazap, E., El Saghir, N.S. et al. (2011). Optimisation of breast cancer management in low-resource and middle-resource countries: Executive summary of the Breast Health Global Initiative consensus, 2010. *Lancet Oncol.* 12 (4): 387–398.

41 Forbes, L.J.L., Warburton, F., Richards, M.A., and Ramirez, A.J. (2014). Risk factors for delay in symptomatic presentation: A survey of cancer patients. *Brit. J. Cancer* 111 (3): 581–588.

42 Pedersen, A.F., Olesen, F., Hansen, R.P. et al. (2013). Coping strategies and patient delay in patients with cancer. *J. Psychosoc. Oncol.* 31 (2): 204–218.

CHAPTER 2

Public health perspectives surrounding cancer prevention and screening: The Ontario edition

Linda Rabeneck[1] and Arlinda Ruco[2]

[1] *Institute for Clinical Evaluative Sciences; Cancer Care Ontario; Department of Medicine, Institute of Health Policy, Management and Evaluation, and Dalla Lana School of Public Health, University of Toronto, Toronto, Canada*
[2] *Institute of Health Policy, Management and Evaluation, University of Toronto; Department of Surgery, St. Michael's Hospital, Canada*

SUMMARY BOX

- Health care is publicly funded and administered at the provincial/territorial level in Canada.

- Cancer Care Ontario (CCO) takes a dual approach to cancer prevention and screening, focusing on initiatives at the policy and individual levels.

- Ontario has three organized province-wide cancer screening programmes (breast, cervical, and colorectal).

- CCO monitors the performance of the screening programmes and publicly reports in the Cancer System Quality Index.

- Cancer screening policy in the province is guided by CCO's Program in Evidence-Based Care, which conducts systematic reviews of new evidence.

Context: Health care in Canada

Canada, a country with ten provinces and three territories, has a population of approximately 35 427 524 [1]. Health care is publicly funded (85% federal and 15% provincial/territorial) and is organized, administered, and delivered at the provincial/territorial level. The Canada Health Act (CHA; passed in 1984) is designed to ensure that all residents have access to medically necessary hospital and physician services. There are five main principles to the Canada Health Act: public administration, comprehensiveness, universality, portability, and accessibility. The Act also establishes conditions related to insured health services

---

Cancer Prevention and Screening: Concepts, Principles and Controversies, First Edition.
Edited by Rosalind A. Eeles, Christine D. Berg, and Jeffrey S. Tobias.
© 2019 John Wiley & Sons, Inc. Published 2019 by John Wiley & Sons, Inc.

and extended health-care services. The provinces and territories must abide by these conditions to receive federal funding under the Canada Health Transfer (CHT). The CHT is the financial support provided by the federal government to assist provinces and territories in the provision of healthcare programmes and services. It is one of the largest major transfers to provinces and payments are made on an equal per capita basis.

In Ontario, Canada's largest province (population approximately 13.6 million) [1], all permanent residents and refugees are entitled to coverage under the Ontario Health Insurance Plan (OHIP). OHIP requires that speciality services be accessed through a referral from a primary care provider. Persons are able to choose their own primary care provider. The majority of physicians are compensated on a fee-for-service model, largely through reimbursement for services provided from OHIP.

What is happening at the federal level?

While provinces and territories are responsible for delivering health care, two federal entities also play important roles. The Public Health Agency of Canada (PHAC), under the same federal health portfolio as Health Canada, is a government agency formed in 2004 responsible for promoting and protecting the health of all Canadians, and preventing and controlling chronic and infectious diseases. The Chief Public Health Officer along with the Agency provides federal leadership and accountability for managing public health emergencies across the nation. Health Canada is the federal department responsible for helping Canadians maintain and improve their health. The department delivers a wide range of surveillance, prevention, control, and research programmes and services, while monitoring the health and safety risks related to the use and sale of drugs, food, chemicals, pesticides, medical devices, and other consumer products.

The Canadian Partnership Against Cancer (CPAC), launched in 2007, is an independent federal organization funded by Health Canada that aims to reduce the burden of cancer and accelerate action on cancer control for all Canadians through coordinated system-level change. The Partnership does not fund the delivery of cancer services. CPAC focuses on multijurisdictional action to attract, connect, and retain key stakeholders to co-create, inform, and lead change in the cancer control continuum, including prevention, screening, system performance, quality control, treatment, and quality of life.

What is happening at the provincial level?
Cancer Care Ontario

Cancer Care Ontario (CCO), originally formed in 1943, is an Ontario government agency that focuses on quality and improvement in cancer prevention, screening, and the delivery of care. CCO is responsible for implementing provincial cancer prevention and screening programmes, planning cancer services, and performance management. CCO is governed by The Cancer Act and is accountable to the Ontario Ministry of Health and Long-Term Care.

The Ontario Cancer Plan

The Ontario Cancer Plan, first released in 2005, was Canada's first provincial cancer plan. A cancer control plan is an organized plan of action to face the cancer burden in all its settings [2]. The Plan is a road map indicating how CCO, health-care professionals and organizations, cancer experts, and the provincial government will work together to reduce the risk of Ontarians developing cancer, while improving the quality of care for current and future patients. The third Ontario Cancer Plan (2011–2015) has six strategic priorities; the two for prevention and screening are:

1 Develop and implement a focused approach to cancer risk reduction; and

2 Implement integrated cancer screening for breast, cervical, and colorectal cancer.

Under each strategic priority there are specific aims, including ensuring that support services are in place so that individuals with abnormal screening test results receive appropriate follow-up care, and ensuring that primary care providers are given the appropriate tools to work with individuals to modify their risks and link them to local initiatives and screening.

Atun et al. [2] carried out a systematic review of National Cancer Control Programmes (NCCP) published between January 2000 and March 2008 in Europe. Using a health systems perspective, they concluded that one of the key shortcomings among the 19 out of 31 European countries with a published NCCP was the lack of information on funding to implement the plan [2]. Subsequently, similar results were reported in a study from the USA [3]. A key strength of the Ontario Cancer Plan is that a budget and funding request is associated with it.

Measuring cancer system performance in Ontario

The Cancer Quality Council of Ontario (CQCO) is an advisory group to CCO and the Ministry of Health and Long-Term Care, established in 2002 to report on cancer system performance in Ontario and make recommendations for improvement. In 2005, in partnership with CCO, the CQCO launched the Cancer System Quality Index (CSQI), a public report published online (http://www.csqi.on.ca/) that tracks Ontario's progress in cancer control and highlights areas for improvement. As of 2014, the CSQI reports on 83 evidence-based quality measures covering every aspect of cancer control, from prevention to survivorship and end-of-life care.

Cancer prevention in Ontario led by CCO

Work at the policy level

The major focus of CCO's work in prevention is at the policy level. Figure 2.1, adapted from the North Karelia study, outlines the importance of policy-level interventions along with those at the individual or behavioural level in addressing the health burden in the population. What the figure shows is that the burden on

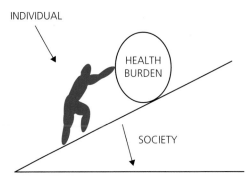

INDIVIDUAL

HEALTH BURDEN

SOCIETY

Figure 2.1 Contributions of individual/behavioural-level and policy/societal-level interventions to addressing the health burden. Source: House of Commons Health Committee 2004 [4].

the individual is lessened with policy (societal) interventions, which decrease the slope of the incline.

In terms of policy work, in collaboration with Public Health Ontario (PHO), CCO published 'Taking Action to Prevent Chronic Disease: Recommendations for a Healthier Ontario' in 2012 [5]. The report lays a foundation for action on the four main risk factors for chronic disease (tobacco control, reduction in alcohol consumption, increase in physical activity, and promotion of healthy eating) by identifying key evidence-based policy interventions intended largely for government action.

The report makes twenty-two recommendations, four for each risk factor addressed in the report and six overarching recommendations that address capacity building and health equity. For example, recommendations regarding alcohol consumption include maintaining and reinforcing socially responsible pricing, ensuring effective controls on alcohol availability, strengthening targeted controls on alcohol marketing and promotion, and increasing access to brief counselling interventions. Examples of overarching recommendations include adopting a whole-of-government approach for the primary prevention of chronic disease, reducing health inequities, and addressing First Nations, Inuit, and Metis (FNIM) health.

In 2004, the Ontario government launched the Smoke-Free Ontario Strategy, an initiative that focuses on public education campaigns, programmes, and policies aimed at preventing Ontarians from starting to smoke, protecting Ontarians from exposure to second-hand smoke, and helping those who smoke to quit. In 2006, the Ontario Smoke-Free Act, comprehensive tobacco control legislation, came into effect. The Act prohibits smoking in all enclosed workplaces and public places, as well as motor vehicles when children are present. Additionally, the Act bans the display of tobacco products prior to purchase. In support of the Smoke-Free Ontario Strategy, CCO administers the Program Training and Consultation Centre (PTCC). PTCC supports the Ontario Smoke-Free Act by building capacity in tobacco control through training, consultation, resource development, and referral services at the local and community level, including Ontario's 36 public health units. Public health units are responsible for

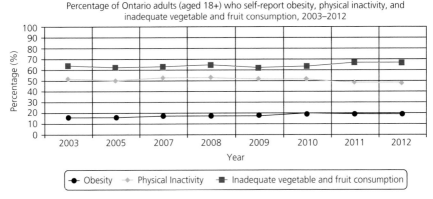

Figure 2.2 Prevalence of selected modifiable risk factors in Ontario adults aged 18 and over, 2003–2012.

administering health promotion and disease prevention programmes to residents in the municipalities and communities they serve.

Cancer prevention indicators in the province are measured and publicly reported in the CSQI. There are approximately 17 prevention indicators, including second-hand smoke exposure in public places, alcohol consumption, cancers attributable to smoking, density of off-premise alcohol retail outlets, and overall outdoor air quality. Figure 2.2 outlines the percentage of Ontario adults aged 18 and over who self-reported obesity, physical inactivity, and inadequate vegetable and fruit consumption between 2003 to 2012, as reported in the CSQI.

CCO is committed to reducing the burden of cancer among Aboriginal communities in Ontario. The term Aboriginal refers to the first inhabitants of the land. In Canada, there are three different Aboriginal communities, including First Nations, Inuit, and Metis (FNIM). Approximately 4.3% of the Canadian population identifies as Aboriginal [6]. In 2012, the Aboriginal Cancer Control Unit developed a three-year Aboriginal Cancer Strategy to combat the lower survival rates for major cancers in FNIM communities compared to the general population [7]. The Strategy outlines six strategic priorities, of which the two for prevention and screening include developing and implementing a province-wide smoking cessation agenda in collaboration with FNIM groups, and establishing screening participation targets for FNIM peoples.

Work at the individual level

In terms of prevention at the individual level, in 2015 CCO launched an online cancer risk assessment tool, MyCancerIQ (https://www.mycanceriq.ca/). The tool allows Ontarians to calculate their risk (average, above average, below average) for four cancers (breast, colorectal, cervix, and lung). Individuals are also able to link to local resources to moderate their risk (e.g. Ontario Breast Screening Program).

Prevention research

CCO supports a variety of research initiatives, including the establishment of the Occupational Cancer Research Centre (OCRC), housed at CCO, in 2009. The Centre aims to fill the gaps in our knowledge of occupation-related cancers and to translate these findings into prevention programmes to control workplace carcinogenic exposures and improve the health of workers. The OCRC is funded by CCO, the Ontario Ministry of Labour, and the Canadian Cancer Society (CCS) – Ontario Division. It is the first centre of its kind in Canada. The OCRC focuses its research on three major areas: identification of causes of cancer in the workplace, surveillance of occupation cancers and workplace exposures, and intervention research to develop and evaluate prevention and exposure reduction strategies.

The Ontario Health Study (OHS) is one of the largest long-term health studies in Canada and investigates risk factors for chronic diseases, including cancer, diabetes, heart disease, and asthma. The project is funded by four organizations: the Ontario Institute for Cancer Research (OICR), CCO, PHO, and CPAC [8]. Since 2010, over 225 000 Ontarians have participated in the study [8]. Participants are asked to complete an online survey and annually update their health questionnaire. Additionally, there is an optional annual follow-up questionnaire in a different area of health, such as mental health, diet, or physical activity. Participants may also be invited to visit an assessment centre where physical measurements and blood and urine samples are collected. The majority of participants in the OHS are between the ages of 40–59 years (20.7% 40–49; 22.9% 50–59) and more than half of participants are women (60.9%) [8]. Data on self-reported rates of chronic disease show a prevalence of 20.5% for high blood pressure and 13.6% for asthma among study participants.

Public Health Ontario

PHO is a government agency that began operations in 2008 and is dedicated to protecting and promoting the health of all Ontarians and reducing inequities in health. PHO's mandate involves providing scientific and technical advice and support to clients, particularly the 36 public health units in Ontario. One example of the work done by PHO includes the Locally Driven Collaborative Projects (LDCP) programme, which aims to strengthen the ability of health units to conduct applied research and programme evaluations, and is delivered through in-person workshops.

Canadian Cancer Society

One of the most prominent community organizations working on cancer prevention is the CCS – Ontario Division. The CCS was officially formed in 1938. As a national, community-based organization, its mission is to eradicate cancer and improve the quality of life of people living with cancer. Strategic priorities of the organization in 2010–2015 include leading research to better prevent cancer, influencing public policy for quality cancer care, supporting programmes that focus on the greatest needs of patients and caregivers, and engaging more

Canadians in the fight against cancer. In 2011–2012, the organization funded more than CAN$46 million in research.

CCO's provincial cancer screening programmes

CCO operates province-wide organized cancer screening programmes for breast, cervical, and colorectal cancer (CRC).

The Ontario Breast Screening Program (OBSP; launched in 1990) provides breast cancer screening for women aged 50–74 years at average risk. The OBSP recommends biannual mammography for these women. Women may self-refer or be referred by their primary care provider. The programme provides high-quality mammograms at sites accredited by the Canadian Association of Radiologists – Mammography Accreditation Program (CAR-MAP). Women who are eligible receive a reminder letter when it is time to return for their next screening mammogram. As reported in the CSQI, in 2011–2012 60% of Ontario screen-eligible women aged 50–74 years were screened for breast cancer, with nearly three-quarters of them screened through the OBSP.

In 2011, CCO launched organized screening for women aged 30–69 years who have been confirmed to be at high risk for breast cancer in its High Risk OBSP. The High Risk OBSP facilitates referrals for genetic assessment and provides annual screening mammography and breast magnetic resonance imaging (MRI) for women who have been confirmed to be at high risk, and facilitates follow-up breast assessment services for women who require extra tests. Women who are considered to be at high risk include those who are known to be carriers of a deleterious gene mutation (*BRCA1* or *BRCA2*); are the first-degree relative of a mutation carrier and have declined genetic testing; are determined to be at greater than or equal to 25% lifetime risk of breast cancer as determined by the IBIS or BOADICEA risk assessment tools; or have received chest radiation before age 30 and at least eight years previously. Results from the first year of operation of the High Risk OBSP have been published [9]. A total of 2290 women were screened, and the cancer detection rates were 10.7 per 1000 for those with an abnormal MRI (or ultrasound) result and a normal mammogram result, and 5.8 per 1000 for those with both an abnormal MRI (or ultrasound) and mammogram result [9].

The Ontario Cervical Cancer Screening Program (OCSP) recommends that women aged 21 years of age or older who are/have been sexually active get screened for cervical cancer every three years using a Pap test. Screening may be discontinued at age 70 provided that there is adequate negative cytology screening history in the previous 10 years. As reported in the CSQI, approximately 64% of eligible women were screened for cervical cancer between 2010 and 2012 (Figure 2.3).

ColonCancerCheck, Canada's first province-wide, population-based CRC screening programme, was launched in Ontario in 2008. The program recommends that all Ontarians aged 50 to 74 years be screened for CRC. For those at average risk, a faecal occult blood test (FOBT) once every two years is recommended. For those at

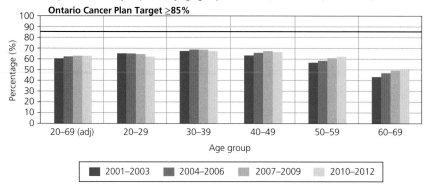

Figure 2.3 Cervical cancer screening Pap test participation rates among Ontario screen-eligible women by age group, 2001–2012.

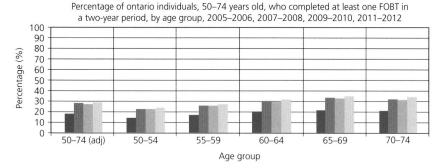

Figure 2.4 Colorectal cancer screening faecal occult blood test (FOBT) participation rates in Ontario by age group, 2005–2012.

increased risk because of a family history of one or more first-degree relatives with a diagnosis of CRC, colonoscopy is advised. Personalized invitation letters are sent to eligible persons to invite them to speak with their family doctor or nurse practitioner about getting screened for CRC. Furthermore, reminder letters are also sent out when it is time to return for screening. Figure 2.4 shows FOBT participation rates in Ontario from 2005 to 2012 by age group as reported in the CSQI. Approximately 30% of the eligible population was screened in 2011–2012. However, in Ontario, opportunistic screening colonoscopy is available as a primary screening test in people at average risk. When use of flexible sigmoidoscopy and colonoscopy for all indications is considered, 42.2% of the target population was overdue for screening in 2012 (Figure 2.5). This may be a more appropriate measure of the extent of

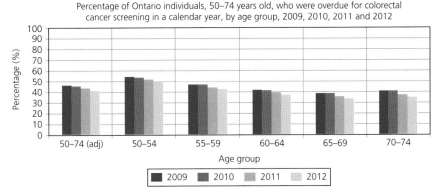

Figure 2.5 Percentage of Ontario individuals, 50–74 years old, who were overdue for colorectal cancer screening by age group, 2009–2012.

screening, as it describes the unmet need. Further results from the programme have been published [10]. The greater cancer detection rate in those at increased risk who undergo screening with colonoscopy suggests that the impact of the programme on colorectal cancer mortality is enhanced through risk stratification [10].

CCO's approach to new evidence for cancer screening

CCO's Program in Evidence-Based Care (PEBC), launched in 1997 and housed at McMaster University (http://fhs.mcmaster.ca/pebc/), convenes multidisciplinary Expert Panels to develop and systematically review scientific evidence to support the development of evidence-based guidelines in the areas of screening, diagnostic assessment, treatment, and supportive care. For example, the PEBC has published guidelines on MRI screening of women at high risk for breast cancer [11], cervical screening [12], and standards for colonoscopy quality assurance [13].

Following publication of the results from the National Lung Screening Trial (NLST) conducted by the US National Cancer Institute, CCO convened an Expert Panel through the PEBC to conduct a systematic review of 8 randomized controlled trials and 13 single-centre studies evaluating lung screening with low-dose computed tomography (CT). The Panel concluded that low-dose CT lung cancer screening is appropriate for individuals aged 55–74 years with a minimum smoking history of at least 30 pack-years [14]. After the initial scan, screening should be conducted annually for two consecutive years, then once every two years after each negative scan. However, the Expert Panel recommended that prior to determining whether to move forward with a population-based screening programme, CCO needs to conduct further work, including a cost-effectiveness analysis and capacity planning [14]. Following release of the PEBC guideline [14], CCO has funded a two-year programme of work that will lay the groundwork for a proposal for a pilot to be submitted to the Ministry of Health and Long-Term Care for funding.

CPAC's role in cancer screening

CPAC has contributed to cancer screening efforts by providing effective and ongoing support for pan-Canadian networks for breast, cervical, CRC, and more recently lung cancer screening. These networks provide an opportunity for experts in the field to share knowledge and explore approaches to screening.

Conclusion

Health care in Canada is publicly funded, and administered, organized, and delivered at the provincial/territorial level. Cancer Care Ontario is responsible for implementing provincial cancer prevention and screening programmes, planning cancer services, and performance management. For cancer prevention, CCO uses a dual approach, focusing on interventions at the policy and individual levels. In cancer screening, CCO operates organized province-wide breast, cervical, and colorectal cancer screening programmes. Cancer screening policy is guided by CCO's Program in Evidence-Based Care. The performance of the cancer system in Ontario is publicly reported in the Cancer System Quality Index.

References

1 Statistics Canada (2014). Table 051-0005 – Estimates of population, Canada, provinces and territories, quarterly (persons). *CANSIM* (database). http://www5.statcan.gc.ca/cansim/a26 ?lang=eng&retrLang=eng&id=0510005&&pattern=&stByVal=1&p1=1&p2=-1&tabMode= dataTable&csid= (accessed 13 August 2014).

2 Atun, R., Ogawa, R., and Martin-Moreno, J.M. (2009). *Analysis of National Cancer Control Programmes in Europe*. London: Imperial College Business School, Imperial College London.

3 Rochester, P., Adams, E., Porterfield, D.S. et al. (2011). Cancer Plan Index: A measure for assessing the quality of cancer plans. *J. Public Health Manag. Pract.* 17 (6): E12–E17.

4 House of Commons Health Committee (2004). Health – Third Report. http://www. publications.parliament.uk/pa/cm200304/cmselect/cmhealth/23/2302.htm(accessed 13 August 2014).

5 Cancer Care Ontario, Ontario Agency for Health Protection and Promotion (Public Health Ontario) (2012). *Taking Action to Prevent Chronic Disease: Recommendations for a Healthier Ontario*. Toronto: Queen's Printer for Ontario.

6 Statistics Canada (2013). National Household Survey (NHS) Aboriginal Population Profile. 2011 National Household Survey. Statistics Canada Catalogue no. 99-011-X2011007. http://www12.statcan.gc.ca/nhs-enm/2011/dp-pd/aprof/index.cfm?Lang=E (accessed 21 November 2014).

7 Cancer Care Ontario (n.d.). Aboriginal Cancer Strategy II. https://www.cancercareontario. ca/sites/ccocancercare/files/assets/CCOACS2.pdf (accessed 2 January 2018).

8 Ontario Health Study (n.d.). https://www.ontariohealthstudy.ca/ (accessed 6 October 2014).

9 Chiarelli, A.M., Prummel, M.V., Muradali, D. et al. (2014). Effectiveness of screening with annual Magnetic Resonance Imaging and mammography: Results of the initial screen from the Ontario high risk breast screening program. *J. Clin. Oncol.* 32 (21): 2224–2230.

10 Rabeneck, L., Tinmouth, J.M., Paszat, L.F. et al. (2014). Ontario's ColonCancerCheck: Results from Canada's first province-wide colorectal cancer screening program. *Cancer Epidemiol. Biomarkers Prev.* 23 (3): 508–515.

11 Warner, E., Messersmith, H., Causer, P. et al. (2008). Systematic review: Using magnetic resonance imaging to screen women at high risk for breast cancer. *Ann. Intern. Med.* 148 (9): 671–679.

12 Murphy, J., Kennedy, E., Dunn, S. et al. (2012). Cervical screening: A guideline for clinical practice in Ontario. *J. Obstet. Gynaecol. Can.* 34 (5): 453–458.

13 Tinmouth, J., Kennedy, E., Baron, D. et al. (2014). Colonoscopy quality assurance in Ontario: Systematic review and clinical practice guideline. *Can. J. Gastroenterol. Hepatol.* 28 (5): 251–274.

14 Roberts, H., Walker-Dilks, C., Sivjee, K. et al. (2013). Screening high-risk populations for lung cancer: Guideline recommendations. *J. Thorac. Oncol.* 8 (10): 1232–1237.

CHAPTER 3

Cancer screening: A general perspective

Otis W. Brawley

American Cancer Society, Georgia, USA

SUMMARY BOX

- The true purpose of a screening test is to decrease mortality from the specific disease being screened for.
- There are three requirements for successful screening:
  - A cancer that can be found in a localized state prior to spread.
  - A test that finds localized disease with some reliability.
  - A treatment that is effective against that localized disease.
- A screening test is assessed by measuring sensitivity, specificity, positive predictive value, and negative predictive value.
- Sensitivity is the probability of a positive result when applied to a person who actually has the disease.
- Specificity is the probability of a negative result in a person who truly does not have the disease.
- Positive predictive value (PPV) is the probability that a subject who screens positive truly has the disease.
- Negative predictive value (NPV) is the probability that a subject who screens negative is actually free of disease.
- The ideal screening test has both high sensitivity and high specificity.
- Subjects should be fully informed of the potential for harm and the potential for benefit. The risk of overdiagnosis and overtreatment must be considered in every screening programme.

Cancer Prevention and Screening: Concepts, Principles and Controversies, First Edition.
Edited by Rosalind A. Eeles, Christine D. Berg, and Jeffrey S. Tobias.
© 2019 John Wiley & Sons, Inc. Published 2019 by John Wiley & Sons, Inc.

Cancer screening by definition is an intervention on asymptomatic individuals with the intent of prompting diagnostic and treatment interventions. It is an effort to reduce suffering and death [1]. The word 'effort' is used, as screening interventions more often than not are unsuccessful at preventing suffering and death. Screening, like all, even minor, health-care interventions, has the potential to cause harm. Most commonly harm is due to screening leading to a harmful diagnostic or treatment intervention. Screening is done on healthy individuals. This means there is a significant obligation to use tests that maximize benefits and minimize harms.

One should adequately assess a screening intervention to determine its benefits and harms and consider the balance of the two before implementing it broadly. This is complicated, as the benefit is reduction in deaths, while the harms associated with screening are usually a different, more qualitative metric. Harms can include emotional distress, mental anguish, and unnecessary morbidity due to unnecessary treatment, but can include premature death. The issue often becomes how many should be inconvenienced to save one life.

Screening is often a political issue, and this is of special concern. Many in the general public and the medical profession do not understand the limitations of cancer screening. People often overestimate the potential for benefit and underestimate its potential for harm. Some assume that every metastatic breast, lung, colon, or prostate cancer is a failure of the patient to get screened or a failure of a doctor to diagnose it. In fact, well-designed clinical trials in almost every cancer studied demonstrate that the majority of those destined to die of a screenable cancer cannot be saved by screening.

A common misconception is that the purpose of a screening test is to increase survival. The true purpose of a screening test is to decrease mortality from the specific disease screened. Indeed, there are examples of screening increasing survival rates without a change in mortality. A poor screening test can even cause an increase in survival with an increase in mortality (risk of death) [2, 3].

On the nature of screening

There are three requirements for successful screening.
1 A cancer that can be found in a localized state prior to spread.
2 A test that finds localized disease with some reliability.
3 A treatment that is effective against that localized disease.
Number 1 has to do with the biological behaviour and nature of the specific cancer. Numbers 2 and 3 have to do with the state of the science and our ability to develop tests and treatments. That is to say, we have some control and influence over elements 2 and 3. We cannot change the nature of a disease. Some cancers are simply not 'screenable' tumours because of their biological behaviour.

Assessing a screening test

A screening test is assessed by measuring sensitivity, specificity, positive predictive value, and negative predictive value [1]; see Table 3.1.

- **Sensitivity** is the probability of a positive result when applied to a person who truly has the disease. A test with high sensitivity detects most disease in a cohort screened. Sensitivity is also referred to as the true positive (TP) rate: TP/TP+FN (false negative).
- **Specificity** is the probability of a negative result in a person who truly does not have the disease. Specificity is sometimes referred to as the true negative (TN) rate: TN/TN+FP (false positive).
- Positive predictive value (PPV) is the probability that a subject who screens positive truly has the disease: TP/TP+FP.
- Negative predictive value (NPV) is the probability that a subject who screens negative is actually free of disease. TN/TN+FN. A high NPV means that few with the disease are missed.

The ideal screening test has both high sensitivity and high specificity. Unfortunately, sensitivity and specificity tend to be negatively associated and the ideal test is rare. Sensitivity and specificity are not dependent on disease prevalence. That being said, when screening a population with a low prevalence of disease, high specificity is more valuable than high sensitivity. This decreases the number of false positive findings requiring additional workup.

The PPV and NPV of a screening test are highly dependent on disease prevalence and are more reactive to specificity versus sensitivity. The classic example is that given a disease with a prevalence of five cases per 1000 (.005), the PPV of a hypothetical screening test increases significantly as specificity goes from 95% to 99.9%, but only marginally as sensitivity goes from 80% to 95% (Table 3.2). Given a disease prevalence of only 1 per 10 000 (.0001), the PPV of the same test is poor even at high sensitivity and specificity (Table 3.3).

Table 3.1 Positive predictive value.

Sensitivity	TP/TP+FN
Specificity	TN/TN+FP
Positive predictive value	TP/TP+FP
Negative predictive value	TN/TN+FN
	TP = True positive
	TN = True negative
	FP = False positive
	FN = False negative

Table 3.2 Positive predictive value given varying sensitivity, specificity, and prevalence.

Disease prevalence		Sensitivity %		
	5/1000	80	90	95
Specificity% 95		7	8	9
99		29	31	32
99.9		80	82	83

Table 3.3 Positive predictive value given varying sensitivity, specificity, and lower prevalence.

Disease prevalence		Sensitivity %		
	1/10 000	80	90	95
Specificity% 95		0.2	0.2	2.0
99		0.8	0.9	0.9
99.9		0.7	8.0	9.0

Assessing benefit from a screening test

The purpose of a screening test is to avert deaths. In a cohort, this is best seen as a decrease in the mortality rate. There is a tendency to think that increasing patient survival, the time from diagnosis to death, is equivalent to 'saving a life' or preventing a cancer death. For a group of screened individuals, this is often portrayed as an increase in the proportion surviving five years, or the five-year survival rate.

Lead-time bias

Lead-time bias is the increase in time from diagnosis due to screening versus what would have been the time of diagnosis due to symptoms [4]. Screening is not beneficial when there is an increase in survival without a prolongation in life. The patient did not live longer, s/he knew they had cancer longer. In the prospective randomized trial of chest X-ray lung cancer screening in the 1960s and 1970s, screening led to an increase in five-year survival rate without a decrease in mortality rate.

Length bias

Length bias is another factor in cancer screening [4]. It has to do with the nature and biological behaviour of the disease. Some cancers are slow growing, others are intermediate, and yet others are fast growing. A regularly scheduled screening programme is more apt to find a slower-growing tumour than a fast-growing tumour, as there are more chances to find the cancer before it is clinically relevant (Figure 3.1).

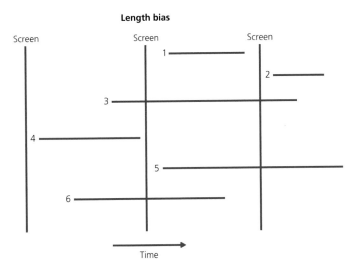

Figure 3.1 Each numbered line represents a patient's course of disease from cancer development to death. The vertical lines represent the potential of routine screening. Horizontal lines
1, 2, and 4 represent patients with disease that would have caused death between scheduled
screens. Patients 3, 5, and 6 had slower-growing tumours that could have been detected by
routine screening. Patient 3 had a tumour that was growing so slowly it was detectable in two
routine screens.

Overdiagnosis

Overdiagnosis is a form of length bias [5]. It occurs when a tumour fulfils all the
histological definitions of cancer, but if left alone would not kill the specific
patient. There are two kinds of overdiagnosis. The first is the cancer that would
never grow, spread, and kill. The second is a cancer that would never grow, spread,
and kill in the specific patient's lifetime. That is to say, a patient might have a
tumour capable of causing death, but the patient, because of age and comorbid
disease, will die of other illness before the tumour can cause harm.

It is often difficult even for the clinician to accept that there are pathologically
diagnosed cancers that will not harm if left alone. It is, perhaps, easier to comprehend this phenomenon by understanding that German pathologists defined our
current histological definitions of cancer in the mid-1800s [6]. They performed
autopsies and were among the first to glass mount and stain tissues and examine
them with a microscope. These physicians created the pathological criteria for
determining a biopsy cancerous. Today we have a number of imaging and diagnostic technologies that allow us to find very small lesions in the breast, prostate,
lung, and other organs. Some small lesions that look like the lesions defined as
cancer are not destined to grow, spread, and kill. These are overdiagnosis lesions.

Overdiagnosis is demonstrated in the long-term follow-up of the Mayo Clinic
lung cancer screening study, which began in the 1960s [3]. This is one of three
lung cancer screening studies cited earlier as demonstrating that survival rates are
not always correlated with decrease in mortality or risk of death. The randomized

study compared an arm screened intensively with chest X-ray and sputum cytology every four months for six years to a control arm receiving 'usual care'. In long-term follow-up of more than 6100 participants, intensive screening diagnosed 585 lung cancers compared with 500 lung cancers in the control arm. After 20 years of follow-up mortality rates were essentially equal, with an 18% excess in lung cancer diagnosis among the intensively screened. This study shows that intensive screening can increase the number of overdiagnosis tumours compared with less intensive screening.

The Quebec Neuroblastoma Screening Project used a urine test to screen 21-day-old children for neuroblastoma from 1989 to 1994 [7]. The result was a dramatic increase in the incidence of neuroblastoma without a change in the mortality rate. After the implementation of screening, researchers determined that there is overdiagnosis in neuroblastoma, as there is a type of neuroblastoma that can be diagnosed and cured, but regresses if left alone. Screening did not alter the natural history of the deadly type of neuroblastoma.

Overdiagnosis of thyroid cancer is demonstrated in the South Korean observation that the age-adjusted incidence of thyroid cancer rose from 5 per 100 000 in 1999 to 70 per 100 000 in 2011, without a significant change in mortality rate. The increase in incidence was linked to increased use of thyroid cancer screening with ultrasound.

It is difficult to diagnose a specific individual as having an indolent cancer. The screening literature suggests that overdiagnosis is seen in the following:
- 10–20% of radiologically detected localized lung cancers.
- 3–40% of mammographically detected localized breast cancers.
- Up to 40% of ultrasound-detected localized thyroid cancers.
- Up to 60% of prostate-specific-antigen-detected localized prostate cancers [8,9].

Today, clinicians are willing to watch some invasive thyroid and prostate cancers based on histological appearance that suggests indolence. Already, genomic profiling of breast and prostate cancers is commercially available and is used to modify the aggressiveness of treatment. There is hope that genomic testing will provide a more objective way of diagnosing and determining the cancers that need to be treated versus the cancers that need to be watched. The combination of histology and genomics is moving us from the mid-nineteenth-century definition of cancer in use today to a twenty-first-century definition of cancer.

The order of evidence of benefit

The strongest assessment of a screening test is a prospective randomized trial with an endpoint of mortality reduction. In the purest form of such a study, people at risk for the disease are enrolled and randomized to be screened or not be screened. These two cohorts are followed and compared over time. Deaths are commonly reported as number of deaths per 1000. Screening is considered effective when the death rate due to the specific cancer is reduced in the intervention arm compared with the control arm, and the differences are statistically significant. This design minimizes the effects of lead-time bias, length bias, and overdiagnosis. Unfortunately, these are large, expensive, long-term trials that are difficult to do and impossible to achieve without some imperfection.

Other commonly employed ways of assessing a screening test in order from strongest to weakest evidence include:

- Evidence obtained from nonrandomized controlled trials.
- Evidence obtained from cohort or case-control studies.
- Evidence from ecological and descriptive studies (e.g. international patterns studies, time series).
- Opinions of respected authorities based on clinical experience, descriptive studies, or reports of expert committees [1].

The population of almost all clinical trials in which participants volunteer to enter has selection bias. This occurs when people different from the population in general enter the trial. The healthy volunteer effect is a common selection bias. People who enter clinical trials are more often interested in health and are healthier than the general population because of this interest. Even the preferred prospective randomized clinical trial is prone to selection bias [10].

Some recently published screening trials have a selection bias effect that is underappreciated. Several European countries do not allow recruitment of subjects to trials followed by randomization to intervention and control arms. A common way of doing trials in these countries is to randomize subjects from voter rolls or census records. Those who are randomized to be screened are approached and asked to participate. Those in the control arm are not aware they are in a trial and may even already have the disease in question [11]. Those selected for the intervention arm have the ability to opt out. This creates the potential for the intervention arm to consist of healthier participants when compared with the control arm. Even further, the screening cohort has disease awareness different from those in the control groups, and if diagnosed may seek treatment at different institutions. This leaves open the possibility of patients diagnosed in the intervention arm receiving better quality of treatment compared with controls.

All these biases favour a finding that screening is better than it actually is. Boyle and colleagues pointed out this bias and its effect when comparing a series of colon cancer screening trials using sigmoidoscopy [12]. This bias is likely a factor in some recent European prostate cancer screening studies.

The population screened

The nature of screening is such that the odds of benefit are highest when aimed at populations with a high risk for disease. One should only screen the general population for diseases that are major causes of death. In some cases, screening can be focused on a population known to be at high risk of the disease, such as screening women of a certain age for breast cancer. Screening the general population for a rare tumour will result in screening many subjects who do not have the disease. A population with a low prevalence of disease is at greater risk of a false positive result. This will lead to wasteful diagnostic testing.

When screening is aimed at a population with a high prevalence of disease, the benefit to harm ratio may be viewed as more favourable even with significant risk of false positive findings. In the future, our ability to define a population at high risk will improve. Already risk calculators have been developed and are being honed to better define candidates at higher risk for breast, lung, and prostate cancer [13].

The magnitude of screening benefit

Most studies that have demonstrated a cancer screening intervention to be effective show that screening can reduce the relative risk of cancer death by 15–35% [14]. This means, for example, that with good screening 15–35% of those destined to die from cancer could be saved from a cancer death [1]. Few people realize that this means that 65–85% of those destined to die from cancer still die, even with high-quality screening. Indeed, most meta-analyses of breast cancer studies suggest that mammography is associated with a 20% risk reduction, meaning that 80% of those destined to die from breast cancer will die despite high-quality screening.

The US National Lung Screening Trial (discussed in detail later in the book) provides an example of how trial data can be misunderstood by the public and even some medical professionals [15]. The trial showed a 20% reduction in risk of death in the low-dose computed tomography (LDCT) arm [16]. That means that the LDCT was not able to prevent 80% of lung cancer deaths among those screened. In the intervention arm with more than 27 000 subjects, screening averted approximately 85 lung cancer deaths, but there were still more than 350 lung cancer deaths in the screened arm. In the case of LDCT where annual screening was done three times, it is possible that continued screening would have increased the relative risk reduction, but cancer screening will rarely prevent most deaths from the disease being screened for. This should not be taken as an argument against lung cancer screening, but an argument that we should appreciate its limitations and not be satisfied with the current technology.

In the European Randomized Study of Prostate Cancer (ERSPC), a 20% reduction in relative risk of death was reported after 13 years of screening [11]. This study result may have been influenced by a selection bias on the intervention arm. Taking the result at face value, the number needed to treat to avert one death was 34. For a cohort of 200 men diagnosed with prostate cancer through screening, this amounts to about 8 deaths prevented after 13 years of screening. The number 200 is used because the death rate associated with prostatectomy in the USA is 0.5%, meaning that for every 200 men treated with radical prostatectomy, one death results as a complication of surgery. Being selective and carefully choosing patients for screening and treatment can reduce the harms associated with screening [17].

Screening in practice

Screening is a public health intervention whose purpose is to decrease cancer mortality and morbidity. Most clinical studies are designed to demonstrate efficacy, meaning that they are an assessment of how or whether the intervention works in a controlled setting. This involves a selected or volunteer cohort in which there may be a 'healthy volunteer effect'. The assessment and treatment may be done in medical facilities that are more skilled in the specific disease than is common for the general population. Effectiveness studies do an assessment of the intervention in real-world circumstances. Effectiveness studies are rare, however, as they tend to be very large and expensive. A prospective study assessing efficacy with follow-up outcomes studies is often the most practical way of estimating the effect of a screening intervention.

Screening is best done through a structured programme that provides oversight of quality of screening and monitors patient follow-up [14]. Screening can be in the context of a physician encounter as part of a regular physical examination, or it can be done in a mass screening effort. In the USA, cancer screening is often done with haphazard scheduling and less than optimal attention to quality. In some cases mass screening is heavily advertised as a one-time effort at public places such as shopping malls or health fairs. These events offer a very uncontrolled intervention with little follow-up.

Mass screening can be done in an organized programme such as a prevention clinic. Some screening clinics screen several hundred patients a day and screen for a number of diseases at one appointment. Common noncancerous diseases screened for at such clinics include macular degeneration, arterial disease, and diabetes. These programmes generally have superior oversight of quality and tracking of patient compliance and patient outcomes.

Conclusion

Cancer screening is an intervention to reduce the risk of death from cancer. Cancer screening should be aimed at those at high risk or for cancers that are common to the population screened. Quality of testing is paramount. Any putative screening test must be assessed carefully, because of the potential for harm in addition to the potential for benefit. Harm can be caused by the test and test result itself; it can also be caused by diagnostic and treatment interventions. Benefit (reduction in cancer mortality) is often difficult to document. Indeed, it is common that the harms of a screening intervention are better proven than the benefits. Subjects should be fully informed of the potential for harm and the potential for benefit.

Cancer overdiagnosis is a real problem in many diseases. The risk of overdiagnosis and overtreatment must be considered in every screening programme. In the future, a definition of cancer that includes histology and genomics may allow us to better determine the malignancies that need treatment because they are a threat to life, versus those that need merely to be watched.

References

1 Croswell, J.M., Ransohoff, D.F., and Kramer, B.S. (2010). Principles of cancer screening: Lessons from history and study design issues. *Semin. Oncol.* 37: 202–215.

2 Marcus, P.M., Bergstralh, E.J., Fagerstrom, R.M. et al. (2000). Lung cancer mortality in the Mayo Lung Project: Impact of extended follow-up. *J. Natl Cancer Inst.* 92: 1308–1316.

3 Marcus, P.M., Bergstralh, E.J., Zweig, M.H. et al. (2006). Extended lung cancer incidence follow-up in the Mayo Lung Project and overdiagnosis. *J. Natl Cancer Inst.* 98: 748–756.

4 Kramer, B.S. (2004). The science of early detection. *Urol. Oncol.* 22: 344–347.

5 Welch, H.G., and Black, W.C. (2010). Overdiagnosis in cancer. *J. Natl Cancer Inst.* 102: 605–613.

6 Virchow, R. (1848). *Vorlesungen über Cellularpathologie in ihrer Begründung auf physiologischer und pathologischer Gewebelehre*. Berlin: August Hirschwald.

7 Woods, W.G., Gao, R.N., Shuster, J.J. et al. (2002). Screening of infants and mortality due to neuroblastoma. *N. Engl. J. Med.* 346: 1041–1046.

8 Welch, H.G., and Albertsen, P.C. (2009). Prostate cancer diagnosis and treatment after the introduction of prostate-specific antigen screening: 1986–2005. *J. Natl Cancer Inst.* 101: 1325–1329.

9 Esserman, L.J., Thompson, I.M., Reid, B. et al. (2014). Addressing overdiagnosis and overtreatment in cancer: A prescription for change. *Lancet Oncol.* 15: e234–e242.

10 Pinsky, P.F., Miller, A., Kramer, B.S. et al. (2007). Evidence of a healthy volunteer effect in the prostate, lung, colorectal, and ovarian cancer screening trial. *Am. J. Epidemiol.* 165: 874–881.

11 Schroder, F.H., Hugosson, J., Roobol, M.J. et al. (2014). Screening and prostate cancer mortality: Results of the European Randomised Study of Screening for Prostate Cancer (ERSPC) at 13 years of follow-up. *Lancet* 384: 2027–2035.

12 Boyle, P., and Autier, P. (1998). Colorectal cancer screening: Health policy or a continuing research issue? *Ann. Oncol.* 9: 581–584.

13 Thompson, I.M., Jr., Leach, R.J., and Ankerst, D.P. (2014). Focusing PSA testing on detection of high-risk prostate cancers by incorporating patient preferences into decision making. *JAMA* 312: 995–996.

14 Smith, R.A., Manassaram-Baptiste, D., Brooks, D. et al. (2015). Cancer screening in the United States, 2015: A review of current American Cancer Society guidelines and current issues in cancer screening. *CA Cancer J. Clin.* 65: 30–54.

15 Wegwarth, O., Schwartz, L.M., Woloshin, S. et al. (2012). Do physicians understand cancer screening statistics? A national survey of primary care physicians in the United States. *Ann. Intern. Med.* 156: 340–349.

16 Church, T.R., Black, W.C., Aberle, D.R. et al. (2013). Results of initial low-dose computed tomographic screening for lung cancer. *N. Engl. J. Med.* 368: 1980–1991.

17 Moyer, V.A. (2012). Screening for ovarian cancer: U.S. Preventive Services Task Force reaffirmation recommendation statement. *Ann. Intern. Med.* 157: 900–904.

CHAPTER 4

The balance of cancer screening risks and benefits

Julietta Patnick

University of Oxford, UK

SUMMARY BOX

- Every screening programme achieves benefits at some cost.
- There are both physical and psychological harms, and some screening programmes have become very controversial regarding the balance of those harms against the benefit achieved.
- Policymakers make these judgements on behalf of the population when deciding whether to recommend screening, but each individual has to make the decision about participation for themselves.
- Breast, cervical, and colorectal screening are considered by most authorities to have a net benefit when applied appropriately.

At one point cancer screening was regarded as a universal good. Cervical screening was the first technique to be developed, and discussions took place about how to persuade women to participate and what factors might make them amenable to persuasion [1]. In recent years, cancer screening has become more controversial, however, with particular concern about the evidence underpinning the programmes offered and overdiagnosis being hotly debated [2, 3]. The potential benefit of screening is the avoidance of the disease, or of dying from the disease. But the harms can include false positives, overdiagnosis, and treatment of lesions and cancers which would never be otherwise diagnosed or cause problems in the patient's lifetime. In addition, there is the anxiety which inevitably accompanies the screening process.

Cancer Prevention and Screening: Concepts, Principles and Controversies, First Edition.
Edited by Rosalind A. Eeles, Christine D. Berg, and Jeffrey S. Tobias.
© 2019 John Wiley & Sons, Inc. Published 2019 by John Wiley & Sons, Inc.

Cervical screening

Cervical cancer may, in the future, be controlled by vaccination against oncogenic types of human papilloma virus (HPV). But for the moment, there are millions of women around the world who have been exposed to the virus and for whom regular screening is most the most appropriate control technique. The traditional method of screening to prevent cervical cancer is cervical cytology, and this is estimated to prevent about 75% of cases of cervical cancer, the efficacy of the technique varying with the woman's age [4].

There are over half a million cases of cervical cancer worldwide each year, and over quarter of a million deaths [5]. Most cases and deaths are in the developing world, where it can be the second most common cancer killer of women. It takes a toll which would be quite unrecognized in those countries where good-quality cervical screening is available and accessible to the majority if not all of the population. The benefit of cervical screening for women in these countries is now unarguable. There may never have been randomized controlled trials as there would be today, but these programmes are undoubtedly saving millions of lives. Vaccination may do the same for the next generation of women in the developing world, but it can still be a struggle to deliver cervical cancer control in that area. Visual Inspection with acetic acid or Lugol's iodine followed by immediate treatment may be suitable in low-resource settings [6].

The physical harms of cervical screening were felt to be few and related only to women who had their cervix treated. The cervix was felt to heal well and the use of colposcopic treatments rather than operative cone biopsies reduced the risks to women who needed treatment. However, evidence has emerged of an increased risk of premature delivery for women whose pregnancies followed treatment for cervical intraepithelial neoplasia (CIN) [7]. This has naturally increased caution about treating and even screening for the youngest women, where the benefit of cervical screening was found to be very low, although the abnormality rate was high and therefore the proportion of women treated was high. In England, this resulted in the raising of the screening start age from 20 to 25, which was not without controversy [8].

HPV testing is now likely to replace cervical cytology in the developed world. This is a more suitable test for a vaccinated population with fewer abnormalities, and is less subjective than cytology. It is more sensitive in terms of identifying the infected and abnormal cervix, but less specific than cytology. So it is likely that cytology would be applied to samples positive for HPV in order to determine which women should be referred immediately and which might just be placed under surveillance. Cytology may be replaced entirely in due course with new molecular techniques. Moving to HPV testing could increase the benefit of cervical screening by preventing more cancers. If applied carefully, it could also reduce harms by allowing less frequent screening for those testing HPV negative. However, the exact management strategies for those women who are HPV positive are not yet fully defined, particularly for those women who are HPV positive but with no evidence of abnormality on their cervix.

Breast screening

Breast cancer is the most common form of cancer for women worldwide. The first screening trial took place in the 1960s in New York [9] and found a 30% reduction in mortality. The next trial was the Swedish Two Counties trial, which has now published 30-year results [10]. This also showed a 30% reduction in mortality. Screening programmes were instituted in Finland and the UK in the late 1980s, and spread throughout the developed world over the next decade [11].

There are about 1.6 million cases of breast cancer diagnosed worldwide and over half a million deaths annually [5]. Survival has improved markedly since the time of the original New York trial. However, breast screening has become increasingly controversial. The New York and Two Counties trials were followed by various other trials, some of which were consistent, but others showed a much lower level of benefit or little benefit at all. The Nordic Cochrane Centre in particular has criticized the quality of many of the original trials, none of which really examined the issue of overdiagnosis which has recently been raised [12]. Estimates of the benefits of breast screening now range down to around a 15% reduction in mortality from 30%, and the estimates of overdiagnosis from 10–30%. These differences in the estimates of the risks and benefits of breast screening come about because of different assessments of the values of the various trials, and because of the different methodologies used by those assessing the estimates.

The context of each screening programme (whether in North America or northern Europe, for example) affects how each screening programme operates, and therefore the benefit-to-risk ratio to which it works, since age groups and frequencies of screening are not consistent. The US Preventative Services Task Force considered the benefits and risks of screening from 39 years. It concluded that the benefits for women aged 39–49 were a 15% reduction in mortality. The degree of benefit then rose with age. The Task Force noted the higher likelihood of a false positive recall among younger women and recommended biennial screening from 50–74 years, with individual decision-making at ages below that [13]. The Canadian Taskforce on Preventative Healthcare estimated that for women aged 50–69 the risk of dying from breast cancer was reduced by 21% if they were screened with two-yearly screening for 11 years, so for each breast cancer death avoided, 'at least 4 women would have part or all of a breast unnecessarily removed and bear the burden of over-diagnosis' [14]. In the UK, the Marmot Review considered women aged 50–69 and calculated that there was a 20% reduction in mortality with three-yearly screening for 20 years, and that for each life saved, there were three women diagnosed with a breast cancer that might not otherwise have been found and treated. It recommended that the UK programmes should continue [15]. The Swiss Medical Board, on the other hand, recommended that no further systematic screening programmes be introduced and that the current ones be reviewed. They argued that for the benefit of 1 or 2 women out of 1000 regularly screened not dying from breast cancer, 100 of those 1000 women would be harmed by unnecessary further investigations and, for some, unnecessary treatments [16].

Colorectal cancer screening

Colorectal cancer is the third most common cancer in men worldwide and the second most common cancer in women. There are about three-quarters of a million cases in men each year, with over 600 000 more cases in men than in women. Incidence is higher in the developed world, but there are more deaths in the developing world. There are just fewer than 700 000 deaths a year worldwide from colorectal cancer [5].

Survival from colorectal cancer varies hugely with stage at diagnosis. In England, five-year survival in men is reported to be 95% from a Dukes A cancer, but less than half from a Dukes C, and only 7% surviving five years with a Dukes D colorectal cancer [17]. However, fewer than 10% of colorectal cancers were found at Dukes A stage in England between 1996 and 2002. Randomized controlled trials for people in middle to older age, working to very similar protocols, took place in Nottingham, England and Funen, Denmark, with a narrower age group trial in Goteborg, Sweden and a large, more complex trial in Minnesota, USA [18–21]. The trials took place in the 1980s and used guaiac-based faecal occult blood testing (FOBT). All trials demonstrated the ability to detect colorectal cancers at an earlier stage than in routine practice with annual or biennial testing, and all demonstrated a mortality reduction after several years of follow-up. There was a variation in different arms of the Minnesota and Goteborg studies where the guaiac was rehydrated, but this led to a very high rate of colonoscopy, with all the risks involved in this examination. The trials overall with biennial testing and unrehydrated guaiac showed about a 16% reduction in mortality in the invited population, about 25% among participants [22]. Given that any adenomas seen were removed from patients testing positive, a reduction in incidence was also sought, but this was only seen in the Minnesota trial and this difference is attributed to the high colonoscopy rate in that trial [23].

With the principle firmly established of screening being able to downstage colorectal cancers sufficiently to reduce mortality, new screening tests for colorectal cancer were sought. Guaiac is a natural substance with an inherent variability and requiring manual interpretation. The test has been estimated to have a sensitivity of 35–55% as a once-only test, although repeat (biennial) testing raises the sensitivity considerably [24]. Newer tests are immunochemical and are often called faecal immunochemical tests (FIT). These have not been used in randomized controlled trials, but comparison exercises with FOBT have been carried out, some of them randomized, which have shown improved sensitivity with FIT and also improved participation rates with a test which appears to be more acceptable to its target population [25]. It is an automated test and is quantitative. This affords the ability to vary the cut-off points according to the desired balance of sensitivity, specificity, and endoscopy capacity for those identified as needing this examination. The immunochemical test is preferred in the European Quality Assurance Guidelines for Colorectal Screening [26].

For those testing positive on either FOBT or FIT, the next stage of the process is endoscopy. This test can both visualize the colon and remove polyps for examination in one procedure. This has led to the suggestion that endoscopy could be the first-line test without the need for any pre-filtering. However, endoscopy is a test which requires considerable patient preparation and has an associated morbidity and mortality rate [27]; furthermore, endoscopy quality and capacity need careful consideration [28, 29]. There have been no trials of colonoscopy as a screening technique, only observational studies, but there have been high-quality trials of flexible sigmoidoscopy as a screening technique. This examination requires less preparation of the patient, reaches those parts of the bowel where most colorectal cancers occur, and has a much-reduced risk of adverse events compared with colonoscopy.

Flexible sigmoidoscopy screening has been shown to reduce the incidence of colorectal cancer. In the UK trial, Atkin showed a 23% reduction in incidence in the intervention group after 11 years of follow-up, and a mortality reduction of 31% [30]. The similar Italian SCORE trial saw a reduction in incidence of 18% and in mortality of 22%, although the latter was not significant [31]. The latter researchers are moving on to a trial to compare flexible sigmoidoscopy screening with computed tomography (CT) colography [32].

The harm that can be done by screening for colorectal cancer is unique, in that it can be quite catastrophic for an asymptomatic individual. Endoscopy is required either as the primary screening test or as its follow-up, and this is accompanied by a morbidity and mortality rate of its own. These can be carefully controlled for in screening programmes, but not avoided altogether [33]. For some patients surgery is required to remove a screen-detected adenoma to which endoscopic access might be difficult or dangerous. Abdominal surgery in people in later middle or old age can also lead to severe consequences and death.

Prostate cancer screening

The cancer screening systems considered so far all have harms associated with them, but the considered opinion of most authorities around the world is that the benefit outweighs the harms. Prostate cancer screening, however, continues to be in the unsatisfactory position of relating to a disease which kills over 300,000 men per year worldwide, for which there is a test, prostate-specific antigen (PSA), which is both acceptable and which is of proven benefit, but where public health authorities consider that the benefits of PSA-based screening for prostate cancer do not outweigh the harms [34].

Over a million men worldwide are diagnosed with prostate cancer each year. Incidence rates vary hugely and are indicative of the amount of PSA testing in a population. The highest incidence rates are seen where PSA testing rates are high [5]. The European Randomized Study of Screening for Prostate Cancer (ERSPC) now has 13 years of follow-up and reports a 21% reduction in mortality [35]. This is calculated to equate to one prostate cancer death avoided for 27 additional prostate cancers detected. The equivalent calculated for breast screening by the UK review was one death avoided for 3 additional breast cancers detected. Furthermore, the consequences of a diagnosis of prostate cancer are not inconsiderable. They can include urinary, bowel, and erectile dysfunction, loss of fertility, and side effects from hormone or chemotherapy. The alternative of watchful waiting can lead to considerable anxiety, and associated repeat biopsies have morbidity from that procedure without a diagnosis of cancer.

Many authorities therefore recommend that men be counselled before PSA testing about the potential harms of the test as well as the potential benefits. The man's decision about whether to undergo testing or not will be informed by his own value system and previous experience, together with any recommendation from his doctor.

Psychological harms of screening

All cancer screening programmes involve an element of anxiety. If the population targeted was not concerned about the cancer being screened for, no one would participate. However, participation brings those anxieties to the fore, and an abnormal result requiring further investigation can lead to anxiety persisting for some time after the 'all clear' has been given [36]. Undoubtedly, having to undergo an investigative procedure after a 'simple' screening test engenders anxiety [37]. For many people, the benefit of 'peace of mind' after a normal result is felt to be the reward for the trial of going through a screening programme, and a reminder that screening tests can be incorrect is not welcome. For those who have had further tests, the anxiety can take some time to abate. Evidence shows, however, that for some people the experience is sufficiently worrying that they do not participate in the screening programme in the next round [36].

Informed decision-making

Consideration of a proposal for participation in cancer screening is generally accompanied by considerable statistical information. The very invitation can induce anxiety as people wrestle to understand the issues and as they have to consider their own susceptibility to cancer of one sort or another. There are studies which show that women want to make their own mind up about breast screening [38] and others which show that women wish to trust the authorities [39]. There is great attention paid to the information offered to accompany a suggestion or invitation to screening [40].

The individual must factor in their own age and health status when considering the statistical risks and benefits of an offer of screening. He/she also brings to bear on the decision over participation not only their understanding of any literature given to them or information imparted by their doctor, but also the values and experiences which influence their lives generally. Similarly, health policymakers apply the values of the society which they reflect or represent in making judgements about which screening tests to recommend. Overall uptake rates are population based, but it is for the individual person to participate or not: it is a dichotomous decision. The individual could decide to opt out of any diagnostic process which might follow, but, once screened, could not decide not to know whether that screen showed a risk of disease or not. The decision about whether risks and benefits come down in favour of offering or participating in a screening test or not is informed by evidence and quality of life indicators, but to a large extent the scales on which risks and benefits are weighed are calibrated in different units. The risk of a cancer being diagnosed and treated which might not otherwise become apparent needs to be weighed against the avoidance of loss of life.

Conclusion

Screening programmes must all balance benefits and harms. For some techniques there is an overwhelming case for benefit or harm, while others are more marginal. Some screening programmes are subject to the opinion of human beings when determining positivity and recall rates. These rates are then affected by cultural and social factors about the tolerance of false positives and false negatives. The person invited for screening has to consider the potential benefit and harm of participating in a screening programme for themselves as an individual, and to bring to bear in that decision their own personal experiences and values. There is no universal right answer.

References

1 Hill, D., Gardner, G., and Rassaby, J. (1985). Factors predisposing women to take precautions against breast and cervix cancer. *J. Appl. Soc. Psychol.* 15 (1): 59–89.

2 Mukhtar, T.K., Yeates, D.R.G., and Goldacre, M.J. (2013). Breast cancer mortality trends in England and the assessment of the effectiveness of mammography screening: Population-based study. *J. R. Soc. Med.* 106 (6): 234–242.

3 Zackrisson, S., Andersson, I., Janzon, L. et al. (2006). Rate of over-diagnosis of breast cancer 15 years after end of Malmö mammographic screening trial: Follow-up study. *BMJ* 332 (7543): 689–692.

4 Sasieni, P., Adams, J., and Cuzick, J. (2003). Benefit of cervical screening at different ages: Evidence from the UK audit of screening histories. *Br. J. Cancer* 89 (1): 88–93.

5 International Agency for Research on Cancer (2012). Globocan 2012: Estimated Cancer Incidence, Mortality and Prevalence Worldwide in 2012. http://globocan.iarc.fr (accessed 20 October 2014).

6 Sankaranarayanan, R., Wesley, R., Thara, S. et al. (2003). Test characteristics of visual inspection with 4% acetic acid (VIA) and Lugol's iodine (VILI) in cervical cancer screening in Kerala, India. *Int. J. Cancer* 106 (3): 404–408.

7 Kyrgiou, M., Koliopoulos, G., Martin-Hirsch, P. et al. (2006). Obstetric outcomes after conservative treatment for intraepithelial or early invasive cervical lesions: Systematic review and meta-analysis. *Lancet* 367: 489–498.

8 Lynch, A. (2008). 'I was told I was too young for a smear test but now I am dying of cervical cancer at just 24'. *Daily Mail*, 10 June. http://www.dailymail.co.uk/health/article-1025334/I-told-I-young-smear-test-I-dying-cervical-cancer-just-24.html (accessed 20 October 2014).

9 Shapiro, S., Venet, W., Strax, P. et al. (1982). Ten- to fourteen-year effect of screening on breast cancer mortality. *J. Natl Cancer Inst.* 69 (2): 349–355.

10 Tabár, L., Vitak, B., Chen, T.H. et al. (2011). Swedish two-county trial: Impact of mammographic screening on breast cancer mortality during 3 decades. *Radiology* 260 (3): 658–663.

11 Ballard-Barbash, R., Klabunde, C., Paci, E. et al. (1999). Breast cancer screening in 21 countries: Delivery of services, notification of results and outcomes ascertainment. *Eur. J. Cancer Prev.* 8 (5): 417–426.

12 Gøtzsche, P.C., and Jørgensen, K.J. (2013). Screening for breast cancer with mammography. *Cochrane Database Syst Rev.* 4 (Art. No.: CD001877). doi: 10.1002/14651858.CD001877.pub5.

13 US Preventive Services Task Force (2009). Screening for breast cancer: U.S. Preventive Services Task Force recommendation statement. *Ann. Intern. Med.* 151 (10): 716–26, W-236.

14 Canadian Task Force on Preventive Health (2011). Breast Cancer – Risks and Benefits, Age 50–69. https://canadiantaskforce.ca/tools-resources/breast-cancer-2/breast-cancer-risks-benefits-age-50-69/ (accessed 2 January 2018).

15 Independent UK Panel on Breast Cancer Screening (2012). The benefits and harms of breast cancer screening: An independent review. *Lancet* 380 (9855): 1778–1786.

16 Swiss Medical Board (2013). Systematisches Mammographie-Screening. http://www.medical-board.ch/fileadmin/docs/public/mb/Fachberichte/2013-12-15_Bericht_Mammographie_Final_Kurzfassung_d.pdf (accessed 20 October 2014).

17 Cancer Research UK (n.d.). Bowel Cancer Survival Statistics. http://www.cancerresearchuk.org/cancer-info/cancerstats/types/bowel/survival/bowel-cancer-survival-statistics#stage (accessed 12 March 2018).

18 Hardcastle, J.D., Chamberlain, J.O., Robinson, M.H. et al. (1996). Randomised controlled trial of faecal-occult-blood screening for colorectal cancer. *Lancet* 348 (9040): 1472–1477.

19 Kronborg, O., Fenger, C., Olsen, J. et al. (1996). Randomised study of screening for colorectal cancer with faecal-occult-blood test. *Lancet* 348 (9040): 1467–1471.

20 Lindholm, E., Brevinge, H., and Haglind, E. (2008). Survival benefit in a randomized clinical trial of faecal occult blood screening for colorectal cancer. *Br. J. Surg.* 95 (8): 1029–1036.

21 Mandel, J.S., Church, T.R., Ederer, F., and Bond, J.H. (1999). Colorectal cancer mortality: Effectiveness of biennial screening for fecal occult blood. *J. Natl Cancer Inst.* 91 (5): 434–437.

22 Hewitson, P., Glasziou, P., Watson. E. et al. (2008). Cochrane systematic review of colorectal cancer screening using the fecal occult blood test (hemoccult): An update. *Am. J. Gastroenterol.* 103 (6): 1541–1549.

23 Church, T.R., Mandel, J.S., Bond, J.H. and Ederer, F. (2003). Colorectal cancer incidence reduction due to polyp removal: Results from the Minnesota trial. *Gastroenterol.* 124 (4, Suppl. 1): A55.

24 Young, G.P., St John, D.J., Winawer, S.J., and Rozen, P. (2002). Choice of fecal occult blood tests for colorectal cancer screening: Recommendations based on performance characteristics in population studies: A WHO (World Health Organization) and OMED (World Organization for Digestive Endoscopy) report. *Am. J. Gastroenterol.* 97 (10): 2499–2507.

25 van Rossum, L.G., van Rijn, A.F., Laheij, R.J. et al. (2008). Random comparison of guaiac and immunochemical fecal occult blood tests for colorectal cancer in a screening population. *Gastroenterol.* 135 (1): 82–90.

26 Segnan, N., Patnick, J., and von Karsa, L., ed. (2011). European Guidelines for Quality Assurance in Colorectal Cancer Screening and Diagnosis. Brussels: European Commission.

27 Rutter, C.M., Johnson, E., Miglioretti, D.L. et al. (2012). Adverse events after screening and follow-up colonoscopy. *Cancer Causes Control* 23 (2): 289–296.

28 Brown, M.L., Klabunde, C.N., and Mysliwiec, P. (2003). Current capacity for endoscopic colorectal cancer screening in the United States: Data from the National Cancer Institute Survey of Colorectal Cancer Screening Practices. *Am. J. Med.* 115 (2): 129–133.

29 Bowel Cancer UK (2014). Early diagnosis: Diagnosing bowel cancer early: right test, right time. www.bowelcanceruk.org.uk/media/173462/1061_bcuk_endoscopy_report.pdf (accessed 22 January 2018).

30 Atkin, W.S., Edwards, R., Kralj-Hans, I. et al.; UK Flexible Sigmoidoscopy Trial Investigators (2010). Once-only flexible sigmoidoscopy screening in prevention of colorectal cancer: A multicentre randomised controlled trial. *Lancet* 375 (9726): 1624–1633.

31 Segnan, N., Armaroli, P., Bonelli. L. et al.; SCORE Working Group (2011). Once-only sigmoidoscopy in colorectal cancer screening: Follow-up findings of the Italian Randomized Controlled Trial – SCORE. *J. Natl Cancer Inst.* 103 (17): 1310–1322.

32 Regge, D., Iussich, G., Senore, C. et al. (2014). Population screening for colorectal cancer by flexible sigmoidoscopy or CT colonography: Study protocol for a multicenter randomized trial. *Trials* 15: 97.

33 Lee, T.J., Rutter, M.D., Blanks, R.G. et al. (2012). Colonoscopy quality measures: Experience from the NHS Bowel Cancer Screening Programme. *Gut* 61 (7): 1050–1057.

34 Moyer, V.A.; U.S. Preventive Services Task Force (2012). Screening for prostate cancer: U.S. Preventive Services Task Force Recommendation Statement. *Ann. Intern. Med.* 157: 120–134.

35 Schröder, F.H., Hugosson, J., Roobol, M.J.; ERSPC Investigators (2014). Screening and prostate cancer mortality: Results of the European Randomised Study of Screening for Prostate Cancer (ERSPC) at 13 years of follow-up. *Lancet* 384 (9959): 2027–2035.

36 Brett, J., Austoker, J., and Ong, G. (1998). Do women who undergo further investigation for breast screening suffer adverse psychological consequences? A multi-centre follow-up study comparing different breast screening result groups five months after their last breast screening appointment. *J. Public Health Med.* 20 (4): 396–403.

37 Brewer, N.T., Salz, T., and Lillie, S.E. (2007). Systematic review: The long-term effects of false-positive mammograms. *Ann. Intern. Med.* 146 (7): 502–510.

38 Hersch, J., Jansen, J., Irwig, L. et al. (2011). How do we achieve informed choice for women considering breast screening? *Prev. Med.* 53 (3): 144–146.

39 Schwartz, L.M., Woloshin, S., Fowler, F.J., Jr, and Welch, H.G. (2004). Enthusiasm for cancer screening in the United States. *JAMA* 291 (1): 71–78.

40 Forbes, L.J., and Ramirez, A.J.; Expert group on Information about Breast Screening (2014). Offering informed choice about breast screening. *J. Med. Screen* 21 (4): 194–200.

CHAPTER 5

Cancer screening issues in black and ethnic minority populations

Otis W. Brawley

American Cancer Society, Georgia, USA

SUMMARY BOX

- Certain populations are at higher risk for certain cancers when compared to others. Common categorizations of populations used in health-care data include area of geographical origin, race, family and genetics, ethnicity and culture, and even socio-economic status and the social deprivation index.

- Area of geographical origin, such as Asian, sub-Saharan African, or European, is perhaps the most common way of categorizing populations.

- Family is another way of categorizing populations. This is correlated with genetic risk. Area of geographical origin is also linked to familial or genetic risk. Perhaps the clearest example is that of the founder Ashkenazi Jewish mutations of the *BRCA1* and *BRCA2* genes.

- Ethnicity and culture involve common behaviour, common lifestyle habits, and common environmental influences.

- Well-intentioned population profiling by race, ethnicity, family history, or social factors can be done to identify populations at high risk for certain cancers. Individuals from these defined populations at high risk are more likely to benefit from screening.

The purpose of cancer screening is to reduce risk of death from cancer. Screening is most appropriately aimed at those at highest risk of having a deadly cancer [1]. Not only are those at highest risk most likely to benefit, the positive predictive value of the screening test is highest among those with the highest prevalence of the disease. The marginal example is that we would never recommend screening all men for breast cancer because of the very low rate of male breast cancer. For a man at high risk for breast cancer due to a genetic mutation or family history, screening is considered reasonable.

There have been significant efforts aimed at identifying individuals at high risk. Common factors used include gender, age, and family history [2, 3]. Some

---

Cancer Prevention and Screening: Concepts, Principles and Controversies, First Edition.
Edited by Rosalind A. Eeles, Christine D. Berg, and Jeffrey S. Tobias.
© 2019 John Wiley & Sons, Inc. Published 2019 by John Wiley & Sons, Inc.

cancers, such as colon cancer, are so common that screening is recommended for all people in the age range generally affected. Some cancers are common in a particular gender and age group, and screening is considered in that group, for instance breast or prostate cancer among people of a certain age [4]. Some organizations look at the same data and choose different ages to start screening.

Certain populations are at higher risk for certain cancers when compared to others. This leads to the question of whether a higher-risk population should be screened while populations at lower risk are not. Defining or profiling populations at risk is complicated and in some cases controversial. Other questions include:

- How much higher should the risk be for screening to be considered?
- Should screening in these populations be held to the same threshold for proof of benefit that is required for screening the general population?

Common categorizations of populations used in health-care data include area of geographical origin, race, family and genetics, ethnicity and culture, and even socio-economic status and the social deprivation index [5].

Many population categorizations, even geographical ones, have unclear boundaries. Area of geographical origin, such as Asian, sub-Saharan African, or European, is perhaps the most common way of categorizing populations. There is some scientific merit to using this category, as some diseases do tend to be associated with certain areas of the world. Migration and co-mingling of populations have made defining populations by area of geographical origin very difficult, however.

Family is another way of categorizing populations. This is correlated with genetic risk. Of course, area of geographical origin is also linked to familial or genetic risk. Perhaps the clearest example is that of the Ashkenazi Jewish mutations in the *BRCA1* and *BRCA2* genes [6]. Three specific mutations are common, but not exclusive, to women of Ashkenazi Jewish families [7, 8]. Population modelling suggests that these mutations have founders in Central and Eastern Europe about 1200 years ago. The mutations are ancestral. They are common to Jewish families due to the influence of segregation caused by area of origin, ethnicity, culture, and other political and social influences.

The concepts of ethnicity and culture as used in academic study are also fluid and without clear boundaries. Ethnicity and culture involve common behaviour, common lifestyle habits, and common environmental influences. Some of these influences can link to risk of disease. Ethnicity can, of course, link to family and genetic inheritance.

Race is a categorization commonly used in the USA [9]. It is a social concept first put forth about 350 years ago. The initial categories were Caucasian, Negroid, and Mongoloid [10]. These had to do with skin colour, facial traits, and presumed geographical area of origin. Race is a flawed, somewhat artificial, concept. Distinct racial groups do not exist. The anthropology community has never accepted race as a 'biological categorization'. That being said, people of the same race do commonly cohabitate. They generally share culture, environment, and genetics.

Just as these ways of categorizing populations are fluid and indistinct, the roles that these categories play in causing and preventing disease are often not singular nor fully defined.

Liver cancer is a common disease among persons originating from Southeast Asia due to endemic hepatitis B, for instance. Liver cancer is also common in western and central Africa due to endemic hepatitis B and large-scale contamination of staple foods, such as maize and groundnuts, with aflatoxin B1, a known environmental carcinogen, produced by mould during inadequate storage of crops. Exposure to aflatoxin is more common among those who are socially deprived [11]. Some researchers have advocated liver cancer screening with ultrasound in these populations [12].

Oesophageal cancer clusters are found in specific regions of southern South America, east and south Africa, and in a geographical belt extending from the Caucasus Mountains eastward to China. In these regions the incidence of oesophageal cancer is up to 20-fold higher than in the USA and Western Europe. Investigations suggest that the cause is both environmental and dietary. Culture is an influence on this cancer [13, 14]. Some studies have advocated screening these populations with endoscopy, even though a randomized controlled trial to demonstrate efficacy has not been attempted.

On the other hand, cervical cancer rates are low in Middle Eastern Arab women [15]. This is thought to be influenced by strict cultural and social behaviours that prevent the spread of the human papilloma virus. It has been argued that cervical screening is a waste of resources in some Middle Eastern countries, but should be emphasized in countries where the death rate from this cancer is high [16].

Once a population at high risk for a disease for which there is a potential screening intervention has been identified, the question becomes: 'Does that screening test work?' or 'Has it been proven that screening and appropriate early treatment reduce risk of death?' At times the question will become: 'Has the screening test been shown to reduce risk of death in any population?' At other times, the appropriate question is: 'Has the test been shown to reduce risk of death in this specific high-risk population?'

Prostate cancer is a disease where all these questions apply. Prostate cancer diagnosis and death are more common among persons originating from sub-Saharan Africa and black people [17]. The reasons are unknown. Some researchers have urged a sort of racial profiling, saying that screening should be offered to men of black African origin if it is offered to any at all.

There are legitimate questions as to whether prostate cancer screening reduces risk of death for any population. Some studies have suggested that prostate cancer is 'a different disease' in African American men versus Caucasian men [18], and some that prostate cancer tends to be more aggressive in African American men. Given the concept of length bias, if screening is beneficial at all, it could be substantially more or substantially less beneficial in African American men compared with Caucasians. This is an especially difficult issue in that the only studies to show that prostate cancer screening is beneficial have been done in largely Caucasian European countries [19]. The race question can only be addressed in a definitive fashion with a prospective randomized controlled trial that is statistically powered to assess the outcome in African Americans and in Caucasians [20]. Such a trial would have to be large, twice the size of a trial addressing the same question in men in general, and would be extremely expensive and last for more than 15 years if it were possible to do. Given the popularity of screening, it is unlikely that one could maintain the integrity of the control group.

US law requires a subset analysis of racial differences in outcome as part of the assessment of US government-funded Phase 3 screening and treatment trials [20]. Such subset analyses by their nature are underpowered to make any factual statement. The lack of statistical power in subset analyses is more challenging than the fact that the racial categories used are socio-political and not biological.

US demographic data show that the age-specific prostate cancer mortality rates are higher among black or African American men age 40–49 years [21]. Some studies have suggested that African American men should start screening at age 40 or 45 years and white or Caucasian men start screening at age 50 or 55 years. Similar arguments are used to advocate screening African American men and women for colon cancer [22]. There are no rules about how to make the decision of the age at which to recommend screening be started in a population. It is certain that the likelihood of benefit is low and the chances of a false positive are higher when the prevalence of disease is low. Exactly when the prevalence of disease is high enough to merit screening is a value judgement and reasonable people can disagree.

It is extremely important to realize the limitations of screening; that is, that no screening test can save all from a cancer death. Indeed, most screening tests, which have been shown to be beneficial, reduce the relative risk of death by 20–30% [1]. This means that 70–80% of those destined to die of the cancer will still die despite high-quality screening. Hence, screening is most effective and saves the most lives when it is focused on the population most likely to die from the disease in question. Even with a higher age-specific mortality rate, a 20% reduction in relative risk among a population at risk from age 40 to 49 will translate into a large number screened for a small absolute number of lives saved.

In the USA, much discussion concerns mass screening or recommendations to screen an entire population, however categorized [1]. Screening for certain cancers is commonly done haphazardly in mass screening centres or at health fairs. Informed decision-making, maintenance of records, follow-up and assurance of compliance with regularly scheduled screening and treatment (if needed) are all challenging. It is most reasonable to make an individualized screening decision within the physician–patient relationship after assessing the specific patient's health status, family and other history, and personal concerns. Also, one should not perform a screening test if quality diagnostics and treatment are not available for someone with a positive screening test.

Screening for most cancers is a procedure in which there are documented harms and a potential for benefit. Perhaps the most important issue is that the health-care provider has a definite obligation to inform the subject/patient about the questions and risks concerning a screening test and to ensure that the patient understands before consenting to testing. It is a fact that many who offer screening are often overly optimistic and enthusiastic about the abilities of screening. It is important to respect an individual's right to self-determination. That is, if a patient says 'no' to screening, that 'no' should be respected.

This ethical issue is especially significant when dealing with racial/ethnic minorities, the less educated, and the poor. Unfortunately, medicine has a long history of abusing and exploiting these vulnerable populations. Making matters worse, many screening tests and resulting treatments are profitable to those offering them, while being of questionable and limited efficacy to those offered them.

A number of professional organizations in the USA, Canada, and Europe have called for informed decision-making and open conversations between the health-care provider and the patient regarding screening [21]. This is especially so when discussing prostate and lung cancer screening, although the trend appears to be moving into breast cancer screening also. Informed decision-making and explaining the complexity of screening, its risk of harm and potential for benefit, are not easy. Tailored messaging and specially designed decision aids are available for some diseases and may be useful.

Conclusion

Well-intentioned population profiling by race, ethnicity, family history, or social factors can be done to identify populations at high risk for certain cancers. Individuals from these defined populations at high risk are more likely to benefit from screening. They might be offered screening when others would not. The decision to offer screening should take into account what is known about the particular screening test and the biology of the disease in the defined population. The limitations of screening should be appreciated. Efficacious screening reduces the risk of death from the specific cancer, but does not reduce the risk to zero. Indeed, most efficacious screening tests have been shown to reduce the relative risk of death by only 20–30%. This can translate into a small absolute benefit. Screening should only be offered when reasonable-quality diagnosis and treatment can be assured. The patient/subject should understand that there are risks and possible benefits associated with screening, and the health-care provider should respect the patient/subject's decision, should s/he decide to refuse the offer of screening.

References

1 Croswell, J.M., Ransohoff, D.F., and Kramer, B.S. (2010). Principles of cancer screening: Lessons from history and study design issues. *Semin. Oncol.* 37: 202–215.

2 Thompson, I.M., Ankerst, D.P., Chi, C. et al. (2006). Assessing prostate cancer risk: Results from the Prostate Cancer Prevention Trial. *J. Natl Cancer Inst.* 98: 529–534.

3 Brawley, O.W. (2012). Risk-based mammography screening: An effort to maximize the benefits and minimize the harms. *Ann. Intern. Med.* 156: 662–663.

4 van Ravesteyn, N., Stout, N., Lee, S. et al. (2012). What level of risk tips the balance of benefits and harms to favor screening mammography starting at age 40? *Ann. Intern. Med.* 156 (9): 609–617.

5 Brawley, O.W. (2003). Population categorization and cancer statistics. *Cancer Metastasis Rev.* 22: 11–19.

6 Berman, D.B., Wagner-Costalas, J., Schultz, D.C. et al. (1996). Two distinct origins of a common BRCA1 mutation in breast-ovarian cancer families: A genetic study of 15 185delAG-mutation kindreds. *Am. J. Hum. Gen.* 58: 1166–1176.

7 Liu, E. (1998). The uncoupling of race and cancer genetics. *Cancer* 83: 1765–1769.

8 Offit, K., Gilewski, T., McGuire, P. et al. (1996). Germline BRCA1 185delAG mutations in Jewish women with breast cancer. *Lancet* 347: 1643–1645.

9 Brawley, O.W. (2010). Toward a better understanding of race and cancer. *Clin. Cancer Res.* 16: 5920–5922.

10 Witzig, R. (1996). The medicalization of race: Scientific legitimization of a flawed social construct. *Ann. Intern. Med.* 125: 675–679.

11 Parkin, D.M., Bray, F., Ferlay, J., and Jemal, A. (2014). Cancer in Africa 2012. *Cancer Epidemiol. Biomarkers Prev.* 23: 953–966.

12 Aghoram, R., Cai, P., and Dickinson, J.A. (2012). Alpha-foetoprotein and/or liver ultra-sonography for screening of hepatocellular carcinoma in patients with chronic hepatitis B. *Cochrane Database Syst. Rev.* 9 (Art. No.: CD002799). doi: 10.1002/14651858.CD002799.pub2.

13 Roshandel, G., Khoshnia, M., Sotoudeh, M. et al. (2014). Endoscopic screening for precancerous lesions of the esophagus in a high risk area in Northern Iran. *Arch. Iran. Med.* 17: 246–252.

14 Golozar, A., Etemadi, A., Kamangar, F. et al. (2016). Food preparation methods, drinking water source, and esophageal squamous cell carcinoma in the high-risk area of Golestan, Northeast Iran. *Eur. J. Cancer Prev.* 25 (2): 123–129.

15 Siegel, R.L., Miller, K.D., and Jemal, A. (2015). Cancer statistics, 2015. *CA Cancer J. Clin.* 65: 5–29.

16 Sankaranarayanan, R., Nene, B.M., Shastri, S.S. et al. (2009). HPV screening for cervical cancer in rural India. *N. Engl. J. Med.* 360: 1385–1394.

17 Hsing, A.W., Yeboah, E., Biritwum, R. et al. (2014). High prevalence of screen detected prostate cancer in West Africans: Implications for racial disparity of prostate cancer. *J. Urol.* 192: 730–735.

18 Fedewa, S.A., Etzioni, R., Flanders, W.D. et al. (2010). Association of insurance and race/ethnicity with disease severity among men diagnosed with prostate cancer, National Cancer Database 2004–2006. *Cancer Epidemiol. Biomarkers Prev.* 19: 2437–2444.

19 Schroder, F.H., Hugosson, J., Roobol, M.J. et al. (2014). Screening and prostate cancer mortality: Results of the European Randomised Study of Screening for Prostate Cancer (ERSPC) at 13 years of follow-up. *Lancet* 384: 2027–2035.

20 Freedman, L.S., Simon, R., Foulkes, M.A. et al. (1995). Inclusion of women and minorities in clinical trials and the NIH Revitalization Act of 1993 – the perspective of NIH clinical trialists. *Control Clin. Trials* 16: 277–285; discussion 86–89, 93–109.

21 Smith, R.A., Manassaram-Baptiste, D., Brooks, D. et al. (2015). Cancer screening in the United States, 2015: A review of current American Cancer Society guidelines and current issues in cancer screening. *CA Cancer J. Clin.* 65: 30–54.

22 Laiyemo, A.O., Doubeni, C., Pinsky, P.F. et al. (2010). Race and colorectal cancer disparities: Health-care utilization vs different cancer susceptibilities. *J. Natl Cancer Inst.* 102: 538–546.

CHAPTER 6

Public awareness of cancer screening

Jane Wardle[†] and Laura A.V. Marlow

Cancer Research UK Health Behaviour Research Centre, Department of Epidemiology & Public Health, UCL, London, UK

SUMMARY BOX

- There is a lack of public awareness that some cancer screening tests can detect 'precancer' and therefore prevent the development of cancer.

- Beliefs such as fear of cancer or fatalism about cancer outcomes can deter screening participation.

- Public perceptions of cancer risk are often inaccurate, but are not related to screening uptake.

- Improvements in risk stratification and an increasing number and complexity of screening tests mean that communication to the public and improving understanding will be a sizeable challenge.

Cancer screening is the term used to describe a range of medical tests designed to identify cancer at an asymptomatic stage or to identify precancerous cell changes. Screening is a significant plank of public health action to reduce cancer deaths, but, unlike developments in cancer treatment, requires the active engagement of the healthy population. The challenge of engaging the public with cancer screening is to promote informed participation in what may be an uncomfortable medical test, with limited specificity and sensitivity, which may yield a distressing clinical outcome. In addition, risk stratification is now actively being considered in order to deliver screening to those most likely to benefit while limiting population exposure to harms. This is likely to entail additional 'prescreening' tests to assess individual risk and provide individual screening recommendations, raising further issues of public education and engagement.

[†] Sadly Professor Jane Wardle died before the publication of this book.

Cancer Prevention and Screening: Concepts, Principles and Controversies, First Edition.
Edited by Rosalind A. Eeles, Christine D. Berg, and Jeffrey S. Tobias.
© 2019 John Wiley & Sons, Inc. Published 2019 by John Wiley & Sons, Inc.

The World Health Organization recommends screening for cervical, breast, and colorectal cancer (CRC), and many countries now offer organized programmes or provide recommendations to clinicians on the appropriate age group, frequency, and modality of testing. Screening for prostate cancer is also widely available, and is covered by Medicare in the USA, although it is not generally recommended by expert groups and is not part of most organized programmes. Screening for lung cancer is likely to be introduced in the near future following evidence of efficacy from clinical trials.

There is an important difference between screening tests that aim to detect cancer before symptoms are manifest and those that aim to detect precancerous changes. Breast, prostate, and lung cancer screening, as well as faecal occult blood testing (FOBT) for CRC, aim to diagnose cancer at an earlier, more treatable, stage. Implementation of these programmes does not prevent the target cancer; on the contrary, such programmes increase recorded incidence, but survival rates are improved. Cervical screening and endoscopic screening for CRC aim to detect precancerous cell changes, so that the affected tissue can be surgically removed to prevent the development of cancer. Implementation of these programmes reduces the incidence of the target cancers, and can therefore be defined as preventive.

The need for high rates of participation in recommended screening programmes in order to deliver the anticipated cost-effective public health benefits now sits alongside a requirement for public understanding of the risks and benefits of cancer screening, making screening participation an issue of considerable interest to social and behavioural scientists.

Awareness of cancer screening

Awareness that cancer screening exists is an important first step to participation [1]. Population-based studies in European countries with organized screening programmes suggest that most people (70–95%) are aware of screening programmes for breast and cervical cancer [2,3]. Awareness of CRC screening is lower in Europe, at around 30–60% [4], but in the USA, where CRC screening has been established for longer, awareness is over 70% for all modalities [5]. As might be expected, these broad figures disguise differences between population subgroups, and awareness is often somewhat lower in ethnic minority or immigrant groups [2,3,5], lower socio-economic status groups [2,5], and younger and older adults [5]; findings that mirror studies of cancer knowledge more generally [6,7].

Awareness of screening is enhanced by written invitations for testing in settings with organized screening programmes, although not surprisingly there are inequalities in both awareness and uptake in relation to levels of health literacy [8]. In settings where screening is offered through a health-care provider, those who have not seen a provider in the last year have lower awareness [5]. Media coverage or advertisements may also influence awareness, and a recent US study found that these were the two most commonly cited sources of information on CRC screening (47% and 39%, respectively) [9]. Media coverage of a trial of endoscopic CRC screening was also found to increase uptake of the FOBT programme in the UK [10].

Beyond simple awareness of the existence of a screening test, people's knowledge about screening is limited. For example, less than half of those who were aware of CRC screening knew the recommended age range or frequency of testing [5]. This may be less of an issue in countries with a routine call–recall programme, but it is important in other environments and could help promote screening readiness. More importantly, public understanding of the purpose of screening tests is limited. For example, in a survey of US women within the cervical screening age range in a Federally Qualified Health Program, only 5% knew that a Pap smear looked exclusively for abnormalities in the cervix and not also for other infections [11]. Recognition of the role of 'precancers' and the potential for prevention is also very limited [12]. When women were asked 'what things do you think affect a woman's chance of getting cervical cancer?', only 6% suggested regular screening [13].

A critical aspect of knowledge about screening is that it is designed for the asymptomatic population. A large-scale survey in the USA identified an association between lack of colorectal symptoms and lower participation in CRC screening [14]. Similarly in the UK, good 'bowel health' was cited as a reason for not feeling at risk of CRC and not thinking that screening was needed [15]. In the years following the introduction of mammography screening, data from the National Health Interview Surveys in the USA (collected in 1987 and 1990) suggested that the most frequently endorsed reason for being unscreened was believing that mammography was unnecessary in the absence of symptoms [16]. The symptom–screening association is no longer clearly demonstrated for breast screening, which may be partly because it is culturally embedded as routine health care. CRC screening, however, is newer (and less easy to discuss) and, as such, needs a more individual decision. If individuals are making the decision about whether they need the test, it is vital that they have correct information; a belief that symptoms are an indicator of the need for screening suggests a lack of understanding of the purpose of screening. It is also interesting to note that perceptions of CRC risk were almost unrelated to CRC findings at screening in a large study [17], suggesting that subjective risk assessments are often inaccurate.

Beliefs relevant to cancer screening

Beliefs about cancer have been widely studied in the screening context, with a particular focus on three factors: perceived risk, fear, and fatalism, as well as specific beliefs about screening.

Perceptions of cancer risk

Cancer risk perceptions relate to the individual's view of their likelihood of getting cancer, either within a given time period or in a lifetime. It appears common sense that risk perceptions are important, and most theoretical models from psychology see perceived risk as an important motivator of health behaviour (e.g. the Extended Parallel Process Model [18]). However, a review of the literature [19] concluded that there was not enough evidence to draw conclusions about the association between perceived risk and screening for cervical or colorectal cancer, although higher perceived risk of breast cancer was modestly associated with participation in mammography. A more recent meta-analysis of perceived risk in breast screening drew a similar conclusion [20], although it pointed to one study suggesting that associations could be stronger for first-time attenders [21]. Even though the results are variable, it is clear that the influence of risk perceptions is much lower than assumed. This has been highlighted in studies where provision of personalized genetic and environmental risk information failed to increase CRC screening uptake among nonattenders [22,23].

These findings need to be viewed in light of the considerable difficulties in measuring perceived risk. In a population-based survey of nearly 7000 US men and women, 60% believed their chance of getting cancer in the future was 'somewhat 'or 'very high', demonstrating recognition of the high incidence of cancer [24]. However, when asked about personal risk compared with others of the same age and sex, people consistently report that their risk is below average, demonstrating what has been called an optimistic bias [25,26]. Interestingly, it is difficult to shift optimistic bias; one large community study showed that providing individual risk information neither modified optimism nor increased intention to screen [27].

Cancer fear

Fear, worry, and anxiety are all terms used to refer to the emotional response to cancer. Historically, cancer was feared because of its terrible prognosis. Advances in early diagnosis and treatment have greatly improved survival rates, yet more than half of the population still say they fear cancer more than any other disease [28], with higher levels of fear in women, younger people, and those from lower socio-economic status or ethnic minority backgrounds [28–30].

Although fear of cancer might be expected to motivate any action designed to reduce the risk of cancer death, studies exploring associations between cancer fear and screening participation show surprisingly mixed results. Some find that higher fear is associated with higher uptake and others find it is associated with lower uptake [29]. One explanation could be a limited range of fear levels within study samples. Two studies have shown a curvilinear association between fear and screening uptake: uptake is lowest for the extremes of low or high fear and highest at medium levels of fear [31,32]. Research carried out in populations who generally have low fear might therefore find that higher fear is associated with higher screening uptake, while studies in populations with generally high fear levels might find that lower fear is associated with higher uptake. Additionally, the type of fear that is being assessed may be important. Fear is a multidimensional concept with cognitive, affective, physiological, and behavioural parameters. Cancer worry may motivate screening as a means of producing reassurance and controlling worrying thoughts. Indeed, worriers may wish to be screened more frequently than is recommended. In contrast, a more visceral discomfort in thinking about cancer could motivate avoidance. People described as 'cancer-phobic' often avoid any exposure to information about cancer, and may even avoid the word 'cancer'. In a recent analysis of CRC screening, worry about cancer was associated with higher intention to be screened, but discomfort thinking about it was associated with lower uptake [33].

Cancer fatalism

The term 'fatalism' refers to the belief that life events are controlled by external forces over which the individual is powerless; although the construct is usually applied only in the context of negative outcomes, so fatalists tend to expect the worst rather than the best. Cancer fatalism has been defined as the belief that a cancer diagnosis is predestined, or that death is inevitable following diagnosis [34]. Cancer fatalism has been associated with nonparticipation in breast and colorectal cancer screening [34]. People who score higher on cancer fatalism are more likely to believe that they will get cancer [35], less likely to believe that screening can help prevent cancer [35], and less likely to participate in screening [34]. Much of the research in this area has focused specifically on fatalism's role in explaining disengagement with cancer screening among ethnic minority groups, particularly those from African American backgrounds [36]. However, more recent studies have examined the wider population, suggesting that fatalistic views can be identified in all ethnic groups, although they tend to be more common in women, and in lower socio-economic status and ethnic minority groups [34,37]. A better exploration of links between fatalism and cancer screening uptake in the general population is needed.

Perceived benefits and harms of cancer screening

In general, people think that routine cancer screening is a good thing; they think that it finds cancer earlier and therefore that lives are saved and treatment is easier, although there are slight differences by socio-economic status [38]. However, although these attitudes are likely to promote screening participation, concern is being expressed that they are too positive, with people overestimating the benefits and underestimating the harms of screening [39,40]. A survey of over 10 000 men and women found that they grossly overestimated the benefits of breast and prostate cancer screening, believing that far more lives were saved than experts estimate to be the case [41]. This is worrying in terms of accuracy of knowledge, although we should be mindful of the fact that screening's benefits are usually estimated at a population level, and most lay people are unfamiliar with levels of risk and benefit that have meaning on a population scale.

The greatest concern has been about the concept of overdiagnosis. By comparing the number of cancers diagnosed at screening with the number of cancer cases seen in the absence of screening, it is clear that some cancers diagnosed at screening must be 'overdiagnosed'; that is, they would never have manifested or resulted in harm. In the case of breast screening, it has been estimated that for every breast cancer death prevented by screening, three cases are 'overdiagnosed' [42], and rates of overdiagnosis in prostate cancer screening are substantially higher.

Clearly, it is important that the public understand the risk of overdiagnosis in order to make informed decisions about screening participation, although the concept is difficult to get across. Several studies find little or no change in attitudes towards screening after evidence is presented for overdiagnosis [43,44]. This may be partly because screening has been strongly promoted for many years and it is hard to change attitudes with simple information. If this is the case, then better public education is clearly vital. But it may also be because the perceived benefit of reassurance that there is no cancer in the body, or even the chance of being saved from cancer death, outweighs the perceived risks of unnecessary treatment. In support of this, a study in which overdiagnosis information was presented verbally, with opportunities to clarify where needed, found that women say they are willing to accept the risk that 'their' cancer may be overdiagnosed in order to avoid being the one with a 'true' cancer and missing out on life-saving treatment; suggesting that they can understand the risk and are willing to take it [40]. However, concern remains that part of the effect is due to broad cultural support for screening, which makes it difficult for women to take a negative stance.

Informed choice

Informed choice is currently operationalized by the combination of knowledge, attitudes, and behaviour, placing emphasis on public understanding of cancer screening as a goal for public health. Knowledge is a prerequisite, but after that, an informed choice is said to have been made if attitudes are positive and the person attends for screening, or attitudes are negative and they do not attend for screening. In practice, knowledge of screening is often poor, even among attenders [11], suggesting that people are participating in procedures they know little about. This illustrates that knowledge is not a prerequisite for participation, and suggests that some of those who are screened do not make an informed choice.

One approach to increasing informed choice is through the use of decision aids. These can encourage involvement in health-care decisions by providing relevant information about the risks and benefits in a format that specifically presents them together, and at the same time alerts individuals to consider their own values. Decision aids have been shown to improve knowledge and reduce decisional conflict, although they do not seem to improve satisfaction with the decision [45]. Decision aids may also reduce uptake, a particular concern in relation to screening tests where there is no issue of overdiagnosis, and particularly in lower literacy who may struggle to understand the material in the

decision aid. In one trial, adults with low educational attainment were randomized to receive a CRC decision aid (interactive workbook and DVD) or standard screening information. Those who received the decision aid had better
knowledge, but their attitudes were less positive and screening uptake was
lower [46].

One criticism of informed choice is that the process is burdensome, and may
be unnecessary when expert committees have reviewed the research data and
endorsed the screening programme [47]. There is also concern that much of the
information needed to understand the risks and benefits of cancer screening is
difficult to comprehend, particularly for people with lower numeracy [48]. One
alternative proposal is that some people may wish to 'consider an offer' to be
screened [47]. This would involve a recommendation to attend screening from a
trusted source, with access to information on why the recommendation has been
made. This approach does not expect people to read detailed technical information, but respects their autonomy by providing sources of further information for
those who want it. It also acknowledges that some people may not want to attend
screening. Consistent with this, the majority of UK adults said that they wanted a
strong recommendation for screening from the National Health Service, but they
also wanted full information to be provided [49].

Intention and action

The traditional focus on knowledge and attitudes is based on the assumption that
human beings make rational conscious choices over matters like screening, and
then act accordingly. However, recognition that many intentions are not actually
translated into action (the 'intention–behaviour gap') has moderated this view
[50]. If intention and action are somewhat independent, then their associations
with knowledge/attitudes may be different. One of the larger studies, carried out
in the context of CRC screening [51], found that factors such as perceived risk and
attitudes were strong predictors of intention, but that among those who intended
to attend, other factors like health status, stress, and social support, which had not
been associated with intention, were the primary predictors of screening uptake.
These results are consistent with the idea that other barriers may emerge when
the time comes to do the test. In some cases the practical difficulties of doing the
test may loom larger at the point of action than they did in advance. For screening
that involves a visit to a health professional, practical factors such as getting an
appointment that fits around other commitments and finding child care are possible barriers [52].

The intention–behaviour gap can also be the result of simple forgetting, in
which case 'cues to action' are important. In the USA, discussion with a health-
care provider and a recommendation to participate in screening are associated
with higher uptake of CRC screening [53]. In organized screening programmes,
there is good evidence that simple mailed reminders increase coverage [54]. In a

multistage study in the USA, a series of reminders were used to increase FOBT uptake. Around 10% of participants returned their kit before being reminded, 40% returned the kit following an automated reminder call/text, and 24% following a second automated reminder. After three months, those who had not returned the kit received a personal phone call, following which a further 8% of kits were returned, raising uptake levels overall from 38% to 82% [55]. The apparent effectiveness of reminders, alongside evidence that the idea of screening attracts widespread community support, suggests that prompting those who have simply 'forgotten' about it is an important aspect of sustaining motivation between deciding to act and actually acting on the decision.

Engagement

A prerequisite of an informed screening decision is individual engagement. An active decision not to attend screening can be entirely appropriate; a person may have a very good reason not to want a cancer diagnosis at that time. However, some nonattenders may be basing their decision on incorrect 'knowledge', or may not have engaged with the screening offer because they lack either the motivation or the capability to understand it. This is likely to be particularly important in relation to novel screening modalities about which there is little general cultural discourse. Many qualitative studies of nonparticipants for CRC screening find that only a minority have definite negative attitudes to the test. Many others have forgotten that they were invited or say that they have not yet decided [56]. Interestingly, despite such interviews being nonpersuasive, participants often say that taking part in the interview made them feel that they would like to participate. This opportunity to discuss CRC screening provides a platform to dispel misconceptions and support screening decisions [57]. In pilot work with community groups in London, educational talks about CRC screening opened up discussion of the topic, improving both awareness and willingness to participate [58]. This is consistent with new survey data showing that the majority of people who did not complete an FOBT said that they had not read the information materials. Considering how best to engage the disengaged is therefore an important goal for screening promotion. Some of the findings with telephone contact or so-called patient navigation take a one-to-one approach to engagement. A recent study that used a stepped approach through written and telephone contact more than doubled CRC screening uptake compared with the usual care condition [55]. The 'screening offer' itself, especially when it consists entirely of mailed written material, is inevitably challenging for sectors of the community with lower health literacy. Research is needed into strategies for achieving awareness of screening – and ultimately informed choices – in population groups who are unable or unwilling to read health-related materials.

The Precaution Adoption Process Model [59] is a framework comprising a series of stages of awareness and action in preventive behaviours, as well as insights into strategies that enhance movement through stages. This could facilitate future research and knowledge translation in the screening area. The particular value of this model compared with many other psychological models is that it provides for 'unaware' and 'unengaged' stages, and these precede the stages where detailed knowledge, attitudes, or choices come into play. It also allows for deciding against action, consistent with informed choice models, as well as continuing beyond a single action into sustained participation, as is needed for most cancer screening programmes.

Conclusion

Understanding what the public know and believe about cancer screening has long been considered important by behavioural scientists working in cancer control. The evidence to date suggests that well-established screening programmes attract strong support regardless of knowledge, but that new screening tests pose a challenge. There is a particular lack of awareness that some screening tests can prevent cancer through identifying and treating precancerous stages. Public recognition of this could play a key role in improving uptake. Cancer screening tests are likely to increase in number and complexity over the coming years, and are likely to involve risk stratification, placing additional demands on people's understanding of the harms and benefits of different types of screening. In the light of moves towards informed choice in screening, public health specialists will be expected to communicate effectively about the tests that are offered, and public knowledge and attitudes are likely to take an increasingly important role in the research and implementation agendas.

References

1 Berkowitz, Z., Hawkins, N.A., Peipins, L.A. et al. (2008). Beliefs, risk perceptions, and gaps in knowledge as barriers to colorectal cancer screening in older adults. *J. Am. Geriatr. Soc.* 56: 307–314.

2 Robb, K., Wardle, J., Stubbings, S. et al. (2010). Ethnic disparities in knowledge of cancer screening programmes in the UK. *J. Med. Screen* 17: 125–131.

3 Carrasco-Garrido, P., Hernandez-Barrera, V., de Lopez, A.A. et al. (2014). Awareness and uptake of colorectal, breast, cervical and prostate cancer screening tests in Spain. *Eur. J. Public Health* 24: 264–270.

4 Keighley, M.R., O'Morain, C., Giacosa, A. et al. (2004). Public awareness of risk factors and screening for colorectal cancer in Europe. *Eur. J. Cancer Prev.* 13: 257–262.

5 Ford, J.S., Coups, E.J., and Hay, J.L. (2006). Knowledge of colon cancer screening in a national probability sample in the United States. *J. Health Commun.* 11 (Suppl. 1): 19–35.

6 Hawkins, N.A., Berkowitz, Z., and Peipins, L.A. (2010). What does the public know about preventing cancer? Results from the Health Information National Trends Survey (HINTS). *Health Educ. Behav.* 37: 490–503.

7 Robb, K., Stubbings, S., Ramirez, A. et al. (2009). Public awareness of cancer in Britain: A population-based survey of adults. *Br. J. Cancer* 101 (Suppl. 2): S18–S23.

8 Kobayashi, L.C., Wardle, J., and von Wagner, C. (2014). Limited health literacy is a barrier to colorectal cancer screening in England: Evidence from the English Longitudinal Study of Ageing. *Prev. Med.* 61: 100–105.

9 Cooper, C.P., Gelb, C.A., and Hawkins, N.A. (2012). How many 'Get Screened' messages does it take? Evidence from colorectal cancer screening promotion in the United States, 2012. *Prev. Med.* 60: 27–32.

10 Lo, S.H., Vart, G., Snowball, J. et al. The impact of media coverage of the Flexible Sigmoidoscopy Trial on English colorectal screening uptake. *J. Med. Screen* 19: 83–88.

11 Hawkins, N.A., Benard, V.B., Greek, A. et al. (2013). Patient knowledge and beliefs as barriers to extending cervical cancer screening intervals in Federally Qualified Health Centers. *Prev. Med.* 57: 641–645.

12 Kavanagh, A.M., and Broom, D.H. (1997). Women's understanding of abnormal cervical smear test results: A qualitative interview study. *BMJ* 314: 1388–1391.

13 Low, E.L., Simon, A.E., Lyons, J. et al. (2012). What do British women know about cervical cancer symptoms and risk factors? *Eur. J. Cancer* 48: 3001–3008.

14 Ioannou, G.N., Chapko, M.K., and Dominitz, J.A. (2003). Predictors of colorectal cancer screening participation in the United States. *Am. J. Gastroenterol.* 98: 2082–2091.

15 Robb, K.A., Miles, A., and Wardle, J. (2007). Perceived risk of colorectal cancer: Sources of risk judgments. *Cancer Epidemiol. Biomarkers Prev.* 16: 694–702.

16 Breem, N., and Kessler, L. (1994). Changes in the use of screening mammography: Evidence from the 1987 and 1990 National Health Interview Surveys. *Am. J. Public Health* 84: 62–67.

17 Robb, K.A., Miles, A., and Wardle, J. (2004). Subjective and objective risk of colorectal cancer (UK). *Cancer Causes Control* 15: 21–25.

18 Witte, K. (1994). Fear control and danger control – a test of the extended parallel process model (Eppm). *Communi Monogr* 61: 113–134.

19 Vernon, S.W. (1999). Risk perception and risk communication for cancer screening behaviors: A review. *J. Natl Cancer Inst. Monogr.* 25: 101–119.

20 Katapodi, M.C., Lee, K.A., Facione, N.C., and Dodd, M.J. (2004). Predictors of perceived breast cancer risk and the relation between perceived risk and breast cancer screening: A meta-analytic review. *Prev. Med.* 38: 388–402.

21 Aiken, L.S., Fenaughty, A.M., West, S.G. et al. (1995). Perceived determinants of risk for breast cancer and the relations among objective risk, perceived risk, and screening behavior over time. *Womens Health* 1: 27–50.

22 Weinberg, D.S., Myers, R.E., Keenan, E. et al. (2014). Genetic and environmental risk assessment and colorectal cancer screening in an average-risk population: A randomized trial. *Ann. Intern. Med.* 161: 537–545.

23 Blumenthal-Barby, J.S., McGuire, A.L., and Ubel, P.A. (2014). Why information alone is not enough: Behavioral economics and the future of genomic medicine. *Ann. Intern. Med.* 161: 605–606.

24 Kowalkowski, M.A., Hart, S.L., Du, X.L. et al. (2012). Cancer perceptions: Implications from the 2007 Health Information National Trends Survey. *J. Cancer Surviv.* 6: 287–295.

25 Robb, K.A., Miles, A., and Wardle, J. (2004). Demographic and psychosocial factors associated with perceived risk for colorectal cancer. *Cancer Epidemiol. Biomarkers Prev.* 13: 366–372.

26 Woloshin, S., Schwartz, L.M., Black, W.C., and Welch, H.G. (1999). Women's perceptions of breast cancer risk: How you ask matters. *Med. Decis. Making* 19: 221–229.

27 Robb, K.A., Campbell, J., Evans, P. et al. (2008). Impact of risk information on perceived colorectal cancer risk: A randomized trial. *J. Health Psychol.* 13: 744–753.

28 Vrinten, C., Van Jaarsveld, C.H., Waller, J. et al. (2014). The structure and demographic correlates of cancer fear. *BMC Cancer* 14: 597.

29 Consedine, N.S., Magai, C., Krivoshekova, Y.S. et al. (2004). Fear, anxiety, worry, and breast cancer screening behavior: A critical review. *Cancer Epidemiol. Biomarkers Prev.* 13: 501–510.

30 McQueen, A., Vernon, S.W., Meissner, H.I., and Rakowski, W. (2008). Risk perceptions and worry about cancer: Does gender make a difference? *J. Health Commun.* 13: 56–79.

31 Andersen, M.R., Smith, R., Meischke, H. et al. (2003). Breast cancer worry and mammography use by women with and without a family history in a population-based sample. *Cancer Epidemiol. Biomarkers Prev.* 12: 314–320.

32 Champion, V.L., Skinner, C.S., Menon, U. et al. (2004). A breast cancer fear scale: Psychometric development. *J. Health Psychol.* 9: 753–762.

33 Vrinten, C., Waller, J., von Wagner, C., and Wardle, J. (2015). Cancer fear: Facilitator and deterrent to participation in colorectal cancer screening. *Cancer Epidemiol. Biomarkers Prev.* 24 (2): 400–405.

34 Powe, B.D., and Finnie, R. (2003). Cancer fatalism: The state of the science. *Cancer Nurs.* 26: 454–465.

35 Miles, A., Voorwinden, S., Chapman, S., and Wardle, J. (2008). Psychologic predictors of cancer information avoidance among older adults: The role of cancer fear and fatalism. *Cancer Epidemiol. Biomarkers Prev.* 17: 1872–1879.

36 Powe, B.D. (1996). Cancer fatalism among African-Americans: A review of the literature. *Nurs. Outlook* 44: 18–21.

37 Niederdeppe, J., and Levy, A.G. (2007). Fatalistic beliefs about cancer prevention and three prevention behaviors. *Cancer Epidemiol. Biomarkers Prev.* 16: 998–1003.

38 Schwartz, L.M., Woloshin, S., Fowler, F.J., Jr., and Welch, H.G. (2004). Enthusiasm for cancer screening in the United States. *JAMA* 291: 71–78.

39 Hersch, J., Jansen, J., Barratt, A. et al. (2013). Women's views on overdiagnosis in breast cancer screening: A qualitative study. *BMJ* 346: f158.

40 Waller, J., Douglas, E., Whitaker, K.L., and Wardle, J. (2013). Women's responses to information about overdiagnosis in the UK breast cancer screening programme: A qualitative study. *BMJ Open* 3: e002703.

41 Gigerenzer, G., Mata, J., and Frank, R. (2009). Public knowledge of benefits of breast and prostate cancer screening in Europe. *J. Natl Cancer Inst.* 101: 1216–1220.

42 Independent UK Panel on Breast Cancer Screening (2012). The benefits and harms of breast cancer screening: An independent review. *Lancet* 380: 1778–1786.

43 Cantor, S.B., Volk, R.J., Cass, A.R. et al. (2002). Psychological benefits of prostate cancer screening: The role of reassurance. *Health Expect.* 5: 104–113.

44 Kattan, M.W., Cowen, M.E., and Miles, B.J. (1997). A decision analysis for treatment of clinically localized prostate cancer. *J. Gen. Intern. Med.* 12: 299–305.

45 O'Connor, A.M., Rostom, A., Fiset, V. et al. (1999). Decision aids for patients facing health treatment or screening decisions: Systematic review. *BMJ* 3192: 731–734.

46 Smith, S.K., Trevena, L., Simpson, J.M. et al. (2010). A decision aid to support informed choices about bowel cancer screening among adults with low education: Randomised controlled trial. *BMJ* 341: c5370.

47 Entwistle, V.A., Carter, S.M., Trevena, L. et al. (2008). Communicating about screening. *BMJ* 337: a1591.

48 Schwartz, L.M., Woloshin, S., Black, W.C., and Welch, H.G. (1997). The role of numeracy in understanding the benefit of screening mammography. *Ann. Intern. Med.* 127: 966–972.

49 Waller, J., Macedo, A., von Wagner, C. et al. (2012). Communication about colorectal cancer screening in Britain: Public preferences for an expert recommendation. *Br. J. Cancer* 107: 1938–1943.

50 Sheeran, P. (2002). Intention–behaviour relations: A conceptual and empirical review. *Eur. Rev. Soc. Psychol.* 12: 1–36.

51 Power, E., Van Jaarsveld, C.H., McCaffery, K. et al. (2008). Understanding intentions and action in colorectal cancer screening. *Ann. Behav. Med.* 35: 285–294.

52 Waller, J., Bartoszek, M., Marlow, L., and Wardle, J. (2009). Barriers to cervical cancer screening attendance in England: A population-based survey. *J. Med. Screen* 16: 199–204.

53 Laiyemo, A.O., Adebogun, A.O., Doubeni, C.A. et al. (2014). Influence of provider discussion and specific recommendation on colorectal cancer screening uptake among U.S. adults. *Prev. Med.* 67: 1–5.

54 Camilloni, L., Ferroni, E., Cendales, B.J. et al. (2013). Methods to increase participation in organised screening programs: A systematic review. *BMC Public Health* 13: 464.

55 Baker, D.W., Brown, T., Buchanan, D.R. et al. (2014). Comparative effectiveness of a multifaceted intervention to improve adherence to annual colorectal cancer screening in community health centers: A randomized clinical trial. *JAMA Intern. Med.* 174: 1235–1241.

56 Hall, N.J., Rubin, G.P., Dobson, C. et al. Attitudes and beliefs of non-participants in a population-based screening programme for colorectal cancer. *Health Expect* 18: 1645–1657.

57 Palmer, C.K., Thomas, M.C., von Wagner, C., and Raine, R. (2014). Reasons for non-uptake and subsequent participation in the NHS Bowel Cancer Screening Programme: A qualitative study. *Br. J. Cancer* 110: 1705–1711.

58 Tai, C.K., Leung, P., Poullis, A., and Curry, G. (2015). Comment on 'Reasons for non-uptake and subsequent participation in the NHS bowel cancer screening programme: A qualitative study'. *Br. J. Cancer* 112: 1834.

59 Weinstein, N.D., Sandman, P.M., and Blalock, S.J. (2008). The precaution adoption process model. In: *Health Behaviour and Health Education*, 4e (ed. K. Glanz, B.K. Rimer, and K. Viswanath), 123–147. San Francisco, CA: Jossey-Bass.

CHAPTER 7

Public understanding of cancer prevention

Jessica Kirby and Sarah Woolnough

Cancer Research UK, London, UK

SUMMARY BOX

- Cancer rates in the UK are rising rapidly, and prevention is critical to helping manage the human and financial costs of cancer.
- Public understanding of cancer prevention is imperfect, but improving.
- Evidence-based interventions to raise understanding and promote healthy behaviour change can be effective, but need careful planning and sustained investment.
- To make information engaging and understandable to people, it should be explained in lay language or visual presentations, be brief and clear, and be relevant to the audience.
- Raising awareness and understanding about cancer prevention is necessary, but not sufficient, for achieving behaviour change and cancer prevention.
- There is a wide range of available information about cancer, of varying quality, so it is important for trusted voices to cut through the noise and bring clarity and evidence to messages on cancer prevention.

Public understanding of prevention

There is a gap between what the public understand to be causes of cancer, and what the evidence shows. Persistent myths about cancer causes, sometimes inflamed and perpetuated by the media, can distract people from evidence-based changes that could actually reduce their risk, while knowledge of proven cancer risk factors (other than smoking) remains low. This contributes to an environment in which many people seek quick fixes to reduce the risk, such as so-called 'superfoods' or vitamin supplements, or look for a single big cause to eliminate, pointing the finger at 'poisonous' plastic bottles or 'E numbers'. When public policy action

---

Cancer Prevention and Screening: Concepts, Principles and Controversies, First Edition.
Edited by Rosalind A. Eeles, Christine D. Berg, and Jeffrey S. Tobias.
© 2019 John Wiley & Sons, Inc. Published 2019 by John Wiley & Sons, Inc.

is directed at corporate activities that do jeopardize public health, such as the marketing of high fat, sugar, and salt foods to children, or alcohol pricing, accusations of 'nanny-statism' abound and can scupper efforts to create a health-promoting environment. But campaigns and information to raise understanding of cancer prevention, and translate this into healthy behaviour change, can and do work. Raising awareness and understanding is an important first step towards promoting healthy behaviour change, and while this cannot achieve behaviour change on its own, it can help create an environment where healthy behaviours are desirable, and where public policy measures to help people make healthy choices are better supported.

To gain a reliable understanding of public knowledge of cancer risk and prevention, UCL and Cancer Research UK researchers developed a validated 'Cancer Awareness Measure' [1], which was then applied in a nationally representative sample of over 2000 UK adults, as well as in an 'ethnic boost' sample of 1500 adults to understand how knowledge varies in these groups. Results from the Cancer Awareness Measure surveys show that, perhaps unsurprisingly, tobacco remains the best-recalled cancer risk factor, with 82% mentioning smoking as a risk factor in the 2017 survey. This highlights how successful sustained, well-funded awareness and behaviour change campaigns can be in embedding public understanding of cancer risk factors. Awareness of other proven risk factors was lower, with alcohol being recalled by only 54%, diet by 36%, and just 15% mentioning the link between obesity and cancer. Although these figures may seem low, recall of these other risk factors has been rising over the years, as charities and health organizations have done more and more to try to help people understand the full range of lifestyle choices that are linked to cancer risk. However, there are significant inequalities within these overall figures – for example, people from more deprived or ethnic minority backgrounds are less likely to be aware of risk factors.

In addition to their knowledge of what can affect cancer risk, people's attitudes towards cancer and cancer prevention can affect how motivated they may be to make healthy choices, sometimes in complex ways. For example, fear of cancer may help motivate people to live more healthily, or it may lead to a 'head in the sand' approach where people do not wish to engage in preventive behaviours. And individuals may simultaneously hold both positive and negative attitudes towards cancer, including prevention [2]. One UK study gave an example of this: 'I am, like most people, actually frightened of it. So ... I tend to dodge thinking about it. But I already take into account things like diet, not smoking, not drinking too much, that kind of thing, keeping my weight down, [and] exercising.'

Fatalistic attitudes towards cancer can materially affect a range of health behaviours relating to cancer, including healthy living. A US study [3] found that people holding more fatalistic attitudes about cancer were less likely to be a non-smoker, to be active, and to eat plenty of fruit and vegetables. In the same study, nearly half agreed that 'It seems like almost everything causes cancer', nearly a third thought 'There's not much people can do to lower their chances of getting cancer', and over 70% agreed 'There are so many recommendations about preventing cancer, it's hard to know which ones to follow.'

Often, enquiries to Cancer Research UK's helplines question why someone who has lived very healthily got cancer, where others who have made different choices do not have the disease. The existence of cases of this nature in people's personal experience serves to undermine belief in the preventability of cancer, potentially leading to a lack of motivation in choosing healthier options that could reduce the risk, and a 'what's the point?' attitude. By clarifying that healthy living is not a guarantee but instead reduces the risk – or stacks the odds in our favour – we can help to combat these fatalistic approaches.

When around 4 out of 10 UK cancer cases may be prevented by healthy lifestyle choices and avoiding risky exposures, it is clear that promoting understanding of what can be done to reduce risk, and cultivating positive attitudes about the preventability of cancer, is and will remain critical to stem the rising tide of new cancer cases. The challenge is to effectively communicate risk information relevant to the whole population, in a way that is helpful for the individual, avoids blame, and acknowledges that prevention is not a guarantee, but leads to a reduction in risk.

There are times when it may not be necessary to link healthy lifestyle behaviours specifically to cancer as an outcome to promote healthy behaviour choices. In certain circumstances, focusing on a more relevant short-term outcome may be more effective. For example, when working on sun protection messaging with young people – especially young women – audience insight demonstrates that concern about the shorter-term effects of the sun on people's appearance is more salient than concern about the risk of skin cancer in a decade or two. As a result, Cancer Research UK's messaging to this audience tends to focus on excess ultraviolet (UV) light leading to premature ageing and coarse, wrinkled, and leathery skin. This has proved to be a more successful and engaging route than focusing on skin cancer messaging. In other circumstances, however, making a link to cancer where people have not previously considered that risk factor in a cancer context can be extremely effective. Obesity, for example, is commonly linked to diabetes and cardiovascular disease, but the cancer link can act as 'new news' to people and raise motivation for healthy behaviour changes. And research shows [4] that when people know about the link between alcohol and cancer, they are more likely to be supportive of public policy measures to help reduce alcohol consumption, such as increasing price, adding health warnings to packaging, and restricting advertising and availability. Understanding the prior knowledge levels, attitudes, and motivations of the audience can help to inform whether making a cancer link is the best way to promote healthy living. Those working to prevent cancers may well be justified in focusing messaging on other health or social impacts of unhealthy behaviours if this leads to changes in behaviour and therefore reduction of cancer risk. The downside of this approach, however, is the loss of the opportunity to build better public knowledge and understanding of cancer prevention in the long run.

What can we do to improve understanding?

Changing people's beliefs and attitudes is difficult; raising awareness and understanding appears to be a more manageable task, and one that many health organizations and governments are actively engaged in tackling. As people learn in many different styles and situations, a range of methods is required to ensure improvements in understanding that can be detected across the whole population.

However daunting the task may seem, there have been improvements in knowledge about cancer prevention between 2014 and 2017, as measured in the Cancer Awareness Measure surveys. At a population level, significant (if sometimes small) increases were seen in recall of obesity (10–15%), and pollution (6–10%) as risk factors for cancer. However, most other risk factors did not see an improvement in recall over this time period, and there is still a clear need to raise awareness of what aspects of lifestyle can affect the risk of cancer.

There are many examples of health promotion activities that have been demonstrated to be successful in raising knowledge and understanding of cancer prevention in the target audiences. Some examples from Cancer Research UK's work are included here as case studies; in addition, there is a wealth of activity to raise understanding of cancer risk and prevention by other charities, local and central public health teams, health departments, and community organizations.

Awareness-raising activity that happens at both a local and national level, and is integrated into settings where people are likely to take messages on board, can be extremely effective. For example, the national smoking cessation campaign 'Stoptober', which began in 2012, was highly effective [5] at raising understanding and promoting behaviour change. The campaign aims to encourage smokers into a mass quit attempt during the month of October, and is based on clear psychological and behavioural principles to promote quit attempts. While it was a national media and social media campaign, it was also locally grounded, in that it linked through to local smoking cessation services and was promoted through general practitioner (GP) surgeries and pharmacies. In the first year, the campaign achieved an additional 350 000 quit attempts, and a 50% increase in quitting compared to other months of the year. The campaign was estimated to have saved over 10 000 discounted life years (DLYs) at a low cost (around £400 per DLY saved). This highly effective campaign shows the benefits of developing insightful campaigns rooted in evidence, and ensuring these are integrated with local services and well funded.

Often, very large increases in awareness and dialogue about prevention or early diagnosis of cancer occur after a high-profile person has been diagnosed with, or died from, cancer. Examples include the actor Michael Douglas discussing potential causes of his throat cancer, after which numerous articles were published in media outlets on the subject of human papilloma virus (HPV) and links to oral and oropharyngeal cancers, a risk factor with low prior public awareness.

In Brazil [6], there were an additional 1.1 million enquiries to smoking cessation services in the month following President Lula da Silva's laryngeal cancer diagnosis, a larger increase than after World No Tobacco Day and other quit-related events, demonstrating associations between cancer preventive behaviours and news about cancer diagnoses of people in the public eye.

In addition to celebrities, there is an important role for trusted voices in the provision of believable and engaging cancer prevention information. Charities clearly have a role in this, as do the media, governments, national health organizations, community health professionals, friends and family, community leaders, and teachers. We all have a role to play in promoting public health, modelling healthy behaviours, and sharing cancer prevention messages within our networks.

It is important to consider people's stage of life and other circumstances when sharing cancer prevention messages. People are more open to new health information, and prepared to make a change, at a range of life stages or events such as pregnancy, hospitalization, disease diagnosis, or after a 'cancer scare' (perhaps a referral for further investigation of a symptom which did not lead to a diagnosis of cancer). Such 'teachable moments' tend to be situations where people have higher perceptions of personal risk, strong positive or negative emotions, or heightened belief that the healthy behaviour would have benefits [7]. They are opportune times to give healthy living messages, and people may be more likely to seek out health information, or make healthy behaviour changes, at these times. There is a wealth of literature identifying teachable moments for cancer prevention, and highlighting the potentially large impact of taking opportunities to share health information at times when it will be better received. For smoking cessation, high quit rates have been found at disease diagnosis, pregnancy, and hospitalization [7]; attendance at cancer screening programmes may also lend itself to promoting a range of healthy behaviours [8], particularly dietary choices.

Cancer diagnosis itself can often function as a teachable moment, and although it may appear at first sight to be 'too late' for prevention information, there is still an important role for healthy living information at and after cancer diagnosis. There is a growing evidence base that healthy living pre- and post-diagnosis, in particular giving up smoking and keeping physically active, can improve outcomes and survival from cancer, as well as improving other health and psychosocial outcomes. In addition, as long-term cancer survival increases, those living with and after cancer may well be at risk of second primary cancers later on. Although there is still a great deal to learn in this area, it appears clear that health professionals should consider what healthy living messages may be appropriate for the patient's situation and encourage appropriate healthy behaviours in patients with and after cancer. The specific teachable moment may be at diagnosis, during treatment, or after completion of treatment [9], and health-care providers should consider the situations of their individual patients, as well as the impact of their cancer treatment, to help them choose the most appropriate time to discuss healthy living messages.

Case study: Online information

The internet is an important source of health information for many people [10]. Health websites, such as WebMD and NHS Choices, receive tens of millions of visitors per month [11,12], and nonspecialist health websites, particularly Wikipedia, are also commonly consulted [13] on health matters. Charity websites are further popular sources of trusted information online.

To service this need to seek out health information, the 'About Cancer' section of the Cancer Research UK website [14] includes prevention information on risk factors for each of 65 cancer types, as well as sections on the risk factors themselves [15], including tips on reducing the risk, inspiration from people who have successfully made a healthy lifestyle change, information on how that risk factor is linked to cancer, and which cancer types are linked. These sections are cross-linked and are arranged within a navigable and relatable information architecture. The information is accredited by The Information Standard, a scheme that ensures information is accurate, up to date, reliable, and user focused. User feedback is collected and acted on, via star rating systems, comment submissions, and cross-site user surveys, and the information is checked and updated regularly. User feedback about the content indicates that it is clear in tone, believable, and persuasive, and users appreciate the trusted source of the information.

Although there is a large demand for online health information, it may well be those who need prevention information most who do not actively seek it out. To engage with those not directly searching for health information, Cancer Research UK carries out a range of other digital engagement activities, including engagement campaigns on social media, targeted digital advertising, and partnerships with other sites. For example, the organization worked with popular beauty vloggers on YouTube to create a series of videos aimed at promoting sun safety messages to their followers. These messages were carried within videos about summer beauty and style, to maximize engagement within the vloggers' YouTube audiences and pass on health messages in an unexpected context outside the Cancer Research UK website, to people who were not deliberately seeking out this information. Over 45 000 people watched enough of the videos to see the health messages.

Case study: The media

Communicating with the public via the mainstream media is one critical way in which Cancer Research UK spreads its messages on cancer prevention. This involves both publicizing health messages through releasing research funded by the organization, and providing expert comment and interpretation on stories from other sources. The primary benefits of communicating via the media are that it reaches large audiences, comes via trusted sources, and is often disruptive; that is, it occurs at a moment when people may not be thinking about health, and can challenge them to think about their own health behaviours and possibly seek medical advice. There is evidence [16] that media coverage of cancer can affect awareness, attitudes, and behaviour.

In interviews with broadcast media outlets, being mindful of health promotion means that spokespeople are able to take opportunities to remind audiences of key preventive behaviours, and using positive, approachable, and empowering language can build belief in the messages and motivation to consider acting. Spokespeople can also ensure they steer the interview so that it will always include prevention messages, and ways to seek more information or advice.

Furthermore, the nature of the stories themselves may make health stories more memorable or motivating. In 2012, to tie in with London Fashion Week, Cancer Research UK encouraged model agencies to sign up to a 'no sunbeds policy' for their models [17]. This used the approach of focusing on a noncancer outcome (appearance) to encourage cut-through and engagement with messages about avoiding sunbed use. The story was engaging to this audience, and the involvement of model agencies built belief in the harmful effects of sunbeds on appearance; the story received wide media coverage.

The provision of balance and context to media stories can be as important as proactive promotion of messages and research. Expert comment, and appropriate influencing, can often encourage journalists to be more balanced, or offer guidance as to the strengths and limitations of the research so they can write a representative story that helps people understand cancer risk, or at least avoids harming understanding. Organizations can also offer balanced reporting directly to the public, such as on blogs. NHS Behind the Headlines is one good example, and Cancer Research UK itself runs a blog covering new research and offering context to news stories if the reporting has not been clear or helpful.

The media environment is complex, and reporting of cancer risk stories is not always consistent, leading to confusion among the public as to what is really linked to cancer risk and how important these risk factors truly are. Cancer Research UK takes its responsibility to provide balanced and accurate stories, and to assist journalists in understanding research and reporting it correctly, very seriously. While it should be recognized that this will not solve the problem entirely, organizations working in this way can begin to have an impact and attempt to bring clarity to the public about cancer prevention.

Case study: The Cancer Awareness Roadshow, a face-to-face intervention

Face-to-face communication remains one of the most effective methods of raising understanding about cancer prevention, and promoting behaviour change. Since 2006, Cancer Research UK has run a Cancer Awareness Roadshow, consisting of up to four mobile units that go into the heart of a community, with a specific focus on reducing health inequalities through targeting more deprived areas and those where there is greatest need. The Roadshow is staffed with trained nurses who are equipped to discuss all areas of cancer prevention and early diagnosis, as well as new and emerging evidence or controversial topics. Supporting written materials are also available, as well as engagement tools such as 'jar of tar', 'pound of fat', and glasses indicating the alcohol content of various drinks. All the information offered by nurses is tailored to the individual's needs and questions. Tools such as body mass index (BMI) measurement and Smokerlyser tests are also available on the Roadshow. The teams work alongside local health partners to signpost people to nearby services, and encourage GP consultations.

Evaluation of this activity has demonstrated that interaction with the Roadshow raises awareness of cancer risk factors in a sustained way, helps reduce fatalistic attitudes towards prevention, raises intentions to live a healthy life, and can even promote behaviour change. After a Roadshow visit, awareness of all tested cancer risk factors significantly rose by between 4% and 10%, and this improved knowledge was sustained at two months post-Roadshow for physical activity, and at seven months post-Roadshow for alcohol. After the Roadshow, agreement with the statement 'I believe there is nothing people can do to reduce their chance of developing cancer' fell significantly from 15% to 10%. There was also a significant increase in intentions to quit smoking, and a significant reduction in cigarette consumption at two- and seven-month follow-up. In addition, 23% of the evaluation sample said they had made improvements in their diet since visiting the Roadshow, 15% said they had increased their level of physical activity, and 7% said they had reduced or quit smoking. Moreover, 90% of visitors say they have learnt more about how to reduce their cancer risk, and most visitors say that the Roadshow has allowed them to access information they would not otherwise have obtained. Over 600 000 people visited the Roadshow between 2006 and 2017.

Case study: Talk Cancer, training for health workers

It is also critical to engage health professionals, health volunteers, and other community health workers in spreading messages about healthy living and cancer prevention, as they may often be in contact with harder-to-reach populations and can act as trusted voices. Talk Cancer training has been offered by Cancer Research UK since 2012, and enables and empowers local front-line health workers and volunteers to raise cancer awareness in their community by increasing their knowledge, confidence, and skills to discuss cancer openly. The format is positive, accessible, and interactive, with trainers leading discussion of cancer risk factors, signs and symptoms, and screening, as well as facilitated sessions to raise trainees' confidence in discussing cancer in their interactions and breaking down negative attitudes about cancer prevention and early diagnosis.

Pre- and post-workshop questionnaires found that awareness of multiple cancer risk factors significantly increased post-training. The most significant changes were the number of trainees recognising that lack of physical activity (45% pre, 84% post) and older age (52% pre, 90% post) increased cancer risk. There were also improvements in knowledge about cancer myths, for example the number of trainees who correctly reported that stress does not cause cancer significantly increased from 24% to 82%, and recognition that antiperspirants do not cause cancer also significantly increased from 36% to 87%. Post-training, participants felt more confident in discussing lifestyle changes that can help to reduce cancer risk (64% pre, 91% post).

Three-month follow-up with participants indicated that they had been incorporating learning from Talk Cancer into their day-to-day roles, with trainees feeling more confident to discuss and initiate conversations about cancer ('I feel more confident in broaching the subject and I feel that I can talk with a bit more knowledge and can offer them advice about changing things') and deal with barriers. Satisfaction with the amount of knowledge gained was at 99% and 96% of trainees were satisfied with the communications skills gained through the workshop.

Communicating risk

Messages involving risk – such as those about cancer prevention – can be difficult to communicate with success in the general population. This is owing in part to low average levels of numeracy and risk literacy, and partly the complex nature of the concepts involved. There are many different methods of expressing messages about risk, and an active research community is bringing academic rigour to the public understanding of risk and how best to achieve this.

Some key principles for successfully communicating risk in verbal or written communication include:

- Simplify the message, language, and sentence structure.
- Use natural frequencies with low numerators (aiming for '1 in x' statements).
- Try to include both absolute and relative risks, or at least avoid including only relative risks.
- As well as numerical information, use words to indicate the qualitative size of the risk (e.g. 'most', 'many', 'few', 'high' etc.), without making value judgements.
- Avoid exaggerating or minimizing the risk.
- Use analogies where appropriate.
- Use the second person ('you') and the active voice ('they did' rather than 'it was done').

Visual communication is also key in giving good understanding of complex risks. Icon arrays, infographics, and diagrams can all be helpful to people who learn visually, though care should be taken to avoid overcomplicating the design or the key message. Often, designing a visual presentation of risk information can help communicators in formulating and prioritizing clear and simple key messages, which further helps with verbal explanations of the risk.

In addition, visual presentations of risk or cancer prevention information can be helpful for engaging on social media and elsewhere online, as they are highly shareable, engaging, and present all the key messages at a glance. An example of an infographic that communicates complex information is given in Figure 7.1. This image conveys the relative contribution of various risk factors to the UK's cancer burden, and is based on data on 'attributable fractions' – the proportion of cancers linked to various causes [18]. The original data are complex and the studies present a large quantity of information, whereas the visual presentation does away with much of the complexity to give an at-a-glance impression of how important each risk factor is, along with clear messages as to what people can do

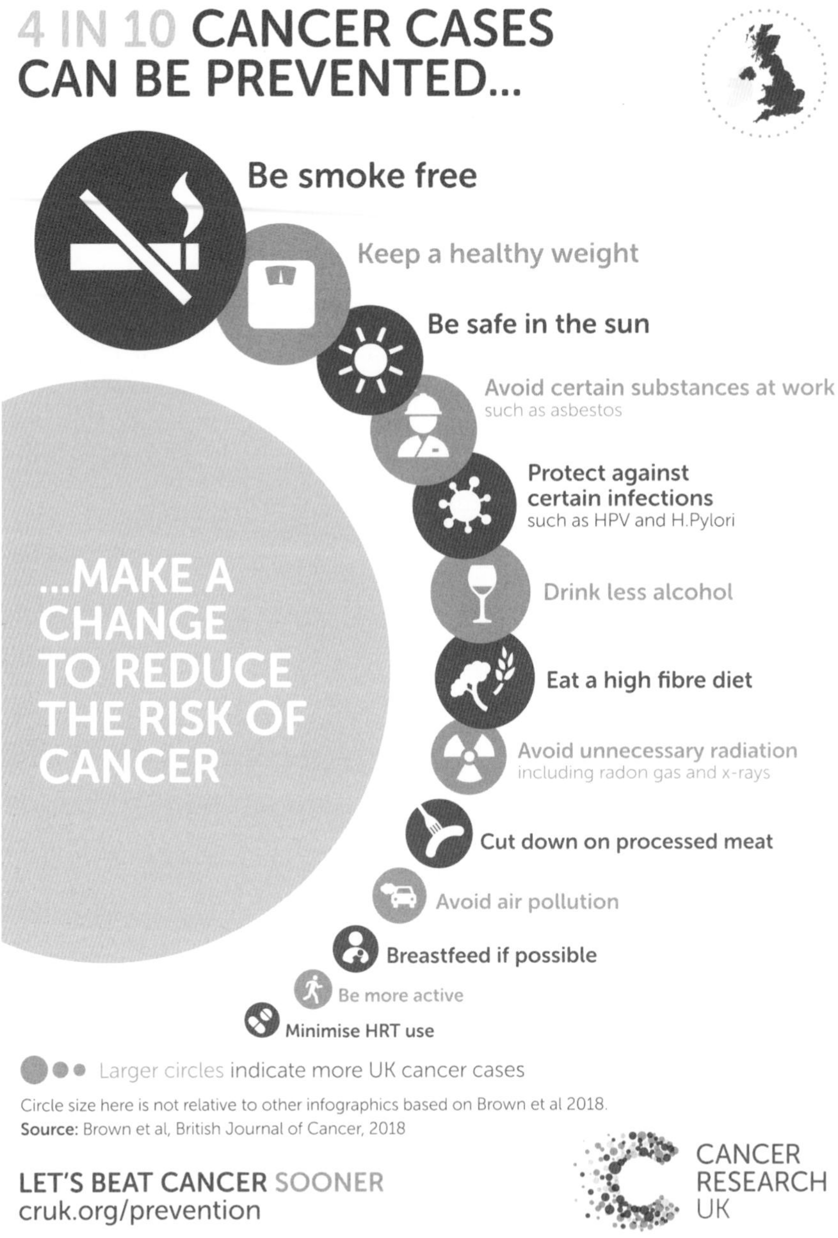

4 IN 10 CANCER CASES CAN BE PREVENTED...

Be smoke free

Keep a healthy weight

Be safe in the sun

Avoid certain substances at work
such as asbestos

Protect against
certain infections
such as HPV and H.Pylori

Drink less alcohol

Eat a high fibre diet

Avoid unnecessary radiation
including radon gas and x-rays

Cut down on processed meat

Avoid air pollution

Breastfeed if possible

Be more active

Minimise HRT use

...MAKE A CHANGE TO REDUCE THE RISK OF CANCER

●●● Larger circles indicate more UK cancer cases

Circle size here is not relative to other infographics based on Brown et al 2018.
Source: Brown et al, British Journal of Cancer, 2018

LET'S BEAT CANCER SOONER
cruk.org/prevention

CANCER
RESEARCH
UK

Figure 7.1 Infographic showing the contributions of cancer risk factors to the burden of cancer in the UK. Based on data from Parkin 2011 [18]. Reproduced with permission from Cancer Research UK.

to reduce the risk. During its development, the infographic was tested with a Cancer Research UK online panel and feedback collected to inform the final design. The key learning from the testing was that the diagram ought to be simplified as far as possible, and this feedback was taken on board to ensure the final version was single-minded and quickly comprehensible.

Conclusion

Although there is still some way to go before the main risk factors for cancer are fully understood by everyone, there have been significant improvements over time in public knowledge of cancer prevention. Work must now continue to ensure that understanding continues to be raised, and that this knowledge is linked through to promoting healthy behaviour change so that healthy lifestyles are the norm. This activity should also help provide support for public policy measures to improve health, further assisting in the promotion of healthy choices and cancer prevention. Communicators should try to provide 'new news' where possible, make information very accessible to combat poor health literacy, provide inspiration and support for healthy behaviour, and try to break down fatalistic attitudes. In addition, with the crowded media environment, it is important to find stories that will achieve cut-through and be relevant and engaging for the audience, as well as being clear sources of trustworthy information.

Improving public understanding of cancer prevention is challenging, but information campaigns are working to raise awareness and promote healthy living. This work lays the foundation for effective behaviour change interventions, and makes these more likely to be successful. Information campaigns and behaviour change interventions should ideally be long term, well funded, and integrated into communities. They need to identify and reduce inequalities in access to health services and information, and they need to carry evidence-based messages from trusted sources, explained in an understandable and accessible way. There is a wealth of accurate information on cancer prevention available to people, both online and in the community at GP surgeries, pharmacies, and dentists, but to ensure that people have equal access to this information, no matter what their social or economic circumstances or backgrounds, we need to actively target health information to those most in need. By achieving better public understanding of prevention, we will be able to help reduce the number of people being diagnosed with cancer in the future.

References

1 Stubbings, S., Robb, K., Waller, J. et al. (2009). Development of a measurement tool to assess public awareness of cancer. *Br. J. Cancer* 101 (Suppl. 2): S13–S17.
2 Robb, K.A., Simon, A.E., Miles, A., and Wardle, J. (2014). Public perceptions of cancer: A qualitative study of the balance of positive and negative beliefs. *BMJ Open* 4 (7): e005434.

3 Niederdeppe, J., and Levy, A.G. (2007). Fatalistic beliefs about cancer prevention and three prevention behaviors. *Cancer Epidemiol. Biomarkers Prev.* 16 (5): 998–1003.

4 Buykx, P., Gilligan, C., Ward, B. et al. (2014). Public support for alcohol policies associated with knowledge of cancer risk. *Int. J. Drug Policy* 26 (4): 371–379.

5 Brown, J., Kotz, D., Michie, S. et al. (2014). How effective and cost-effective was the national mass media smoking cessation campaign 'Stoptober'? *Drug Alcohol Depend.* 135: 52–58.

6 Ayers, J.W., Althouse, B.M., Noar, S.M., and Cohen, J.E. (2014). Do celebrity cancer diagnoses promote primary cancer prevention? *Prev. Med.* 58: 81–84.

7 McBride, C.M., Emmons, K.M., and Lipkus, I.M. (2003). Understanding the potential of teachable moments: The case of smoking cessation. *Health Educ. Res.* 18 (2): 156–170.

8 Senore, C., Giordano, L., Bellisario, C. et al. (2012). Population based cancer screening programmes as a teachable moment for primary prevention interventions: A review of the literature. *Front. Oncol.* 2: 45.

9 Rabin, C. (2009). Promoting lifestyle change among cancer survivors: When is the teachable moment? *Am. J. Lifestyle Med.* 3 (5): 369–378.

10 Fox, S. (2011). The Social Life of Health Information. Washington, DC: Pew Research Center.

11 NHS (2014). NHS Choices performance and statistics. http://www.nhs.uk/ABOUTNHSCHOICES/PROFESSIONALS/DEVELOPMENTS/Pages/Trafficreports.aspx (accessed 29 October 2014).

12 eBizMBA (2014). Top 15 most popular health websites. http://www.ebizmba.com/articles/health-websites (accessed 29 October 2014).

13 Laurent, M.R., and Vickers, T.J. (2009). Seeking health information online: Does Wikipedia matter? *J. Am. Med. Inform. Assoc.* 16 (4): 471–479.

14 Cancer Research UK (2014). About cancer. http://www.cancerresearchuk.org/about-cancer/ (accessed 27 October 2014).

15 Cancer Research UK (2014). Healthy living. http://www.cancerresearchuk.org/cancer-info/healthyliving/ (accessed 29 October 2014).

16 Portnoy, D.B., Leach, C.R., Kaufman, A.R. et al. (2014). Reduced fatalism and increased prevention behavior after two high-profile lung cancer events. *J. Health Commun.* 19 (5): 577–592.

17 Cancer Research UK (2012). Leading UK model agencies sign up to 'No Sunbed' policy. http://www.cancerresearchuk.org/about-us/cancer-news/press-release/leading-uk-model-agencies-sign-up-to-no-sunbed-policy (accessed 29 October 2014).

18 Brown, K.F., Rumgay, H., Dunlop, C. et al. (2018). The fraction of cancer attributable to modifiable risk factors in England, Wales, Scotland, Northern Ireland, and the United Kingdom in 2015. *Br. J. Cancer.* https://doi.org/10.1038/s41416-018-0029-6.

CHAPTER 8

Cervical cancer screening: An exemplar of a population screening programme, and cervical cancer prevention

Albert Singer[1] and Ashfaq Khan[2]

[1] Institute for Women's Health, UCL, London, UK
[2] Whittington Hospital; UCL Medical School, London, UK

SUMMARY BOX

- Dramatic reductions in the incidence of invasive cervical cancer in developed countries have occurred during the last four decades, mainly due to screening with exfoliative cytology.
- Both meta-analysis and cross-sectional studies have suggested that HPV testing has a higher sensitivity than cytology in detecting high-grade cervical precancer.
- Cryotherapy or cold coagulation of all women who are HPV positive and/or who have been diagnosed with disease by VIA (visual inspection with acetic acid) could be an option for the developing world.
- The introduction of self-collection may well be a way forward to involve women who are reluctant to participate in the screening programme.

Probably one of the best exemplars of a population screening programme is that in relation to cervical cancer screening. Results over the last half-century with this programme have been spectacular. There is no other comparable screening programme with such success.

Medical screening is defined as a public health service in which members of a defined population, who do not necessarily perceive they are at risk or are already affected by a disease, are offered a test to identify those individuals who are more likely to be helped than harmed by further tests or treatment to reduce the risk of disease or its complications.

Cancer Prevention and Screening: Concepts, Principles and Controversies, First Edition.
Edited by Rosalind A. Eeles, Christine D. Berg, and Jeffrey S. Tobias.
© 2019 John Wiley & Sons, Inc. Published 2019 by John Wiley & Sons, Inc.

Table 8.1 How to improve different components of a successful screening programme.

	To maximize benefit	To minimize harm
Coverage	Invite, remind, convenient, pleasant	Informed choice, prevent overscreening
Test	Identify disease, accurate, repeatable	Don't mislabel healthy, quality control
Triage	Failsafe, identify those needing treatment	Avoid anxiety, avoid overtreatment
Treatment	Failsafe effective treatment	Minimize; side effects
Recall	Before new cancers develop	As infrequently as possible

By definition, therefore, cervical cancer is an appropriate disease for screening because:

- Cervical intraepithelial neoplasia (CIN) is regarded as a premalignant epithelial lesion which progresses in about 30% of cases over a 30-year period, through the stages of CIN2 and CIN3 (high-grade squamous intraepithelial lesion or HSIL, Bethesda Classification) to invasive cancer [1].
- Most CIN lesions (low-grade squamous intraepithelial lesion or LSIL, Bethesda Classification) will regress naturally.
- With modern screening, small and earlier lesions that are less likely to progress in the immediate future are found, making them easier to treat and cure.
- Clinically treating the known precancer stages of CIN2 and CIN3 will prevent their possible progression to cancer [2,3].

The aims, therefore, of cervical cancer screening are twofold: the first is to prevent cancer by identifying and treating asymptomatic (precancerous, CIN2, CIN3) lesions; and the second to reduce cervical cancer mortality by preventing cervical cancer or diagnosing cervical cancer in the very early invasive cancer stages, while these lesions are still curable.

Cervical cancer screening, like any other screening programme, has its benefits, but also it has the potential to cause harm. In Table 8.1, the requirements to maximize the benefits and minimize the harm that may be caused by screening are listed.

How do we screen for cervical precancer?

The primary method of screening for cervical precancer over the last 70 years has been exfoliative cytology. However, over the last 10–15 years, human papilloma virus (HPV) testing, or a combination of exfoliative cytology and HPV testing, known as co-testing, has become important and the principal diagnostic technique [4,5]. Recent evidence indicates that HPV testing is slowly replacing cytology in many centres.

A positive screening test with either cytology or HPV testing will demand further investigations (triage), with the follow-up options or triage depending on the nature of the screening results. The value and the place of biomarkers in screening and diagnosis have now become recognized as a potential future modality. In the following review, both exfoliative cytology and HPV testing will be considered in detail, and the advantages and disadvantages of both will be discussed.

Prevention of invasive cervical cancer: The impact of cytological screening

Dramatic reductions in the incidence of invasive cervical cancer in developed countries have been evident during the last four decades. Much of this reduction is in relation to incidence and mortality rates, which reflect the widespread availability of exfoliative cytology screening. For example, in North America, the incidence of cervical cancer has decreased by 75% and mortality has decreased by 74% since the implementation of Papanicolaou (Pap) cervical exfoliative cytological screening in 1949 [6]. The decline in cervical cancer over the years 1975 to 2008 from 14.79 to 6.43 per 100 000 women, as measured by the age-adjusted incidence rate for cervical cancer, represented a 57% decrease. Interestingly, within this reduction was a 75% reduction in the incidence in Afro-Caribbean women as compared to white women [7].

Probably some of the most spectacular falls in the incidence of cervical cancer have occurred in Scandinavian countries [8] (Figure 8.1). The national screening programme in Finland, which commenced in the 1950s, lowered the rate of cervical cancer to only 5.5 cases per 100 000 women. In Sweden, a similar drop occurred. In Norway, however, where a screening programme was only instituted in 1995, the reduction was much smaller and the rate of cervical cancer is three

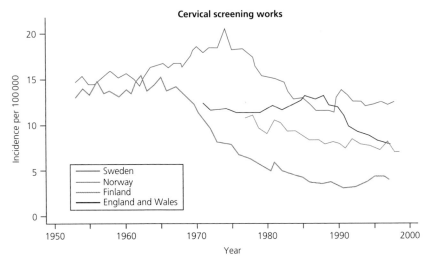

Figure 8.1 Effect of cervical screening on the incidence of cancer. Source: NORDCAN database (Association of Nordic Cancer Registries, version 4.06.2011).

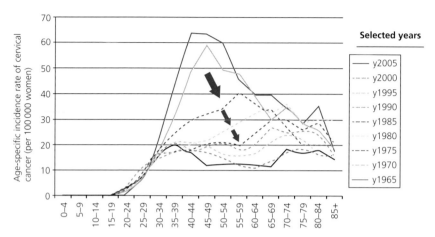

Figure 8.2 Age-specific incidence of cervical cancer in Scandinavian countries between 1965 and 2005. Source: NORDCAN database (Association of Nordic Cancer Registries, version 4.06.2011).

times higher (15.6 per 100 000) than in Finland. The Nordic data also demonstrate the significant impact on women aged 30–60 years, as shown in Figure 8.2.

In comparison to the Scandinavian countries, a number of other organized screening programmes developed using the call and recall follow-up system. In England, until 1994, there was a system of opportunistic screening which had very little impact on cervical cancer rates. It was only in 1988, when the call and recall system was instituted with payment to general practitioners for screening at least 80% of their eligible patients, that the rates started to decrease. Indeed, by 1994, the coverage rate for women aged 25–64 rose from 45% to 85% and has remained at about this level ever since. Consequently, since 1990, there has been a dramatic and continuing reduction in the incidence and mortality from cervical cancer (Figure 8.3). This reduction has occurred simultaneously with this high coverage [9].

Not all countries have adopted cervical screening, or when a programme has been instigated it has been poorly administered. An excellent exemplar of this situation is illustrated in the International Agency for Research on Cancer (IARC) figures for Lithuania versus Finland. Figure 8.4 shows the impact or not that screening has produced. In Finland, where screening has been employed for many years, the rate of cervical cancer has fallen dramatically, whereas in neighbouring Lithuania, where no screening has been employed, there has been a rise in disease incidence.

Even when screening programmes are employed, there are significant problems. There seems to be very little effect on cervical cancer incidence before the age of 30, as demonstrated by nearly identical incidence rates for women below this age in well-screened populations such as in the UK and in a country where minimal screening has occurred, such as in Brazil [10]. It has also been shown that in some developed countries, where screening is considered adequate,

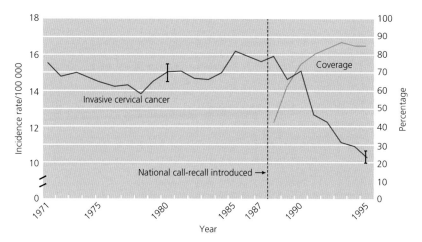

Figure 8.3 Age-standardized incidence of invasive cervical cancer and coverage of screening in the UK, 1971–1975. Source: Quinn 1999 [9]. Reproduced by permission of British Medical Journal Publishing Group.

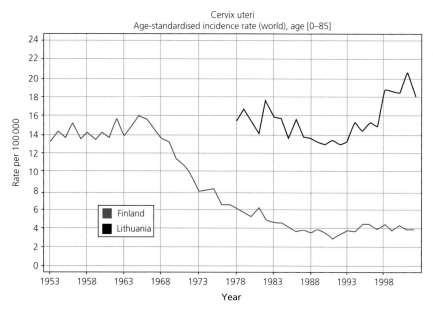

Figure 8.4 Age-standardized incidence of cervical cancer: Comparison between two European countries, Finland and Lithuania. Source: IARC 2001. Reproduced by permission of The International Agency for Research on Cancer (IARC), World Health Organisation.

cervical cancer incidence is actually higher for young women aged 15–44 than for age-matched women in less developed countries. Identical rates below age 30 years also indicate similar exposure. These identical rates for women aged 30 and under may be explained as indicating similar levels of exposure to HPV, which is the aetiological agent of cervical cancer, in screened and unscreened populations. For women aged over 45 who live in less developed countries, cervical cancer incidence is more than double that found in developed countries, and after age 30, the shape of the incidence curve is purely dependent on the amount of screening that takes place, as is shown in Figure 8.4.

Adenocarcinoma of the cervix seems to be increasing worldwide, and although there have been dramatic reductions in invasive squamous cell cancer of the cervix, the same cannot be said for invasive adenocarcinoma. In the USA there was nearly a 30% increase in the age-standardized incidence rates for adenocarcinoma between 1976 and 2000 [11]. Bray et al. [12] noted a rate of 0.5% per year in Denmark, Sweden, and Switzerland, with higher rates for Slovenia. Part of the reason may be explained by the fact that early glandular lesions are less likely to be detected by exfoliative cytology. Increasing use of the oral contraceptive pill and the prevalence of HPV 16 and 18 infections, which are linked to the aetiology of adenocarcinomas, may also account for the increase.

It is important to note, when discussing the dramatic falls in incidence of invasive cervical cancer, that some reduction was already noted before the introduction of cervical cancer screening campaigns. Kessler [13] commented that the incidence of invasive cancer in the late 1940s was 33 per 100 000 for white women and 70 per 100 000 for black women, but by 1969 this incidence had dropped to 16.5 and 35.7, respectively, in these two groups. This occurred before the introduction of widespread cytological screening and probably reflected improvement in lifestyle in the general population, which includes a reduction in smoking incidence in women.

The effect of screening seems to be less effective in a younger cohort of women. This was shown dramatically by Sasieni et al. in 2009 (Figure 8.5) [14]. The other debate is about at what age screening should start. In the UK, screening is not undertaken under the age of 25, because it is felt that the incidence of cervical cancer is very low in these women, at 2.5 per 100 000 per year, and nationally only 1.7% of cervical cancers occur in the 20–25 age group. The high prevalence of HPV infection means that many of these lesions are of low risk and most are reversible, and 1 in 6 smears reported as abnormal is associated with highly reversible atypical squamous cells of undetermined significance (ASCUS, borderline type). Indeed, lesions treated under the age of 25 may prevent cancer developing later, but again, about 60% of low-grade lesions in young women will be self-cleared and will not progress to high-grade CIN [15,16].

Factors influencing the success of a screening programme

The Pap smear has been described by Koss as a triumph and a tragedy [17]. The reason for this is that it has a very poor sensitivity, which can range between 40% and 75% with variability in relation to sampling and reading areas in the cervix. Frequent repeat screening is necessary because of this low sensitivity, which in turn leads to compliance problems. Overall cumulative specificity is poor at under 85%, with approximately 6% of adequate smears being abnormal on each

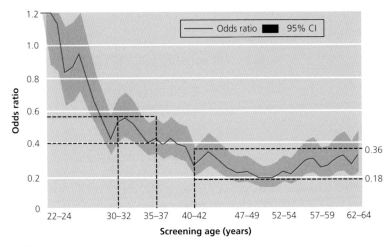

Figure 8.5 Odds ratio for developing invasive cervical cancer stage IA or worse (in the next five-year interval) in those screened in a given (three-year) age band compared with those not screened in that age band (or in two previous years). Odds ratios plotted for overlapping age bands. Broken lines indicate risk of developing cervical cancer at ages 33–40 and 43–65. Odds ratios and confidence intervals are truncated at 1.2. The figure is based on 4012 cases (including 437 in women under age 30) and 7889 controls. Source: Sasieni 2009 [14]. Reproduced by permission of British Medical Journal Publishing Group.

screening round. There seems to be an excellent single-test specificity of 95%, which allows it to be a very effective triage component when dealing with a positive HPV test, as will be shown later. Also, the test is certainly not prognostic. With this lack of sensitivity, the question has been asked as to how one can improve this. The introduction of liquid-based cytology (LBC) testing gave hope that there would be an improvement in sensitivity. When LBC technology was introduced into the UK screening programme, the rate of unsatisfactory smears fell from 9% to 2.5% over a four-year period, but the change did very little for improvement in sensitivity [18]. Indeed, in 2008, a meta-analysis of studies using LBC showed that it is neither more sensitive nor more specific for detection of high-grade CIN compared with a conventional Pap test [19].

One method of improving the screening programme would be if women who do not get regular screening with Pap smears and who are particularly vulnerable to cervical cancer could be enticed into participating in the screening programme. The introduction of self-collection may well be a way forward in this respect. In the USA, women who have never been screened have an estimated lifetime risk of developing cervical cancer in the region of 3.7% (3748 cases per 100 000 women). Cox showed that with annual cytological screening, the lifetime risk in this group drops to 0.4% or 0.3% (305 cases per 100 000 women) [20]. This lack of screening is found in many cases, and Andrae et al. [21] showed that in Sweden, 64% of Swedish women diagnosed with cervical cancer had not been screened recently.

The introduction of self-collection, which has been used in the Netherlands for a number of years, is primarily aimed at such women. However, though they have enthusiastically taken it up, its major advantage has been in the collection of samples for HPV DNA sampling and not for exfoliative cytology. A comparison study between HPV and cytology in a community-based study in Mexico using a self-collection system showed the distinct advantage of HPV over Pap smears [22]. This topic will be discussed later when examining the use of HPV in screening.

One of the factors contributing to the success of the screening programme in many countries has been its restriction to every three years. Sasieni et al. [14] showed that the effectiveness of cervical screening varied with age (Figure 8.6). In his population-based case-control study, he prospectively recorded data which showed that the duration of protection increases with age. He showed that at three years since the last negative smear, there was considerable increase in risk of cervical cancer, so that three years is the optimum time for a repeat smear.

Finally, one of the other successes in relation to the screening programme is coverage. It is one of the most important aspects of screening and at least 75–80% of the eligible population should be screened. The degree of coverage in the UK screening programme stands at 78% for 25–64-year-old women screened [23], which means that the rate of cervical cancer has been able to be reduced using exfoliative cytology, notwithstanding that this technique has limited sensitivity in respect of screening. With the introduction of automated screening, which was driven originally by the need to reduce the labour required for manual screening rather than improvement in sensitivity, it has been found in a number of studies that automated cytology does provide more rapid, accurate, standardized screening, while also reducing labour and cost [24]. In a study by Wilbur et al. in 2009, the sensitivity for high-grade lesions was increased by 19% and for low-risk lesions by nearly 10% [25]. In this clinical trial, an advanced imaging automated

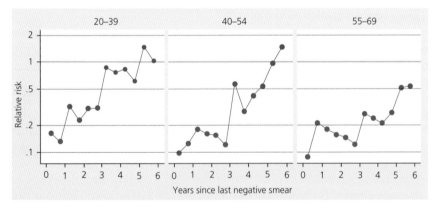

Figure 8.6 Population-based study showing that the duration of protection increases with age in an organized cervical screening programme. Source: Sasieni 2009 [14]. Reproduced by permission of British Medical Journal Publishing Group.

system was used with quality-controlled rescreening, and was compared with routine manual screening. There was a small, statistically significant decrease in specificity. However, in those with ASCUS+ (the plus indicating the presence of HPV), sensitivity and specificity were comparable between the two study arms and the authors concluded that the use of this system might be expected to improve accuracy for the 'clinically important entities without increasing equivocal case detection'. Further developments in this field are anticipated.

Molecular-based cervical screening technologies

HPV has been recognised for the last 20 years as being the major cause of cervical neoplasia [26]. In 2007, IARC concluded that there was 'strong epidemiological evidence' that HPV types 16 and 18 are carcinogenic in humans and cause invasive cervical cancer [27]. Since that time, overwhelming evidence has shown that certain HPV types are oncogenic. A major causal role was initially attributed to HPV types 16 and 18 based on strong epidemiological evidence [28]. Muñoz et al. [29] and Bosch et al. [30], in trials conducted under the auspices of IARC, have designated a further 10 HPV types as oncogenic. The strength of the causality of association of HPV with cervical cancer is based on our understanding of the molecular biology of HPV and its epidemiology. This has enabled molecular-based technologies to be at the forefront of screening for cervical cancer.

It is evident that the molecular testing of exfoliated cervical cells for the presence of HPV DNA has significant clinical utility as a screening test for identifying cervical cancer precursors. Both meta-analysis and cross-sectional studies have suggested that HPV testing has a higher sensitivity than cytology in detecting high-grade cervical precancer (CIN2–3; (Figures 8.7 and 8.8). The high negative predictive value (NPV) of HPV DNA testing has enormous potential clinical usage and importance. This has now been used as a primary screening test, either as an adjunct or as a stand-alone component.

The use of HPV DNA further highlights the contention that screening for cervical cancer is a leading if not *the* leading exemplar in respect of general screening for cancer. An example of this has been the study by Cuzick et al. [31] of over 60 000 North American and European women, in which cytology was used as a primary screen and where high-risk HPV DNA testing (Hybrid Capture 2, Qiagen, Gaithersburg MD) was run in parallel and showed that high-risk HPV DNA was found to be more sensitive for the detection of CIN2+ (96.1%) than cytology (53%). However, cytology was more specific at 96.3% compared with 90.7% for high-risk HPV DNA for women under 35, although it was similar for women over 35. Figures 8.7 and 8.8 show the sensitivity and specificity of HPV DNA testing when compared with exfoliative cytology. Sixteen controlled trials are listed. The superiority of HPV testing can be seen over cytology in terms of sensitivity; however, the reverse is seen for specificity, where cytology comes out at 5% higher than HPV DNA. Oversensitivity of HPV DNA and the higher specificity of cytology

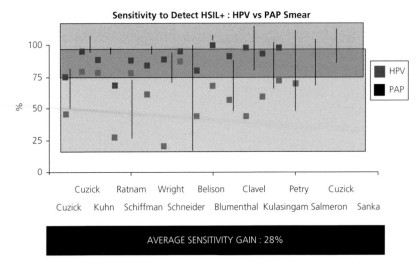

Figure 8.7 Sensitivity of HPV DNA test to detect HSIL/CIN2+ in comparison to Pap smear in different studies.

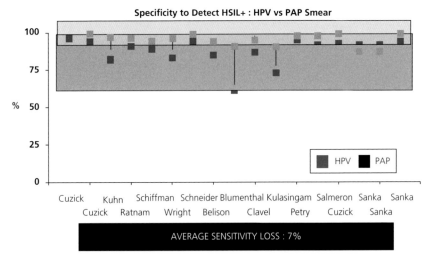

Figure 8.8 Specificity of HPV DNA test to detect HSIL/CIN2+ in comparison to Pap smear in different studies.

can be used to advantage in trials, and in screening where HPV is used exclusively and cytology, because of its better specificity, is employed to triage.

In a recent analysis by Ronco et al. [32] of 17 000 women in four large European trials, who were screened with either HPV DNA or cytology and followed for a median time of 6.5 years, it was shown that HPV-based screening provided a 60–70% greater protection against invasive cervical cancer than cytology. Data from these large-scale randomized trials support the usage of HPV screening in women aged over 30 and at five-year intervals.

In summary, the practical and clinical value of HPV DNA testing and its advantages over cytology are significant. For example, HPV DNA testing is more sensitive than cytology and allows screening to be done less frequently. It is more reproducible than cytology and reduces interim intra-laboratory variations, and it identifies women at risk for developing CIN2–3 and cervical cancer. With the rationalization and centralization of technology, it allows testing to be done that serves the screening of large populations.

Algorithms employing HPV DNA in primary screening

By using the data discussed, it is possible to establish a number of algorithms which employ both HPV DNA testing and the inclusion of other methods as triage indicators, such as cytology and biomarkers. Cytology identifies many women with low-grade abnormalities, and HPV in these instances can also be used as a reflex test in conjunction with cytology to identify those who are HPV negative and who have a benign cervical abnormality. The negative predictive value for HPV testing is high (in the range of 98–99%) and therefore selects those women who do not need further investigation and can be referred back to routine screening. However, there are those who are HPV positive and cytologically abnormal, and they are directed along a course which entails colposcopy and other investigations [4,5].

One of the problematic aspects of primary cervical HPV screening is that of the HPV-positive woman with negative cytology at triage. This group has a twofold increased risk of having an HPV infection than the normal population of women, and if HPV persists, then a number of further investigations can be used: colposcopy, genotyping biomarkers of p16/Ki-67 dual-stain cytology, or methylation markers.

The value of biomarkers in triage

There are many instances when triage is employed in relation to abnormalities in cytology, the presence of a positive HPV test such as in primary screening, or in other instances, such as women with a positive HPV test but negative cytology. These situations lend themselves to new and contemporary technologies of triage.

In women with a positive HPV in primary screening, the value of cytology can be exploited. Although cytology provides moderate sensitivity in detecting CIN2+, its specificity is high and is a satisfactory marker for triage, in that it identifies, using other markers such as HPV, P16INK4a, or dual staining, those women who need further investigation. Various studies over the last decade [33–35] have attested to the efficacy of this method. Women with normal cytology are tested with HPV genotyping [34] in the algorithm used by Bulkmans et al. in the Netherlands [33], and the finding of type 16, 18, 31, 33, or 45 meant a repeat in

12 months. Those with types other than 16, 18, 31, 33, and 45 were retested at 24 months. This programme for screening women with HPV followed by direct triage of reflex cytology and HPV genotyping has been in progress for many years. However, to this scheme can now be added P16INK4a, dual staining, and DNA methylation classifiers [35–37].

By 2012, an in-depth understanding of the molecular events leading to neo-plastic transformation of HPV-infected human cells had been described, and involved the cyclin-dependent kinase inhibitor p16INK4a, which was shown to be substantially overexpressed in virtually all HPV-transformed cells [35]. This finding opened novel avenues in diagnostic histopathology to substantially improve the diagnostic accuracy of cervical cancer and its precursor lesions. Furthermore, it provided a novel technical platform to substantially improve the accuracy of cytology-based cancer early detection programmes [38].

It soon became obvious that p16 overexpression is a marker for CIN2 or worse, or for development of CIN2 or worse within three years in HPV-positive women, especially those aged 35–60 years. It soon became obvious that HPV-positive, p16-positive women needed immediate colposcopy and, if the colposcopic assessment was negative, then annual follow-up could be at 12-monthly intervals. In those women who were HPV positive but p16 negative, immediate colposcopy could be avoided, and they could be safely managed with repeat screening at 2–3-year intervals [35,36].

Another triaging technique used with Pap-negative/HPV-positive screened women relied on p16/Ki-67 dual-stained cytology, which furthermore will signific-antly increase sensitivity compared to cytology, with a slight decrease in specific-ity [39]. This approach can significantly reduce false negatives with only a minimal increase in false positives, thus reducing the incidence of cervical cancer.

Gustinucci et al. [40] examined 6272 women who were recruited in a popula-tion-based screening using HPV DNA as the primary test; 396 were positive and were tested for cytology and biomarkers, which included cytology, E6/E7 mRNA, and p16INK4a-Ki-67. All tests were performed on the same sample. Cytology-positive women were referred to colposcopy; cytology-negative women were referred to one-year HPV retesting. The endpoint was CIN2+ at baseline or follow-up. The high sensitivity of combined strategies probably allows longer intervals in HPV-positive, triage-negative women. In an earlier study by Gustinucci et al. [35], the sensitivity, specificity, PPV, and NPV confirmed the importance of the utiliza-tion of p16INK4a-Ki-67 in the categories of ASCUS and LSIL after triage with a high-risk HPV (hrHPV) test. In the ASC-H (atypical squamous cells cannot exclude HSIL) and HSIL-CIN3 lesions, p16INK4a-Ki-67 was shown to be an excellent marker for picking up CIN2+ lesions, especially in cases with cytohistological screening discordance.

Bergeron [36] and Badiga et al. [41] both showed the clinical usefulness and efficiency of triaging women with ASCUS or LSIL by Pap cytology and p16/Ki-67 dual-stained cytology testing in a prospective, pan-European study. The high posi-tive predictive value of dual-stained cytology for the presence of high-grade CIN helps to reduce the number of unnecessary colposcopy referrals. Badiga et al. [41] also showed that specimens that were positive for p16INK4A expression were 5.3 and 16.6 times more likely to be diagnosed as CIN2 and CIN3 lesions, respectively, compared to CIN1 lesions.

Recently, Tjalma et al. [39] showed the impact on women's health and the cervical cancer screening budget of primary HPV screening with dual-stain cytology triage. Using Belgium as his model, he evaluated the cost-effectiveness of diagnostic cytology using the CINtec® PLUS Cytology test or dual-stain cytology triage in screening. In this approach, precancerous cells are more likely to be immediately identified during the first screening visit. This reduces both the number and frequency of follow-up visits required. After two cycles (six years), the prevalence of CIN and cervical cancer was decreased significantly in the screened population. At a population level, the research showed that these shifts can reduce the screening budget by 21%, resulting in savings of €5.3 million a year in Belgium. The authors concluded that diagnostic cytology benefits all stakeholders involved in cervical cancer screening.

Consensus guidelines for the management of abnormal cervical cancer screening tests and cancer precursors

Massad et al. in 2012 [5] produced guidelines which were a follow-up to a similar set of guidelines produced in 2006. The goal of the consensus meeting attended by 47 experts was to provide revised evidence-based consensus guidelines in respect of CIN adenocarcinoma in situ. The consensus was based on a literature review, but also on data from 1.4 million women who had undergone screening using co-testing (HPV DNA plus cytology) in the Kaiser Permanente Northern California Medical Care Plan. The authors focused on analysis of outcome risks from this huge database of women who were followed for eight years, providing evidence on risk after abnormal tests.

There were also updates from previous consensus guidelines. The present guidelines discuss using genotyping to triage in the case of HPV positivity, as well as also triaging HPV-positive women with HPV type 16 or 18 to earlier colposcopy only after negative cytology: colposcopy is indicated for all women with HPV and ASCUS cytology, regardless of genotyping results. The serial cytology option for ASCUS incorporates cytology at 12 months, not 6 or 12 months, and then, if negative, cytology every three years. HPV-negative and ASCUS results should be followed with co-testing at three years rather than five years, and HPV-negative and ASCUS results are insufficient to allow exit from screening at age 65. The pathway to long-term follow-up of untreated and treated CIN2+ is more clearly defined by incorporating co-testing.

These new guidelines stress that more strategies exist that incorporate co-testing to reduce follow-up visits. Pap-only strategies are now limited to women younger than 30 years, but co-testing has expanded even to women younger than 30 years in some circumstances. Women aged 21–24 years are managed conservatively. However, recently Castle et al. showed that code testing with both cytology and HPV testing did not improve cancer detection to any great degree in comparison with HPV testing alone [42].

As women aged 65 and older represent 14% of the US population and have nearly 20% of new cases of cervical cancer, there is a discrepancy among various groups as to when to stop screening. Many authorities have argued that continuing to screen women in this older age group with a history of several recent normal Pap results would not appear to offer much additional protection. As well as this factor, the epithelial effect of ageing, due to declining oestrogen production, results in confusing cellular changes that are difficult to differentiate from those related to HPV in neoplasia. However, the guidelines as to when to discontinue screening vary between different groups. The American College of Surgeons (ACS), the American College of Obstetrics and Gynecology (ACOG), and the US Preventive Services Task Force (USPSTF) all have differing views [4,5,43]. ACS recommends a 70-year limit, whereas ACOG recommends between 65 and 70 years, and USPSTF recommends against routine screening after age 65. It is obvious that those women exposed to HPV beyond the age of 65 or 70 are unlikely to develop cervix cancer within their remaining lifetime.

Another dilemma in screening with HPV is as to which assay should be used. Several new ones have been developed for hrHPV testing. A comparison by Cuzick et al. [44] of six of the major ones concluded that a positivity rate in cytology-negative specimens was similar for the DNA-based test, but lower for the hrHPV E6-E7 mRNA (APTIMA), and suggests that this latter test maintains a high sensitivity compared with DNA tests, but with better specificity. The APTIMA HPV test, which identifies the RNA of 14 high-risk HPV types, was compared with hybrid capture HC2 (hrHPV DNA) for the triage of women with minor cellular abnormality. Although the results were similar for detection of CIN2+, APTIMA proved to be as sensitive but more specific than HC2 for detecting cervical precancer [45]. Furthermore, in 2014 the US Food and Drug Administration (FDA) approved the first HPV test for primary cervical cancer screening, an HPV DNA test (cobas) to be used alone, to allow for the assessment of the need for women to undergo additional diagnostic testing for cervical cancer. The test can provide information about the patient's risk for developing cervical cancer in the future. The cobas HPV test detects DNA from 14 hrHPV types, but it specifically identifies types 16 and 18 while concurrently detecting 12 other types. It is fitting that the cobas HPV test is part of the ATHENA trial, from which Wright et al. concluded in 2011 [46] that women who were HPV 16 positive have a 13% risk of having CIN2 or greater, compared with only a 4.6% risk among women who have one of the other 12 high-risk types [5]. An important conclusion from this ATHENA trial was that the absolute risk of CIN2+ in a screened population of women 30 years of age and older who had normal cytology was 1.2%. The prevalence of HPV positivity for hrHPV was 6.7%; for HPV 16, 1%; and for HPV 18, 0.5%. The estimated absolute risk of CIN3 + was 9.8% for women who were HPV 16–18 positive, compared with only 0.3% for women who were hrHPV negative. The trial also concluded that 1 in 10 women with normal cytology but HPV 16 and/or HPV 18 positive has CIN3+. From a clinical point of view, these data support referral to colposcopy of all women with normal cytology who are HPV 16 and/or HPV 18 positive.

Finally, a review by Gage et al. [47], examining cervical precancer and cancer in respect of a negative HPV test, concluded that the three-year risks following an HPV-negative result were lower than the three-year risks following a Pap-negative result and the five-year risks following a HPV-negative/Pap-negative co-test. Their conclusion was that 'these findings suggest that primary HPV testing merits consideration as an overall alternative for cervical screening'. Recently, Canfell et al. [48] have completed a randomised controlled trial of primary HPV testing versus cytology screening for cervical cancer in HPV unvaccinated and vaccinated women aged 25–69 years in Australia where they showed that primary HPV screening was associated with a significantly increased detection of CIN 2–3 compared to cytology, in a population where high vaccine uptake was reported in women aged 33 or younger who were offered a vaccination.

Risk assessment to guide cervical screening strategies

A study by Zhao et al. in 2016 [49] introduced the concept of risk assessment of the various screening modalities so far described in this review, and is a most significant contribution to the screening strategies at present employed. These researchers described a technique for evaluating the risk of CIN3+ in a large population of (Chinese) women, examining three different cervical screening methods (cytology, HPV testing, and visual inspection with acetic acid or VIA) and evaluating the immediate risk of CIN3+ for these different screening results, which were derived from individual and combined tests. They developed a unique and novel statistical method that was specifically designed for this purpose, called Mean Risk Stratification (MRS), and used it to compare the three tests. Their data were derived by examination of a pooled analysis of 17 cross-sectional population studies of 30 371 Chinese women who had been screened with all three methods. The tissue diagnosis was derived from a combination of colposcopically directed biopsies of abnormal tissue or by random 4-quadrant biopsies in women with no colposcopically obvious abnormal tissue. They concluded that 'comparing risks of CIN3 and cervical cancer (CIN3+) for different results can inform test choice and management guidelines'.

The results and conclusions from their study were that the three tests combined powerfully and distinguished the risk for CIN3+. When the three screening tests were compared, the following were shown:

- HPV status most strongly stratified CIN3+ risk.
- In HPV-positive women, cytology was the most useful second test.
- In HPV-positive women, the CIN3+ risks associated with cytology were 0.9% for negative cytology, 3.6% for ASCUS, 6.3% for LSIL, and 38.5% for HSIL1.

• In HPV-negative women, the immediate risks of CIN3+ ranged from 0.01% for negative cytology, 0.00% for ASCUS, and 1.1% for LSIL, to 6.6% for HSIL1.
• VIA results did not meaningful stratify CIN3+ risk among HPV-negative women with negative or ASCUS cytology. Positive VIA substantially elevated CIN3+ risk for all other, more positive combinations of HPV and cytology compared with a negative VIA.

Because all three screening tests had independent value in defining the risk of CIN3+, different combinations can be optimized as pragmatic strategies in different resource settings.

Male Circumcision and Cervical Cancer

Since Hutchinson reported in 1855 that circumcision might prevent syphilis studies have suggested that circumcision may reduce the risk of penile cancer, and common sexually transmitted diseases, including human immunodeficiency virus (HIV) infection [50–52]. Increasingly, evidence from randomized controlled trials and other clinical studies have demonstrated that male circumcision reduces the risks of the acquisition and transmission not only of HIV, but also HPV, and thus has a potential role in preventing cervical cancer; HPV being the major cause of cervical cancer.

Castellsague et al. in 2002 [50] in a large study of men, the partners of women with cervical cancer and a control group without cervix cancer showed that penile HPV was detected in 166 of the 847 uncircumcised men (19.6%) and in 16 of the 292 circumcised men (5.5%). After adjustment for age at first intercourse, lifetime number of sexual partners, and other potential confounders, circumcised men were less likely than uncircumcised men to have HPV infection (odds ratio, 0.37). Monogamous women whose male partners had six or more sexual partners and were circumcised had a lower risk of cervical cancer than women whose partners were uncircumcised (adjusted odds ratio, 0.42). Results were similar in the subgroup of men in whom circumcision was confirmed by medical examination. Therefore, factors that reduce the probability of acquiring or transmitting HPV among men or women may reduce the risk of disease associated with these infections such as cervical cancer.

Bosch et al. in 2007 [53] have conducted an extensive search of nine literature databases in respect of HPV infection and cervical cancer. Their analysis generated 112 eligible publications, of which 60 reported quantitative biomedical health outcomes and 57 were included. Of these, most studies were observational and nine were randomized controlled trials. Women were from populations in Africa, North America, South America, Asia, and Europe. Their ages spanned from either 15 or 18 years through to either 49 or 65 years. Strong, consistent evidence was found for protection against cervical cancer (eight of nine studies involving women in multiple non-African settings) and cervical pre-cancer (four of five studies involving women in Africa and other continents. Among women who had a high-risk sexual partner (defined as one who had ≥6 sexual partners and first intercourse before the age of 17 years), cervical cancer was 82% less prevalent if that partner was circumcised than if he was uncircumcised. Reduction of cervical cancer risk from circumcision was 50% for women whose male partner had an intermediate risk index. The authors speculated that infected cervicovaginal secretions including those containing HPV might be retained under the foreskin of the uncircumcised male.

However, Van Howe in 2007 [54] argued that the medical literature does not support the claim that circumcision reduces the risk for genital HPV infection. However Castellsagué et al. (2007) [55] rebutted their findings as "biased, inaccurate and a misleading meta analysis".

The literature as of 2017, summarised by Grund et al. [51] and Morris [52], have convincingly shown that male circumcision reduces the risk of HPV acquisition in men due to heterosexual exposure and in turn reduces the risk in their female consorts of developing cervical cancer.

Conclusions

It can safely be said without much contradiction that the cervical cancer screening programme is an exemplary population screening programme, from its earliest beginnings as a pure exfoliative cytological test to the recent molecular-based technologies, which are now recognized by the FDA for primary screening in a programme of continual refinement and development. The exciting molecular-based technologies, especially in the field of biomarkers, will usher in a new era to increase the accuracy of cervical screening.

In the developing world, where incidence and mortality rates are highest, it is difficult to implement cervical screening programmes of any complexity because of lack of resources. However, newly developed rapid HPV DNA tests can provide results in two hours, and immediate treatment by cryotherapy or cold coagulation of all women who are HPV positive and/or who have been diagnosed with disease by VIA could be an effective alternative approach. The recent development of a risk assessment protocol will aid the delivery of rational screening programmes based on an objective measure of the available screening technologies available at this time.

References

1 Ostör, A.G. (1993). Natural history of cervical intraepithelial neoplasia: A critical review. *Int. J. Gynecol. Pathol.* 12 (2): 186–192.

2 Melnikow, J., Nuovo, J., Willan, A.R. et al. (1998). Natural history of cervical squamous intraepithelial lesions: A meta-analysis. *Obstet. Gynecol.* 92 (4, Pt 2): 727–735.

3 Holowaty, P., Miller, A.B., Rohan, T., and To, T. (1999). Natural history of dysplasia of the uterine cervix. *J. Natl Cancer Inst.* 91 (3): 252–258.

4 Saslow, D., Solomon, D., Lawson, H.W. et al.; ACS-ASCCP-ASCP Cervical Cancer Guideline Committee (2012). American Cancer Society, American Society for Colposcopy and Cervical Pathology, and American Society for Clinical Pathology screening guidelines for the prevention and early detection of cervical cancer. *CA Cancer J. Clin.* 62 (3): 147–172.

5 Massad, L.S., Einstein, M.H., Huh, W.K. et al.;2012 ASCCP Consensus Guidelines Conference (2013). 2012 updated consensus guidelines for the management of abnormal cervical cancer screening tests and cancer precursors. *J. Low Genit. Tract Dis.* 17 (5, Suppl. 1): S1–S27.

6 National Cancer Institute (n.d.). Surveillance, Epidemiology, and End Results Program. https://seer.cancer.gov (accessed 3 January 2018).

7 National Cancer Institute (2014). SEER Cancer Statistics Review (CSR) 1975–2011. http://seer.cancer.gov/csr/1975_2011/ (accessed 21 November 2014).

8 Hristov, L., and Hakama, M. (1997). Effect of screening for cancer in Nordic countries on deaths, cost, and quality of life up till 2017. *Acta Oncol. Suppl.* 9: 1–60.

9 Quinn, M., Babb, P., Jones, J., and Allen, E. (1999). Effect of screening on the incidence of and the mortality from cancer of the cervix in England: Evaluation based on routinely collected statistics. *BMJ* 318: 904–908.

10 Bosch, X., and de Sanjose, S. (2003). Human papillomavirus and cervical cancer burden: An assessment of causality. *J. Nat. Cancer Instit. Monogr.* 31: 3–13.

11 Wang, S.S., Sherman, M.E., Hildesheim, A. et al. (2004). Cervical adenocarcinoma and squamous cell carcinoma incidence trends among white women and black women in the United States for 1976–2000. *Cancer* 100 (5): 1035–1044.

12 Bray, F., Carstenson, B., Moller, H. et al. (2005). Incidence trends of adenocarcinoma of the cervix in 13 European countries. *Cancer Epidemiol. Biomarkers Prev.* 14: 2191–2199.

13 Kessler, I.I. (1974). Cervical cancer epidemiology in historical perspective. *J. Reprod. Med.* 12 (5): 173–185.

14 Sasieni, P., Castanon, A., and Cuzick, J. (2009). Effectiveness of cervical screening with age: Population based case-control study of prospectively recorded data. *BMJ* 339: b2968.

15 Castanon, A., Leung, V.M., Landy, R. et al. (2013). Characteristics and screening history of women diagnosed with cervical cancer aged 20–29 years. *Br. J. Cancer* 109 (1): 35–41.

16 Patel, A., Galaal, K., Burnley, C. et al. (2012). Cervical cancer incidence in young women: A historical and geographic controlled UK regional population study. *Br. J. Cancer* 106 (11): 1753–1759.

17 Koss, L.G. (1989). The Papanicolaou test for cervical cancer detection: A triumph and a tragedy. *JAMA* 261 (5): 737–743.

18 Sasieni, P., Fielder, H., and Rose, B. (2006). Liquid-based versus conventional cervical cytology. *Lancet* 367 (9521): 1481.

19 Arbyn, M., Bergeron, C., Klinkhamer, P. et al. (2008). Liquid compared with conventional cervical cytology: A systematic review and meta-analysis. *J. Obstet. Gynecol.* 111 (1): 167–177.

20 Cox, J.T. (1999). Management of cervical intraepithelial neoplasia. *Lancet* 353: 857–858.

21 Andrae, B., Kemetli, L., Sparen, P. et al. (2008). Screening preventable cervical cancer risks: Evidence from a nationwide audit in Sweden. *J. Nat. Cancer Inst.* 100: 622–629.

22 Lazcano-Ponce, E., Lorincz, A.T., Cruz-Valdez, A. et al. (2011). Self-collection of vaginal specimens for human papillomavirus testing in cervical cancer prevention (MARCH): A community-based randomised controlled trial. *Lancet* 378 (9806): 1868–1873.

23 NHS Cervical Screening Programme (2013). Statistics for the NHS Cervical Screening Programme. http://webarchive.nationalarchives.gov.uk/20150506045933/http://www.cancerscreening.nhs.uk//cervical/statistics.html (accessed 3 January 2018).

24 Sherman, M.E. (2003). Chapter 11: Future directions in cervical pathology. *J. Natl Cancer Instit. Monogr.* 31: 80–88.

25 Wilbur, D.C., Black-Shaffer, W.S., Luff, R.D. et al. (2009). The Becton Dickenson Focal Point GS imaging system: Clinical trials demonstrate the improved sensitivity in the detection of important cervical lesions. *Am. J. Clin. Path.* 132 (5): 767–775.

26 Schiffman, M., Castle, P.E., Jeronimo, J. et al. (2007). Human papillomavirus and cervical cancer. *Lancet* 370: 890–907.

27 IARC Working Group on the Evaluation of Carcinogenic Risks to Humans (2007). Human Papillomaviruses. *IARC Monographs on the Evaluation of Carcinogenic Risks to Humans*, vol. 90. Lyon: International Agency for Research on Cancer.

28 Khan, M.J., Castle, P.E., Lorincz, A.T. et al. (2005). The elevated 10-year risk of cervical precancer and cancer in women with human papillomavirus (HPV) type 16 or 18 and the possible utility of type-specific HPV testing in clinical practice. *J. Natl Cancer Inst.* 97 (14): 1072–1079.

29 Muñoz, N., Bosch, F.X., de Sanjosé, S. et al.; International Agency for Research on Cancer Multicenter Cervical Cancer Study Group (2003). Epidemiologic classification of human papillomavirus types associated with cervical cancer. *N. Engl. J. Med.* 348 (6): 518–527.

30 Bosch, F.X., Burchell, A.N., Schiffman, M. et al. (2008). Epidemiology and natural history of human papillomavirus infections and type-specific implications in cervical neoplasia. *Vaccine* 26 (Suppl. 10): K1–K16.

31 Cuzick, J., Clavel, C., Petry, K.U. et al. (2006). Overview of the European and North American studies on HPV testing in primary cervical cancer screening. *Int. J. Cancer* 119 (5): 1095–1101.

32 Ronco, G., Dillner, J., and Elfström, K.M.; International HPV Screening Working Group (2014). Efficacy of HPV-based screening for prevention of invasive cervical cancer: Follow-up of four European randomised controlled trials. *Lancet* 383 (9916): 524–532.

33 Bulkmans, N.W., Berkhof, J., Rozendaal, L. et al. (2007). Human papillomavirus DNA testing for the detection of cervical intraepithelial neoplasia grade 3 and cancer: 5-year follow-up of a randomised controlled implementation trial. *Lancet* 370 (9601): 1764–1772.

34 Luttmer, R., Berkhof, J., Dijkstra, M.G. et al. (2015). Comparing triage algorithms using HPV DNA genotyping, HPV E7 mRNA detection and cytology in high-risk HPV DNA-positive women. *J. Clin. Virol.* 67: 59–66.

35 Gustinucci, D., Passamonti, B., Cesarini, E. et al. (2012). Role of p16(INK4a) cytology testing as an adjunct to enhance the diagnostic specificity and accuracy in human papillomavirus-positive women within an organized cervical cancer screening program. *Acta Cytol.* 56 (5): 506–514.

36 Bergeron, C., Ikenberg, H., Sideri, M. et al. (2015). Prospective evaluation of p16/Ki-67 dual-stained cytology for managing women with abnormal Papanicolaou cytology: PALMS study results. *Cancer Cytopathol.* 123 (6): 373–381.

37 Brentnall, A., Vasiljević, N., Scibior-Bentkowska, D. et al. (2014). A DNA methylation classifier of cervical precancer based on human papillomavirus and human genes. *Int. J. Cancer* 135 (6): 1425–1432.

38 Grabe, N., Lahrmann, B., Pommerencke, T. et al. (2010). A virtual microscopy system to scan, evaluate and archive biomarker enhanced cervical cytology slides. *Oncol.* 32 (1–2): 109–119.

39 Tjalma, W.A., Kim, E., and Vandeweyer, K. (2017). The impact on women's health and the cervical cancer screening budget of primary HPV screening with dual-stain cytology triage in Belgium. *Eur. J. Obstet. Gynecol. Reprod. Biol.* 212: 171–181.

40 Gustinucci, D., Giorgi Rossi, P., Cesarini, E. et al. (2016). Use of cytology, E6/E7 mRNA, and p16INK4a-Ki-67 to define the management of human papillomavirus (HPV)-positive women in cervical cancer screening. *Am. J. Clin. Pathol.* 145 (1): 35–45.

41 Badiga, S., Chambers, M.M., Huh, W. et al. (2016). Expression of p16INK4A in cervical precancerous lesions is unlikely to be preventable by human papillomavirus vaccines. *Cancer* 122 (23): 3615–3623.

42 Castle, P.E., Kinney, W.K., Xue, X. et al. (2017). Effect of several negative rounds of human papillomavirus and cytology co-testing on safety against cervical cancer: An observational cohort study. *J. Natl. Cancer Inst.* doi: 10.1093/jnci/djx225. [Epub ahead of print].

43 Moyer, V.A., LeFevre, M.L., Siu, A.L. et al.; U.S. Preventive Services Task Force (2012). Screening for cervical cancer: U.S. Preventive Services Task Force recommendation statement. *Ann. Intern. Med.* 156: 880–891.

44 Cuzick, J., Cadman, L., Mesher, D. et al. (2013). Comparing the performance of six human papillomavirus tests in a screening population. *Br. J. Cancer* 108 (4): 908–913.

45 Arbyn, M., Roelens, J., Cuschieri, K. et al. (2013). The APTIMA HPV assay versus the Hybrid Capture 2 test in triage of women with ASC-US or LSIL cervical cytology: A meta-analysis of the diagnostic accuracy. *Int. J. Cancer* 132 (1): 101–108.

46 Wright, T.C., Jr, Stoler, M.H., Sharma, A. et al.; ATHENA (Addressing THE Need for Advanced HPV Diagnostics) Study Group (2011). Evaluation of HPV-16 and HPV-18 geno-typing for the triage of women with high-risk HPV+ cytology-negative results. *Am. J. Clin. Pathol.* 136 (4): 578–586.

47 Gage, J.C., Schiffman, M., Katki, H.A. et al. (2014). Reassurance against future risk of pre-cancer and cancer conferred by a negative human papillomavirus test. *J. Natl Cancer Inst.* 106 (8).

48 Canfell, K., Caruana, M., Gebski, V. et al. (2017). Cervical screening with primary HPV testing or cytology in a population of women in which those aged 33 years or younger had previously been offered HPV vaccination: Results of the Compass pilot randomised trial. *PLoS Med.* 14 (9).

49 Zhao, F.-H., Hu, S.-Y., Zhang, Q. et al. (2016). Risk assessment to guide cervical screening strategies in a large Chinese population. *Int. J. Cancer* 138: 2639–2647.

50 Castellsague, X., Bosch, F.X., Munoz, N. et al. (2002). International Agency for Research on Cancer Multicenter Cervical Cancer Study G. Male circumcision, penile human papillomavirus infection, and cervical cancer in female partners. *N. Engl. J. Med.* 346: 1105–111.

51 Grund, J.M., Bryant, T.S., Jackson, I. et al. (2017). Association between male circumcision and women's biomedical health outcomes: a systematic review. *Lancet Glob Health.* 5: e1113–e1122.

52 Morris, B.J., and Hankins, C.A. (2017). Effect of male circumcision on risk of sexually trans-mitted infections and cervical cancer in women. *Lancet Glob Health* 5 (11): e1054–e1055.

53 Bosch, F.X., Albero, G., and Castellsague, X. (2007). Male circumcision, human papillomavirus and cervical cancer: from evidence to intervention. *J. Infect.* 54 (5): 490–6.

54 Van Howe, R.S. (2007). Human papillomavirus and circumcision: a meta-analysis. *J. Infect.* 55 (1): 91–3.

55 Castellsagué, X., Albero, G., Clèries, R., and Bosch, F. X. (2007). Human papillomavirus and circumcision: a meta-analysis: Comment on a biased, inaccurate and misleading meta-analysis. *J. Infect.* 93–6. Epub Apr 11.

CHAPTER 9

Prevention of and screening for anal cancer

Andrew E. Grulich[1], Richard J. Hillman[2], and Isobel M. Poynten[1]

[1] Kirby Institute, University of New South Wales, Sydney, Australia
[2] HIV, Immunology and Infectious Diseases, St Vincent's Hospital, Sydney, Australia

SUMMARY BOX

- Anal cancer is a generally uncommon cancer which is highly concentrated among gay and bisexual men, women with previous human papillomavirus-related anogenital disease, solid organ transplant recipients, and people with HIV.

- Adolescent human papillomavirus vaccination will eventually lead to substantial reductions in incidence, but the full effect is several decades away.

- Other prevention approaches are required in the interim.

- Human papillomavirus vaccination of adults may be of help, but will not reduce incidence in those with current chronic human papillomavirus infection.

- Screening using cytology, coupled with ablative treatment of high-grade intra-epithelial cancer precursors, has been proposed, but has not been proven to reduce cancer incidence.

- Digital anorectal examination of the highest-risk individuals, HIV-positive gay and bisexual men, has been advocated to diagnose cancers at an early stage, when treatments are more effective.

Squamous cell cancer of the anus (hereafter referred to as anal cancer) is a generally uncommon cancer that is second only to cervical cancer in the closeness of its association with infection with high-risk types of human papillomavirus (HPV). In a recent meta-analysis, HPV could be detected in 84% of cases [1]. Given the known limitations of HPV detection techniques using stored tissues, it may be that HPV is a necessary cause of anal cancer, as it is for cervical cancer [2]. In a recent Australian series, HPV could be detected in 96% of anal cancer cases [3]. The most common HPV type detected is HPV16, which can be detected in 70–80% of cases [1, 3, 4].

Cancer Prevention and Screening: Concepts, Principles and Controversies, First Edition.
Edited by Rosalind A. Eeles, Christine D. Berg, and Jeffrey S. Tobias.
© 2019 John Wiley & Sons, Inc. Published 2019 by John Wiley & Sons, Inc.

Table 9.1 Relative risk and incidence of anal cancer described in the general population and in various subgroups of the population.

Population	Relative risk	Approximate annual incidence (per 100 000)
General population	1 (referent)	1–2
Women with previous anogenital HPV disease	5	5–10
Organ transplant recipients	5	5–10
HIV-negative gay and bisexual men	5–20	5–40
HIV-positive men (except gay and bisexual men) and women	10	15–20
HIV-positive gay and bisexual men	50	50–100

The annual incidence of anal cancer is between 1 and 2 per 100 000 in most populations for which data are available. In all published reports of time trends from Europe, North America, and Australia, incidence has been increasing for several decades, and it continues to increase to this day [5]. In Denmark, where earlier data are available, incidence has been increasing since the 1960s [6]. Incidence increases with age, with about 50% of cases occurring in people aged older than 65 years [5].

A key feature of the epidemiology of anal cancer is that incidence is very heavily concentrated in certain population subgroups (Table 9.1). In women, incidence is raised about 5-fold after the diagnosis of cervical intra-epithelial disease or cervical cancer [7, 8], and is raised about 20-fold after vulvar carcinoma [8], demonstrating a tendency for HPV-related anogenital neoplasia to present at more than one site in an individual. HPV-related cancers occur at increased rates in people with immune deficiency, reflecting the role of immune function in controlling HPV infection and its consequences. Incidence of anal cancer is raised about 5-fold in solid organ transplant recipients who receive pharmaceutical immune suppression [9, 10]. People with HIV have the dual risk factors of increased exposure to HPV and immune dysfunction, and thus have the highest rates of HPV-associated cancer, including anal cancer, of any population. Anal cancer incidence among people with HIV is increased 10–15-fold in women, heterosexual men, and injecting drug users, and is increased even more, by around 50-fold, in gay and bisexual men with HIV [11]. Some large cohort studies of HIV-positive gay and bisexual men have reported annual incidence rates of over 100/100 000 [12]. Although male homosexuality has been consistently associated with increased risk of anal cancer in case-control studies, the degree to which risk is raised in HIV-negative gay and bisexual men is uncertain. A meta-analysis identified only two cohort studies of anal cancer incidence in HIV-negative gay and bisexual men, with an annual incidence of about 5 per 100 000 [12].

Primary prevention

Given the closeness of the association with HPV infection, prevention of anal infection with high-risk HPV types should offer protection against anal cancer.

Vaccination

Two randomized controlled trials have demonstrated substantial efficacy of available HPV vaccines in preventing anal cancer precursors. The bivalent HPV vaccine, which protects against HPV16 and 18 only, reduced the rate of anal HPV 16 or 18 detection by 84% over three years of follow-up in women who did not have infection with these types at baseline [13]. The quadrivalent HPV vaccine, which protects against HPV16, 18, 6 and 11, reduced the risk of anal high-grade squamous intra-epithelial lesions (HSIL) related to these HPV types in men who have sex with men by 78% over three years of follow-up in a per-protocol analysis [14]. These data demonstrate that widespread HPV vaccination should lead to substantial declines in anal cancer incidence in the cohort of adolescents and young adults who currently receive the HPV vaccine.

Since 2007, many countries have begun to offer routine vaccination to school-aged girls. Countries with high HPV vaccine uptake in girls, such as Australia, have seen enormous declines in the incidence of HPV-associated genital warts in women [15], and in the prevalence of detectable cervical infection with high-risk HPV types [16]. In addition, substantial declines in genital warts have also been demonstrated in young heterosexual men. Since these declines were seen well before the commencement of male vaccination, this is believed to be due to herd immunity [15]. In contrast to the declines seen in heterosexual men, declines in HPV-related genital warts have not been seen in gay and bisexual men [15]. These data suggest that the population with the highest rates of HPV-related morbidity, gay and bisexual men, will only be protected if males as well as females are vaccinated. Currently, only a few countries recommend routine vaccination of boys, and only in Australia is there public funding for universal HPV vaccination for school-aged boys [17]. An alternative is to target HPV vaccination at young adult gay and bisexual men. The UK Department of Health Joint Committee on Vaccination and Immunisation recently released an interim statement recommending a targeted HPV vaccination programme aiming to vaccinate men who have sex with men aged 16–40 years attending genitourinary medicine clinics [18]. In the USA, the Advisory Committee on Immunization Practices has recommended that men who have sex with men aged up to 26 should receive HPV vaccination [19]. In Australia, in addition to publicly funded vaccination of school-aged boys, targeted vaccination of adult gay and bisexual men is recommended [20], but is not publicly funded.

Modification of behaviour and other exposures

HPV is the most prevalent of all sexually transmitted infections. This, coupled with the fact that it may be transmitted sexually on fingers [21] and from ano-genital skin, means that modification of sexual behaviour is not as successful in reducing incidence as it can be for some other sexually transmitted infections, which are predominantly transmitted via bodily fluids such as semen and cervical secretions. Some studies have demonstrated that condoms provide a widely vary-ing degree of partial protection against genital HPV infection [22]. In gay and bisexual men, receptive condomless anal intercourse has been reported to increase the risk of anal HPV detection [23, 24].

As is the case for cervical cancer, tobacco exposure is associated with increased risk of anal cancer [5]. It is therefore plausible that smoking cessation may reduce the risk of anal cancer.

In people with HIV, severe present or past immune deficiency, as measured by low nadir CD4 positive lymphocyte count, has been associated with increased anal cancer risk [5]. In this population, early initiation of HIV therapy to avoid severe immune deficiency may be associated with lower anal cancer risk.

Secondary prevention

Screening and treatment for cancer precursors

In many respects, the natural history of anal HPV infection and anal HSIL resem-bles that of cervical HPV infection and cervical HSIL. It is believed that chronic, established high-risk HPV infection leads to anal HSIL and, in a small proportion of cases, to invasive cancer. This has led some researchers to propose a Papanicolaou (Pap) smear-based screening programme in the highest-risk population, gay and bisexual men with or without HIV [25]. Population-based implementation of cervical Pap screening in women has been associated with sustained, dramatic reductions in cervical cancer incidence. However, there is as yet no evidence that anal Pap screening leads to a decline in anal cancer inci-dence at an individual or population level, and the impetus for screening has largely been based on reasoning by analogy [26]. There are currently no national guidelines which recommend anal Pap smear screening in any population. In this context, it is critical to consider areas of similarity and difference between the natural history, screening for, and therapy of high-risk HPV infection and HSIL in the cervix and the anus.

Differences in the epidemiology of high-risk HPV infection in the cervix and anus

In women, incidence and prevalence of cervical high-risk HPV infection peak in adolescence, and rapidly decline after the age of 25 [27]. During adolescence, about 90% of cervical high-risk HPV infections clear without the need for therapy [28, 29]. Pap screening is generally not recommended in this young population, where both incidence and clearance of high-risk HPV are common. At older ages, when screening occurs, prevalent high-risk HPV detection is much more likely to represent chronic established HPV infection of carcinogenic potential. The higher incidence of cervical high-risk HPV infection in the young reflects differences in sexual behaviour with age. Young women aged less than 25 years are much more likely to report multiple sexual partners than older women. Among heterosexual women aged over 30 years, fewer than 5% report more than one sexual partner in the past year [30]. Thus, at these older ages, new self-limiting high-risk HPV infections are relatively uncommon, and a large proportion of detectable high-risk HPV reflects chronic infection.

There are relatively few studies of anal high-risk HPV infection, and most of these have been in gay and bisexual men. Compared with cervical high-risk HPV infection in women, studies in gay and bisexual men show that the prevalence of anal high-risk HPV infection is very high. In addition, in this population anal high-risk HPV prevalence remains elevated across the adult age range, including well past 50 years of age [31, 32]. Prevalence of high-risk HPV is higher in HIV-positive (74%) than HIV-negative gay and bisexual men (37%) [12]. In contrast to heterosexual women, the majority of gay and bisexual men report multiple sexual partners at all ages [33]. The continued exposure to new sexual partners is likely to be reflected in high rates of acute high-risk HPV infection. The natural history of anal high-risk HPV infection is poorly described, and the proportion of infections which clear without the need for therapy has been little studied. It seems plausible, however, that a high proportion of detected high-risk HPV infection in older adult gay and bisexual men is due to acute infection or transient detection, rather than long-term chronic infection of carcinogenic potential. This pattern reflects high numbers of sexual partners, and persists across the age ranges.

In comparison to gay and bisexual men, the prevalence of anal HPV is lower in women, but is still over 20% in several studies [21]. While anal sex is clearly a risk factor in some women, it is also thought that sexual behaviours that do not involve penile-anal penetration may transmit HPV to the anus [21].

Differences in progression rates of established cervical and anal HSIL

Few follow-up studies of untreated cervical HSIL have been reported, but one New Zealand study reported a rate of progression to cervical cancer of about 0.8 per 100 person years [34]. Based on a cross-sectional comparison of anal HSIL prevalence and cancer incidence, a large meta-analysis estimated progression rates from anal HSIL to cancer of 1 in 600 per year in HIV-positive gay and bisexual men, and about 1 in 4000 per year in HIV-negative men [12]. The prevalence of anal HSIL is so high in this population (29% in the HIV positive and 22% in the HIV negative in this meta-analysis) that it is clear that the great majority of HSIL does not progress to anal cancer. Longitudinal studies with careful observation of anal HSIL are required to confirm these estimates, both in gay and bisexual men and in other high-risk populations.

Performance characteristics of anal cancer screening tests

The performance characteristics of the anal cancer screening test are less well studied than the cervical Pap or HPV screening tests. The sensitivity of anal cytology is estimated to be similar to that of cervical cytology, but the specificity is considerably lower [35]. This is probably at least partially because a lower cytological threshold for the anal referral test (high-resolution anoscopy) than for the cervical referral test (colposcopy) is generally chosen. In addition, as already described, gay and bisexual men have a much higher HPV incidence than women in the general population. This means that a larger proportion of HPV-related disease is likely to be acute and self-limiting than is the case in women, leading to a higher rate of false positives and a lower positive predictive value. In addition, the diagnostic test, high-resolution anoscopy, is technically more demanding than its colposcopic equivalent. The highly involuted surface of the anal mucosa means it is easier to miss a HSIL lesion than is the case in the cervix [36].

Different characteristics of treatment of anal and cervical HSIL

The aim of treatment of cervical HSIL is to completely remove the lesion and the entire transformation zone using a technique such as loop excision. Removal of the entire transformation zone is not possible in the anus because of unacceptable morbidity, including severe pain and risk of anal stenosis. Related to the inability to remove the entire transformation zone, treatment of anal HSIL is not as effective as treatment of cervical HSIL. A meta-analysis estimated recurrence rates of 5% and 15% after a single treatment of cervical HSIL [37]. In comparison, there are few large studies of anal HSIL recurrence after treatment, but the largest randomized trial estimated a mean recurrence rate at 72 weeks of 67% [38]. A recent Cochrane review concluded there was insufficient evidence of HSIL treatment efficacy [39].

Early detection and treatment of cancer

Survival from anal cancer is highly dependent on stage of diagnosis. US registry data from 1988 to 1993 showed that five-year survival was 71% for those with Stage 1 (localized) disease, but declined to 23% for those with Stage 4 (metastatic) disease [40]. The size of the primary tumour is also closely related to survival. In the USA, based on anal cancer cases diagnosed between 1988 and 2001, relative survival increased from 45% when the primary tumour had a largest diameter of more than 5 cm to 80% when it was less than or equal to 2 cm [41]. A small French series of 69 people with tumours of less than or equal to 1 cm at diagnosis reported five-year overall survival of 94%, with 85% colostomy-free survival [42].

Given the much-improved survival when anal cancer is diagnosed early, there has been substantial interest in the use of digital anorectal examination as a screening test to diagnose anal cancer early. This technique is recommended as a screening test in European and US clinical guidelines for the management of people with HIV [43], but it is explicitly acknowledged that this is based only on 'expert opinion'. There have been no studies of the test performance characteristics of digital anorectal examination in the diagnosis of anal cancer, and no evidence that it will reduce cancer morbidity or mortality. Based on limited data, the test appears to be acceptable to gay and bisexual men living with HIV [44].

Conclusion

Anal cancer is a condition that is highly concentrated among certain population groups and is an uncommon cancer in the general population. The prevention response should be tailored to those groups at highest risk. Incidence is highest in gay and bisexual men, particularly those with HIV, and most research has been performed in this population. However, incidence is also substantial in women with previous HPV-related anogenital disease and in organ transplant recipients. HPV vaccination of adolescents, before sexual exposure to HPV, is clearly the most effective preventive intervention against anal cancer, but this will take decades to have an impact on adult cancer rates. Concerns that HPV vaccine efficacy will be lessened in previously exposed individuals have impeded the wider introduction to adults, although some guidelines do now recommend vaccination of adult gay and bisexual men up to age 26. For older gay and bisexual men, much research has investigated the role of screening and treatment of precursor lesions. The utility of screening is unproven and treatment efficacy appears to be limited, with considerable side effects and disease recurrence. In addition, delivering treatment to those who are truly at risk has been a challenge, as 30–40% of gay and bisexual men in many studies have HSIL, the presumed intra-epithelial cancer precursor. Developing a biomarker that identifies those people with anal HSIL who are at most risk of progression to cancer, and focusing treatment on this group, is a promising research direction. In 2014, a randomized trial comparing topical or ablative treatment with active monitoring in preventing anal cancer in HIV-positive patients with HSIL began recruitment. The study will recruit over 5000 participants, with a primary end-point of anal cancer, and is scheduled to report in 2022 [45]. In the meantime, and while studies of biomarkers to identify those at highest risk of cancer are also under way, many experts recommend using digital anorectal examination as a screening test.

Acknowledgements

This work was supported by a Cancer Council NSW Strategic Research Partnership Grant (#13–11) and a National Health and Medical Research Council Program Grant (# 568971).

References

1 De Vuyst, H., Clifford, G.M., Nascimento, M.C. et al. (2009). Prevalence and type distribution of human papillomavirus in carcinoma and intraepithelial neoplasia of the vulva, vagina and anus: A meta-analysis. *Int. J. Cancer* 124 (7): 1626–1636.

2 Daling, J.R., Madeleine, M.M., Johnson, L.G. et al. (2004). Human papillomavirus, smoking, and sexual practices in the etiology of anal cancer. *Cancer* 101 (2): 270–280.

3 Hillman, R.J., Garland, S.M., Gunathilake, M.P. et al. (2014). Human papillomavirus (HPV) genotypes in an Australian sample of anal cancers. *Int. J. Cancer* 135 (4): 996–1001.

4 Hoots, B.E., Palefsky, J.M., Pimenta, J.M., and Smith, J.S. (2009). Human papillomavirus type distribution in anal cancer and anal intraepithelial lesions. *Int. J. Cancer* 124 (10): 2375–2383.

5 Grulich, A.E., Poynten, M., Machalek, D.A. et al. (2012). The epidemiology of anal cancer. *Sex. Health* 9: 504–508.

6 Frisch, M., Melbye, M., and Moller, H. (1993). Trends in incidence of anal cancer in Denmark. *BMJ Clin Res.* 306 (6875): 419–422.

7 Edgren, G., and Sparen, P. (2007). Risk of anogenital cancer after diagnosis of cervical intraepithelial neoplasia: A prospective population-based study. *Lancet Oncol.* 8 (4): 311–316.

8 Saleem, A.M., Paulus, J.K., Shapter, A.P. et al. (2011). Risk of anal cancer in a cohort with human papillomavirus-related gynecologic neoplasm. *Obstet. Gynecol.* 117 (3): 643–649.

9 Grulich, A.E., van Leeuwen, M.T., Falster, M.O., and Vajdic, C.M. (2007). Incidence of cancers in people with HIV/AIDS compared with immunosuppressed transplant recipients: A meta-analysis. *Lancet* 370 (9581): 59–67.

10 Madeleine, M.M., Finch, J.L., Lynch, C.F. et al. (2013). HPV-related cancers after solid organ transplantation in the United States. *Am. J. Transplant.* 13 (12): 3202–3209.

11 Chaturvedi, A.K., Madeleine, M.M., Biggar, R.J., and Engels, E.A. (2009). Risk of human papillomavirus-associated cancers among persons with AIDS. *J. Natl Cancer Inst.* 101 (16): 1120–1130.

12 Machalek, D.A., Poynten, M., Jin, F. et al. (2012). Anal human papillomavirus infection, and associated neoplastic lesions in homosexual men: Systematic review and meta-analysis. *Lancet Oncol.* 13: 487–500.

13 Kreimer, A.R., Gonzalez, P., Katki, H.A. et al. Efficacy of a bivalent HPV 16/18 vaccine against anal HPV 16/18 infection among young women: A nested analysis within the Costa Rica Vaccine Trial. *Lancet Oncol.* 12 (9): 862–870.

14 Palefsky, J.M., Giuliano, A.R., Goldstone, S. et al. HPV vaccine against anal HPV infection and anal intraepithelial neoplasia. *New Engl. J. Med.* 365 (17): 1576–1585.

15 Ali, H., Donovan, B., Wand, H. et al. (2013). Genital warts in young Australians five years into national human papillomavirus vaccination programme: National surveillance data. *BMJ Clin. Res.* 346: f2032.

16 Tabrizi, S.N., Brotherton, J.M., Kaldor, J.M. et al. (2014). Assessment of herd immunity and cross-protection after a human papillomavirus vaccination programme in Australia: A repeat cross-sectional study. *Lancet Infect. Dis.* 14 (10): 958–966.

17 Brill, D. (2013). Australia launches national scheme to vaccinate boys against HPV. *BMJ Clin. Res.* 346: f924.

18 United Kingdom Joint Committee on Vaccination and Immunisation Public Health England (2014). JCVI interim position statement on HPV vaccination of men who have sex with men (MSM). https://www.gov.uk/government/uploads/system/uploads/attachment_data/file/373531/JCVI_interim_statement_HPV_vacc.pdf (accessed 3 January 2018).

19 Markowitz, L.E., Dunne, E.F., Saraiya, M. et al. (2014). Human papillomavirus vaccination. *MMWR Recomm. Rep.* 63 (RR-05): 1–30.

20 Australian Technical Advisory Group on Immunisation (2014). *The Australian Immunisation Handbook*, 10e. Canberra: Australian Government Department of Health.

21 Nyitray, A.G. (2012). The epidemiology of anal human papillomavirus infection among women and men having sex with women. *Sex. Health* 9 (6): 538–546.

22 Hariri, S., and Warner, L. (2013). Condom use and human papillomavirus in men. *J. Infect. Dis.* 208 (3): 367–369.

23 Hu, Y., Qian, H.Z., Sun, J. et al. (2013). Anal human papillomavirus infection among HIV-infected and uninfected men who have sex with men in Beijing, *China. J. Acquir. Immune Defic. Syndr.* 64 (1): 103–114.

24 Nyitray, A.G., Carvalho da Silva, R.J., Baggio, M.L. et al. (2011). Age-specific prevalence of and risk factors for anal human papillomavirus (HPV) among men who have sex with women and men who have sex with men: The HPV in men (HIM) study. *J. Infect. Dis.* 203 (1): 49–57.

25 Palefsky, J.M., Holly, E.A., Hogeboom, C.J. et al. (1997). Anal cytology as a screening tool for anal squamous intraepithelial lesions. *J. Acquir. Immune Defic. Syndr. Hum. Retrovirol.* 14 (5): 415–422.

26 Arbyn, M., de Sanjose, S., Saraiya, M. et al. (2012). EUROGIN 2011 roadmap on prevention and treatment of HPV-related disease. *Int. J. Cancer* 131 (9): 1969–1982.

27 Bruni, L., Diaz, M., Castellsague, X. et al. (2010). Cervical human papillomavirus prevalence in 5 continents: Meta-analysis of 1 million women with normal cytological findings. *J. Infect. Dis.* 202 (12): 1789–1799.

28 Schiffman, M., Wentzensen, N., Wacholder, S. et al. (2011). Human papillomavirus testing in the prevention of cervical cancer. *J. Nat. Cancer Inst.* 103 (5): 368–383.

29 Case, A.S., Rocconi, R.P., Straughn, J.M., Jr. et al. (2006). Cervical intraepithelial neoplasia in adolescent women: Incidence and treatment outcomes. *Obstet. Gynecol.* 108 (6): 1369–1374.

30 Badcock, P.B., Smith, A.M., Richters, J. et al. (2014). Characteristics of heterosexual regular relationships among a representative sample of adults: The Second Australian Study of Health and Relationships. *Sex. Health* 11 (5): 427–438.

31 Chin-Hong, P.V., Vittinghoff, E., Cranston, R.D. et al. (2004). Age-specific prevalence of anal human papillomavirus infection in HIV-negative sexually active men who have sex with men: The EXPLORE study. *J. Infect. Dis.* 190 (12): 2070–2076.

32 Vajdic, C.M., van Leeuwen, M.T., Jin, F. et al. (2009). Anal human papillomavirus genotype diversity and co-infection in a community-based sample of homosexual men. *Sex. Transm. Infect.* 85 (5): 330–335.

33 Poynten, I.M., Grulich, A.E., and Templeton, D.J. (2013). Sexually transmitted infections in older populations. *Curr. Opin. Infect. Dis.* 26 (1): 80–85.

34 McCredie, M.R., Sharples, K.J., Paul, C. et al. (2008). Natural history of cervical neoplasia and risk of invasive cancer in women with cervical intraepithelial neoplasia 3: A retrospective cohort study. *Lancet Oncol.* 9 (5): 425–434.

35 Roberts, J.M., and Thurloe, J.K. (2012). Comparison of the performance of anal cytology and cervical cytology as screening tests. *Sex. Health* 9 (6): 568–573.

36 Palefsky, J.M. (2012). Practising high-resolution anoscopy. *Sex. Health* 9 (6): 580–586.

37 Wright, T.C., Jr., Massad, L.S., Dunton, C.J. et al. (2007). 2006 consensus guidelines for the management of women with cervical intraepithelial neoplasia or adenocarcinoma in situ. *J. Low. Genit. Tract Dis.* 11 (4): 223–239.

38 Richel, O., de Vries, H.J., van Noesel, C.J. et al. (2013). Comparison of imiquimod, topical fluorouracil, and electrocautery for the treatment of anal intraepithelial neoplasia in HIV-positive men who have sex with men: An open-label, randomised controlled trial. *Lancet Oncol.* 14 (4): 346–353.

39 Macaya, A., Munoz-Santos, C., Balaguer, A., and Barbera, M.J. (2012). Interventions for anal canal intraepithelial neoplasia. *Cochrane Database Syst. Rev.* 12 (Art. No.: CD009244). doi: 10.1002/14651858.CD009244.pub2.

40 Myerson, R.J., Karnell, L.H., and Menck, H.R. (1997). The National Cancer Data Base report on carcinoma of the anus. *Cancer* 80 (4): 805–815.

41 Madeleine, M.M. and Newcomer, L.M. (2007). Cancer of the anus. In: *SEER Survival Monograph: Cancer Survival among Adults: US SEER Program, 1988–2001, Patient and Tumor Characteristics* (ed. L.A.G. Ries, J.L. Young, Jr, G.E. Keel et al.), 43–48. Bethesda, MD: National Cancer Institute, Surveillance Epidemiology and End Results Research Program, National Institutes of Health.

42 Ortholan, C., Ramaioli, A., Peiffert, D. et al. (2005). Anal canal carcinoma: Early-stage tumors< or =10 mm (T1 or Tis): Therapeutic options and original pattern of local failure after radiotherapy. *Int. J. Radiat. Oncol. Biol. Phys.* 62 (2): 479–485.

43 Ong, J.J., Chen, M., Grulich, A.E., and Fairley, C.K. (2014). Regional and national guideline recommendations for digital ano-rectal examination as a means for anal cancer screening in HIV positive men who have sex with men: A systematic review. *BMC Cancer* 14: 557.

44 Read, T.R., Vodstrcil, L., Grulich, A.E. et al. (2013). Acceptability of digital anal cancer screening examinations in HIV-positive homosexual men. *HIV Med.* 14 (8): 491–496.

45 AIDS Malignancy Clinical Trials Consortium (2014). Topical or Ablative Treatment in Preventing Anal Cancer in Patients With HIV and Anal High-Grade Squamous Intraepithelial Lesions. https://clinicaltrials.gov/ct2/show/NCT02135419 (accessed 3 January 2018).

CHAPTER 10

The prevention of breast cancer

Anthony Howell[1,2], Michelle N. Harvie[1], Sacha J. Howell[1,2],
Louise S. Donnelly[1], and D. Gareth Evans[1,2,3]

[1]*Genesis Breast Cancer Prevention Centre, University Hospital of South Manchester NHS Trust, Wythenshawe, UK*
[2]*The Christie NHS Foundation Trust & Institute of Cancer Sciences, University of Manchester, UK*
[3]*Manchester Centre for Genomic Medicine, St Mary's Hospital, Manchester Academic Health Sciences Centre
(MAHSC), Institute of Human Development, University of Manchester, UK*

SUMMARY BOX

- It is now feasible to prevent a proportion of breast cancers using preventive therapy
  (chemoprevention), lifestyle change, and risk-reducing breast and ovarian surgery.

- There is considerable work to be done before all at-risk women can be offered preventive therapy, and *all* middle-aged and older women who are overweight or obese and
  who do not take regular exercise also have help to make lifestyle changes.

- It is important to emphasize the breast cancer risks of excess alcohol.

- Currently tamoxifen is the only approved preventive therapy available for premenopausal women, and is given for five years. In postmenopausal women, NICE guidelines
  indicate that five years' treatment with either tamoxifen 20 g/day or raloxifene 60 mg/
  day may be considered.

- Studies of other agents are in progress.

Randomized controlled trials of preventive therapy and observational studies of
lifestyle change and risk-reducing surgery indicate that breast cancer risk may be
reduced by between 25% and 90–95% in appropriate groups of women [1, 2].
However, our knowledge of the relative effectiveness of these approaches for
breast cancer prevention far exceeds our ability to apply them to the women at
risk in the general population.

In many health services, mechanisms are in place for referral of women with
a strong family history of breast cancer to specialist clinics for advice, and for estimating the probability of a genetic cause of breast cancer within families [3]. The
discovery and rapid application of testing for mutations in the *BRCA1* and *BRCA2*
genes were major drives for setting up widespread clinical referral systems for

Cancer Prevention and Screening: Concepts, Principles and Controversies, First Edition.
Edited by Rosalind A. Eeles, Christine D. Berg, and Jeffrey S. Tobias.
© 2019 John Wiley & Sons, Inc. Published 2019 by John Wiley & Sons, Inc.

these groups of women. Now multiple other gene mutations and single nucleo-tide polymorphisms related to breast cancer risk have been discovered, and the process of determining how best to apply such new knowledge in the clinic is in progress [4].

Between 20% and 54% of women who develop breast cancer have a family history of the disease [5]. This may or may not be due to familial risk factors such as mutations in high-penetrance genes that account for around 5% of breast can-cer, or more polygenic inheritance of moderate-risk alleles or lower-risk common variants that make up most of the rest of the estimated 27–30% of breast cancer due mainly to hereditary factors [1, 2]. Much of the remainder of the recent increased breast cancer incidence is related to nonmodifiable factors such as nulli-parity or late age of first pregnancy, and modifiable factors such as lack of breast-feeding, weight gain, and lack of exercise. Despite our knowledge of such factors, many women develop breast cancer in the absence of them, suggesting that some risks remain to be uncovered or may be related to chance. An estimate of the proportion of breast cancer related to differences in reproductive habits was given by Beral and her colleagues [6]. They estimated that all of the increase in breast cancer in Western women compared with African women was related to reduc-tion in family size and lack of breast-feeding. In Iceland there was a fourfold increase in the risk of sporadic breast cancer and breast cancer related to the Icelandic founder *BRCA2* mutation between 1920 and 2000 [7]. Such a rapid change in risk is most likely to be epigenetic, related to lifestyle and unspecified environmental factors. In the context of this and other studies, it is also important to understand that lifestyle factors may influence the penetrance of genetic changes.

Nongenetic, nonfamilial breast cancer is not usually appreciated by women or many of their clinicians, partly because it is multifactorial and partly because mechanisms are not in place to detect and act on nongenetic risks. Clinical genet-ics services rightly focus efforts on establishing the veracity of family histories in determining the probabilities of mutations in families and pre- and post-mutation test counselling. However, clinics have been established, largely associated with Breast Units, to assess women at lower levels of increased risk (defined as moder-ate risk 17–29% lifetime risk in National Institute for Health and Care Excellence [NICE] guidelines) and to provide risk counselling and information concerning preventive measures. Although nongenetic factors are usually assessed in such clinics, initial referral is often precipitated by a woman's family history of breast cancer. Furthermore, referrals are usually in women under the age of 50, since familial risk is predominantly thought to reside in this group, and the main inter-vention of early breast screening in moderate-risk women is between 40 and 49 years of age (Figure 10.1a) [8]. In the UK, management of women with a family history of breast cancer is the subject of guidelines produced by NICE in 2004/2006 and updated more recently [8]. The guidelines cover the assessment of familial risk and management of the woman at risk concerning genetic testing, screening, and preventive approaches, and are important for family practitioners, clinicians,

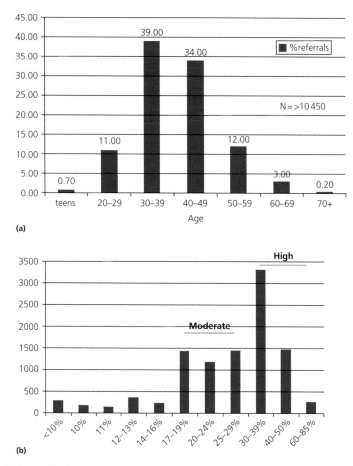

Figure 10.1 Age distribution (a) and breast cancer risk (b) of women referred to the Genesis Breast Cancer Risk and Prevention Clinic in Manchester, UK.

and nurses who run clinics for women at nongenetic risk, and for geneticists and genetics counsellors in genetics centres.

Estimation of risk of breast cancer

The UK NICE guidelines indicate that women at high risk of breast cancer (greater than or equal to 30% lifetime risk) should be 'offered' preventive treatment with tamoxifen, anastrazole or raloxifene, and that women at moderate risk (greater than or equal to 1 in 6 lifetime risk or greater than 3% 10-year risk aged 40 years) should be 'considered' for five years of therapy. In the USA, the NCI Gail Risk Model (Breast Cancer Risk Assessment Tools or BCRAT) is used; one cut-off for indicating higher risk is a 1.66% 5-year risk (3.32% 10-year risk) [9], which approximates the NICE moderate-risk guideline from age 40. Based on risk–benefit tables developed by Freedman et al. [10], the US Preventive Services Task Force (USPSTF) [11] concludes that women with an estimated 5-year breast cancer risk of 3% or more are likely to have more benefit than harm, but the balance depends on age, ethnicity, the preventive therapy used, and whether or not the woman at risk has a uterus [11]. NICE gives thresholds for chemoprevention in terms of 10-year and lifetime risks. To be at moderate risk, the 10-year risk thresholds are 3–8% for women age 40–50 and 5–8% for those above age 50. For high risk the threshold is above 8% 10-year risk at any age [8].

There are several potential models for estimating breast cancer risk in the clinic. Ideally (very much an ideal) each model should be validated in the population attending a particular clinic or in a particular region. We have found that the Gail Model and risk models based wholly on family history (Claus, BRCAPRO) underpredict in our own familial risk population in the northwest of England (Table 10.1) [12]. Two models which combine family history, reproductive risk factors, and weight give a reasonably accurate prediction of risk. One is the Tyrer–Cuzick model, developed for risk prediction for entry into the International Breast Intervention Studies (IBIS). It asks for a three-generation family history and for information concerning lifestyle factors such as age of first pregnancy and body mass index (BMI). The second model is a modification of the Claus tables concerning family history to include lifestyle factors: this gives an accurate prediction of risk in our original report, and in a more recent, larger study with over 8000 women who developed over 400 breast tumours in the Manchester clinic [13].

Younger women with a family history of breast cancer are a population selected for a risk factor (Family history!). The distribution of risks in more than 10 000 women referred to our regional family history clinic are shown in Figure 10.1b based on estimates of family and lifestyle risk using the modification

Table 10.1 Comparison of the effectiveness of models to predict the breast cancers which occurred during follow up of 1900 women in the Genesis Breast Cancer Risk and Prevention Clinic in Manchester. Comparison is made of expected and observed cancers. (Gareth Evans personal communication).

	Observed (O)	Expected (E)	E/O	95% CI
Gail	64	44.3037	0.69	0.54 to 0.90
Claus	64	48.5565	0.76	0.59 to 0.99
Ford	64	42.2790	0.66	0.52 to 0.86
Tyrer–Cuzick	64	69.5653	1.09	0.85 to 1.41
Manual	64	77.9232	1.22	0.95 to 1.58

CI, confidence interval.

of the Claus model [13]. Most women were, as expected, at moderate or high risk as defined by the NICE criteria. Some were found on attendance and further estimation to be at lower risk and not followed further. The predominance of younger women is shown in Figure 10.1a, where only 15.2% of referrals were over the age of 50.

Moderate and high risk of breast cancer does not stop at the age of 50. Indeed, by far the majority of breast cancers are diagnosed in women over 50 years old. A major question is how to detect older women at higher risk as a result of a family history, but also those with lifestyle and other factors who may be at high risk even without a family history and have no knowledge of their risks. In order to approach this problem, we elected to determine risks of breast cancer in the context of the UK National Health Service Breast Screening Programme (NHSBSP), where women undergo mammography every three years between the ages of 50 and 70 (PROCAS Study: Prediction of Cancer at Screening [5]). Women are sent risk factor questionnaires before and consented at screening. In this context, it is also possible to assess the effect of mammographic density and single nucleotide polymorphisms (SNPs) in addition to the Tyrer–Cuzick model risk based on standard risk factors. Figure 10.2 shows the distribution of 10-year risks of breast cancer in a subgroup of women in the PROCAS study. Using the Tyrer–Cuzick model, about 10% of women were at moderate risk and a further 3% at high risk. Adding additional risk factors such as mammographic density and 18 risk SNPs tended to increase the numbers of women at high and low risk; with all risk factors included, about 12% of women were at moderate risk and about 6% at high risk. Interestingly, 94% of the over 58 000 women entered into the study wished to

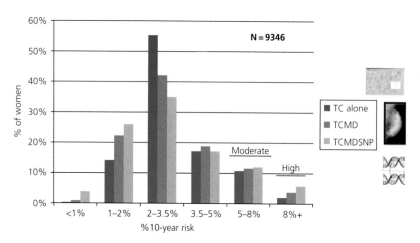

Figure 10.2 Distribution of 10-year breast cancer risks in the UK National Health Service Breast Screening Programme, determined using the Tyrer–Cuzick model and with the addition of visually assessed mammographic density (MD) and 18 single nucleotide polymorphisms (SNPs) related to risk of breast cancer.

know their risk of breast cancer. Thus the PROCAS study gives an indication of how risk factors might be collected and risk information given to older women.

Clinical breast cancer prevention

After explaining risk in the clinic, it is then important to decide on the most appropriate screening schedule and modality (in the UK, NICE guidelines indicate annual screening by mammography from 40–60 years of age) and to consider which preventive approaches may be suitable.

Preventive therapy (chemoprevention)

Currently tamoxifen is the only approved preventive therapy available for premenopausal women and is given for five years. In postmenopausal women, NICE guidelines indicate that five years' treatment with either tamoxifen 20 mg/day or raloxifene 60 mg/day may be considered [14]. Since the gynaecological toxicity of tamoxifen far outweighs the minimal gynaecological issues seen with raloxifene, tamoxifen is usually given to those who have had a prior hysterectomy and raloxifene to those with an intact uterus [15–17].

The effectiveness of tamoxifen has been assessed in four and raloxifene in two randomized placebo-controlled trials [14] (Figure 10.3). Five years of treatment with tamoxifen resulted in a 33% (hazard ratio [HR] 0.67; 95% confidence interval [CI] 0.59–0.76) reduction in breast cancer risk. For raloxifene, the MORE/CORE trial (the MORE trial was for four years and continued for a further four years in the CORE extension, so a total of eight years of treatment) resulted in an overall 66% (HR 0.34; 95% CI 0.22–0.50) reduction in risk [15] and the RUTH trial resulted in a 44% (HR 0.56; 95% CI 0.38–0.83) reduction in risk [16]. The STAR randomized trial directly compared the two selective oestrogen receptor modulators (SERMs). It demonstrated that raloxifene was less effective than tamoxifen after seven years of follow-up: the risk ratio (RR; raloxifene: tamoxifen) for invasive breast cancer was 1.24 (95% CI 1.05–1.47) and for noninvasive disease was 1.22 (95% CI 0.95–1.59) [17].

Since raloxifene is poorly absorbed (around 2%) and has a short half-life (27 hours), absolute compliance may be more important than with tamoxifen. It is possible that longer-term use of raloxifene is indicated [18]. In the extension CORE trial of raloxifene versus placebo use for an average treatment period of eight years, the reduction in risk was greater (HR 0.34) in the second four years (CORE) compared with that in the MORE trial over the first four years (HR 0.41) [15].

The tamoxifen trials were performed in women at increased risk, usually by virtue of a family history of breast cancer (with the exception of the Italian trial, where women were entered at any risk and many were at low risk because of an oophorectomy at a young age). The MORE/CORE trial was performed in women with osteoporosis thought to be at low risk of breast cancer because of low

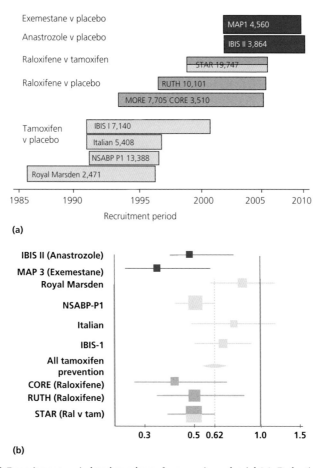

Figure 10.3 Recruitment period and numbers of women in each trial (a). Reduction in breast cancer risks (b). CORE, Continued Outcomes of Raloxifene; IBIS, International Breast Intervention Study; MAP3, Mammary Prevention 3; NSABP, National Surgical Adjuvant Breast Project; STAR, Study of Tamoxifen and Raloxifene.

oestrogen concentrations; however, the average Gail score was 1.9% higher than the 1.66% five-year risk criterion used in many studies and in the clinic [19]. The RUTH trial was performed in women at risk of or with cardiovascular disease; however, 40% of women entered had Gail risk scores of greater than 1.66% five-year risk. Thus most studies of preventive therapy have been performed in women at elevated risk and are largely relevant to women at increased risk detected in the general population.

When explaining the risk reduction to women at high and moderate risk of breast cancer, it seems reasonable to suggest an overall 40% reduction in breast cancer risk, and to indicate that raloxifene is somewhat less effective than tamoxifen. Compared with the NSABP P1 trial where the reduction of risk was 50%, the effects in both the IBIS I and Royal Marsden (RM) trials were lower. In both of these studies additional HRT was allowed in women who had severe hot flushes. In IBIS I (but not the RM trial), addition of HRT to tamoxifen resulted in abrogation of its effectiveness (HR 0.87 [95% CI 0.64–1.19] vs nonusers 0.55 [0.42–0.72]; p = 0·03) [20]. It is also important to give some indication of the duration of effect of SERMs. The long-term effect of five years of tamoxifen treatment was reported In the IBIS I trial. It showed risk reduction for invasive breast cancer of 29% for years 0–10 from randomization, which was similar to the reduction of 31% in the period beyond 10 years [20]. Risk reduction was greater in women entered because of a diagnosis of atypical ductal hyperplasia, with a 70% risk reduction in the NSABP P1 trial and 60% in the IBIS I trial [21]. Both tamoxifen and raloxifene maintain bone density and reduce cholesterol, although the latter has not been formally shown to be useful in terms of reduction of cardiovascular events [16].

Side effects of preventive therapy

It is clearly highly important to detail the expected toxicity of each drug to women at elevated risk deciding whether to have treatment or not. In premenopausal women, tamoxifen is the only available therapy. It is important to emphasize potential changes in menses, but also that, uncommonly, fibroids and ovarian cysts may enlarge, cause pain, and may result in the need for gynaecological interventions. Endometrial cancer is not induced by tamoxifen in premenopausal women. In postmenopausal women there is an increase in endometrial cancer. In the IBIS I trial, during the five-year treatment period, 4 of 3575 women in the controls and 15 of 3579 women in the treated women developed endometrial cancer, a 3.76-fold increase, but still an uncommon occurrence. Importantly, however, five women in the tamoxifen group died from endometrial cancer (four within the first 10 years), compared with none in the placebo group (p = 0.06). At other periods of follow-up (5–10 and over 10 years), there was no significant increase in endometrial cancer [20]. It therefore seems wise to avoid tamoxifen for breast cancer prevention in postmenopausal women with a uterus and to consider using raloxifene or an aromatase inhibitor instead. In the MORE trial there was no difference in the development of endometrial cancer between raloxifene and the control, and in the extension CORE trial there was a nonsignificant reduction in endometrial cancer [19]. The toxicity of raloxifene is different from tamoxifen, since with raloxifene there is an increase in ankle swelling and aches in the legs. Both drugs increase the risk of deep vein thrombosis and pulmonary embolism 2–3-fold. As yet tamoxifen has shown no significant effect on breast cancer–specific survival or death without a prior diagnosis of breast cancer. In IBIS 1 tamoxifen was associated with a nonsignificant and small increase in deaths (166 controls and 182 tamoxifen) [20]. However, it would be important to garner specific mortality risks in women aged under 50 years old, the main target for tamoxifen, where endometrial cancer risks are minimal and thrombo-embolic events less common. In the MORE trial there was a nonsignificant 37% reduction in deaths, and in the CORE trial a nonsignificant 23% reduction in deaths in women treated with raloxifene [19]. In the RUTH trial there was a nonsignificant reduction in deaths on raloxifene and a significant reduction in noncardiovascular, noncancer deaths [16].

Specially designed decision aids for each drug and for women at moderate and high risk should be used for women contemplating treatment [22, 23]. We encourage women to read the decision aid at home and to come back to the clinic if they wish to go ahead with treatment. Treatment may be initiated in secondary care and continued in primary care, since family physicians are wary of taking prime responsibility for treatment, partly because they do not feel they have been trained sufficiently, and some refuse to prescribe on the basis that, in the UK at least, neither drug is licensed for prevention, despite being endorsed for use by NICE [24]. In the USA, tamoxifen obtained Food and Drug Administration (FDA) approval for preventive use in 1998 and raloxifene in 2007. The equivalent body in the UK, the Medicines and Healthcare Products Regulatory Agency (MHRA), only accepts applications for a new licence from the pharmaceutical industry, which, in turn, is not interested in obtaining a licence for drugs it originally developed but are now off patent.

Other preventive agents
Other SERMs

The breast cancer preventive effectiveness of two other SERMs, lasofoxafine and arzoxafine, has been assessed in randomized controlled trials. Compared with placebo, 0.5 mg of lasofoxifene significantly reduced the risk of total breast cancer by 79% (HR 0.21; 95% CI 0.08–0.55), maintained bone density, and reduced the risk of coronary heart disease (CHD) events, regardless of the presence or absence of risk factors for cardiovascular disease (CVD). The spectrum of activity for lasofoxifene makes it an attractive preventive agent, but, at present, the manufacturer is not developing it further for prevention [25]. Arzoxifene prevents fractures and reduces the incidence of invasive breast cancer in postmenopausal women (56% relative reduction in risk; HR 0.44, 95% CI 0.26–0.76, p<.001), but is also not being developed further [26].

Aromatase inhibitors

Aromatase inhibitors (AIs) are superior to tamoxifen for preventing relapse and reducing the incidence of contralateral breast cancer after primary surgery for breast cancer [27]. Both exemestane and anastrozole have now been tested in randomized placebo-controlled trials in postmenopausal women at increased risk of breast cancer. Exemestane reduced relapse by 65% after a median follow-up of 36 months, and anastrozole reduced relapse by 50% after a median follow-up of 7 years [28, 29]. As expected, women taking AIs have more joint aches and flushes than controls and it also results in a reduction of bone density. The latter is prevented by the use of bisphosphonates [30]. In 2017 NICE guidelines have approved anastrazole to be offered as first line to post menopausal women at high risk. If they are prescribed, it is important to emphasize the bone toxicity and also an increase in rarer conditions, such as carpal tunnel syndrome and stroke. There was no reduction in deaths at this early stage, but interestingly a significant reduction in cancers overall, from 4% in the controls to 2% in women treated with anastrozole (HR 0.58, 95% CI 0.39–0.85) [29].

Antiprogestins

Antiprogestins may be useful for prevention, since animal data indicate that they inhibit the oestrogen/progesterone-induced increase in normal breast epithelial proliferation and carcinogenesis. In humans the antiprogestin mifepristone was shown to inhibit the progesterone-induced increase in proliferation seen in the luteal phase of the menstrual cycle [31]. Several new antiprogestins are becoming available and are entering early clinical trials for breast cancer prevention (e.g. Ullipristal acetate).

Bisphosphonates

Two cohort studies in women with osteoporosis have reported a 30% lower breast cancer incidence in users versus nonusers of bisphosphonates. Furthermore, these studies suggested that bisphosphonates may have a greater effect in oestrogen receptor–negative breast cancer. However, there was no significant reduction in another study [32]. Overall, bisphosphonates are well tolerated. Since they are used to prevent bone loss in women taking aromatase inhibitors, there is a need to determine whether the combination has a higher preventive effect than either drug alone.

Metformin

Metformin is widely used to treat type 2 diabetes and works by targeting the enzyme AMP-activated protein kinase (AMPK), which induces muscles to take up glucose from the blood. Cohort studies in women with type 2 diabetes have shown a possible reduced risk of breast cancer with metformin. Small preoperative biomarker studies indicate some reduction in proliferation indices in breast cancers. An adjuvant trial in breast cancer is currently in progress, and if positive may lead to prevention studies with the agent [32].

Aspirin

Aspirin has consistently been shown to be preventive in epidemiological and interventional studies for a number of cancers. Evidence from case-control and cohort studies indicates a reduction of breast cancer risk by about 10% for aspirin and possibly a little more for ibuprofen. Given the long-term effect of aspirin on cancer risk, further insight is best derived from a longer follow-up of current trials. Similar results have been found with other nonsteroidal anti-inflammatory drugs (NSAIDs) and COX-2 inhibitors.

Oestrogen receptor–negative tumours

Oestrogen receptor–negative tumours remain a challenge for prevention, and new targets will be needed to prevent these tumours. There is interest in the epidermal growth factor receptor (EGFR) family, including agents targeting HER2, such as trastuzumab and joint HER1/HER2 inhibitors, although these agents are too toxic for prevention. NSAIDs, COX-2 inhibitors, retinoids, rexinoids, and statins may have the capacity to protect against both receptor-positive and receptor-negative tumours. Similarly, agents such sulphoraphane, derived from cruciferous vegetables, and low-dose antibiotics also hold promise [32].

Uptake of preventive therapy

Since tamoxifen was accepted by the FDA in 1998, the uptake for breast cancer prevention in the USA has been variable. Uptake in other countries is not well described, possibly because of regulatory restrictions. In a study in Manchester of all premenopausal women at moderate or high risk of breast cancer attending for annual screening, there was an overall 10% uptake. It was highest (17%) in women at high non-*BRCA* risk and lowest in women with *BRCA1/2* mutations [23], suggesting a benefit of increasing risk until genetic determinism takes over. A review of uptake in most other studies is shown in Table 10.2. The lowest uptake (0.2%) was seen when women were contacted by letter by investigators who they did not know. The highest uptakes were seen in specialist risk clinics. In all health services there are difficulties in identifying women at moderate and increased risk outside of clinical trials. This is particularly so in postmenopausal women, since premenopausal women are referred to risk and prevention clinics. A better indication of uptake will come when most women at high and moderate risk are identified and offered chemoprevention in a systematic and sympathetic way, by specially trained clinicians and nurses and using appropriate decision aids.

Lifestyle change

The lifestyle factors which are potentially reversible include weight gain, lack of exercise, and excess alcohol consumption. An important consideration for lifestyle change and prevention of breast cancer is that the factors which enhance breast cancer risk also increase the risk of some other cancers, heart disease, diabetes, and dementia. Moreover, weight is linked to 12 other cancers, including endometrial, gall bladder, renal, rectal, postmenopausal breast, pancreatic, thyroid, colon, and oesophageal cancers, leukaemia, multiple myeloma, non-Hodgkin lymphoma, malignant melanoma [33], type 2 diabetes, and CVD. Sedentary lifestyle is also linked to colorectal and endometrial cancer, diabetes, CVD, and dementia [34], while alcohol is also linked to oral/pharyngeal, oesophageal (squamous), laryngeal, colorectal, liver, stomach, gall bladder, pancreas, and lung cancer [35]. Knowledge of the general disease-preventive effects of lifestyle change

Table **10.2** Comparison of the uptake of tamoxifen for chemoprevention in the Manchester study (Donnelly et al) with most other reported studies in the literature.

Non-trial, non-BRCA1/2		
Surgical practice—4 surgeons	2/47 (4.7)	Port *et al*, 2001
Post-biopsy. Referred to general practice	1/89 (1.1)	Taylor and Tagucbi, 2005
Referred to surgical service	57/137 (42.0)	Tchou *et al*, 2004
High-risk clinic	37/158 (29.0)	Bober *et al*, 2004
High-risk clinic	15/48 (31.0)	Layeequr Rahman and Crawford, 2009
High-risk clinic	136/1279 (10.6)	Donnelly *et al*—this study
Health-care systems	3/652 (0.5)	Fagerlin *et al*, 2010
Population (US) 2000	27/10 601 (0.25)	Waters *et al*, 2010
2005	8/10 690 (0.03)	Waters *et al*, 2010
2010	32/9 906 (0.32)	Waters *et al*, 2012
Non-trial, BRCA1/2		
International study	76/1135(5.5)	Metcalfe *et al*, 2008
Multicentre study (Canada)	17/270(6.0)	Metcalfe *et al*, 2007
High-risk clinic	7/170 (4.1)	Donrelly *et al*—this study
Trial recruitment		
IBIS-I	32/278 (11.5)	Elvans *et al*, 2001
IBIS-I	273/2278(12.0)	Elvans *et al*, 2010
STAR	35/158 (27.0)	Bober *et al*, 2004
STAR	19 747/91 325 (21.6)	McCaskill-Stevens *et al*, 2013
PI	13 954/57 641 (24.2)	Fisher *et al*, 2005

Abbreviations: IBIS-I=International Breast Cancer Intervention Study I; STAR=Study of Tamoxifen and Raloxifene.

may enhance uptake in women at elevated risk of breast cancer, but, since most women are at some degree of breast cancer risk, lifestyle change may be suggested for the whole population irrespective of degree of breast cancer risk.

Weight control

Most of the evidence that weight is related to breast cancer and that weight loss reduces breast cancer risk comes from observational studies. Weight gain of more than 20 kilos between the age of 18 to above 50 resulted in a doubling of breast cancer risk [36]. In the only large randomized trial performed by the Women's Health Initiative investigators, a comparison was made between reducing the fat content of the diet and not [37]. The diet was not designed to reduce weight, but there was a modest weight reduction overall of 3%, and there was a near significant 9% reduction in risk (risk ratio [RR] 0.91, 95% CI 0.83–1.01, p=.07) [37].

Two major observational studies suggest that sustained weight loss reduces the risk of postmenopausal breast cancer. Within the Iowa women's health study, maintained weight loss of over 5% after the menopause reduced risk by over 25% compared with women who continued to gain weight [38], while other studies reported a 60% reduction in risk with a greater than 15% weight loss [39]. However, the data on weight loss and reduction in breast cancer risk are not conclusive in all trials [40].

Because of the very large numbers of women required to perform a randomized trial of energy restriction, it seems reasonable to advocate weight control on the basis of the data available, and other data which indicate reduction in risk of diabetes and in cardiovascular risk markers.

Exercise

Objective measurements of physical activity in the 2008 Health Survey for England [41] indicate that only 4% of adult women are meeting current exercise guidelines of 150 minutes of moderate or 75 minutes of vigorous physical activity (PA) per week. The WCRF/AICR Expert Report [42] described the evidence for an inverse association between PA and breast cancer risk as 'probable' and 'limited – suggestive' for post- and premenopausal women, respectively. A review of 73 observational studies indicated that moderate to vigorous PA reduces breast cancer risk by an average of 25% in pre- and postmenopausal women compared with inactive women [43]. The strongest inverse associations with breast cancer risk were observed for recreational PA, lifetime PA, postmenopausal PA, and participation in moderate to vigorous PA. There was also evidence of dose–response relationships, with higher volumes of PA associated with greater risk reduction, but with the most pronounced reductions in risk being observed in lean versus obese women. The optimal level of PA for breast cancer risk reduction is unclear, however, and may be greater than the current recommendation of 150 minutes per week for general health. A major limitation of observational studies is the heterogeneity of self-report questionnaires that have been used to measure PA. The use of more objective measures, such as seven-day accelerometry, would provide more robust PA data. There is a clear need for randomized controlled trials which include clinical end-points or biomarkers on the causal pathway, but designing such trials is challenging because of the large sample size required and the expense of collecting long-term follow-up data.

Alcohol

It is estimated that breast cancer risk is increased by 7–10% for each additional 10 g (one-unit increase) in intake of alcohol per day (a unit is half a pint of 4% strength beer or cider, or 25 ml of 40% strength spirits, and only 80 ml of 12%

strength wine). Increased risk is thought to be related to acetaldehyde-induced DNA strand deletions, chromosomal aberrations and DNA adducts, downregulation of the tumour-suppressor gene *BRCA1*, and increased oestrogen and prolactin receptor activity. Data suggest that alcohol intake before first-term pregnancy is particularly associated with cumulative risk [44]. Unresolved questions include the specific effects of binge drinking, whether dietary folate intake can reduce excess risk of higher alcohol intake, and interactions with genes involved in alcohol metabolism/detoxification and folate metabolism [45]. Light drinking (10 g/day) is linked to breast cancer risk; however, zero alcohol intake is not recommended, as light drinking is consistently linked to reductions in overall (17%) [46] and cardiovascular (20%) mortality [47].

Lifestyle programmes for breast cancer risk reduction
The question then becomes how a lifestyle programme might be applied to the general population of pre- and postmenopausal women or high-risk women. Behaviour change is difficult to achieve and maintain. Successful lifestyle disease prevention programmes, for example the Diabetes Prevention Programme [48], have been labour intensive and involved around 40 hours of health-care professional contact per patient, and are therefore not feasible within the health service. Further research is required on ways to engage women to join and adhere to lifestyle behaviour change programmes. It is clear that there is great difficulty in applying weight control in primary care [49]. The time of breast screening is a potentially teachable moment, but there is currently little direct evidence to support this assertion [50].

Lifestyle change may be possible among women at increased breast cancer risk referred to risk and prevention clinics. Qualitative work in our unit, however, suggests that breast cancer risk is not a primary driver for weight control in this group of women. Key motivators for weight loss were often more immediate concerns of appearance, well-being, and self-esteem [51]. Another approach is to advise weight control in the context of national breast screening programmes, since approximately 70% of women aged 47–73 years attend for screening.

Risk-reducing surgery

Risk-reducing mastectomy (RRM) reduces the risk of breast cancer by 90–95% with a skin-sparing mastectomy approach [52, 53]. This appears to be equally effective in *BRCA1/2* mutation carriers. NICE guidelines recommend discussion of RRM with women at high risk (30% + lifetime risk) of breast cancer. Uptake varies, from as little as 1.8–2.5% in the lowest category of the high-risk group compared to an uptake of over 50% by seven years after positive testing for *BRCA1/2* in a study in northwest England [54]. However, uptake is very variable across Europe and North America, with very low uptake in Southern Europe and Poland [55]. Although risk-reducing oophorectomy prior to the natural menopause has been associated with around a 50% reduction in breast cancer risk in *BRCA1/2* mutation carriers [56], there is now some doubt about the degree of short-term risk reduction once adequate left censoring of data is carried out [57]. Risk-reducing surgery has nonetheless been associated with an overall reduction in mortality of *BRCA1/2* carriers unaffected at the time of ascertainment [58].

Conclusion

This chapter gives a brief guide to the current status of breast cancer prevention, with a major focus in the UK and the work from the Manchester Clinic. It indicates that there is considerable work to be done before all at-risk women can be offered preventive therapy, and *all* middle-aged and older women who are overweight or obese and who do not take regular exercise also have help to make lifestyle changes. In addition, it is important to broadcast the message concerning the breast cancer risks of excess alcohol.

A major problem is implementation of what we know could work. Currently most preventive efforts are understandably focused on the present referral pattern from primary care, which is predominantly younger women with a family history of breast cancer. This leaves the majority of women at risk over 50 without access, partly because of the mistaken belief that family history applies only to risk in young women; partly because of the understandable lack of knowledge of risk estimation and the impact of lifestyle risk factors on breast cancer risk by both women and their doctors; and finally because of new developments in understanding of other risk factors such as mammographic density and SNPs, which are only just being introduced to enhance risk prediction above that provided by family history and lifestyle factors. We argue that if we can deliver preventive options, this should have a marked effect on the overall prevention of breast cancer.

References

1 Howell, A., Anderson, A.S., Clarke, R.B. et al. (2014). Risk determination and prevention of breast cancer. *Breast Cancer Res.* 16 (5): 446.
2 Pruthi, S., Heisey, R.E., and Beyers, T.B. (2015). Chemoprevention for breast cancer. *Ann. Surg. Oncol.* 22: 3230–3235.
3 Evans, D.G., Cuzick, J., and Howell, A. (1996). Cancer genetics clinics. *Eur. J. Cancer* 32A (3): 391–392.
4 Easton, D.F., Pharoah, P.D., Antoniou, A.C. et al. (2015). Gene-panel sequencing and the prediction of breast-cancer risk. *N. Engl. J. Med.* 372 (23): 2243–2257.
5 Evans, D.G., Brentnall, A.R., Harvie, M. et al. (2014). Breast cancer risk in young women in the national breast screening programme: Implications for applying NICE guidelines for additional screening and chemoprevention. *Cancer Prev. Res.* 7 (10): 993–1001.
6 Collaborative Group on Hormonal Factors in Breast Cancer (2002). Breast cancer and breast-feeding: Collaborative reanalysis of individual data from 47 epidemiological studies in

30 countries, including 50302 women with breast cancer and 96973 women without the disease. *Lancet* 360 (9328): 187–195.

7 Tryggvadottir, L., Sigvaldason, H., Olafsdottir, G.H. et al. (2006). Population-based study of changing breast cancer risk in Icelandic BRCA2 mutation carriers, 1920–2000. *J. Natl Cancer Inst.* 98 (2): 116–122.

8 National Collaborating Centre for Cancer (2013). Classification and Care of People at Risk of Familial Breast Cancer and Management of Breast Cancer and Related Risks in People with a Family History of Breast Cancer. *NICE Clinical Guidelines*, No. 164.

9 Visvanathan, K., Hurley, P., Bantug, E. et al. (2013). Use of pharmacologic interventions for breast cancer risk reduction: American Society of Clinical Oncology clinical practice guideline. *J. Clin. Oncol.* 31 (23): 2942–2962.

10 Freedman, A.N., Yu, B., Gail, M.H. et al. (2011). Benefit/risk assessment for breast cancer chemoprevention with raloxifene or tamoxifen for women age 50 years or older. *J. Clin. Oncol.* 29: 2327–2333.

11 Moyer, V.A. (2013). Medications to decrease the risk for breast cancer in women: Recommendations from the U.S. Preventive Services Task Force recommendation statement. *Ann. Intern. Med.* 159: 698–708.

12 Amir, E., Evans, D.G., Shenton, A. et al. (2003). Evaluation of breast cancer risk assessment packages in the family history evaluation and screening programme. *J. Med. Genet.* 40 (11): 807–814.

13 Evans, D.G., Ingham, S., Dawe, S. et al. (2014). Breast cancer risk assessment in 8,824 women attending a family history evaluation and screening programme. *Fam. Cancer* 13 (2): 189–196.

14 Cuzick, J., Sestak, I., Bonanni, B. et al.; SERM Chemoprevention of Breast Cancer Overview Group (2013). Selective oestrogen receptor modulators in prevention of breast cancer: An updated meta-analysis of individual participant data. *Lancet* 381 (9880): 1827–1834.

15 Martino, S., Cauley, J.A., Barrett-Connor, E. et al.; CORE Investigators (2004). Continuing outcomes relevant to Evista: Breast cancer incidence in postmenopausal osteoporotic women in a randomized trial of raloxifene. *J. Natl Cancer Inst.* 96 (23): 1751–1761.

16 Barrett-Connor, E., Mosca, L., Collins, P. et al.; Raloxifene Use for The Heart (RUTH) Trial Investigators (2006). Effects of raloxifene on cardiovascular events and breast cancer in postmenopausal women. *N. Engl. J. Med.* 355 (2): 125–137.

17 Vogel, V.G. (2009). The NSABP Study of Tamoxifen and Raloxifene (STAR) trial. *Expert Rev. Anticancer Ther.* 9 (1): 51–60.

18 Maximov, P.Y., Lee, T.M., and Jordan, V.C. (2013). The discovery and development of selective estrogen receptor modulators (SERMs) for clinical practice. *Curr. Clin. Pharmacol.* 8 (2): 135–155.

19 Recker, R.R., Mitlak, B.H., Ni, X., and Krege, J.H. (2011). Long-term raloxifene for postmenopausal osteoporosis. *Curr. Med. Res. Opin.* 27 (9): 1755–1761.

20 Cuzick, J., Sestak, I., Cawthorn, S. et al.; IBIS-I Investigators (2015). Tamoxifen for prevention of breast cancer: Extended long-term follow-up of the IBIS-I breast cancer prevention trial. *Lancet Oncol.* 16 (1): 67–75.

21 Cuzick, J., Sestak, I., and Thorat, M.A. (2015). Impact of preventive therapy on the risk of breast cancer among women with benign breast disease. *Breast* 24 (Suppl. 2): S51–S55.

22 Juraskova, I., Butow, P., Bonner, C. et al. (2014). Improving decision making about clinical trial participation: A randomised controlled trial of a decision aid for women considering participation in the IBIS-II breast cancer prevention trial. *Br. J. Cancer* 111 (1): 1–7.

23 Donnelly, L.S., Evans, D.G., Wiseman, J. et al. (2014). Uptake of tamoxifen in consecutive premenopausal women under surveillance in a high-risk breast cancer clinic. *Br. J. Cancer* 110 (7): 1681–1687.

24 Kaplan, C.P., Haas, J.S., Perez-Stable, E.J. et al. (2005). Factors affecting breast cancer risk reduction practices among California physicians. *Prev. Med.* 41: 7–15.

25 Ensrud, K., LaCroix, A., Thompson, J.R. et al. (2010). Lasofoxifene and cardiovascular events in postmenopausal women with osteoporosis: Five-year results from the Postmenopausal Evaluation and Risk Reduction with Lasofoxifene (PEARL) trial. *Circulation* 122 (17): 1716–1724.

26 Cummings, S.R., McClung, M., Reginster, J.Y. et al. (2011). Arzoxifene for prevention of fractures and invasive breast cancer in postmenopausal women. *J. Bone Miner. Res.* 26 (2): 397–404.

27 Early Breast Cancer Trialists' Collaborative Group (EBCTCG); Dowsett, M., Forbes, J.F., Bradley, R. et al. (2015). Aromatase inhibitors versus tamoxifen in early breast cancer: Patient-level meta-analysis of the randomised trials. *Lancet* 386 (10001): 1341–1352.

28 Goss, P.E., Ingle, J.N., Alés-Martínez, J.E. et al.; NCIC CTG MAP.3 Study Investigators (2011). Exemestane for breast-cancer prevention in postmenopausal women. *N. Engl. J. Med.* 364 (25): 2381–2391.

29 Cuzick, J., Sestak, I., Forbes, J.F. et al.; IBIS-II investigators (2014). Anastrozole for prevention of breast cancer in high-risk postmenopausal women (IBIS-II): An international, double-blind, randomised placebo-controlled trial. *Lancet* 383 (9922): 1041–1048.

30 Sestak, I., Singh, S., Cuzick, J. et al. (2014). Changes in bone mineral density at 3 years in postmenopausal women receiving anastrozole and risedronate in the IBIS-II bone sub-study: An international, double-blind, randomised, placebo-controlled trial. *Lancet Oncol.* 15 (13): 1460–1468.

31 Engman, M., Skoog, L., Söderqvist, G., and Gemzell-Danielsson, K. (2008). The effect of mifepristone on breast cell proliferation in premenopausal women evaluated through fine needle aspiration cytology. *Hum. Reprod.* 23 (9): 2072–2079.

32 Sestak, I., and Cuzick, J. (2015). Update on breast cancer risk prediction and prevention. *Curr. Opin. Obstet. Gynecol.* 27 (1): 92–97.

33 Renehan, A.G., Tyson, M., Egger, M. et al. (2008). Body-mass index and incidence of cancer: A systematic review and meta-analysis of prospective observational studies. *Lancet* 371 (9612): 569–578.

34 Liu, L., Shi, Y., Li, T. et al. (2015). Leisure time physical activity and cancer risk: Evaluation of the WHO's recommendation based on 126 high-quality epidemiological studies. *Br. J. Sports Med.* 50 (6): 372–378.

35 Bagnardi, V., Rota, M., Botteri, E. et al. (2015). Alcohol consumption and site-specific cancer risk: A comprehensive dose-response meta-analysis. *Br. J. Cancer* 112 (3): 580–593.

36 Huang, Z., Hankinson, S.E., Colditz, G.A. et al. (1997). Dual effects of weight and weight gain on breast cancer risk. *JAMA* 278: 1407–1411.

37 Prentice, R.L., Caan, B., Chlebowski, R.T. et al. (2006). Low-fat dietary pattern and risk of invasive breast cancer: The Women's Health Initiative. Randomized Controlled Dietary Modification Trial. *JAMA* 295: 629–642.

38 Harvie, M., Howell, A., Vierkant, R.A. et al. (2005). Association of gain and loss of weight before and after menopause with risk of post-menopausal breast cancer in the Iowa women's health study. *Cancer Epidemiol. Biomarkers Prev.* 14: 656–661.

39 Eliassen, A.H., Colditz, G.A., Rosner, B. et al. (2006). Adult weight change and risk of post-menopausal breast cancer. *JAMA* 296: 193–201.

40 Teras, L.R., Goodman, M., Patel, A.V. et al. (2011). Weight loss and postmenopausal breast cancer in a prospective cohort of overweight and obese US women. *Cancer Causes Control* 22 (4): 573–579.

41 Health and Social Care Information Centre (2012). Health Survey for England. http://www.hscic.gov.uk/catalogue/PUB13218 (accessed 3 January 2018).

42 Hastert, T.A., Beresford, S.A., Patterson, R.E. et al. (2013). Adherence to WCRF/AICR cancer prevention recommendations and risk of post-menopausal breast cancer. *Cancer Epidemiol. Biomarkers Prev.* 22: 1498–1508.

43 Lynch, B.M., Neilson, H.K., and Friedenreich, C.M. (2011). Physical activity and breast cancer prevention. *Recent Results Cancer Res.* 186: 13–42.

44 Scoccianti, C., Lauby-Secretan, B., Bello, P.Y. et al. (2014). Female breast cancer and alcohol consumption: A review of the literature. *Am. J. Prev. Med.* 46 (3, Suppl. 1): S16–S25.

45 Chen, P., Li, C., Li, X. et al. (2014). Higher dietary folate intake reduces the breast cancer risk: A systematic review and meta-analysis. *Br. J. Cancer* 110 (9): 2327–2338.

46 Di, C.A., Costanzo, S., Bagnardi, V. et al. (2006). Alcohol dosing and total mortality in men and women: An updated meta-analysis of 34 prospective studies. *Arch. Intern. Med.* 166 (22): 2437–2445.

47 Ronksley, P.E., Brien, S.E., Turner, B.J. et al. (2011). Association of alcohol consumption with selected cardiovascular disease outcomes: A systematic review and meta-analysis. *BMJ* 342: d671.

48 Knowler, W.C., Fowler, S.E., Hamman, R.F. et al. (2009). 10-year follow-up of diabetes incidence and weight loss in the Diabetes Prevention Program Outcomes Study. *Lancet* 374 (9702): 1677–1686.

49 Hartmann-Boyce, J., Johns, D.J., Jebb, S.A. et al.; Behavioural Weight Management Review Group (2014). Behavioural weight management programmes for adults assessed by trials conducted in everyday contexts: Systematic review and meta-analysis. *Obes. Rev.* 15 (11): 920–932.

50 Anderson, A.S., Mackison, D., Boath, C., and Steele, R. (2013). Promoting changes in diet and physical activity in breast and colorectal cancer screening settings: An unexplored opportunity for endorsing healthy behaviors. *Cancer Prev. Res.* 6 (3): 165–172.

51 Wright, C.E., Harvie, M., Howell, A. et al. (2015). Beliefs about weight and breast cancer: An interview study with high risk women following a 12 month weight loss intervention. *Hered. Cancer Clin. Pract.* 13 (1): 1.

52 Evans, D.G., Baildam, A.D., Anderson, E. et al. (2009). Risk reducing mastectomy: Outcomes in 10 European Centres. *J. Med. Genet.* 46 (4): 254–258.

53 Hartmann, L.C., Schaid, D.J., Woods, J.E. et al. (1999). Efficacy of bilateral prophylactic mastectomy in women with a family history of breast cancer. *N. Engl. J. Med.* 340 (2): 77–84.

54 Evans, D.G., Lalloo, F., Ashcroft, L. et al. (2009). Uptake of risk reducing surgery in unaffected women at high risk of breast and ovarian cancer is risk, age and time dependent. *Cancer Epid. Biomarkers Prev.* 18 (8): 2318–2324.

55 Metcalfe, K.A., Birenbaum-Carmeli, D., Lubinski, J. et al.; Hereditary Breast Cancer Clinical Study Group (2008). International variation in rates of uptake of preventive options in BRCA1 and BRCA2 mutation carriers. *Int. J. Cancer* 122 (9): 2017–2022.

56 Rebbeck, T.R., Kauff, N.D., and Domchek, S.M. (2009). Meta-analysis of risk reduction estimates associated with risk-reducing salpingo-oophorectomy in BRCA1 or BRCA2 mutation carriers. *J. Natl Cancer Inst.* 101 (2): 80–87.

57 Heemskerk-Gerritsen, B.A., Seynaeve, C., van Asperen, C.J. et al.; Hereditary Breast and Ovarian Cancer Research Group Netherlands (2015). Breast cancer risk after salpingo-oophorectomy in healthy BRCA1/2 mutation carriers: Revisiting the evidence for risk reduction. *J. Natl Cancer Inst.* 107 (5): djv033.

58 Ingham, S.L., Sperrin, M., Baildam, A. et al. (2013). Risk-reducing surgery increases survival in BRCA1/2 mutation carriers unaffected at time of family referral. *Breast Cancer Res. Treat.* 142 (3): 611–618.

CHAPTER 11

Breast cancer: Population and targeted screening

Fiona J. Gilbert[1], Fleur Kilburn-Toppin[1], Valérie D.V. Sankatsing[2], and Harry J de Koning[2]

[1] University of Cambridge, School of Clinical Medicine; University Hospitals NHS Foundation Trust, Addenbrooke's Hospital, Cambridge, UK
[2] Department of Public Health, Erasmus Medical Centre, Rotterdam, The Netherlands

---

SUMMARY BOX

- Meta-analyses of the randomized controlled trials of mammography screening show a reduction in breast cancer mortality of approximately 20% in women invited to screening. A benefit of mammography screening is supported by numerous observational studies.

- The evidence for the benefit of screening below age 50 and above age 70 is less conclusive than the evidence for the benefit of screening between ages 50 and 69.

- There are considerable similarities between organized screening programmes in Europe with respect to the minimum target age range (50–69) and the screening interval (biennial).

- Coverage by invitation and participation rates differ substantially between European screening programmes.

- Digital breast tomosynthesis with either 2D or synthetic mammography has increased sensitivity (2–27%) and improved specificity (11–15%) when used in screening.

- Magnetic resonance imaging remains the most sensitive technique for the detection of breast cancer, particularly in younger women (under 50 years) and in women with dense breasts.

Evidence for the benefit of breast cancer screening

Randomized controlled trials

Randomized controlled trials (RCTs) are generally believed to provide the most accurate evidence for the efficacy of mammography screening, in terms of breast cancer mortality reduction. Nine RCTs of mammography screening have been

---

conducted, of which seven were population based (New York health insurance plan [HIP], Malmö Mammographic Screening Trial, Swedish Two County, Stockholm, Göteborg, Edinburgh, and UK Age trial), meaning that personal invitations were sent to women based on registry data. The other two trials were volunteer based (Canadian National Breast Screening Study-1 and -2), meaning that no formal invitations based on registries were used. The trials were consistent in comparing women randomized to be invited to mammography screening with women randomized to the control arm who were not invited to mammography screening, and in using breast cancer mortality as the end-point. There are, however, considerable differences between the trials with regard to (among others) the targeted age group, the screening interval, the follow-up period, the number of screening rounds, compliance, and the type of randomization. The Canadian trial for women aged 50–59 (Canadian National Breast Screening Study-2) included annual physical examination by trained nurses in the control arm, which has been shown to be effective in causing a stage shift and probably in reducing breast cancer mortality [1]. This trial thereby differed from the other mammography screening trials without any form of screening in the control arm.

Several meta-analyses of the RCTs of breast cancer have been conducted. The Cochrane collaboration published an update of its systematic review on mammography screening in 2013, in which the results of a fixed-effect meta-analysis were reported [2]. The Edinburgh trial was excluded from the analysis because of inadequate randomization, leading to incomparable groups with regard to socio-economic status. After 13 years of follow-up, the combined risk ratio (RR) estimate for the seven trials was 0.81 (95% CI 0.74–0.87), corresponding to a 19% reduction of breast cancer mortality, for women invited to screening compared to women not invited to screening aged 40–74 at entry.

The independent UK Panel on Breast Cancer Screening conducted a meta-analysis, again excluding the Edinburgh trial, including 13 years of follow-up and using a random-effects analysis [3]. The combined RR was estimated to be 0.80 (95% CI 0.73–0.89), corresponding to a breast cancer mortality relative risk reduction of 20% (95% CI 11–27%).

In the meta-analysis of the US Preventive Task Force, a RR of 0.85 (95% CI 0.75–0.96) was estimated for women aged 39–49, a RR of 0.86 (95% CI 0.75–0.99) for women aged 50–59, and a RR of 0.68 (95% CI 0.54–0.87) for women aged 60–69 at entry [4].

The RCTs of mammography screening were conducted in the 1970s and 1980s. The value and relevance of these RCTs today have been questioned with respect to improvements in imaging techniques, the screening process, and breast cancer treatment since the start of the trials. Another issue is that the results of the trials are based on the comparison of breast cancer mortality rates in invited women (including those who attend and those who do not attend screening) to a control group, rather than breast cancer mortality rates in women who actually attend screening. Thus, the overall concern addresses the applicability of the estimated RR reduction in breast cancer mortality from the trials to existing screening programmes.

Observational studies

In addition to the trials, numerous observational studies have been conducted to estimate the effectiveness of screening on breast cancer mortality.

Cohort studies estimate the effect of invitation to screening or the effect of attending screening. Breast cancer mortality reduction estimates from cohort studies for women screened between age 50 and 69 range from circa 15% to 40% [5–10].

Case-control studies estimate the effect of actual exposure to screening. A meta-analysis of recently conducted case-control studies found a combined odds ratio (OR) for breast cancer mortality of 0.52 (95% CI 0.42–0.65) in screened versus unscreened women aged 50 and older, after adjustment for self-selection [11]. The combined OR for invited versus uninvited women was 0.69 (95% CI 0.57–0.83), which is not substantially different from the results of the meta-analyses of the RCTs.

Observational studies are more prone to bias than RCTs, and adequate control of these biases by design or analysis is difficult. In the majority of case-control studies, a greater breast cancer mortality reduction associated with screening is reported than in the RCTs. However, adjustment of the combined RR estimate of the RCTs for lack of compliance and the presence of contamination of the control group with screening resulted in a risk estimate that approaches the combined risk estimate of the case-control studies. Demissie et al. [12] concluded that use of case-control studies to evaluate the effect of screening, if conduction of an RCT is not feasible (any longer), is appropriate.

Evidence for the benefit of screening women under age 50

The impact of screening on breast cancer mortality may be different for women aged 40–49 because of several factors associated with younger age, including a lower breast cancer incidence, a lower sensitivity of mammography due to greater breast density, and possibly more aggressive tumour growth. Meta-analyses of the results of the RCTs, in which women aged 40–49 at entry were included, report a statistically significant breast cancer mortality reduction of 15–17% [4,13]. However, methodologically these analyses are flawed by an age creep; that is, the benefit of screening, observed in the group of women aged 40–49 at randomization, may be (partially) attributable to early detection of breast cancer by screening these women at age 50 and older.

The largest (Swedish) cohort study on women aged 40–49 years that compared breast cancer mortality between women invited and not invited to screening showed an RR estimate of 0.74 (95% CI 0.66–0.83) for women invited to screening [14]. The RR for women attending screening was 0.71 (95% CI 0.62–0.80).

Evidence for the benefit of screening women above age 70

The only trial that invited women over 70 years of age was the Swedish Two County trial. Women aged 70–74 at entry were invited for two screening rounds. There was no statistically significant effect found in the evaluation of the trial for women aged 70–74 at entry in Kopparberg (RR 0.76, 95% CI 0.44–1.33) [15]. Participation rates in women aged 70–74 were reported to be relatively low.

Otto et al. [16] conducted a case-control study to assess the effectiveness of population-based screening in the Netherlands. The OR for the association between the risk of breast cancer death and attending either of three screenings prior to breast cancer diagnosis, for women aged 70–75 years, was 0.16 (95% CI 0.09–0.29).

Balance of benefits and harms

Whether mammography screening is justifiable and whether the benefits of screening (breast cancer mortality reduction) outweigh the harms associated with screening (e.g. false-positive findings and overdiagnosis) have been debated frequently, despite the evidence from the RCTs. First, the benefit of mammography screening, in terms of breast cancer mortality reduction, has been questioned.

Second, questions regarding the magnitude of the harms of screening have been raised. Overdiagnosis, screen detection of a cancer that would never have presented clinically during a woman's lifetime (in the absence of screening), is often considered the most adverse outcome of breast cancer mammography screening. The absolute number of overdiagnosed cases reflects the excess of cancers diagnosed in women who are invited to screening (or attend screening), relative to women who are not invited to screening (or do not attend screening). As an overdiagnosed cancer is detected only in the presence of screening, treatment of an overdiagnosed cancer will not improve disease prognosis and life expectancy, and is therefore considered to be harmful.

Overdiagnosis can be assessed from the RCTs; however, in order to estimate the extent of overdiagnosis adequately, sufficiently long follow-up is crucial. If follow-up is not sufficient, some of the cancers that would have appeared later in the control group are not taken into account, and the number of excess cancers only detected because of screening (excess cancers in the intervention group relative to the control group after x years of follow-up) is overestimated. The level of overdiagnosis may differ between trials because of differences in screening interval, the age group enrolled, and possible contamination of the control group with screening. Furthermore, many different denominators (perspectives) are used for the calculation of overdiagnosis rates from the trials or from observational data, resulting in a wide range of overdiagnosis estimates [17]. De Gelder et al. [17] compared seven different methods to estimate the magnitude of overdiagnosis, and concluded that estimated overdiagnosis rates varied by a factor of 3.5, using these different measures. According to the independent UK panel, there is no single best perspective with regard to calculating overdiagnosis rates, but an adequate calculation should take into account ductal carcinoma *in situ* (DCIS) [3]. The panel argues that the best data from which to estimate overdiagnosis rates are obtained from RCTs in which the control group was not invited for screening at the end of the trial, as screening of the control group after the end of an RCT will most likely also result in overdiagnosis (and therefore in an underestimation of overdiagnosis in the intervention group). The panel concluded that in three of the RCTs, the control group was certainly not invited for screening at the end of the trial [3,18–20]. Analysis of the data from these trials combined resulted in an estimated overdiagnosis rate (excess cancers as a proportion of cancers diagnosed) for women invited to screening of around 11% during their lifetime and approximately 19% during the screening period. The panel stated that data obtained from the three RCTs are limited in size, and the estimate of overdiagnosis is therefore surrounded with more uncertainty than the estimate of breast cancer mortality reduction.

Overdiagnosis can also be estimated from observational studies. As discussed earlier, observational studies are subject to biases associated with the comparability between the screened and unscreened (or invited and noninvited) groups. These biases will also affect estimates of the extent of overdiagnosis. Estimates of overdiagnosis from observational studies, conducted in European countries, vary widely; however, adjusting for both underlying risk of breast cancer and lead-time reduces the range of estimates to 1–10% [21].

The ideal follow-up time to assess overdiagnosis is from the time screening ceases until death. For obvious reasons, this is not feasible in practice. However, life-long follow-up can be simulated via a mathematical model. Using the Dutch MISCAN model, the overdiagnosis rate (expressed as the excess cancers as a proportion of all predicted cancers in a situation without screening) was estimated to be 2.8% in women aged 0–100, five years after screening was fully implemented [17]. The overdiagnosis rate was considerably higher during the implementation period of the screening programme (11.4%), which illustrates that sufficiently long follow-up is essential.

Implementation of mammography screening in different countries

Organized screening programmes

In many countries, breast cancer screening is conducted routinely through an organized screening programme. Organized screening requires a clear policy with respect to the target age categories, the screening interval, and the screening method [22]. Between organized screening programmes in Europe, there is large consistency regarding these policy aspects on a minimum age range of 50–69 years to invite, a screening interval of two years, the use of mammography as the screening method, and double reading [23]. The agreement on the age range of 50–69 stems from the results of the RCTs, as this age group was targeted in most of the trials and the evidence for the benefit of screening was most clear in this group. In the trials that conducted screening at three-year intervals, higher interval cancer rates were present [22]. Despite this evidence, women are screened once every three years in the UK and Malta (Table 11.1).

Coverage by invitation and participation rates are highly variable between European organized screening programmes. Giordano et al. [23] report that coverage by invitation varies from 50.9% to full coverage, and participation rate from 19.4% to 88.9%. Half of the European screening programmes had a participation rate that was higher than 70%, which is considered the acceptable level of participation in the European Union (EU) Guidelines. Eleven European organized screening programmes have reported maximum recall rates, ranging from 1% (the Netherlands) to 7% (UK) for subsequent screening rounds [22]. Differences in the discussed aspects between screening programmes may cause variations in the effectiveness of the programmes. The aspects of screening policies in European countries are summarized in Table 11.1. Women under age 50 years are invited in twelve European screening programmes, and five of these programmes invite women from age 40.

In Canada, organized breast cancer screening programmes are present in all provinces. These programmes all invite women in the age range 50–69; however, some programmes offer screening to a wider age range [25]. A recently published study of breast cancer mortality among participants in seven Canadian breast cancer screening programmes, using an incidence-based mortality approach, reported that the average breast cancer mortality rate was 40% lower (95% CI 33–48%) among participants, relative to expected mortality based on rates in nonparticipants [26]. The target age range varied between the different programmes, with a maximum age range of 40–79 years (annual screening 40–49, biennial screening 50+). Average breast cancer mortality reduction was only moderately influenced by age at entry into the screening programme (range 35–44%).

In Australia, the upper age limit of screening is currently extended from age 69 to 74 years, based on international recommendations for BreastScreen Australia [27]. Although the organized screening programme in Australia is targeted specifically at women aged 50–74, women from age 40 and women aged 75 and older are allowed to attend screening.

Opportunistic screening

Screening conducted outside of a screening programme is referred to as opportunistic screening. In countries in which the health-care system is supported by the government, opportunistic screening does occur, but is relatively rare [22]. On the

Table 11.1 Characteristics of breast cancer screening programmes in the European Union.

Country	Start age (years)	Stop age (years)	Interval (years)	Attendance (%)	Primary test
Austria	40	–	2	57	Mammography
Belgium	50	69	2	61	Mammography
Bulgaria	45	69	–	NA	Mammography
Croatia	50	69	2	63	Mammography
Cyprus	50	69	2	56	Mammography
Czech Republic	45	69	2	70	Mammography
Denmark	50	69	2	73	Mammography
Estonia	50	65	2	51	Mammography
Finland	50	69	2	85	Mammography
France	50	74	2	52	Mammography
Germany	50	69	2	54	Mammography
Greece	40	50/64	2	NA	Mammography
Hungary	45	65	2	54	Mammography
Ireland	50	64	2	78	Mammography
Italy	45/50	69/74	2	69	Mammography
Latvia	50	69	2	37	Mammography
Lithuania	50	69	2	NA	Mammography
Luxembourg	50	69	2	64	Mammography
Malta	50	59	3	55	Mammography
Netherlands	50	74	2	80	Mammography
Poland	50	69	2	39	Mammography
Portugal	45	69	2	63	Mammography
Romania	40	–	1	14	Mammography
Slovakia	40	–	2	NA	Mammography
Slovenia	50	69	2	76	Mammography
Spain	45/50	64/69	2	67	Mammography
Sweden	40	74	2	70	Mammography
UK	47	70	3	73	Mammography

Attendance (%) represents the proportion of the target population that has been screened; NA, data not available.
Source: Altobelli 2014 [24].

contrary, opportunistic screening is the most common form of breast cancer screening in the USA, where screening is usually conducted on recommendation of a physician. In the absence of a national screening programme, there is no national standard regarding screening aspects in the USA; however, recommendations with respect to the target age categories and screening interval are provided by the US Preventive Services Task Force (USPSTF) and the American Cancer Society. These recommendations are updated regularly. In 2009, the USPSTF recommended biennial screening for women aged 50–74 [28]. With respect to screening before age 50, it stated: 'The decision to start regular, biennial screening mammography before the age of 50 years should be an individual one and take patient context into account, including the patient's values regarding specific benefits and harms.' The USPSTF decided that the additional benefits and harms of screening women aged 75 or older were not clear due to lack of evidence for this age group.

Individualized screening

In most countries, organized screening programmes invite all women in a specific age group (often 50–69 years), regardless of their risk for breast cancer. A woman's individual risk for breast cancer, dependent on the presence or absence of risk factors (e.g. breast density, family history of breast cancer), may be of influence on the balance between benefits and harms associated with screening. An alternative to offering one screening strategy to all women is a risk-based approach, in which the aspects of a screening strategy, including the target age range, the screening interval, and possibly the screening method, are adjusted to different risk groups. In Italy, a tailored breast screening trial is conducted in which women aged 45–49 at entry in the intervention group are offered a screening strategy based on their breast density [29].

Apart from risk factors for breast cancers, comorbid conditions may also affect the balance of benefits and harms of screening. A recently published collaborative modelling study (including breast, prostate, and colorectal cancer screening) reported that comorbid conditions negatively affect the balance of benefits and harms, and suggested that screening of individuals with (severe) comorbid conditions should stop earlier than screening of average-health individuals to maintain a similar balance [30].

New technologies in breast cancer screening

Digital breast tomosynthesis

Digital breast tomosynthesis (DBT) is a three-dimensional (3D) imaging modality in which tomographic images of the breast are reconstructed from multiple low-dose projection images acquired by moving the X-ray tube over a limited angular range. This range varies by manufacturer, but the exposure used for each projection image is relatively small, so that the overall mean glandular dose for DBT is comparable to that of conventional two-dimensional (2D) imaging. The tomosynthesis projection images are processed by reconstruction algorithms to produce a pseudo-3D tomographic image of the breast, typically with a 1 mm slice thickness. Conventional 2D images are usually acquired at the same time, and readers are able to scroll vertically through the tomographic images as well as compare them with corresponding 2D images. The image quality of DBT is highly dependent on system geometry and the choice of optimal image acquisition, reconstruction, and display parameters [31–33].

DBT has the potential to overcome the primary limitation of standard 2D mammography that arises from overlapping fibroglandular breast tissue, improving diagnostic accuracy by differentiating benign and malignant features, and increasing lesion conspicuity, particularly in dense breasts. Several publications, primarily from USA-based studies, have reported superiority of full-field digital mammography (FFDM) plus DBT (combo imaging) compared to 2D alone in terms of increased sensitivity and specificity and in reader performance [34–38], but variations in study methodology and the use of DBT systems with different technical configurations have resulted in conflicting results [39–41].

More rigorous evaluation of DBT in large-scale prospective trials and optimization of the performance of DBT in terms of image acquisition, reconstruction with synthetic 2D images, and the development of CAD algorithms have shown promising results. The Oslo Tomosynthesis Screening Trial reported a 27% increase in cancer detection rate across all breast densities, and a 15% decrease in false-positive recall rate using DBT in combination with 2D mammography compared with 2D mammography alone [42]. The population-based STORM screening study comparing sequential 2D reading and combined DBT and 2D reading reported a 34% increase in cancer detection across all age groups and breast densities, and the potential to reduce the false-positive recall rate by 17% [43]. Reading time doubled, however. The Malmö breast tomosynthesis screening trial is conducting a paired analysis of the sensitivity and specificity of DBT compared with 2D in a population-based screening programme in Sweden. Preliminary results indicated a 15% increase in sensitivity with DBT compared to 2D mammography, but with a slight (3%) increase in recall rates [44]. A large, US retrospective study by Friedewald et al. [45], comparing performance measures before and after the introduction of DBT + 2D screening, reported a 29% increase in cancer detection rate. Results from the TOMMY trial, a large, retrospective reading study, show a modest 2% improvement in cancer detection rate for DBT + 2D compared with 2D alone, but a clear improvement of 11% in specificity [46,47].

Observers have suggested that DBT is unlikely to be used as a stand-alone imaging modality, as a 2D mammogram is required for optimal microcalcification assessment [31,48,49]. However, the use of DBT in combination with 2D requires an approximate doubling of radiation exposure. It is possible to generate a synthetic 2D image from a single DBT scan [50]. The accuracy of

DBT + synthetic 2D is currently being evaluated within the OSLO trial [51] and this, together with results comparing DBT + synthetic 2D with DBT + 2D and 2D alone due to be published from the TOMMY trial [46,47] and results from a recent study by Zuley et al. [52], demonstrate that synthetic images are of acceptable diagnostic quality, and that conventional 2D exposure can be potentially eliminated.

Automated whole-breast ultrasound

Although mammography is the only imaging modality to have proven to decrease breast cancer mortality in screening the general population, one of its limitations lies in the imaging of the 40% of women classified as having 'dense breasts'. Women with dense breast tissue have a 4–6-fold increased risk of breast cancer, partly due to independent risk factors for breast cancer, but also due to the decreased sensitivity of mammography in this cohort of women. With the advent of the 'Are You Dense' campaign in the USA requiring radiologists to inform women of their breast density and suggest alternative screening options, there has been even further interest in developing screening methods to address this particular issue. Magnetic resonance imaging (MRI) has been recommended as a screening tool for women with dense breasts, but it has its drawbacks in terms of cost, accessibility, and contra-indications for certain patients.

Many studies have demonstrated that ultrasound is a good screening tool for women with dense breast tissue, and is appealing due to its accessibility, relative low cost, patient tolerance, and lack of ionizing radiation. Berg et al. [53] demonstrated that 55% more cancers were detected in women with dense breasts using hand-held ultrasound and mammography than mammography alone. However, there are drawbacks to using hand-held ultrasound as a screening tool, namely the radiologist time required to perform the examination, significant operator dependence, and relatively low positive predictive value. A recent technological advance which aims to address some of these issues is automated whole-breast ultrasound (ABUS). Various types of equipment are currently available, with ultrasound performed mechanically to eliminate operator dependence. In some systems a large transducer panel is placed over the breast with gentle compression, allowing the whole breast to be imaged in the same time it takes to perform a whole-breast ultrasound using the hand-held method. Images can be stored and reviewed by a radiologist at any time, with the added benefit of reconstructing the raw data into 3D images. The coronal view unique to ABUS has been suggested to be particularly good for detecting areas of distortion, which are often associated with malignancy [54]. The wide field of view also allows multiple masses and large lesions to be displayed in a single view.

Multiple studies have demonstrated equal or greater lesion detectability with ABUS than with hand-held imaging [55]. Kelly et al. [56] demonstrated that ABUS increased the cancer detection rate from 3.8 per 1000 with mammography alone to 7.2 per 1000 using both modalities. The many benefits of automated scanning include the ability to produce consistent reproducible images which do not require significant radiologist time to acquire. However, limitations to the technique include radiologist time taken to review images, and the concern regarding false positives and high recall rates. Nevertheless, this may improve with increasing radiologist experience, and with prior imaging to compare to rather than just with a single baseline scan in most current studies. Other limiting factors include lack of ability to examine the axilla, and inability to perform colour Doppler and elastography. Even so, the increasing requirements for better imaging in women with high-density breasts mean that ABUS is likely to evolve into a useful adjunct to mammography in widespread screening.

Contrast-enhanced digital mammography

The introduction of digital mammography has led to the ability to develop new technological advances in breast imaging. Contrast-enhanced digital mammography (CEDM) is based on a similar principle to MRI, utilizing the fact that leaky basement membranes in vessels in malignancy make tissues more permeable to contrast material that is injected intravenously, and results in tumour enhancement. Despite its proven value in allowing earlier detection of malignancy, particularly in women with dense breasts, MRI has numerous drawbacks, including cost and availability, which has led to investigation into the potential uses of CEDM.

Two main techniques are available, temporal CEM and spectral or dual-energy CEM (CESM), both of which require the injection of approximately 1.5 ml/kg of iodine-based contrast medium. In the temporal technique, the breast is compressed initially while a nonenhanced masked image is taken prior to contrast injection with compression, and a series of post-contrast images are obtained over a period of three to five minutes. The noncontrast image is then subtracted from the contrast image. Although only a few small studies have been performed using this method, the results are promising. Diekmann et al. [57] demonstrated that this method improved the sensitivity of cancer detection, particularly in women with dense breasts. However, the limitations to this method are that motion artefact can prove problematic, particularly due to the period of time the women is required to be imaged, and also only one breast can be imaged at a time [58].

Contrast-enhanced spectral imaging obtains high- and low-energy images after the administration of intra-venous (IV) contrast. A standard mammographic image as well as a high-energy image containing information on lesion enhancement are obtained, and these can be added together to eliminate background breast parenchyma and demonstrate areas of contrast enhancement within the breast. Studies by Dromain [59] demonstrated that CESM has higher sensitivity than conventional mammography (93% vs 78%), with no loss of specificity. CESM has also been compared with MRI [60,61], demonstrating equally accurate breast cancer detection rates with MRI and CESM as well as good lesion size agreement, but with fewer false positives for CESM, which are an issue in screening.

The drawbacks to CESM include higher radiation dose (54% greater than standard mammography at 2.65 mGy) [62], as well as the use of IV contrast medium and the time taken to perform the examination. Other factors include the enhancement of benign lesions such as fibroadenomas and radial scars, which require biopsy confirmation, and that temporal enhancement curves have not proven as accurate as MRI temporal curves. There is also the issue of not currently being able to perform biopsy with this method. These factors may limit its use as a screening tool; however, given the ability of CEDM to combine anatomical and physiological characteristics and its high diagnostic accuracy even in lower-prevalence groups [63], it is likely to be used in imaging women referred from screening or as an alternative to MRI screening in higher-risk groups.

MRI

MRI has demonstrated superior sensitivity to both mammography and ultrasound in the detection of breast cancer, and is now routinely used for multiple indications, including the screening of women at high risk of breast cancer. Its use in more widespread screening has been limited by a number of factors, namely prolonged imaging time, cost, availability, and false-positive rates [64]. Kuhl et al. [65] have proposed an abbreviated MRI protocol to overcome some of these problems. This consists of a 3D maximum-intensity projection (MIP) image and a first post-contrast T1-weighted image (FAST), disposing of further sequences that are mostly used for lesion characterization. These authors demonstrate that in a cohort of asymptomatic women with intermediate to slightly high rate of breast cancer risk with negative mammographic imaging, MIP analysis alone has a sensitivity and negative predictive value of 98.9%, which can be increased to 100% with the associated FAST images. Moreover, 61% of studies were negative on MIP images which can be read in less than 3 seconds, with the additional use of FAST imaging on the remainder making the reading time still less than 30 seconds, comparable with mammographic reading time. Combined with the lack of radiation and high sensitivity, this rapid MRI protocol makes for promising advances in the use of MRI in more widespread screening [66]. With regard to false positives, all screening trials so far have used the same protocol as for diagnostic imaging, and the number may diminish with increased radiologist training. Currently there is only indirect evidence that screening with MRI may affect survival, and further prospective multicentre trials are required to see if abbreviated MRI imaging may be successfully used as a screening modality.

Breath testing

Molecular biomarkers are being increasingly investigated for the detection of early malignancy. Breath analysis is an appealing potential screening method, being noninvasive and relatively easy to use. Exhaled human breath contains a large number of volatile organic compounds (VOC), some of which are produced endogenously from the body's metabolism and may be detected by various methods, including gas chromatography and mass spectrometry. It is proposed that due to increased oxidative stress caused by malignancy, alkanes and alkane derivatives are produced by reactive oxygen species (ROS), causing lipid peroxidation of cell membranes. The detection of VOCs in exhaled human breath is already used in a clinical setting for the detection of *Helicobacter pylori* ($^{13}CO_2$) and asthma (nitric oxide). Numerous potential biomarkers for the detection of breast cancer have been proposed [67] and have shown promising results in the detection of malignancy [68], but these are not necessarily specific for breast malignancy in particular, and only relatively small patient studies have been performed as yet. Larger, standardized trials are required to see if this method could be used as a potential adjunct to screening mammography.

Conclusion

There is clear evidence of benefit from undertaking screening in women between 50–69 years of age with some evidence of benefit from 40–49 and from 70–74 years of age. The mortality reduction is estimated to be around 20%. The risk of an over diagnosis in a women attending screening is between 11–20% although some groups have given higher estimates using different methodologies. There is increasing recognition that screening with mammography is less effective in women with dense breasts and alternative techniques such as Digital Breast Tomosynthesis, Contrast Enhanced Mammography, Fast Magnetic Resonance Imaging or supplementary whole breast ultrasound are all being investigated. Policy makers should consider the evidence from these trials and explore the feasibility of a more risk stratified approach.

References

1 Rijnsburger, A.J., van Oortmarssen, G.J., Boer, R. et al. (2004). Mammography benefit in the Canadian National Breast Screening Study-2: A model evaluation. *Int. J. Cancer* 110 (5): 756–762.

2 Gotzsche, P.C., and Jorgensen, K.J. (2013). Screening for breast cancer with mammography. *Cochrane Database Syst. Rev.* 6 (Art. No.: CD001877). doi: 10.1002/14651858.CD001877.pub5.

3 Marmot, M.G., Altman, D.G., Cameron, D.A. et al. (2013). The benefits and harms of breast cancer screening: An independent review. *Br. J. Cancer* 108 (11): 2205–2240.

4 Nelson, H.D., Tyne, K., Naik, A. et al. (2009). Screening for breast cancer: An update for the U.S. Preventive Services Task Force. *Ann. Intern. Med.* 151 (10): 727–37, W237–W242.

5 Moss, S.M.; UK Trial of Early Detection of Breast Cancer Group (1999). 16-year mortality from breast cancer in the UK Trial of Early Detection of Breast Cancer. *Lancet* 353 (9168): 1909–1914.

6 Olsen, A.H., Njor, S.H., Vejborg, I. et al. (2005). Breast cancer mortality in Copenhagen after introduction of mammography screening: Cohort study. *BMJ* 330 (7485): 220.

7 Sarkeala, T., Heinavaara, S., and Anttila, A. (2008). Organised mammography screening reduces breast cancer mortality: A cohort study from Finland. *Int. J. Cancer* 122 (3): 614–619.

8 Kalager, M., Zelen, M., Langmark, F., and Adami, H.O. (2010). Effect of screening mammography on breast-cancer mortality in Norway. *N. Engl. J. Med.* 363 (13): 1203–1210.

9 Hofvind, S., Ursin, G., Tretli, S. et al. (2013). Breast cancer mortality in participants of the Norwegian Breast Cancer Screening Program. *Cancer* 119 (17): 3106–3112.

10 Weedon-Fekjaer, H., Romundstad, P.R., and Vatten, L.J. (2014). Modern mammography screening and breast cancer mortality: Population study. *BMJ* 348: g3701.

11 Broeders, M., Moss, S., Nystrom, L. et al. (2012). The impact of mammographic screening on breast cancer mortality in Europe: A review of observational studies. *J. Med. Screen.* 19 (Suppl. 1): 14–25.

12 Demissie, K., Mills, O.F., and Rhoads, G.G. (1998). Empirical comparison of the results of randomized controlled trials and case-control studies in evaluating the effectiveness of screening mammography. *J. Clin. Epidemiol.* 51 (2): 81–91.

13 Magnus, M.C., Ping, M., Shen, M.M. et al. (2011). Effectiveness of mammography screening in reducing breast cancer mortality in women aged 39-49 years: A meta-analysis. *J. Womens Health* 20 (6): 845–852.

14 Hellquist, B.N., Duffy, S.W., Abdsaleh, S. et al. (2011). Effectiveness of population-based service screening with mammography for women ages 40 to 49 years: Evaluation of the Swedish Mammography Screening in Young Women (SCRY) cohort. *Cancer* 117 (4): 714–722.

15 Tabar, L., Vitak, B., Chen, H.H. et al. (2000). The Swedish Two-County Trial twenty years later: Updated mortality results and new insights from long-term follow-up. *Radiol. Clin. North Am.* 38 (4): 625–651.

16 Otto, S.J., Fracheboud, J., Verbeek, A.L. et al. (2012). Mammography screening and risk of breast cancer death: A population-based case-control study. *Cancer Epidemiol. Biomarkers Prev.* 21 (1): 66–73.

17 de Gelder, R., Heijnsdijk, E.A., van Ravesteyn, N.T. et al. (2011). Interpreting overdiagnosis estimates in population-based mammography screening. *Epidemiol. Rev.* 33 (1): 111–121.

18 Miller, A.B., To, T., Baines, C.J., and Wall, C. (2000). Canadian National Breast Screening Study-2: 13-year results of a randomized trial in women aged 50–59 years. *J. Natl Cancer Inst.* 92 (18): 1490–1499.

19 Miller, A.B., To, T., Baines, C.J., and Wall, C. (2002). The Canadian National Breast Screening Study-1: Breast cancer mortality after 11 to 16 years of follow-up. A randomized screening trial of mammography in women age 40 to 49 years. *Ann. Intern. Med.* 137 (5, Part 1): 305–312.

20 Zackrisson, S., Andersson, I., Janzon, L. et al. (2006). Rate of over-diagnosis of breast cancer 15 years after end of Malmo mammographic screening trial: Follow-up study. *BMJ* 332 (7543): 689–692.

21 Puliti, D., Duffy, S.W., Miccinesi, G. et al. (2012). Overdiagnosis in mammographic screening for breast cancer in Europe: A literature review. *J. Med. Screen.* 19 (Suppl. 1): 42–56.

22 International Agency for Research on Cancer (2002). Volume 7: Breast cancer screening. In: *IARC Handbooks of Cancer Prevention* (ed. H. Vainio and F. Bianchini). Lyon: IARC Press.

23 Giordano, L., von Karsa, L., Tomatis, M. et al. (2012). Mammographic screening programmes in Europe: Organization, coverage and participation. *J. Med. Screen.* 19 (Suppl. 1): 72–82.

24 Altobelli, E., and Lattanzi, A. (2014). Breast cancer in European Union: An update of screening programmes as of March 2014. *Int. J. Oncol.* 45 (5): 1785–1792.

25 Canadian Partnership against Cancer (2013). Organized Breast Cancer Screening Programs in Canada: Report on Program Performance in 2007 and 2008. https://content.cancerview.ca/download/cv/prevention_and_screening/screening_and_early_diagnosis/documents/organizedbreastcancerpdf?attachment=0 (accessed 3 January 2018).

26 Coldman, A., Phillips, N., Wilson, C. et al. (2014). Pan-Canadian study of mammography screening and mortality from breast cancer. *J. Natl Cancer Inst.* 106 (11): dju261.

27 BreastScreen Australia Program (n.d.). http://www.cancerscreening.gov.au/internet/screening/publishing.nsf/Content/breast-screening-1 (accessed 20 October 2014).

28 Force USPST (2009). Screening for breast cancer: U.S. Preventive Services Task Force recommendation statement. *Ann. Intern. Med.* 151 (10): 716–726, W236.

29 Paci, E., Mantellini, P., Giorgi Rossi, P. et al. (2013). Tailored Breast Screening Trial (TBST). *Epidemiol. Prev.* 37 (4–5): 317–327.

30 Lansdorp-Vogelaar, I., Gulati, R., Mariotto, A.B. et al. (2014). Personalizing age of cancer screening cessation based on comorbid conditions: Model estimates of harms and benefits. *Ann. Intern. Med.* 161 (2): 104–112.

31 Dobbins, J.T., III (2009). Tomosynthesis imaging: At a translational crossroads. *Med. Phys.* 36: 1956–1967.

32 Sechopoulos, I. (2013). A review of breast tomosynthesis. Part I. The image acquisition process. *Med. Phys.* 40: 014301.

33 Sechopoulos, I. (2013). A review of breast tomosynthesis. Part II. Image reconstruction, processing and analysis, and advanced applications. *Med. Phys.* 40: 014302.

34 Gur, D., Abrams, G.S., Chough, D.M. et al. (2009). Digital breast tomosynthesis: Observer performance study. *Am. J. Roentgenol.* 193: 586–591.

35 Rafferty, E.A., Park, J.M., Philpotts, L.E. et al. (2013). Assessing radiologist performance using combined digital mammography and breast tomosynthesis compared with digital mammography alone: Results of a multicenter, multireader trial. *Radiology* 266: 104–113.

36 Skaane, P., Bandos, A.I., Gullien, R. et al. (2013). Comparison of digital mammography alone and digital mammography plus tomosynthesis in a population-based screening program. *Radiology* 267: 47–56.

37 Haas, B., Kalra, V., Geisel, J. et al. (2013). Comparison of tomosynthesis plus digital mammography and digital alone for breast cancer screening. *Radiology* 269: 694–700.

38 Rose, S.L., Tidwell, A.L., Bujnoch, L.J. et al. (2013). Implementation of breast tomosynthesis in a routine screening practice: An observational study. *Am. J. Roentgenol.* 200: 1401–1408.

39 Alakhras, M., Bourne, R., Rickard, M. et al. (2013). Digital tomosynthesis: A new future for breast imaging? *Clin. Radiol.* 68: 225–236.

40 Houssami, N., and Skaane, P. (2013). Overview of the evidence on digital breast tomosynthesis in breast cancer detection. *Breast* 22: 101–108.

41 Screening Section, Department of Health and Ageing (2013). Digital breast tomosynthesis: Overview of the evidence and issues for its use in screening for breast cancer. Australia: Commonwealth of Australia.

42 Skaane, P., Bandos, A.I., Gullien, R. et al. Comparison of digital mammography alone and digital mammography plus tomosynthesis in a population-based screening program. *Radiology* 267: 47–56.

43 Ciatto, S., Houssami, N., Bernardi, D. et al. (2013). Integration of 3D digital mammography with tomosynthesis for population breast-cancer screening (STORM): A prospective comparison study. *Lancet Oncol.* 14: 583–589.

44 Malmö Breast Tomosynthesis Screening Trial (MBTST) (2010). https://clinicaltrials.gov/ct2/show/NCT01091545 (accessed 10 February 2015).

45 Friedewald, S.M., Rafferty, E.A., Rose, S.L. et al. (2014). Breast cancer screening using tomosynthesis in combination with digital mammography. *JAMA* 311 (24): 2499–2507.

46 Gilbert, F.J., Tucker, L., Gillan, M.G.C. et al. (2015). The accuracy of digital breast tomosynthesis in detecting breast cancer subgroups in a UK retrospective reading study (TOMMY Trial). *Radiology* 277 (3): 697–706.

47 Gilbert, F.J., Tucker, L., Gillan, M.G.C. et al. (2015). TOMMY trial: A comparison of TOMosynthesis with digital MammographY in the UK NHS Breast Screening Programme. *Health Technol. Assess.* 19 (4): i–xxv, 1–136.

48 Das, M., Gifford, H.C., O'Connor, J.M., and Glick, S.J. (2009). Evaluation of a variable dose acquisition technique for microcalcification and mass detection in digital breast tomosynthesis. *Med. Phys.* 36: 1976–1984.

49 Nishikawa, R.M., Reiser, I., and Seifi, P. (2007). A new approach to digital breast tomosynthesis for breast cancer screening. *Proc. SPIE Medical Imaging* 6510: 65103C-65108.

50 Gur, D., Zuley, M.L., Anello, M.I. et al. (2012). Dose reduction in digital breast tomosynthesis (DBT) screening using synthetically reconstructed projection images: An observer performance study. *Acad. Radiol.* 19: 166–171.

51 Skaane, P., Bandos, A.I., Eben, E.B. et al. (2014). Two-view digital breast tomosynthesis screening with synthetically reconstructed projection images: Comparison with digital breast tomosynthesis with full-field digital mammographic images. *Radiology* 271 (3): 655–663.

52 Zuley, M.L., Guo, B., Catullo, U.J. et al. (2014). Comparison of two dimensional synthesised mammograms versus original digital mammograms alone and in combination with tomosynthesis images. *Radiology* 271 (3): 664–671

53 Berg, W.A., Blume, J.D., Cormack, J.B. et al. (2008). Combined screening with ultrasound and mammography vs mammography alone in women at elevated risk of breast cancer. *JAMA* 299 (18): 2151–2163.

54 Kaplan, S.S. (2014). Automated whole breast ultrasound. *Radiol. Clin. North Am.* 52 (3): 539–546.

55 Lin, X., Wang, J., Han, F. et al. (2012). Analysis of eighty-one cases with breast lesions using automated breast volume scanner and comparison with handheld ultrasound. *Eur. J. Radiol.* 81 (5): 873–878.

56 Kelly, K.M., Dean, J., Comulada, W.S., and Lee, S.J. (2010). Breast cancer detection using automated whole breast ultrasound and mammography in radiographically dense breasts. *Eur. Radiol.* 20 (3): 734–742.

57 Diekmann, F., Freyer, M., Diekmann, S. et al. (2011). Evaluation of contrast-enhanced digital mammography. *Eur. J. Radiol.* 78: 112–121.

58 Jochelson, M. (2014). Contrast-enhanced digital mammography. *Radiol. Clin. North Am.* 52 (3): 609–616.

59 Dromain, C., Thibault, F., Muller, S. et al. (2011). Dual-energy contrast-enhanced digital mammography: Initial clinical results. *Eur. Radiol.* 21 (3): 565–574.

60 Fallenberg, E.M., Dromain, C., Diekmann, F. et al. (2014). Contrast-enhanced spectral mammography versus MRI: Initial results in the detection of breast cancer and assessment of tumour size. *Eur. Radiol.* 24 (1): 256–264.

61 Jochelson, M.S., Dershaw, D.D., Sung, J. et al. (2013). Bilateral contrast-enhanced dual energy mammography: Feasibility and comparison with conventional digital mammography and MR imaging in women with known breast carcinoma. *Radiology* 266 (3): 743–751.

62 Badr, S., Laurent, N., Régis, C. et al. (2014). Dual-energy contrast-enhanced digital mammography in routine clinical practice in 2013. *Diagn. Interv. Imaging* 95 (3): 245–258.

63 Lobbes, M.B., Lalji, U., Houwers, J. et al. (2014). Contrast-enhanced spectral mammography in patients referred from the breast cancer screening programme. *Eur. Radiol.* 24 (7): 1668–1676.

64 Mahoney, M.C., and Newell, M.S. (2013). Screening MR imaging versus screening ultrasound: Pros and cons. *Magn. Reson. Imaging Clin. N. Am.* 21 (3): 495–508.

65 Kuhl, C.K., Schrading, S., Strobel, K. et al. (2014). Abbreviated breast magnetic resonance imaging (MRI): First postcontrast subtracted images and maximum-intensity projection – a novel approach to breast cancer screening with MRI. *J. Clin. Oncol.* 32 (22): 2304–2310.

66 Morris, E.A. (2014). Rethinking breast cancer screening: Ultra FAST breast magnetic resonance imaging. *J. Clin. Oncol.* 32 (22): 2281–2283.

67 Li, J., Peng, Y., and Duan, Y. (2013). Diagnosis of breast cancer based on breath analysis: An emerging method. *Crit. Rev. Oncol. Hematol.* 87 (1): 28–40.

68 Phillips, M., Beatty, J.D., Cataneo, R.N. et al. (2014). Rapid point-of-care breath test for biomarkers of breast cancer and abnormal mammograms. *PLoS One* 9 (3): e90226.

CHAPTER 12

Prostate cancer prevention

Evan Kovac[1], Andrew J. Stephenson[1], Margaret G. House[2], Eric A. Klein[1], and Howard L. Parnes[2]

[1]Glickman Urological and Kidney Institute, Cleveland Clinic, Cleveland, OH, USA
[2]National Cancer Institute, Rockville, MD, USA

SUMMARY BOX

- Prostate cancer is a prevalent disease among men over the age of 50. The risk of developing, living with, and having treatment for the disease can be a major source of anxiety and/or morbidity to the patient and of significant cost to the health-care system. Primary prevention of prostate cancer, therefore, would seem to be an attractive option to many men.

- To date, several randomized, placebo-controlled trials have been completed with the aim of finding the ideal combination of an effective preventive therapy with minimal side effects.

- Two recently completed trials evaluating the 5-ARIs exhibited promising results. PCPT and REDUCE both showed an approximate 25% reduction in prostate cancer in two different risk populations. While both trials reported an increased risk of high-grade cancer, subsequent analyses suggest that the increased risk is likely explained, at least in part, by detection bias introduced by the 5-ARIs. Both 5-ARIs now carry a black-box warning stating that their use could cause aggressive prostate cancer. This warning has likely caused primary care physicians and urologists to shy away from prescribing these agents, and deterred their use for chemoprevention.

- Vitamins and minerals such as vitamin E and selenium showed promise as prostate cancer primary prevention agents, based on secondary analyses of cancer prevention trials conducted in the mid-1990s. Unfortunately, when subjected to rigorous evaluation through randomized, double-blind, placebo-controlled trials, the theorized benefit was lost, and it was even shown that vitamin E increases the risk of prostate cancer when taken alone.

- While the ideal prostate cancer primary prevention strategy has not yet been elucidated, ongoing evaluation of approved and novel agents continues.

Cancer Prevention and Screening: Concepts, Principles and Controversies, First Edition.
Edited by Rosalind A. Eeles, Christine D. Berg, and Jeffrey S. Tobias.
© 2019 John Wiley & Sons, Inc. Published 2019 by John Wiley & Sons, Inc.

Prostate cancer is the most prevalent noncutaneous malignancy among men, accounting for 43% of all diagnosed cancers [1]. An estimated 1 in 7 men will be diagnosed with prostate cancer in their lifetime, while approximately 1 in 38 will die from the disease [2]. Following the introduction of prostate-specific antigen (PSA) testing in the 1980s, the incidence of prostate cancer increased dramatically, and continues to rise in many countries [3]. An estimated 220 800 cases of prostate cancer will be diagnosed in the USA in 2015 [2], with a mean age at diagnosis of 66 years [2]. Once diagnosed, treatment strategies vary widely, depending on patient factors, physician practices, and their respective preferences.

Management of prostate cancer can be expectant, as exemplified by a watchful waiting strategy, or aggressive, as in radical prostatectomy or radiation therapy. In recent years, active surveillance has been favoured over watchful waiting as an expectant management strategy for men with a life expectancy of 10 or more years [4]. A diagnosis of prostate cancer may be the source of considerable anxiety to the patient and his family irrespective of prognosis and proposed management, and represents a substantial cost to the health-care system. Preventing the disease altogether is a preferable route. This chapter will endeavour to provide an evidence-based summary with regard to prevention of prostate cancer, with a focus on chemoprevention.

Rationale for prostate cancer prevention

Given its high prevalence, long natural history, and the nonmodifiable nature of the major risk factors, prostate cancer is an obvious choice as a target for prevention. The disease and its treatment are associated with substantial morbidity, including urinary obstruction and bleeding from locally advanced prostate cancer; urinary incontinence, erectile dysfunction, and radiation proctitis from definitive local therapy; and bone pain from metastatic disease. In addition, the process of prostate carcinogenesis often begins 20–30 years before the appearance of cancer [5], thus providing a window for intervention before clinically important cancer develops. Accordingly, the prevention of prostate cancer has garnered much attention over the last two decades. The goal of any prevention strategy is to reduce the incidence of a given cancer, thus reducing both disease and treatment-related morbidity and mortality, as well as alleviating the cost burden on the health-care system. An ideal prevention strategy would employ lifestyle modifications or pharmacological or natural agents to inhibit, delay, or reverse the process of carcinogenesis [6], reserving interventions with the greatest potential for toxicity for those at highest risk for developing the disease.

Risk factors

Age, race, and genetics are the most important prostate cancer risk factors. Among all cancers, prostate cancer exhibits the greatest age-risk increase among men in the seventh decade [7]. In the USA, black men of African ancestry have a 1.58

relative risk of developing prostate cancer and a 2.44 relative risk of dying of the disease [8]. Men with a first-degree relative with prostate cancer are at a 2.48 times greater risk of developing the disease than a man with a negative family history [9].

While one's age, race, or genetic predisposition to develop prostate cancer cannot be altered, several modifiable risk factors have been linked to the development of the disease. The chemoprevention trials (to be discussed later) allowed for secondary analyses due to their large patient cohorts. As a result of these Phase 3 studies, the roles of several environmental prostate cancer risk factors have been clarified.

Chronic inflammation of the prostate

A link has been established between men with chronic inflammatory conditions of the urinary tract, such as frequent urinary tract infections (UTIs) and chronic prostatitis, and a slight increased risk of prostate cancer [10,11], although other researchers argue that the association between inflammation and prostate cancer risk is mainly theoretical [12]. Several organisms have been implicated in this association, with the main suspects being human papillomavirus, cytomegalovirus, and *Trichomonas vaginalis* (*T. vaginalis*) [11,13]. The common denominator among men with frequent UTIs, chronic prostatitis, and prostate cancer may be chronic inflammation of the prostate, leading to a pro-neoplastic environment. Furthermore, despite reporting an insignificant overall prostate cancer risk increase, the Physicians' Health Study showed a statistically significant association between *T. vaginalis* seropositivity and aggressive prostate cancer phenotypes [14]. Yet four post-hoc studies from the Prostate Cancer Prevention Trial (PCPT) demonstrated null associations between human herpesvirus type 8 (HHV-8), cytomegalovirus (CMV), human papillomavirus (HPV) types 16, 18, and 31, and *T. vaginalis* and prostate cancer risk (15–18). Currently, the role of chronic inflammatory conditions of the prostate, such as frequent UTIs or chronic prostatitis, and the development of prostate cancer is incompletely defined and warrants more research. Presently, a cause-and-effect relationship between chronic prostatic inflammation and prostate cancer has not been proven, and currently represents an association only. Epidemiological and clinical studies performed to date have not lent strong support for anti-inflammatory agents such as aspirin [19], celecoxib [20], and sulindac sulfone (B.J. Nelson, personal communication, 2006) for prostate cancer prevention. Thus, prostate cancer preventive strategies that target patients with recurrent prostatic inflammatory and infectious processes have yet to be defined.

Smoking

As opposed to urothelial carcinoma, where smoking exhibits a major carcinogenic effect, its role in the development of prostate cancer is less clear. Epidemiological studies have shown a modest increased risk of prostate cancer among smokers, especially in non-Hispanic white men [21]. However, correlations between duration and intensity of smoking and prostate cancer risk have yet to be established.

Retrospective studies have also suggested an association between smoking and prostate cancer outcomes. The most recent data, a retrospective analysis of 7191 men with known smoking status treated with radical prostatectomy (RP), showed a twofold increase in biochemical recurrence among both current smokers and former smokers who had quit within 10 years of surgery. However, these data are not adjusted for preoperative and postoperative stage and grade [22]. In another analysis of 1450 prostate cancer patients, current smokers had a statistically significant, 2.5-fold increase in metastases (the primary study end-point), but not in biochemical recurrence, after adjustments for pre- and postoperative pathological features [23]. In a retrospective cohort study of 1416 RP patients, a statistically significant, 2.3-fold increased risk of combined PSA and clinical recurrence, independent of stage and grade, was observed among men still smoking one year after surgery. Notably, recurrence rates were not significantly increased among men who reported smoking five years before, or who had quit within one year of RP [24]. Although these data are not entirely consistent, the emerging evidence supports a role for smoking cessation to reduce prostate cancer recurrence among men undergoing potentially curative therapy.

Obesity

Previous epidemiological reports have described an increased risk of aggressive prostate cancer in obese men [25]. An analysis of PCPT showed an increased risk of high-grade (HG) prostate cancer, and an inverse risk of low-grade (LG) prostate cancer, in men with a body mass index (BMI) over 30 [26]. Recently, a secondary analysis of patients who were enrolled in the Reduction by Dutasteride of Prostate Cancer Events (REDUCE) trial confirmed the findings of PCPT [27]. Thus, multiple retrospective epidemiological analyses have found a link between obesity and the development of HG prostate cancer. Avoiding or reversing obesity, although difficult for many people, may be an effective way of reducing the risk of HG disease.

Chemoprevention

The ideal chemopreventive agent should be formulated for oral administration, widely available, inexpensive, nontoxic, and, most importantly, should reduce the risk of the target disease with minimal risks or side effects. Over the past 20 years, research has focused on the use of novel agents, drugs previously approved for other indications, and micronutrients for prostate cancer risk reduction. During this time, the National Cancer Institute (NCI) has supported numerous preclinical and clinical trials of so-called bioactive foods, including lycopene, selenium, pomegranate fruit extract, soy isoflavones, vitamins C, D, and E, multivitamins, green tea catechins, and di-indolyl-methane (DIM). The rationale for studying these agents has come largely from epidemiological literature [28]. The NCI has also supported large clinical trials of hormonal therapy for prevention of the two most common hormonally dependent malignancies, prostate and breast cancer.

5-Alpha-Reductase Inhibitors (5-ARIs)

The 5-ARIs are a class of drugs originally approved to treat men with lower urinary tract symptoms (LUTS) due to benign prostatic hyperplasia (BPH). They exert their effect by blocking the action of the enzyme 5-alpha-reductase, the principle catalyst in the conversion of the male hormone testosterone (T) to its most potent form, dihydrotestosterone (DHT). DHT is the main prostatic androgen, and binds the intracytoplasmic androgen receptor (AR) with much greater affinity than T. Once bound to AR, the steroid–receptor complex is translocated to the nucleus, where it activates androgen-response elements [29].

The rationale for investigating 5-ARIs for prostate cancer prevention stems from population-based studies demonstrating that men with a congenital deficiency of 5-alpha-reductase do not develop prostate cancer. Other work has demonstrated that Japanese men, a population with low incidences of prostate cancer, express lower levels of 5-alpha-reductase activity compared to age-matched white and African American men [30].

Two 5-ARIs have been extensively investigated in the role of prostate cancer prevention: finasteride and dutasteride. Finasteride is a potent inhibitor of the type 2 isoform of 5-alpha-reductase, while dutasteride effectively blocks the action of both type 1 and type 2 isoforms. Numerous physiological effects are noted in men treated with either drug. Most notably, both drugs effectively shrink the prostate by approximately 25–30% and reduce serum PSA levels by approximately 50% after six months of use [31]. However, when adjusting for this PSA decline by a factor of two, the sensitivity of PSA testing is maintained [32].

Prostate Cancer Prevention Trial (PCPT)

The PCPT was a randomized, double-blind, placebo-controlled trial that, between 1993 and 1996, randomized 18 882 men 55 years of age or older with a normal digital rectal exam (DRE) and a serum PSA level of 3.0 ng/ml or lower to treatment with finasteride (5 mg per day) or placebo for seven years. The primary end-point was the prevalence of prostate cancer during the study period. Secondary objectives included the effects of finasteride on grade and stage, performance characteristics of PSA and DRE for prostate cancer detection, and toxicity. Finasteride reduces serum PSA levels by about 50%. Therefore, adjusted PSA values were reported to participants and their physicians in order to preserve the blind and to equalize the number of biopsies performed on the two study arms. Patients were recommended to undergo prostate biopsy if the adjusted PSA exceeded 4.0 ng/ml or for an abnormal DRE during follow-up. In order to reduce biases in prostate cancer detection that could have been introduced by the effects of finasteride on PSA and gland size, all participants were asked to undergo a prostate biopsy on completion of the seven-year study, if they had not previously been diagnosed with prostate cancer. Despite its large size, the PCPT was not adequately powered to assess the effects of finasteride on prostate cancer-specific or overall mortality, as it was neither large enough nor of sufficiently long duration.

At study termination, 24.4% of patients in the placebo arm were diagnosed with prostate cancer, versus 18.4% in the treatment arm, translating to a 6% absolute and 24.8% relative reduction in prostate cancer (p<0.001). Reductions in cancer risk were consistent across all risk groups (age, race/ethnicity, family history, and entry PSA). Against the backdrop of these promising findings was the secondary analysis revealing more HG cancers (defined as Gleason score [GS] greater than or equal to 7) diagnosed in the finasteride group (6.4% vs 5.1%, p<0.001). Sexual side effects were more common by a small but statistically significant amount, while urinary symptoms were significantly less common among men taking finasteride [33].

Several interesting findings are derived from PCPT. Since all study participants were intended to have an end-of-study biopsy, regardless of serum PSA level or DRE finding, we gained valuable insight into the prevalence of indolent prostate cancer in the general population. With approximately 25% of all biopsies revealing prostate cancer in the placebo group, we confirmed previous observations that prostate cancer may represent an indolent entity with little to no potential to cause harm during a man's lifetime.

The increased incidence of HG prostate cancer in men on the finasteride arm of the PCPT has generated much controversy. While it is biologically plausible that finasteride could have caused *de novo* HG disease by reducing intra-prostatic androgens, the early separation of the HG curves and the observation that the relative risk of HG disease did not increase during the seven-year trial argued against this hypothesis [33]. An alternative explanation is that finasteride may have increased the detection of HG disease by introducing two forms of bias: PSA bias and biopsy bias.

PSA bias

In a post-hoc analysis of the PCPT, finasteride significantly improved the performance of PSA for the detection of HG prostate cancer [34]. For example, the sensitivity for detecting GS greater than 7 disease was 53% on the finasteride arm, but only 39.2% on the placebo arm, holding specificity constant at 90.5%. Therefore, PSA appears to be a more sensitive marker for HG prostate cancer among men taking finasteride, which may have biased the study towards more detection of HG cancer on the finasteride arm [34]. The relative inability of finasteride to suppress PSA production by HG tumours is consistent with the primary finding of the PCPT; that is, inhibition of LG, but not HG, tumours by finasteride.

Biopsy bias

The 5-ARIs ameliorate the symptoms of BPH by reducing prostate gland size. In fact, a 24.1% relative reduction in median prostate volume, documented by ultrasound, was observed on the finasteride arm of the PCPT [33]. This reduction in gland size could have introduced biopsy bias by increasing the likelihood that a focus of HG cancer, if present, would have been detected in the smaller, finasteride-treated glands. This hypothesis is supported by an analysis of PCPT patients who underwent radical prostatectomies, the gold standard for determining GS: men with HG disease at prostatectomy were significantly more likely to have had HG cancer detected by prostate biopsy if they had been on finasteride (70% versus 51%, p=0.01) [35].

Examination of pathological surrogates of disease extent in PCPT prostate biopsies provided additional evidence of detection bias [36]. Among men with GS 7–10 cancers, evaluation of biopsy specimens revealed fewer involved cores (34% vs 38%, p=0.02), less bilateral disease (22.8% vs 30.6%, p=0.05), and a decrease in perineural invasion (14.2% vs 20.3%, p=0.07) among men on the finasteride arm. These findings, which have been corroborated in the subset of men with GS 8–10 prostate cancer [36], suggest that HG cancers were more likely to be detected earlier in their course in men receiving finasteride, thus contributing to the observed increase in HG disease.

In a recent, follow-up analysis of PCPT extending up to 18 years, nearly identical overall survival rates were observed between the placebo and treatment groups (78.2% vs 78.0%, respectively) with an unadjusted hazard ratio (HR) for death in the finasteride group of 1.02 (95% confidence interval [CI] 0.97–1.08; p=0.46) [37]. However, due to the small impact of screen-detected prostate cancer on overall mortality, this analysis had extremely low power to detect differences in overall survival. For this reason, the absence of a significant difference in overall survival is not particularly helpful in sorting out the HG issue. An analysis of prostate cancer-specific mortality, which will have considerably more statistical power, is being planned.

Reduction by Dutasteride of Prostate Cancer Events Trial (REDUCE)

REDUCE evaluated the ability of the 5-ARI dutasteride, an inhibitor of both isoforms of 5-alpha-reducatase, to inhibit prostate cancer among an at-risk population of men. Dutasteride has a more profound inhibitory effect on both serum and intraprostatic DHT levels than finasteride [38], and these observations suggested that this 'dual inhibitor' might confer even greater protection against prostate cancer than finasteride. In a multicentre, randomized, double-blind, placebo-controlled fashion, men aged 55–75 with a PSA level of 2.5–10.0 ng/ml and one negative prostate biopsy (6–12 cores) within six months of enrolment were randomized to receive either dutasteride 0.5 mg daily or placebo. Subjects underwent a 10-core prostate biopsy at two and four years after enrolment. The primary end-point was a comparison of the number of prostate cancers detected in the two study arms. Secondary end-points included GS, disease extent on biopsy, and the presence of HG intraepithelial neoplasia or atypical small acinar proliferation. In total, 6729 men were enrolled. Similar to PCPT, a relative risk reduction of 22.8% was noted in the dutasteride arm over four years (p < .001). As in PCPT, risk was reduced across all prespecified sub-groups, including age, family history, and PSA level. In addition, dutasteride reduced the incidence of acute urinary retention, in line with previous findings when the drug was given to men with BPH. At two and four-year biopsies, no statistically significant increase in GS 7–10 cancers was found in patients receiving daily dutasteride. However, a significantly increased number of patients were diagnosed with GS 8–10 cancers during years 3 and 4 (p = 0.003) [39]. Similar to PCPT, the question of whether these findings are a true biological effect or a result of sampling bias arises. In a reanalysis performed by the US Food and Drugs Administration (FDA) using the 'modified' Gleason score, as was done in the PCPT, rather than the original scoring method, the overall increase in GS 8–10 cancers, for instance in years 1 through 4, observed on dutasteride did reach statistical significance (1.0% vs 0.5%, relative risk [RR] 2.06, 95% CI 1.13–3.75) [40]. For comparison, the seven-year period prevalence of GS 8–10 cancer in PCPT was 1.8% on finasteride versus 1.1% on placebo (RR 1.70, 95% CI 1.23–2.34) [40].

In 2010, the FDA convened to assess the efficacy of the 5-ARIs in reducing prostate cancer risk in men. After reviewing all prostate biopsy specimens from both PCPT and REDUCE, they reported an increased risk of GS 8–10 tumours across both trials, at a relative risk of 1.7 (95% CI 1.2–2.3). In their conclusions, the FDA recommended against the routine use of 5-ARIs for the prevention of prostate cancer, citing an unfavourable risk-to-benefit ratio [40]. From a cost standpoint, however, several models have shown that 5-ARIs are cost-effective in men who are at an increased risk of prostate cancer [41].

Do the 5-ARIs make the grade?

Although a small increase in HG prostate cancer due to the 5-ARIs cannot be ruled out, it is important to note that the effect of these agents on cancer grade represents a secondary finding, based on prostate biopsies with all of their limitations. Conversely, it is clear that both finasteride and dutasteride decrease the prevalence of LG prostate cancer, and that their use could help reduce overtreatment, the most important adverse consequence of screening. Therefore, it is reasonable to inform men being screened for this disease that the 5-ARIs have been shown to reduce the risk of LG disease (thus reducing the likelihood of detecting, and subsequently treating, insignificant cancers) and may help detect HG disease earlier, when it is more likely to be curable. These considerations must be weighed against the possibility that these agents could potentially cause *de novo* HG prostate cancer in a small minority of men. The use of 5-ARIs for prostate cancer prevention would be especially appropriate in men with LUTS, as these drugs are approved for this indication. Finally, men who are concerned about sexual side effects can be reassured that in PCPT, a very large, randomized, placebo-controlled trial, finasteride had a minimal impact on sexual functioning that diminished over time [42].

Metformin

The oral biguanide metformin is a widely prescribed insulin sensitizer for diabetics. Previous studies on the mechanism of action of metformin as an anti-neoplastic agent have shown anti-tumour action through activation of cell-cycle regulatory protein mammalian Target of Rapamycin (mTOR) [43]. In addition, a multicentre Phase 2 trial showed a significant PSA response in men with castrate-resistant, chemotherapy-naive prostate cancer that were treated with metformin [44]. These findings have prompted the investigation of metformin as a prostate cancer chemopreventive agent, yielding mixed results.

In a retrospective analysis, Randazzo et al. [45] studied the effect of metformin on serum PSA levels, free-to-total PSA ratio, prostate cancer incidence and grade, and overall survival in men enrolled in a large PSA screening trial (ERSPC). Of the 4314 men analysed, 150 (3.5%) used metformin. No differences in PSA levels, prostate cancer incidence, and grade were observed between men who were on metformin and those who were not.

In a large, retrospective, case-control study of 119 315 men with diabetes, no association was found between metformin use and the risk of overall, LG, or HG prostate cancer [46]. However, in the subgroup of 3837 diabetics in this cohort who subsequently developed prostate cancer, a significant cumulative reduction in both all-cause and prostate cancer–specific mortality was observed [47]. Interestingly, the prostate cancer–specific mortality reduction increased with increasing duration of metformin use, whereas the association with all-cause mortality declined over time.

Preston et al. [48] conducted a retrospective case-control study of patients in the Danish Cancer Registry. Metformin exposure was determined using redeemed prescription records. Controlling for those who received PSA screening, metformin exposure was associated with an overall prostate cancer diagnosis risk reduction of 16% when compared with diabetics on other oral hypoglycemic agents.

Finally, a recent meta-analysis of metformin use and overall cancer risk in diabetics showed that while metformin use was associated with 31% risk reduction of overall cancer mortality, no differences were found for prostate cancer specifically [49].

In summary, while metformin possesses many interesting potential anti-tumour properties, the data do not currently support its use as a chemopreventive agent. While the epidemiological data are mixed, adjustments for BMI and time-related biases tend to reduce the statistical significance of any protective effect [50]. If there is a benefit among diabetics, it is not clear that this extends to the nondiabetic population. Studies are ongoing to better define the potential role of this compound for the prevention of prostate and other cancers.

Statins

HMG-CoA-reductase inhibitors (statins), a class of drugs used to treat hypercholesterolemia, are among the most commonly prescribed medications worldwide. Urologically, they have been shown to reduce serum PSA levels [51], and have even been shown to inhibit prostate cancer growth in vitro [52]. While the mechanism of these effects remains unclear, it is postulated that statins may exert their anti-prostate cancer effects via both cholesterol-mediated and noncholesterol-mediated pathways. While this class of agents may have chemopreventive potential, the extraordinarily high prevalence of current usage is likely to make accrual to large-scale clinical trials of these drugs challenging.

In a Danish population-based case-control study of over 42 000 men, statin use was associated with a 6% lower risk of prostate cancer compared with non-use. The risk reduction was not duration or statin-type dependent, although statin use was associated with a 10% risk reduction of advanced prostate cancer overall, increasing to 22% with greater than 10 years of statin use [53].

In a screened population, Platz et al. [54] reviewed 9457 men in the placebo arm of PCPT and their associated prostate cancer risk based on statin use. During seven years of follow-up, statin use was not shown to reduce the risk of LG or HG prostate cancer. The inclusion of only screened men suggests that statins do not prevent early prostate cancer. However, the results were at risk of detection bias, given that statins also reduce serum PSA levels. These findings in a screened population were confirmed by a secondary analysis performed on patients enrolled in the REDUCE study [55].

The most compelling epidemiological data in support of statins as a chemopreventive agent comes from the Health Professional Follow-up Study. During 276 939 person-years of follow-up, this prospective, cohort study reported a RR of 0.51 for advanced disease and 0.39 for metastatic or fatal disease in participants who reported current statin use on biennial questionnaires [56].

In summary, statins are a commonly prescribed and generally well-tolerated class of medications that may reduce the risk of advanced and fatal prostate cancer. No significant effect has been shown in a screened population, which could be related to detection bias due to the effect of these agents on lowering serum PSA levels. Alternatively, it is possible that the potential benefits of statins may be obscured by the overdiagnosis of indolent disease introduced by screening. However, if these agents did decrease the risk of developing fatal prostate cancer, one would expect to see a reduction of HG disease in a screened population.

Dietary supplements

Selenium and vitamin E

In 1994, the alpha-Tocopherol, beta-Carotene Cancer Prevention Study Group published its findings on the effect of vitamin E and beta-carotene supplementation on the incidence of lung cancer and other cancers. This randomized, double-blind, placebo-controlled primary prevention trial did not find a reduction in the incidence of lung cancer among those who received vitamin E, but in a secondary analysis did find a 32% reduction in prostate cancer incidence [57].

Then, in 1997, the Nutrition Prevention of Cancer Study Group published the results of a multicentre, double-blind, randomized, placebo-controlled cancer prevention trial in which 1312 patients were randomized to receive 200 mcg of selenium per day or placebo. The primary end-point was development of non-melanoma skin cancer. While the primary result showed a 14% nonsignificant increase in the incidence of skin cancer, which with subsequent follow-up became statistically significant, a secondary analysis revealed an impressive 65% reduction in prostate cancer incidence over a mean follow-up of 4.5 years [58].

These two studies formed the basis for the Selenium and Vitamin E Cancer Prevention Trial (SELECT).

SELECT was a multicentre, randomized, double-blind, placebo-controlled trial which recruited 35 533 men from 427 institutions from across North America. Patients were assigned to one of four groups: selenium, vitamin E, selenium plus vitamin E, and placebo. African American men over the age of 50 and all other men over the age of 55 with a serum PSA level of 4 ng/ml or less and a normal DRE were eligible for inclusion and randomization. Annual PSA tests and DREs were not mandatory, since the benefits of this screening were (and still are) under debate when the trial opened, and community standards regarding prostate cancer screening were expected to evolve over the course of this planned 7–12-year trial. The primary end-point of SELECT was the clinical incidence of prostate cancer. The large sample size provided 96% power to detect a 25% decrease in prostate cancer for either of the single agents versus placebo, and 89% power to detect a 25% decrease for selenium plus vitamin E versus an active single agent. Secondary end-points included lung, colon, and total cancer incidence, cardiovascular events, death from any cause, and toxicity. In addition, four prospectively conducted sub-studies addressing the usefulness of selenium and vitamin E in the prevention of macular degeneration, chronic obstructive lung disease, Alzheimer's disease, and colon polyps were performed in men already accrued to the parent study.

Although the planned follow-up period was 12 years, the study was discontinued at the second interim analysis at 7 years due to convincing data that neither selenium nor vitamin E when used alone or in combination reduced the risk of prostate cancer in this population [59]. A subsequent report on this trial was published with 54 464 additional person-years of follow-up. Surprisingly, men randomized to the vitamin E–only arm had a significantly increased risk of prostate cancer when compared with placebo (hazard ratio [HR] 1.17, 99% CI 1.004–1.36, p = .008) [60]. Consequently, neither supplement is recommended as a prostate cancer chemopreventive agent.

Despite its initial promise and subsequent disappointment as a primary chemopreventive agent, selenium was further examined in a secondary prevention role. In a double-blind, randomized, placebo-controlled trial, the Southwest Oncology Group (SWOG) randomized 423 men with high-grade prostatic intraepithelial neoplasia (HGPIN) to 200 mcg/day of selenomethionine or placebo over a three-year period. The primary end-point was progression of HGPIN to prostate cancer. The three-year prostate cancer rates between the two groups were nearly identical (35.6% in the selenium group, 36.6% in the placebo group, p=0.73). Furthermore, no differences in grade were noted between the two groups. While a subset analysis showed a slightly reduced risk of prostate cancer with selenium supplementation in patients with low baseline selenium levels (RR 0.82, 95% CI 0.40–1.69), this risk reduction did not approach statistical significance [61].

More recent analyses of SELECT considered patient outcomes based on baseline plasma selenium levels. In one such analysis, selenium supplementation had no preventive effect in men with low baseline selenium levels (under the 60th percentile of toenail selenium), while selenium supplementation increased the risk of HG prostate cancer in men with high baseline selenium levels by 91%. Meanwhile, vitamin E supplementation increased the risk of both LG and HG prostate cancer in men with lower selenium status [62].

A separate analysis of prostate cancer risk in SELECT patients demonstrated that vitamin E supplementation increased the risk of prostate cancer regardless of baseline plasma levels of alpha-tocopherol (the predominant form of vitamin E in supplements). In addition, baseline vitamin E levels were not independently associated with prostate cancer risk in the absence of supplementation. However, selenium supplementation was associated with an increased risk of prostate cancer among men with the highest baseline vitamin E levels. Of particular concern is that this observation was driven by a twofold increase in the risk of HG disease [63]. While these findings suggest a biological interaction between vitamin E and selenium in prostate cancer carcinogenesis, the underlying mechanism remains unknown.

The results of SELECT underscore several principles. First, the observed 17% increase in prostate cancer in the vitamin E arm suggests that a drug or supplement may exert an effect even after the intervention is stopped, highlighting the need for extended follow-up of these patients. Secondly, consumers should be wary of health claims that vitamins and minerals are innocuous, in the absence of well-designed, randomized trials to assess the true benefits or harms of a particular over-the-counter supplement.

Prostate cancer prevention clinical trials

Trial end-points

One consequence of the long natural history of prostate cancer is that many years are required to determine whether a putative prevention agent has an effect on cancer incidence. Therefore, early-phase clinical trials designed to provide preliminary evidence of efficacy must rely on intermediate biomarker end-points [64–66]. While serum-based biomarkers (e.g. PSA) can provide useful information, tissue is required to determine whether an agent achieves measurable levels in the prostate gland, and to assess the effect of an intervention on pathways and mechanisms recognized as hallmarks of carcinogenesis, such as cellular proliferation (Ki-67), apoptosis (TUNEL), and angiogenesis (VEGF) [67,68]. However, it should be emphasized that there are no validated surrogates for the end-point of true interest, clinically relevant prostate cancer [69], and that large, Phase 3 trials with cancer incidence end-points are required to demonstrate cancer prevention efficacy.

Study design

This reliance on intermediate biomarker end-points, as opposed to more objective clinical end-points such as tumour shrinkage, necessitates that even early-phase prevention trials be rigorously controlled. This principle was nicely illustrated by a placebo-controlled study in the 1990s of a synthetic retinoid derivative, fenretinide, in which modulation of prostate tissue-based biomarkers was observed following the administration of the active agent, but was also seen post placebo. This unexpected finding, presumably due to a nonspecific effect of the prostate biopsy itself on the biomarker end-point, underscores the need for a placebo control group when relying on biomarker end-points [70].

Study cohorts

Cohort selection for prevention agent development clinical trials is predominantly driven by the need to obtain prostate tissue for assessment of the most important – that is, tissue-based – study end-points. Several clinical settings in which prostate tissue is obtained as part of the standard of care have led to the identification of so-called informative cohorts for prostate cancer prevention agent development. These include men with high-grade intra-prostatic neoplasia (HGPIN cohort); men with a negative prostate biopsy following an elevated PSA (negative biopsy cohort); men with a diagnosis of prostate cancer who have elected to be treated with prostatectomy (pre-prostatectomy cohort); and men with low- or intermediate-risk prostate cancer who have elected to be followed expectantly (active surveillance cohort). The NCI has supported cancer prevention agent development clinical trials in all of these cohorts.

HGPIN cohort

In 2001, Sakr and Partin [71] proposed that HGPIN was an important intermediary in the development of prostate cancer. They noted the high frequency with which HGPIN is detected in prostate biopsies containing invasive cancer, its relatively high prevalence in young African American men, and the degree to which the two entities share molecular and genetic abnormalities, including loss of 8P, 10q, and 16q, and gain of 7q31 and 8q. However, the degree to which HGPIN represents a true pre-malignant lesion and the extent to which it is predictive for subsequent invasive prostate cancer are controversial [72]. Increased prostate sampling, as urologists have moved from sextant (6-core) biopsies to extended template (12-core) biopsies, appears has been associated with a decrease in prostate cancer incidence among men with HGPIN, raising the possibility that this lesion is an indicator of the presence of prostate cancer, rather than a true risk factor for the future development of the disease.

In the largest clinical trial in this cohort performed to date, 1590 men with HGPIN but no invasive cancer (median number of cores examined 12) were randomized to receive either toremifene (an anti-oestrogen) or placebo for three years. After undergoing yearly prostate biopsies for up to three years, the cumulative rate of prostate cancer was 34.7% (placebo) versus 32.3% (toremifene), p=0.39 [73]. While the investigators argued that the 'high likelihood' of subsequent invasive prostate cancer in this cohort supported the continued inclusion of men with HGPIN in cancer prevention trials, and that these men 'require surveillance by periodic biopsy', the actual cancer rates on the placebo arm at years 1, 2, and 3 were only 17.9%, 12.9%, and 13.6%, precisely what would be expected for men of similar median age (65 years) and mean PSA (4.2 ng/dl), irrespective of the presence or absence of HGPIN [74]. For this reason, the HGPIN cohort may not be as informative as previously believed for the purpose of prostate cancer agent development.

Negative biopsy cohort

Men with prior negative prostate biopsies, performed to evaluate an elevated PSA or a suspicious digital rectal examination, comprise the so-called negative biopsy cohort. As men in this category have historically been advised to undergo repeat prostate biopsies due to concerns that cancer may have been missed by the initial biopsy, this cohort appeared to fulfil the 'informative cohort' requirement of providing prostate tissue as part of routine management.

The largest study ever undertaken in this cohort, the so-called Negative Biopsy Trial, randomized 699 participants from 20 urology practices in the USA and two hospitals in New Zealand to receive high-selenium yeast (200 mcg/day/day or 400 mcg/day/day) or a matching placebo [75]. Men on this study were followed with PSA tests every six months, and the decision regarding whether and when to have a repeat prostate biopsy was left up to each patient and his urologist. With an overall median follow-up of three years, only 10.6% (74 men) of the study population had a positive follow-up prostate biopsy, and no significant differences were observed between the placebo group (11.3%) and the active intervention groups (10.3% and 10.0% for 200 mcg/day and 400 mcg/day Se-yeast, respectively, p=0.88).

Analogous to the situation in men with HGPIN, the cancer detection rate during surveillance was highly dependent on the number of cores obtained at the time of the baseline biopsy: 16.8% subsequent positive prostate biopsies among those whose initial biopsy was less than or equal to six cores versus 9.3% if more than six cores were initially sampled. It is noteworthy that only 42% of the study participants ever had a follow-up biopsy, indicating that a substantial proportion decided not to undergo a repeat biopsy. The widespread adoption of extended-template biopsies, in which at least 10 prostate tissue cores are routinely sampled at the time of prostate biopsy, raises questions regarding the usefulness of the negative biopsy cohort for prostate cancer prevention agent development clinical trials.

Active surveillance cohort

Prostate cancer screening results in the diagnosis and treatment of many cancers not destined to become clinically apparent during a man's lifetime [76,77]. Accumulating experience over the past two decades with active surveillance (AS), also referred to as 'delayed intervention with curative intent' [78], in men with favourable-risk, localized prostate cancer has provided the basis for growing acceptance of this approach in selected patients with newly diagnosed prostate cancer regardless of life expectancy [78–82].

In 2011 the US National Institutes of Health (NIH) held a State-of-the-Science Conference on the role of AS in the management of men with low-risk prostate cancer [83]. After consideration of a systematic review of the literature as well as presentations from 22 experts in pertinent fields, such as urology, pathology, and cancer prevention and control, the panel concluded that AS 'should be offered' to patients with low-risk prostate cancer, and that more than 100 000 men a year diagnosed in the USA would be candidates for this approach. However, as AS has become more widely accepted by both patients and urologists, so too has the need to develop effective strategies to delay or inhibit disease progression in order to reduce the ultimate need for definitive therapy with surgery or radiation. While follow-up strategies vary, the term AS (as opposed to the older term, watchful waiting) implies that subsequent prostate biopsies will be performed, thus providing the necessary tissue for evaluation of biomarker end-points in prevention agent development clinical trials. For this reason, men being followed on AS represent ideal candidates for inclusion in such trials, as well as for evaluating the usefulness of genomics and other strategies to predict the natural history of this heterogeneous disease.

One such completed trial, Reduction by Dutasteride of Clinical Progression Events in Expectant Management (REDEEM), evaluated the efficacy and safety of daily dutasteride versus placebo on prostate cancer progression in men diagnosed with low-risk disease and who elected to be entered in an active surveillance program [84]. Over the three years of the trial, the incidence of prostate cancer progression, as defined by GS upgrading or initiation of medical/surgical management, was markedly lowered in the intervention arm (HR 0.62, 95% CI 0.43–0.89, $p = 0.009$). The results of REDEEM provided evidence of the anti-tumour effects of 5-ARIs in tissues that have already malignantly transformed, in addition to their anti-carcinogenic effects seen in presumably normal tissues, as shown in REDUCE.

Sparked by the promising results of REDEEM, a randomized, placebo-controlled study of oral aspirin and vitamin D3, alone or in combination, in men enrolled in active surveillance for low-risk prostate cancer is currently under way [85]. Its aim is to evaluate the effects of each supplement, individually and in combination, in preventing disease progression in an active surveillance cohort. While the results will not be known for several years, these agents may prove effective in preventing the negative consequences of disease progression and/or subsequent definitive treatment in men already diagnosed with prostate cancer.

As noted in Table 12.1, NCI-sponsored studies of soy isoflavones, lycopene, omega-3 fatty acids, and selenium have been conducted in this cohort, with

Table 12.1 US National Cancer Institute–sponsored prostate cancer prevention trials.

Study Description	Cohort	Intervention	End-points	Sample Size	Findings/Status
Randomized, placebo-controlled trial of PSA-TRICOM	Active surveillance	PSA-TRICOM-V (priming dose) Day 0; PSA-TRICOM-F (boosts) Days 14, 28, 56, 84, 112, and 140	1 Change in CD4 and CD8 staining in prostate tissue 2 PD-L1 prostate tissue staining; PSADT	90	In development
Randomized, placebo-controlled trial of pomegranate fruit extract	Active surveillance	Pomegranate fruit extract (1000 mg/day) × 1 year	1 Plasma IGF-1 2 PSADT; TUNEL; PCNA	30	Accrual ongoing
Randomized, placebo-controlled trial of nutritional supplements (MENS)	Active surveillance	Lycopene (30 mg/day) vs n-3 fatty acids (1 gm/day) × 3 months	1 IGF-1 and COX-2 gene expression 2 Global gene expression; tumour progression	85	No change in IGF-1 or COX-2 gene expression in prostate tissue; no significant associations between individual genes and dietary or supplemental intake of omega-3 fatty acids or lycopene [87]
Randomized, placebo-controlled trial of soy isoflavones	Active surveillance	Soy isoflavones (80 mg/day) × 3 months	1 Isoflavone levels; PSA 2 T; E; SHBG	53	Increased plasma isoflavones on the isoflavone arm; no effect on PSA, T, E, or SHBG [88]
Randomized, placebo-controlled trial of soy protein and isoflavones	High-risk prostate cancer, post-RP	Soy protein (20 g/day) and genistein (24 mg/day) × 2 years	1 Two-year PSA failure rate 2 Time to PSA failure	169	No change in PSA levels [92]
Randomized, placebo-controlled trial of soy isoflavones	Pre-RP, brachytherapy, or cryotherapy	Genistein (150, 300, 600 mg/day) × 2–6 weeks	1 Oxidative stress (ODD) 2 Plasma and tissue isoflavone levels	34	No change in oxidative stress biomarkers observed (O. Kucuk, personal communication, 2006)
Randomized, placebo-controlled trial of selenium	Elevated PSA/ negative biopsy	Se-yeast (200, 400 mcg/day) up to 5 years	1 Prostate cancer 2 PSAV 3 Prostate cancer progression; alkaline phosphatase; chromogranin A	699	No change in prostate cancer incidence or PSAV [75]

Study design	Population	Intervention	Endpoints	N	Results
Randomized, placebo-controlled trial of selenium	Active surveillance	Se-yeast (200, 800 mcg/day) up to 5 years	1 PSAV 2 Bcl-2; Ki-67	140	No change in PSAV [86]
Randomized, placebo-controlled trial of selenium	Healthy men	Se-yeast (240, 350 mcg/day) Se-met (200 mcg/day) × 9 months	1 Plasma and urine selenium concentration; oxidative stress biomarkers (urine 8-OHdG and 8-iso-PGF$_2^\alpha$ and blood GSH) 2 DHT, T, PSA	69	Significant reductions in urinary biomarkers of oxidative stress on Se-yeast arm only [93]
Randomized, placebo-controlled trial of finasteride and selenium (2 × 2 factorial)	Pre-RP	Se-met (400 mcg/day), Finasteride (5 mg/day) × 3–5 weeks	1 PSA gene expression 2 TUNEL; caspase-3	55	Analysis pending [94] (C. Ip, personal communication, 2008)
Randomized, placebo-controlled trial of selenium	Pre-RP	Se-met (200 mcg/day) × 14–31 days	1 Selenium tissue levels 2 Serum and seminal vesicle selenium levels; PSA	68	22% increase in prostate tissue selenium concentration on the selenium arm [95]
Randomized, placebo-controlled trial of selenium	HGPIN	Se-met (200 mcg/day) × 3 years	1 Prostate cancer incidence 2 TUNEL; Ki-67	423	No decrease in prostate cancer incidence [61] (J. Marshall, personal communication, 2008)
Randomized, placebo-controlled trial of green tea catechins	Pre-RP	Green tea catechins (800 mg EGCG/day) × 3–6 weeks	1 Tissue catechin levels 2 Clusterin; MMPs; IGFs; 8-OH-dG	50	Low to undetectable prostate tissue catechin levels; no change in tissue biomarkers of proliferation, apoptosis, and angiogenesis [96]
Randomized, placebo-controlled trial of green tea catechins	HGPIN or ASAP	Green tea catechins (400 mg EGCG/day) × 12 months	1 Prostate cancer rates at 1 year 2 Prostate cancer+ASAP at 1 year	97	Analysis pending

Continued

Table 12.1 Continued

Study Description	Cohort	Intervention	End-points	Sample Size	Findings/Status
Randomized, placebo-controlled trial of DIM	Pre-RP	DIM (100, 200 mg/day) × 3–4 weeks	1 Tissue DIM levels 2 Ki-67; TUNEL; caspase-3	45	Analysis pending
Randomized, placebo-controlled trial of cholecalciferol and genistein	Pre-RP	Cholecalciferol (200,000 IU) × 1 dose and genistein (600 mg/day) × 3–4 weeks	1 Cholecalciferol serum and tissue bioavailability 2 VDR tissue levels	15	Analysis pending
Randomized, open-label trial of 1α-hydroxyvitamin D2	Pre-RP	1α-hydroxyvitamin D2 (10 mcg/day) × 4–6 weeks	1 MIB-1 and TUNEL prostate tissue staining 2 Microvessel density; vitamin D receptor expression	31	No significant changes in biomarkers [97]
Nonrandomized trial of sulindac sulfone (historical and concurrent controls)	Pre-RP	Sulindac sulfone (375 mg/day) × 4 weeks	1 Bcl-2; Bax; TUNEL; Par-4; M30; PTEN 2 PSA; HGPIN; MIB-1; DNA ploidy	105	No significant changes in biomarkers (B.J. Nelson, personal communication, 2006)
Randomized, placebo-controlled trial of celecoxib	Pre-RP	Celecoxib (400 mg BID) × 4–6 weeks	1 Tissue PG levels 2 COX-2; mRNA expression; DNA oxidation; p27; p21; PCNA; Ki-67; PSA	64	No significant changes in biomarkers [20]
Randomized, placebo-controlled trial of finasteride	Pre-RP	Finasteride (5 mg/day) × 4–6 weeks	1 Effect of finasteride on IHC markers associated with high grade 2 Ki-67; caspace-3	204	Analysis pending
Randomized, placebo-controlled trial of finasteride pre-biopsy	Intermediate risk of prostate cancer based on PCPT calculator, scheduled for prostate biopsy	Finasteride (5 mg/day) × 3 months	1 sensitivity and specificity of PSA and DRE for prostate cancer detection 2 PCA3; % [-2]proPSA; and TMPRSS2:ERG for biopsy outcome	274	Ongoing

Trial	Population	Intervention	Biomarkers/endpoints	N	Results
Randomized, placebo-controlled trial of DFMO	Positive family history with negative biopsy	DFMO (500 mg/day) × 1 year	1 Prostate polyamines levels (putrescine, spermine, and spermadine) 2 PSA	81	Decreased putrescine levels on DFMO arm; no significant effect on other polyamines or PSA [98]
Randomized, placebo-controlled trial of toremifene	Pre-RP	Toremifene (40 mg/day) × 3–6 weeks	1 HGPIN Index 2 Bcl-2, Ki-67, cd31 3 DHT, T, PSA, E	52	No effect in HGPIN or other biomarkers (B.J. Nelson, personal communication, 2006)
Randomized, placebo-controlled trial of metformin	Pre-RP	Metformin ER (500 mg/day week one, 1000 mg/day week two, then 1500 mg/day) × 4–12 weeks	1 Tissue metformin levels 2 Proliferation; apoptosis; angiogenesis; AMPK; mTOR; cell cycle regulation	20	Analysis pending
Randomized trial of telephone counselling (MEAL)	Active surveillance	Telephone counselling to increase cruciferous vegetable intake × 2 years	1 Clinical progression 2 PSADT; QOL; dietary change	386	Ongoing

8-iso-PGF$_{2\alpha}$, 8-iso-prostaglandin-F$_{2\alpha}$; AMPK, 5′ adenosine monophosphate-activated protein kinase; ASAP, atypical small acinar proliferation; Bax, a pro-apoptotic gene; Bcl-2, an anti-apoptotic proto-oncogene; BID, bis in die (twice a day); Caspase-3, caspases are critical effectors of apoptosis; CD4, cluster of differentiation 4; CD8, cluster of differentiation 8; cd31, membrane protein, cell–cell interactions, adhesion; COX, cyclooxygenase; DFMO, α-difluoromethylornithine; DHT, dihydrotestosterone; DIM, 3,3-diindolylmethane; DNA, deoxyribonucleic acid; DRE, digital rectal exam; E, estradiol; EGCG, epigallocatechin-3-gallate; ER, extended release; ERG, gene involved in chromosomal translocations; GSH, glutathione; HGPIN, high-grade prostatic intraepithelial neoplasia; IGF, insulin-like growth factor; IHC, immunohistochemistry; Ki-67, a marker of cellular proliferation; M30, a marker of apoptosis; MIB-1, a monoclonal antibody that detects the Ki-67 antigen; MMP, matrix metalloproteinase; mRNA, messenger ribonucleic acid; mTOR, mammalian target of rapamycin; ODD, oxidative DNA damage; p21, a cyclin-dependent kinase, cell cycle control; p27, a cyclin-dependent kinase inhibitor, cell cycle control; Par-4, protease-activated receptor 4; PCA3, prostate cancer gene 3; PCNA, proliferating cell nuclear antigen; PCPT, Prostate Cancer Prevention Trial; PD-L1, programmed death ligand-1; PG, prostaglandin; [−2] proPSA, a truncated form of proPSA, a subform of free PSA that is associated with cancer; PSA, prostate-specific antigen; PSADT, prostate-specific antigen doubling time; PSAV, prostate-specific antigen velocity; PTEN, a tumor suppressor gene; QOL, quality of life; RP, radical prostatectomy; Se-met, selenomethionine; Se-yeast, selenium yeast; SHBG, sex hormone binding globulin; T, testosterone; TMPRSS, transmembrane protease, serine 2 gene; TUNEL, terminal deoxynucleotidyl transferase (TdT)-mediated dUTP nick-end labelling; VDR, vitamin D receptor.

little evidence of benefit to date [86–88]. A double-blind, placebo-controlled trial evaluating the role of a polyphenol-rich supplement (POMI-T) on PSA progression in men diagnosed with clinically localized prostate cancer and enrolled in either active surveillance (60%) or watchful waiting (40%) demonstrated favourable and statistically significant PSA kinetics in the intervention arm over a six-month period [89]. While the results of this trial suggest that this concoction is biologically active, more clinically meaningful outcomes, such as metastases-free survival, disease-specific survival, and overall survival, were not measured, thus limiting the conclusions of this trial. A trial of pomegranate fruit extract (PFE) in men on AS was recently begun on the strength of the TRAMP mouse data [90] and the observation that PFE appeared to prolong PSA doubling time in men with biochemical failure following definitive therapy [91].

A multicentre, placebo-controlled trial of PSA-TRICOM, a Poxviral-based PSA-targeted vaccine, in the AS cohort is currently in development to assess the effect of six months of vaccine therapy on immune end-points (CD4, CD8, and PD-L1 immunohistochemical staining) in prostate tumour tissue. The rationale for this 'prevention of progression' trial is the increase in overall survival observed as a secondary end-point among men who were randomized to receive active vaccine versus an empty vector control group, in a preliminary study conducted in 125 men with asymptomatic or minimally symptomatic castrate-resistant prostate cancer (mCRPC). The results of a confirmatory trial, which recently met its accrual goal of 1200 men with mCRPC, to definitively address the impact of this vaccine on overall survival are anxiously anticipated.

Pre-prostatectomy cohort

Men with localized prostate cancer planning to undergo definitive surgery represent another potentially informative cohort, and the majority of prostate cancer prevention agent development trials supported by the NCI's Division of Cancer Prevention over the past decade have been conducted in this cohort. Study agents (or placebos) are administered for up to six weeks in this model, the period of time between the diagnostic biopsy and prostatectomy. Despite the short duration of drug/day exposure, valuable information can be obtained regarding distribution of the candidate agent in prostate tissue and the effect of the study drug/day on tissue-based biomarkers, as the entire gland will become available following prostatectomy. Most of the drug/days currently in Phase 2 testing in the NCI prostate cancer chemoprevention agent development programme have been evaluated in this cohort (Table 12.1).

Chemoprevention clinical trial programme

The Prostate and Urologic Cancers Research Group in the NCI's Division of Cancer Prevention has sponsored a number of Phase 1 and 2 chemoprevention trials that are completed or currently under way. A complete list of these trials is included in Table 12.1.

Conclusion

Prostate cancer is a prevalent disease among men over the age of 50. The risk of developing, living with, and having treatment for the disease can be a major source of anxiety and/or morbidity to the patient and of significant cost to the health-care system. Primary prevention of prostate cancer, therefore, would seem to be an attractive option to many men. To date, several randomized, placebo-controlled trials have been completed with the aim of finding the ideal combination of an effective preventive therapy with minimal side effects.

Two recently completed trials evaluating the 5-ARIs exhibited promising results. PCPT and REDUCE both showed approximately a 25% reduction in prostate cancer in two different risk populations. While both trials reported an increased risk of high-grade cancer, subsequent analyses suggest that the increased risk is likely explained, at least in part, by detection bias introduced by the 5-ARIs. Both 5-ARIs now carry a black-box warning stating that their use could cause aggressive prostate cancer. This warning has likely caused primary care physicians and urologists to shy away from prescribing these agents, and deterred their use for chemoprevention. Vitamins and minerals such as vitamin E and selenium showed promise as prostate cancer primary prevention agents, based on secondary analyses of cancer prevention trials conducted in the mid-1990s. Unfortunately, when subjected to rigorous evaluation through randomized, double-blind, placebo-controlled trials, the theorized benefit was lost, and it was even shown that vitamin E increases the risk of prostate cancer when taken alone. While the ideal prostate cancer primary prevention strategy has not yet been elucidated, ongoing evaluation of approved and novel agents continues.

References

1 DeSantis, C.E., Lin, C.C., Mariotto, A.B. et al. (2014). Cancer treatment and survivorship statistics, 2014. *CA Cancer J. Clin.* 64 (4): 252–271.

2 American Cancer Society (2016). About prostate cancer and key statistics. https://www.cancer.org/content/dam/CRC/PDF/Public/8793.00.pdf (accessed 3 January 2018).

3 Ferlay, J., Shin, H.R., Bray, F. (2010). Estimates of worldwide burden of cancer in 2008: GLOBOCAN 2008. *Int. J. Cancer* 127 (12): 2893–2917.

4 Han, C.S., Parihar, J.S., and Kim, I.Y. (2013). Active surveillance in men with low-risk prostate cancer: Current and future challenges. *Am. J. Clin. Exp. Urol.* 1 (1): 72–82.

5 Umar, A., Dunn, B.K., and Greenwald, P. (2012). Future directions in cancer prevention. *Nat. Rev. Cancer* 12 (12): 835–848.

6 Hong, W.K., and Sporn, M.B. (1997). Recent advances in chemoprevention of cancer. *Science* 278 (5340): 1073–1077.

7 Armitage, P., and Doll, R. (1954). The age distribution of cancer and a multi-stage theory of carcinogenesis. *Br. J. Cancer* 8 (1): 1–12.

8 Merrill, R.M., and Sloan, A. (2012). Risk-adjusted incidence rates for prostate cancer in the United States. *Prostate* 72 (2): 181–185.

9 Kicinski, M., Vangronsveld, J., and Nawrot, T.S. (2011). An epidemiological reappraisal of the familial aggregation of prostate cancer: A meta-analysis. *PLoS One* 6 (10): e27130.

10 Gurel, B., Lucia, M.S., Thompson, I.M., Jr. et al. (2014). Chronic inflammation in benign prostate tissue is associated with high-grade prostate cancer in the placebo arm of the prostate cancer prevention trial. *Cancer Epidemiol. Biomarkers Prev.* 23 (5): 847–856.

11 Sutcliffe, S., and Platz, E.A. (2008). Inflammation and prostate cancer: A focus on infections. *Curr. Urol. Rep.* 9 (3): 243–249.

12 Sfanos, K.S., Isaacs, W.B., and De Marzo, A.M. (2013). Infections and inflammation in prostate cancer. *Am. J. Clin. Exp. Urol.* 1 (1): 3–11.

13 Sutcliffe, S., Neace, C., Magnuson, N.S. et al. (2012). Trichomonosis, a common curable STI, and prostate carcinogenesis: A proposed molecular mechanism. *PLoS Pathog.* 8 (8): e1002801.

14 Stark, J.R., Judson, G., Alderete, J.F. et al. (2009). Prospective study of Trichomonas vaginalis infection and prostate cancer incidence and mortality: Physicians' Health Study. *J. Natl Cancer Inst.* 101 (20): 1406–1411.

15 Sutcliffe, S., Alderete, J.F., Till, C. et al. (2009). Trichomonosis and subsequent risk of prostate cancer in the Prostate Cancer Prevention Trial. *Int. J. Cancer* 124 (9): 2082–2087.

16 Sutcliffe, S., Till, C., Gaydos, C.A. et al. (2012). Prospective study of cytomegalovirus serostatus and prostate cancer risk in the Prostate Cancer Prevention Trial. *Cancer Causes Control* 23 (9): 1511–1518.

17 Sutcliffe, S., Till, C., Jenkins, F.J. et al. (2015). Prospective study of human herpesvirus type 8 serostatus and prostate cancer risk in the placebo arm of the Prostate Cancer Prevention Trial. *Cancer Causes Control* 26 (1): 35–44.

18 Sutcliffe, S., Viscidi, R.P., Till, C. et al. (2010). Human papillomavirus types 16, 18, and 31 serostatus and prostate cancer risk in the Prostate Cancer Prevention Trial. *Cancer Epidemiol. Biomarkers Prev.* 19 (2): 614–618.

19 Algra, A.M., and Rothwell, P.M. (2012). Effects of regular aspirin on long-term cancer incidence and metastasis: A systematic comparison of evidence from observational studies versus randomised trials. *Lancet Oncol.* 13 (5): 518–527.

20 Antonarakis, E.S., Heath, E.I., Walczak, J.R. et al. (2009). Phase II, randomized, placebo-controlled trial of neoadjuvant celecoxib in men with clinically localized prostate cancer: Evaluation of drug-specific biomarkers. *J. Clin. Oncol.* 27 (30): 4986–4993.

21 Shahabi, A., Corral, R., Catsburg, C. et al. (2014). Tobacco smoking, polymorphisms in carcinogen metabolism enzyme genes, and risk of localized and advanced prostate cancer: Results from the California Collaborative Prostate Cancer Study. *Cancer Med.* 3 (6): 1644–1655.

22 Rieken, M., Kluth, L., Fajkovic, H. et al. (2015). Association of cigarette smoking and smoking cessation with biochemical recurrence in patients treated with radical prostatectomy for prostate cancer. 15th European Association of Urology conference, Madrid, Spain.

23 Moreira, D.M., Aronson, W.J., Terris, M.K. et al. (2014). Cigarette smoking is associated with an increased risk of biochemical disease recurrence, metastasis, castration-resistant prostate cancer, and mortality after radical prostatectomy: Results from the SEARCH database. *Cancer* 120 (2): 197–204.

24 Joshu, C.E., Mondul, A.M., Meinhold, C.L. et al. (2011). Cigarette smoking and prostate cancer recurrence after prostatectomy. *J. Natl Cancer Inst.* 103 (10): 835–838.

25 Discacciati, A., and Wolk, A. (2014). Lifestyle and dietary factors in prostate cancer prevention. *Recent Results Cancer Res.* 202: 27–37.

26 Gong, Z., Neuhouser, M.L., Goodman, P.J. et al. (2006). Obesity, diabetes, and risk of prostate cancer: Results from the prostate cancer prevention trial. *Cancer Epidemiol. Biomarkers Prev.* 15 (10): 1977–1983.

27 Vidal, A.C., Howard, L.E., Moreira, D.M. et al. (2014). Obesity increases the risk for high-grade prostate cancer: Results from the REDUCE study. *Cancer Epidemiol. Biomarkers Prev.* 23 (12): 2936–2942.

28 Parnes, H.L., House, M.G., Kagan, J. et al. (2004). Prostate cancer chemoprevention agent development: The National Cancer Institute, Division of Cancer Prevention portfolio. *J. Urol.* 171 (2, Part 2): S68–S74; discussion S5.

29 Steers, W.D. (2001). 5alpha-reductase activity in the prostate. *Urology* 58 (6, Suppl. 1): 17–24.

30 Ross, R.K., Bernstein, L., Lobo, R.A. et al. (1992). 5-alpha-reductase activity and risk of prostate cancer among Japanese and US white and black males. *Lancet* 339 (8798): 887–889.

31 Andriole, G.L., and Kirby, R. (2003). Safety and tolerability of the dual 5alpha-reductase inhibitor dutasteride in the treatment of benign prostatic hyperplasia. *Eur. Urol.* 44 (1): 82–88.

32 Andriole, G.L., Marberger, M., and Roehrborn, C.G. (2006). Clinical usefulness of serum prostate specific antigen for the detection of prostate cancer is preserved in men receiving the dual 5alpha-reductase inhibitor dutasteride. *J. Urol.* 175 (5): 1657–1662.

33 Thompson, I.M., Goodman, P.J., Tangen, C.M. et al. (2003). The influence of finasteride on the development of prostate cancer. *N. Engl. J. Med.* 349 (3): 215–224.

34 Thompson, I.M., Chi, C., Ankerst, D.P. et al. (2006). Effect of finasteride on the sensitivity of PSA for detecting prostate cancer. *J. Natl Cancer Inst.* 98 (16): 1128–1133.

35 Lucia, M.S., Epstein, J.I., Goodman, P.J. et al. (2007). Finasteride and high-grade prostate cancer in the Prostate Cancer Prevention Trial. *J. Natl Cancer Inst.* 99 (18): 1375–1383.

36 Lucia, M.S., Darke, A.K., Goodman, P.J. et al. (2008). Pathologic characteristics of cancers detected in the Prostate Cancer Prevention Trial: Implications for prostate cancer detection and chemoprevention. *Cancer Prev. Res.* 1 (3): 167–173.

37 Thompson, I.M., Jr., Goodman, P.J., Tangen, C.M. et al. (2013). Long-term survival of participants in the prostate cancer prevention trial. *N. Engl. J. Med.* 369 (7): 603–610.

38 Tindall, D.J., and Rittmaster, R.S. (2008). The rationale for inhibiting 5alpha-reductase isoenzymes in the prevention and treatment of prostate cancer. *J. Urol.* 179 (4): 1235–1242.

39 Andriole, G.L., Bostwick, D.G., Brawley, O.W. et al. (2010). Effect of dutasteride on the risk of prostate cancer. *N. Engl. J. Med.* 362 (13): 1192–1202.

40 Theoret, M.R., Ning, Y.M., Zhang, J.J. et al. (2011). The risks and benefits of 5alpha-reductase inhibitors for prostate-cancer prevention. *N. Engl. J. Med.* 365 (2): 97–99.

41 Kattan, M.W., Earnshaw, S.R., McDade, C.L. et al. (2011). Cost effectiveness of chemoprevention for prostate cancer with dutasteride in a high-risk population based on results from the REDUCE clinical trial. *Appl. Health Econ. Health Policy* 9 (5): 305–315.

42 Moinpour, C.M., Darke, A.K., Donaldson, G.W. et al. (2007). Longitudinal analysis of sexual function reported by men in the Prostate Cancer Prevention Trial. *J. Natl Cancer Inst.* 99 (13): 1025–1035.

43 Leone, A., Di Gennaro, E., Bruzzese, F. et al. (2014). New perspective for an old antidiabetic drug: Metformin as anticancer agent. *Cancer Treat. Res.* 159: 355–376.

44 Rothermundt, C., Hayoz, S., Templeton, A.J. et al. (2014). Metformin in chemotherapy-naive castration-resistant prostate cancer: A multicenter phase 2 trial (SAKK 08/09). *Eur. Urol.* 66 (3): 468–474.

45 Randazzo, M., Beatrice, J., Huber, A. et al. (2015). Influence of metformin use on PSA values, free-to-total PSA, prostate cancer incidence and grade and overall survival in a prospective screening trial (ERSPC Aarau). *World J. Urol.* 33 (8): 1189–1196.

46 Margel, D., Urbach, D., Lipscombe, L.L. et al. (2013). Association between metformin use and risk of prostate cancer and its grade. *J. Natl Cancer Inst.* 105 (15): 1123–1131.

47 Margel, D., Urbach, D.R., Lipscombe, L.L. et al. (2013). Metformin use and all-cause and prostate cancer-specific mortality among men with diabetes. *J. Clin. Oncol.* 31 (25): 3069–3075.

48 Preston, M.A., Riis, A.H., Ehrenstein, V. et al. (2014). Metformin use and prostate cancer risk. *Eur. Urol.* 66 (6): 1012–1020.

49 Decensi, A., Puntoni, M., Goodwin, P. et al. (2010). Metformin and cancer risk in diabetic patients: A systematic review and meta-analysis. *Cancer Prev. Res.* 3 (11): 1451–1461.

50 Gandini, S., Puntoni, M., Heckman-Stoddard, B.M. et al. (2014). Metformin and cancer risk and mortality: A systematic review and meta-analysis taking into account biases and confounders. *Cancer Prev. Res.* 7 (9): 867–885.

51 Chang, S.L., Harshman, L.C., and Presti, J.C., Jr. (2010). Impact of common medications on serum total prostate-specific antigen levels: Analysis of the National Health and Nutrition Examination Survey. *J. Clin. Oncol.* 28 (25): 3951–3957.

52 Wang, C., Tao, W., Wang, Y. et al. (2010). Rosuvastatin, identified from a zebrafish chemical genetic screen for antiangiogenic compounds, suppresses the growth of prostate cancer. *Eur. Urol.* 58 (3): 418–426.

53 Jespersen, C.G., Norgaard, M., Friis, S. et al. (2014). Statin use and risk of prostate cancer: A Danish population-based case-control study, 1997–2010. *Cancer Epidemiol.* 38 (1): 42–47.

54 Platz, E.A., Tangen, C.M., Goodman, P.J. et al. (2014). Statin drug use is not associated with prostate cancer risk in men who are regularly screened. *J. Urol.* 192 (2): 379–384.

55 Freedland, S.J., Hamilton, R.J., Gerber, L. et al. (2013). Statin use and risk of prostate cancer and high-grade prostate cancer: Results from the REDUCE study. *Prostate Cancer Prostatic Dis.* 16 (3): 254–259.

56 Platz, E.A., Leitzmann, M.F., Visvanathan, K. et al. (2006). Statin drugs and risk of advanced prostate cancer. *J. Natl Cancer Inst.* 98 (24): 1819–1825.

57 The Alpha-Tocopherol, Beta Carotene Cancer Prevention Study Group (1994). The effect of vitamin E and beta carotene on the incidence of lung cancer and other cancers in male smokers. *N. Engl. J. Med.* 330 (15): 1029–1035.

58 Clark, L.C., Combs, G.F., Jr., Turnbull, B.W. et al. (1996). Effects of selenium supplementation for cancer prevention in patients with carcinoma of the skin: A randomized controlled trial. Nutritional Prevention of Cancer Study Group. *JAMA* 276 (24): 1957–1963.

59 Lippman, S.M., Klein, E.A., Goodman, P.J. et al. (2009). Effect of selenium and vitamin E on risk of prostate cancer and other cancers: The Selenium and Vitamin E Cancer Prevention Trial (SELECT). *JAMA* 301 (1): 39–51.

60 Klein, E.A., Thompson, I.M., Jr., Tangen, C.M. et al. (2011). Vitamin E and the risk of prostate cancer: The Selenium and Vitamin E Cancer Prevention Trial (SELECT). *JAMA* 306 (14): 1549–1556.

61 Marshall, J.R., Tangen, C.M., Sakr, W.A. et al. (2011). Phase III trial of selenium to prevent prostate cancer in men with high-grade prostatic intraepithelial neoplasia: SWOG S9917. *Cancer Prev. Res.* 4 (11): 1761–1769.

62 Kristal, A.R., Darke, A.K., Morris, J.S. et al. (2014). Baseline selenium status and effects of selenium and vitamin E supplementation on prostate cancer risk. *J. Natl Cancer Inst.* 106 (3): djt456.

63 Albanes, D., Till, C., Klein, E.A. et al. (2014). Plasma tocopherols and risk of prostate cancer in the Selenium and Vitamin E Cancer Prevention Trial (SELECT). *Cancer Prev. Res.* 7 (9): 886–895.

64 Greenwald, P. (2001). From carcinogenesis to clinical interventions for cancer prevention. *Toxicology* 166 (1–2): 37–45.

65 Bostwick, D.G., and Qian, J. (2001). Effect of androgen deprivation therapy on prostatic intraepithelial neoplasia. *Urology* 58 (2, Suppl. 1): 91–93.

66 Kelloff, G.J., Sigman, C.C., Hawk, E.T. et al. (2001). Surrogate end-point biomarkers in chemopreventive drug development. *IARC Scientific Publications* 154: 13–26.

67 Hanahan, D., and Weinberg, R.A. (2011). Hallmarks of cancer: The next generation. *Cell* 144 (5): 646–674.

68 De Marzo, A.M., Marchi, V.L., Epstein, J.I., and Nelson, W.G. (1999). Proliferative inflammatory atrophy of the prostate: Implications for prostatic carcinogenesis. *Am. J. Pathol.* 155 (6): 1985–1992.

69 Sooriakumaran, P. (2006). Management of prostate cancer. Part 1: Chemoprevention. *Expert Rev. Anticancer Ther.* 6 (3): 419–425.

70 Urban, D., Myers, R., Manne, U. et al. (1999). Evaluation of biomarker modulation by fenretinide in prostate cancer patients. *Eur. Urol.* 35 (5–6): 429–438.

71 Sakr, W.A., and Partin, A.W. (2001). Histological markers of risk and the role of high-grade prostatic intraepithelial neoplasia. *Urology* 57 (4, Suppl. 1): 115–120.

72 Ploussard, G., Plennevaux, G., Allory, Y. et al. (2009). High-grade prostatic intraepithelial neoplasia and atypical small acinar proliferation on initial 21-core extended biopsy scheme: Incidence and implications for patient care and surveillance. *World J. Urol.* 27 (5): 587–592.

73 Taneja, S.S., Morton, R., Barnette, G. et al. (2013). Prostate cancer diagnosis among men with isolated high-grade intraepithelial neoplasia enrolled onto a 3-year prospective phase III clinical trial of oral toremifene. *J. Clin. Oncol.* 31 (5): 523–529.

74 UT Health Science Center SA (2006). Prostate Cancer Prevention Trial Risk Calculator Version 2.0. http://deb.uthscsa.edu/URORiskCalc/Pages/uroriskcalc.jsp (accessed 26 January 2015).

75 Algotar, A.M., Stratton, M.S., Ahmann, F.R. et al. (2013). Phase 3 clinical trial investigating the effect of selenium supplementation in men at high-risk for prostate cancer. *Prostate* 73 (3): 328–335.

76 Smith, P.H. (1990). The case for no initial treatment of localized prostate cancer. *Urol. Clin. N. Am.* 17 (4): 827–834.

77 Lu-Yao, G.L., Albertsen, P.C., Moore, D.F. et al. (2009). Outcomes of localized prostate cancer following conservative management. *JAMA* 302 (11): 1202–1209.

78 Carter, H.B., Kettermann, A., Warlick, C. et al. (2007). Expectant management of prostate cancer with curative intent: An update of the Johns Hopkins experience. *J. Urol.* 178 (6): 2359–2364; discussion 64–65.

79 Klotz, L., Vesprini, D., Sethukavalan, P. et al. (2015). Long-term follow-up of a large active surveillance cohort of patients with prostate cancer. *J. Clin. Oncol.* 33 (3): 272–277.

80 Xia, J., Trock, B.J., Cooperberg, M.R. et al. (2012). Prostate cancer mortality following active surveillance versus immediate radical prostatectomy. *Clin. Cancer Res.* 18 (19): 5471–5478.

81 Welty, C.J., Cowan, J.E., Nguyen, H. et al. (2014). Extended followup and risk factors for disease reclassification in a large active surveillance cohort for localized prostate cancer. *J. Urol.* 193 (3): 807–811.

82 Singer, E.A., Kaushal, A., Turkbey, B. et al. (20120. Active surveillance for prostate cancer: Past, present and future. *Curr. Opin. Oncol.* 24 (3): 243–250.

83 Ganz, P.A., Barry, J.M., Burke, W. et al. (2011). NIH State-of-the-Science Conference Statement: Role of active surveillance in the management of men with localized prostate cancer. *NIH Consensus and State-of-the-Science Statements* 28 (1): 1–27.

84 Fleshner, N.E., Lucia, M.S., Egerdie, B. et al. (2012). Dutasteride in localised prostate cancer management: The REDEEM randomised, double-blind, placebo-controlled trial. *Lancet* 379 (9821): 1103–1111.

85 Centre for Cancer Prevention (2015). PROVENT: A randomised, double blind, placebo controlled feasibility study to examine the clinical effectiveness of aspirin and/or Vitamin D3 to prevent disease progression in men on active surveillance for prostate cancer. ISRCTN91422391. http://www.isrctn.com/ISRCTN91422391 (accessed 3 January 2018).

86 Stratton, M.S., Algotar, A.M., Ranger-Moore, J. et al. (2010). Oral selenium supplementation has no effect on prostate-specific antigen velocity in men undergoing active surveillance for localized prostate cancer. *Cancer Prev. Res.* 3 (8): 1035–1043.

87 Chan, J.M., Weinberg, V., Magbanua, M.J. et al. (2011). Nutritional supplements, COX-2 and IGF-1 expression in men on active surveillance for prostate cancer. *Cancer Causes Control* 22 (1): 141–150.

88 Kumar, N.B., Krischer, J.P., Allen, K. et al. (2007). A Phase II randomized, placebo-controlled clinical trial of purified isoflavones in modulating steroid hormones in men diagnosed with localized prostate cancer. *Nutr. Cancer* 59 (2): 163–168.

89 Thomas, R., Williams, M., Sharma, H. et al. (2014). A double-blind, placebo-controlled randomised trial evaluating the effect of a polyphenol-rich whole food supplement on PSA progression in men with prostate cancer: The U.K. NCRN Pomi-T study. *Prostate Cancer Prostatic Dis.* 17 (2): 180–186.

90 Adhami, V.M., Siddiqui, I.A., Syed, D.N. et al. (2012). Oral infusion of pomegranate fruit extract inhibits prostate carcinogenesis in the TRAMP model. *Carcinogenesis* 33 (3): 644–651.

91 Paller, C.J., Ye, X., Wozniak, P.J. et al. (2013). A randomized phase II study of pomegranate extract for men with rising PSA following initial therapy for localized prostate cancer. *Prostate Cancer Prostatic Dis.* 16 (1): 50–55.

92 Ozten-Kandas, N., and Bosland, M.C. (2011). Chemoprevention of prostate cancer: Natural compounds, antiandrogens, and antioxidants – in vivo evidence. *J. Carcinog.* 10: 27.

93 Phillips, J.G., Aizer, A.A., Chen, M.H. et al. (2014). The effect of differing Gleason scores at biopsy on the odds of upgrading and the risk of death from prostate cancer. *Clin. Genitourin Cancer* 12 (5): e181–e187.

94 Wu, Y., Zu, K., Warren, M.A. et al. (2006). Delineating the mechanism by which selenium deactivates Akt in prostate cancer cells. *Mol. Cancer Ther.* 5 (2): 246–252.

95 Sabichi, A.L., Lee, J.J., Taylor, R.J. et al. (2006). Selenium accumulation in prostate tissue during a randomized, controlled short-term trial of l-selenomethionine: A Southwest Oncology Group Study. *Clin. Cancer Res.* 12 (7, Part 1): 2178–2184.

96 Nguyen, M.M., Ahmann, F.R., Nagle, R.B. et al. (2012). Randomized, double-blind, placebo-controlled trial of polyphenon E in prostate cancer patients before prostatectomy: Evaluation of potential chemopreventive activities. *Cancer Prev. Res.* 5 (2): 290–298.

97 Gee, J., Bailey, H., Kim, K. et al. (2013). Phase II open label, multi-center clinical trial of modulation of intermediate endpoint biomarkers by 1alpha-hydroxyvitamin D2 in patients with clinically localized prostate cancer and high grade pin. *Prostate* 73 (9): 970–978.

98 Simoneau, A.R., Gerner, E.W., Phung, M. et al. (2001). Alpha-difluoromethylornithine and polyamine levels in the human prostate: Results of a phase IIa trial. *J. Natl Cancer Inst.* 93 (1): 57–59.

CHAPTER 13

Population screening for prostate cancer

Richard J. Bryant[1], Monique J. Roobol[2], and Freddie C. Hamdy[1]

[1] *Nuffield Department of Surgical Sciences, Oxford Cancer Research Centre, University of Oxford; Department of Urology, Oxford University Hospitals NHS Foundation Trust, Oxford, UK*
[2] *Erasmus University Medical Center, Rotterdam, Netherlands*

SUMMARY BOX

- Screening for prostate cancer with repeat PSA-testing has been demonstrated to reduce mortality and the metastatic burden of this disease in European studies, but causes unnecessary over-detection and over-treatment.

- Screening with a single PSA-test followed by transrectal ultrasound guided biopsies failed to demonstrate survival advantage at an average 10-year follow-up in a large UK-based study.

- In view of the adverse balance of risks versus benefits, PSA screening for prostate cancer is not currently a recommended public health policy for the general population.

- There are early data which suggest that targeted prostate-specific antigen (PSA) screening in men with rare germline mutations which confer higher prostate cancer risks (particularly *BRCA2* mutation carriers) identifies a higher proportion of intermediate- and high-risk prostate cancer than population PSA screening programmes. This is addressed further in Chapter 27.

- It is possible that in the near future refinements to the screening protocol, such as targeted screening of high-risk individuals and incorporation of new adjuncts such as kallikrein markers and pre-biopsy multiparametric magnetic resonance imaging, may improve the ratio of risks to benefits from screening, such that its uptake may become acceptable from a public health perspective.

Screening for prostate cancer (PCa) remains one of the most controversial issues in urological practice. Although the last few years have seen robust data emerge from the European Randomized Study of Screening for Prostate Cancer (ERSPC) suggesting a clear survival benefit for prostate-specific antigen (PSA)–based PCa screening [1,2], the benefit-to-risk ratio has not yet become acceptable for it to be adopted as public health policy. More recently, results from the Cluster

---

Cancer Prevention and Screening: Concepts, Principles and Controversies, First Edition.
Edited by Rosalind A. Eeles, Christine D. Berg, and Jeffrey S. Tobias.
© 2019 John Wiley & Sons, Inc. Published 2019 by John Wiley & Sons, Inc.

randomized trial of PSA-testing for Prostate cancer (CAP) showed no evidence of survival benefit at a median of 10-y follow-up using a single PSA-test followed by transrectal ultrasound (TRUS) guided biopsies [3]. Further refinements to screening strategies are needed for it to become acceptable to the general population and health-care providers. This chapter outlines several of the issues pertinent to screening for this common malignancy, and summarizes the available and rapidly emerging new evidence along with potential refinements that may enhance its acceptability in the future.

Screening

Screening is defined by the World Health Organization as 'the use of simple tests across a healthy population to identify individuals who have a disease but as yet have no symptoms'. The aim of any screening programme is to identify a disease during its early stages when it can be cured by treatment. Early PCa can be diagnosed using PSA testing followed by a prostate biopsy, and it can be cured by a number of interventions, including radical prostatectomy, radical radiotherapy, brachytherapy, and a number of emerging minimally invasive focal or partially ablative therapies. However, despite the successes of radical intervention for early localized PCa, there are concerns regarding the 'overdetection' and 'overtreatment' of 'low-risk' PCa cases which are unlikely to pose a threat to life if left undiagnosed or untreated [4]. Indeed, in the USA there has been a call to stop PCa screening based on the potential harms such a programme may cause [5]. A significant challenge for any population-based PCa screening programme is to identify 'clinically significant' or 'high-risk' early, curable cases of PCa in men who are likely to benefit from radical treatment, without overdetecting 'indolent' or 'low-risk' cases which may be subject to 'overtreatment' with no survival benefit, but with intervention-associated morbidity [6,7] such as erectile dysfunction and urinary incontinence.

In 1968, Wilson and Jungner [8] identified several criteria which need to be met by any screening programme in order for it to be acceptable in the general population (Table 13.1). Each of these criteria is discussed below with particular emphasis on PCa.

Table 13.1 Requirements of a screening programme.

- The disease is an important health problem
- The natural history of the disease is well known
- The disease can be recognized at an early stage
- Treatment of the disease at an early stage is advantageous
- A suitable diagnostic test exists
- The diagnostic test is acceptable
- Adequate facilities exist to deal with any abnormalities detected by the test
- Screening is done at repeated intervals when the onset is insidious
- The chance of harm from screening is less than the chance of benefit
- The cost of screening is balanced against the benefits

The malignancy should be an important health problem

PCa is the most commonly diagnosed malignancy in men in the Western world, and the second leading cause of male cancer-related death. In Europe alone during 2012, 416 732 new PCa cases were diagnosed, and 92 247 men died from this disease [9]. Since the introduction of PSA testing in the 1980s [10], there has been a large rise in the incidence of PCa due to increased detection of the latent pool of largely asymptomatic cases. In recent years, improvements in the mortality rates from PCa have been observed [11]; however, while part of this improvement may be due to earlier detection of cases, other factors such as increasingly effective therapies and resources to treat this condition may have contributed to improved outcomes [12]. Concerns have been raised recently regarding other complex issues such as overdetection of PCa and overtreatment [4]. Each of these issues has implications for the introduction of a population-based PCa screening programme. It is therefore clear that PCa is an important health problem in several respects, including the frequency of diagnosis, the variable risks of progression of individual cases, and the importance of tailoring treatment to the individual.

The natural history of PCa needs to be well understood

In recent years, understanding of the natural history of PCa has improved, but less is known about the natural history of screen-detected cases. The majority of PCa cases detectable through PSA-based screening represent low- or intermediate-risk disease from within the reservoir of latent PCa in the general population of adult men. The vast majority of these screen-detected cases may never become lethal during an individual's lifetime. However, there is compelling evidence from the ERSPC trial that PSA-based screening for PCa can yield a significant survival benefit, albeit at the cost of exposing large numbers of men to screening and radical treatment for each life saved. The contemporary challenge is for screening programmes to detect exclusively the 'clinically significant' or 'high-risk' cases of PCa, which may need treatment in order to prevent PCa-associated deaths, while avoiding the detection of 'clinically insignificant' or 'indolent' cases, which currently constitute overdetection or overdiagnosis. These clinically insignificant cases could either be managed conservatively through strategies such as active surveillance, without having adverse effects on quality of life, or preferably not be detected, thereby reducing the anxiety of a cancer diagnosis in men who are very unlikely to come to harm from their relatively indolent malignancy.

PCa is a very heterogeneous malignancy, and it is becoming increasingly apparent that our definition of significant versus insignificant PCa is inadequate [13]. Indeed, PCa patients may harbour several independent foci of PCa [14], one of which might be the 'index lesion' [15], and it is crucial that any PCa screening programme identifies this particular focus of disease, with less emphasis on the more indolent lesions. Moreover, although in recent years a great deal of research effort has identified germline mutations and single-nucleotide polymorphisms, some of which are reported to be associated with clinically aggressive or significant disease, little has yet reached standard clinical practice. New data now suggest that the original definition of insignificant PCa warrants re-evaluation [13]. A landmark recent case report using whole-genome sequencing of metachronous lesions in one individual patient suggests that our ability to accurately assign a risk category to cases of localized disease through histological evaluation of biopsied material, PSA, and clinical examination may be suboptimal [16], given that the clone of metastatic lethal cells in this case arose in a small low-grade focus of PCa rather than within a larger adjacent higher-grade focus (which would ordinarily have been defined as the index lesion). This suggests that our understanding of the natural history of PCa is not sufficiently adequate for clinicians to safely reassure all men with apparent low-risk disease based on PSA, histology of biopsy specimens, and digital rectal examination (DRE), that they do not need radical intervention. Longstanding assumptions about the natural history of localized PCa and its evolution to metastatic disease are now being challenged through cutting-edge studies of novel molecular signatures, and warrant further investigation.

Effective treatments for PCa should be available

The recently published Melbourne Consensus Statement on Prostate Cancer Testing has advocated that the processes of PCa diagnosis and intervention need to be uncoupled, in recognition of the fact that many men with PCa do not necessarily need active treatment [7]. Men with early localized PCa have a number of management options, including active surveillance for low-volume, low-risk disease and therapeutic intervention for clinically significant disease. Despite the available evidence suggesting that active surveillance is a safe alternative to radical therapy for men with low-volume, low-risk disease, this option continues to be underused in several countries, including the US [17,18], because of the lack of reliable protocols. Active treatment options for clinically significant PCa include radical prostatectomy, radical radiotherapy, or brachytherapy, and several novel therapies currently undergoing clinical evaluation, such as focal therapy or partial ablation of the prostate, which appear to be promising but require further careful evaluation before widespread uptake. In the UK, the ProtecT (Prostate Testing for Cancer and Treatment) trial is currently the world's largest ongoing RCT testing treatment effectiveness of the three treatment options in PSA-detected disease. A 10-year median follow-up, clinical outcomes have shown that active monitoring (a surveillance programme) or radical treatment in localized prostate cancer have similar disease-specific survivals (~99%) irrespective of treatment allocated at 10-y median follow-up [19]. However, radical treatments reduced the rate of disease progression and metastasis by half compared with active monitoring, 55% of men on active monitoring received a radical intervention, and 44% avoided side-effects of treatments [20]. The CAP trial (Cluster randomised triAl of PSA testing for Prostate cancer), within which ProtecT is embedded, is a UK-wide primary care–based RCT investigating the clinical and cost-effectiveness of PSA testing of men aged 50–69 years [21]. Over 415 000 men from 573 primary care practices across the UK have been successfully recruited into CAP, making it the largest study of PSA-based PCa screening to date. Findings at 10-y median follow up showed no difference in survival using a single PSA-test followed by TRUS biopsies. Low-risk disease detection was higher in the intervention group than in the controls, but the single PSA-test failed to identify many of the lethal prostate cancers. This demonstrates the inadequacy of a single PSA test as a screening tool, warranting different approaches to the prostate cancer diagnostic pathway, such as the addition of imaging in the form of multparametric magnetic resonance imaging prior to biopsy.

The forthcoming PREFERE clinical trial aims to confirm the noninferiority of cancer-specific survival after external-beam radiotherapy, brachytherapy, or active surveillance compared with radical prostatectomy for men with 'early intermediate' PCa [22]. The best currently available published evidence from observational studies suggests that radical surgery might confer a survival advantage compared with radical radiotherapy in clinically significant disease [23], and it is known that high-volume PCa surgeons are associated with better oncological outcomes than their low-volume counterparts [24]. While there is clear evidence that radical surgery significantly improves disease-specific mortality when compared with watchful waiting for clinically detected PCa [25], this finding may not be applicable to screen-detected PCa, which generally comprises lower-volume and lower-risk cases than those detected clinically. The emerging concept of focal therapy, or partial ablation of the prostate, using new technologies such as high-intensity focused ultrasound, radiofrequency ablation, cryotherapy, and vascular-targeted therapy, is gaining popularity and may represent an acceptable alternative to radical intervention in men with an index lesion who do not wish to undergo active surveillance [15]. In the future it is possible that the best hopes for cure of men with clinically significant localized PCa, without causing overtreatment, will be through precision medicine with thorough and accurate molecular profiling of each individual focus of PCa, in order to determine its potential aggressiveness and predict its behaviour if left untreated, followed by selection of the optimal clinical management based on validated risk calculators.

The screening test should be acceptable

An ideal screening test should be safe and acceptable to perform well in large numbers of asymptomatic individuals, and should have high sensitivity, specificity, positive predictive, and negative predictive values. PSA testing of asymptomatic individuals has been in clinical use since the late 1980s [10] and is widespread in the USA and many other Western countries. While PSA has a reasonable sensitivity, it lacks specificity and therefore is not a perfect screening test for PCa [26,27]. Ideally, due to the variations in the PSA test result, patients should undergo a repeat test in order to confirm that the PSA is truly elevated before they undergo a prostate biopsy [28]. The Prostate Cancer Prevention Trial demonstrated that there is no true 'normal' threshold for PSA below which a risk of PCa can be excluded [29]. Conversely, a raised PSA does not always imply the presence of a focus of PCa, but might occur due to a number of benign pathologies, such as benign prostatic hyperplasia or a urinary tract infection [30]. While the ERSPC used a threshold of 3 ng/ml in the setting of a large RCT of population-based screening, the ideal threshold of PSA for such a public health programme remains unclear. Moreover, the optimal screening interval for individuals within such a programme remains to be determined. Despite these caveats, recent data support the conception that PSA testing in men in young middle age might identify individuals with the greatest risk of developing life-threatening PCa many decades later, and in whom focused intensive screening in later years may yield the greatest benefits, while, equally importantly, it may reassure others at low risk of lethal PCa that they may be suitable for less frequent testing [31]. Clearly, there is no 'one-size-fits-all' approach for screening large populations of asymptomatic men, and individual algorithms are likely to represent the way ahead.

Tests other than standard PSA, such as urinary PCA3 ribonucleic acid measurement, may be available for screening; however, this particular test requires a DRE and prostate massage [32], and is unlikely to be acceptable to the general male population for use as a screening test. In recent years, evidence has emerged to suggest that a combination of four kallikreins (free PSA, intact PSA, total PSA, and human kallikrein 2), with or without concomitant DRE, may be more accurate than standard PSA testing in identifying clinically significant PCa, and that simultaneously these assays have the capability to reduce the number of negative biopsies by approximately one half [30]. The Prostate Health Index (phi), which uses the formula ([-2]proPSA/freePSA x √totalPSA), has been Food and Drug Administration (FDA) approved for PCa diagnosis, and may also help to identify clinically significant cases while reducing overdetection [30]. The use of such tests within a screening programme may make it more acceptable than is currently the case using PSA testing alone, and requires formal evaluation in prospective studies.

While previous research has focused on the identification of a single biomarker or panel of tests to replace PSA testing, it has become increasingly clear that such an approach is unlikely to find a better test for some considerable time, at least within the context of a PCa screening programme. Promising data have been published regarding the use of nomograms as risk prediction tools, combining the use of a number of different markers along with age and DRE findings. It is likely that the use of combinations of biomarkers, utilizing the advantages of each of their individual positive characteristics, will be the way forward for the foreseeable future, rather than attempting to replace PSA as the best test for screening.

When considering the acceptability of PCa screening, it should be remembered that potential identified abnormalities such as a raised PSA, 4-kallikrein, or phi assay, or an abnormal DRE, may potentially lead to a prostate biopsy, which with associated risks of complications [33,34]. There is increasing enthusiasm for the use of pre-biopsy multiparametric magnetic resonance imaging (mpMRI) in order to identify or exclude significant lesions [35], and MRI-transrectal ultrasound (TRUS) fused image-guided biopsies [36]. This could also help the development of effective focal or partially ablative therapy with organ preservation if the tumour and patient characteristics are suitable [37]. Two recent studies demonstrated the superiority of targeted biopsies of mpMRI-detected lesions over conventional transrectal ultrasound guided biopsy protocols. Both studies, PROMIS and PRECISION have demonstrated that when mpMRI lesions only are targeted, as many as 28% of men with a raised PSA can avoid a biopsy, over-detection of low-risk cancers is reduced, and the diagnosis of significant cancer is increased, compared with TRUS-guided systematic biopsies. This will produce a paradigm shift in the prostate cancer diagnostic pathway, and is likely to contribute to a significant reduction in over-detection of low-risk disease, although a small proportion of men with higher-risk disease may escape the diagnosis with unknown consequences [38,39].

Adequate facilities should be available to deal with any abnormalities detected

Men with an abnormality detected at the initial PCa screening evaluation will need to undergo further investigations, and full facilities and expertise will be required to deal with such investigations, and to treat the conditions diagnosed. To date, the next investigation following an abnormal PSA test has usually been a TRUS-guided prostate biopsy, which is usually performed under local anaesthesia and antibiotic cover. The performance of population-based PSA testing followed by TRUS biopsy has been examined in several multicentre prospective RCTs. With recent data on the superiority of mpMRI, it is evident that TRUS-guided biopsies as a reflex intervention following a raised PSA will become antiquated. Resources will be required to deal adequately with false negative biopsies and an increase in mpMRI scans. Screening protocols will have to manage lesions such as multifocal high-grade prostatic intraepithelial neoplasia or atypical small acinar proliferation, both of which are known to be associated with concomitant foci of adenocarcinoma of the prostate [40].

The benefits of screening should exceed the harms

A key aim of PCa screening is to reduce morbidity and mortality and to improve quality of life of men with this malignancy. There is evidence, however, that screening for PCa may cause harm (Table 13.2). One commonly described effect of PCa screening is the overdetection of a large number of cases of clinically low-risk disease. In recent years it has been recommended that these cases might be safely managed by active surveillance, keeping the patient within a closely monitored 'window of curability', while avoiding side effects of radical treatment [41] such as erectile dysfunction and urinary incontinence. The conception of active surveillance is based on the assumption that such cases of low-risk, low-volume PCa are very unlikely to progress, and that if this occurs it can be detected by PSA surveillance and regular repeat prostate biopsies. Very few men on an active surveillance programme die from PCa [41], although over time, reported series suggest that over one-third of men on active surveillance protocol decide to undergo active treatment for a variety of reasons, not necessarily related to disease progression.

Table 13.2 Effects of prostate cancer (PCa) screening.

Benefits	Adverse effects
• Prevention of PCa-related deaths	• Need to attend screening and associated anxiety
• Gain of life-years for those with curable and/or treatable disease	• False-positive results and unnecessary biopsies and biopsy-related morbidity
• Reduction in the number of prostate biopsies with a negative result outside screening	• Increase in life-years and extended morbidity post-diagnosis without an increase in survival ('lead-time bias')
• Prevention of advanced metastatic PCa	• Potential 'overdetection' of 'indolent low-risk' PCa, possibly resulting in men receiving unnecessary treatment for lesions which might otherwise have never become harmful
• Avoidance of morbidity and expense of late-stage treatment (e.g. adverse systemic effects of androgen-deprivation therapy)	• Labelling an asymptomatic man with indolent 'low-risk' PCa as a 'cancer patient'
• Reassurance of a 'negative' test or 'low-risk' estimation of 'clinically significant' disease	• Potential exposure to radical 'overtreatment'
• Psychological advantage of avoiding radical treatment	• False reassurance of a 'negative' screening test result, leading to failure to present when symptoms occur, and subsequent delayed diagnosis
	• Economic costs associated with the screening process and with treating the additional PCa cases identified

It is important that men are appropriately informed of the issues and uncertainties regarding PCa screening, and that they do not undergo testing without formal counseling. It is also important not to screen men who are unlikely to benefit, such as the elderly [42], or those with other advanced malignancies or limited life expectancy [43]. It may be more appropriate to use higher PSA cut-off levels for older men [44,45] and, while it has been suggested that screening should perhaps be stopped at the age of 70 years [1,6], the key aspect is a man's life expectancy, and less than 10 years is generally considered to be a reasonable point at which to discontinue screening. The quality-of-life effects of PCa screening have been evaluated [46] and, based on recent calculations, 56 quality-adjusted life years are gained from screening per 1000 men screened through protocols of repeat PSA-testing. It has been estimated that without PCa screening there would be a threefold increase in the rates of diagnosis of metastatic PCa [47], while other evidence suggests that screening has led to a 70% reduction in advanced disease in the USA [48]. At present, however, the introduction of a population PSA-based PCa screening programme is unjustified due to the potential overdetection and possible overtreatment of diagnosed cases. Before PCa screening can be introduced by health-care providers, further evaluation of the associated costs, screening protocols, and quality-of-life issues is required.

Future developments

The fact that the ERSPC has clearly demonstrated that PCa screening can reduce the future development of advanced metastatic disease [2] is a strong argument for the introduction of screening. It is likely that the screening process will be further refined through the risk stratification of men at the introduction of the screening process, taking into consideration factors such as family history, race, life expectancy, and baseline PSA level [49], with the subsequent screening protocol modified for individuals based on these risk factors. Other improvements in PSA-based screening may be brought about by incorporating multivariate risk prediction tools [50,51], given that it is now clear that PSA is both a diagnostic and a prognostic marker [31,52]. The frequency with which men may need to be screened may also be influenced by their initial PSA test result within a screening programme protocol [6,53]. Other developments in the contemporary PCa diagnosis pathway, such as the introduction of mpMRI, are also likely to have a significant impact on the exact algorithm of a PCa screening protocol and need formal evaluation. Other future developments are likely to influence the ratio of risks and benefits in favour of the introduction of screening in due course [54]. There are recent data that combine the use of genetic markers and biomarkers in a population-based cohort in Sweden (the Stockholm III Study), which has reduced the numbers of biopsies needed and increased the proportion of high-risk cancers detected [55].

Conclusion

PCa screening remains a topical and controversial public health issue. Although it is clear that PSA-based PCa screening can save lives and reduce the burden of advanced metastatic disease, in its present form PSA-based testing is unsuitable for population-based screening. Refinements to the PCa screening programme [53], along with novel adjuncts such as the use of additional kallikrein markers, targeted screening, and the introduction of mpMRI, may improve the performance of a screening protocol such that the benefits may be increased and the risks reduced. Meanwhile, a well-informed man should consider carefully the potential consequences of a PSA test, the uncertainties surrounding its treatment, and the trade-off between early detection, side-effects of interventions and possible benefits in improving survival and disease progression.

References

1 Schroder, F.H., Hugosson, J., Roobol, M.J. et al. (2014). Screening and prostate cancer mortality: Results of the European Randomised Study of Screening for Prostate Cancer (ERSPC) at 13 years of follow-up. *Lancet* 384 (9959): 2027–2035.

2 Schroder, F.H., Hugosson, J., Carlsson, S. et al. (2012). Screening for prostate cancer decreases the risk of developing metastatic disease: Findings from the European Randomized Study of Screening for Prostate Cancer (ERSPC). *Eur. Urol.* 62 (5): 745–752.

3 Martin, R.M. et al. (2018). Effect of a Low-Intensity PSA-Based Screening Intervention on Prostate Cancer Mortality: The CAP Randomized Clinical Trial. *JAMA* 319: 883–895, doi:10.1001/jama.2018.0154.

4 Loeb, S., Bjurlin, M.A., Nicholson, J. et al. (2014). Overdiagnosis and overtreatment of prostate cancer. *Eur. Urol.* 65 (6): 1046–1055.

5 Moyer, V.A.; Force USPST (2012). Screening for prostate cancer: U.S. Preventive Services Task Force recommendation statement. *Ann. Intern. Med.* 157 (2): 120–134.

6 Heidenreich, A., Bastian, P.J., Bellmunt, J. et al. (2014). EAU guidelines on prostate cancer. Part 1: Screening, diagnosis, and local treatment with curative intent – update 2013. *Eur. Urol.* 65 (1): 124–137.

7 Murphy, D.G., Ahlering, T., Catalona, W.J. et al. (2014). The Melbourne Consensus Statement on the early detection of prostate cancer. *BJU Int.* 113 (2): 186–188.

8 Wilson, J.M., and Jungner, Y.G. (1968). Principles and practice of mass screening for disease [in Spanish]. *Bol. Oficina Sanit. Panam.* 65 (4): 281–393.

9 Ferlay, J., Steliarova-Foucher, E., Lortet-Tieulent, J. et al. (2013). Cancer incidence and mortality patterns in Europe: Estimates for 40 countries in 2012. *Eur. J. Cancer* 49 (6): 1374–1403.

10 Stamey, T.A., Yang, N., Hay, A.R. et al. (1987). Prostate-specific antigen as a serum marker for adenocarcinoma of the prostate. *N. Engl. J. Med.* 317 (15): 909–916.

11 Siegel, R., DeSantis, C., Virgo, K. et al. (2012). Cancer treatment and survivorship statistics, 2012. *CA Cancer J. Clin.* 62 (4): 220–241.

12 Etzioni, R., Tsodikov, A., Mariotto, A. et al. (2008). Quantifying the role of PSA screening in the US prostate cancer mortality decline. *Cancer Causes Control* 19 (2): 175–181.

13 Van der Kwast, T.H., and Roobol, M.J. (2013). Defining the threshold for significant versus insignificant prostate cancer. *Nature Rev. Urol.* 10 (8): 473–482.

14 Arora, R., Koch, M.O., Eble, J.N. et al. (2004). Heterogeneity of Gleason grade in multifocal adenocarcinoma of the prostate. *Cancer* 100 (11): 2362–2366.

15 Ahmed, H.U. (2009). The index lesion and the origin of prostate cancer. *N. Engl. J. Med.* 361 (17): 1704–1706.

16 Haffner, M.C., Mosbruger, T., Esopi, D.M. et al. (2013). Tracking the clonal origin of lethal prostate cancer. *J. Clin. Invest.* 123 (11): 4918–4922.

17 Cooperberg, M.R. (2014). Progress in management of low-risk prostate cancer: How registries may change the world. *Eur. Urol.* 67 (1): 51–52.

18 Cooperberg, M.R., Broering, J.M., and Carroll, P.R. (2010). Time trends and local variation in primary treatment of localized prostate cancer. *J. Clin. Oncol.* 28 (7): 1117–1123.

19 Hamdy, F.C., Donovan, J.L., Lane J.A. et al. for the ProtecT Study Group (2016). 10-year outcomes after monitoring, surgery, or radiotherapy for localized prostate cancer. *N. Engl. J. Med.* 375: 1415–1424.

20 D'Amico, A.V. (2016). Treatment or monitoring for early prostate cancer. *N. Engl. J. Med.* 375: 1482–1483.

21 Turner, E.L., Metcalfe, C., Donovan, J.L. et al. (2014). Design and preliminary recruitment results of the Cluster randomised triAl of PSA testing for Prostate cancer (CAP). *Br. J. Cancer* 110 (12): 2829–2836.

22 Wiegel, T., Stockle, M., and Bartkowiak, D. (2014). PREFEREnce-based randomized evaluation of treatment modalities in low or early intermediate-risk prostate cancer. *Eur. Urol.* 67 (1): 1–2.

23 Sooriakumaran, P., Nyberg, T., Akre, O. et al. (2014). Comparative effectiveness of radical prostatectomy and radiotherapy in prostate cancer: Observational study of mortality outcomes. *BMJ* 348: g1502.

24 Vickers, A., Savage, C., Bianco, F. et al. (2011). Cancer control and functional outcomes after radical prostatectomy as markers of surgical quality: Analysis of heterogeneity between surgeons at a single cancer center. *Eur. Urol.* 59 (3): 317–322.

25 Bill-Axelson, A., Holmberg, L., Ruutu, M. et al. (2005). Radical prostatectomy versus watchful waiting in early prostate cancer. *N. Engl. J. Med.* 352 (19): 1977–1984.

26 Catalona, W.J., Partin, A.W., Slawin, K.M. et al. (1998). Use of the percentage of free prostate-specific antigen to enhance differentiation of prostate cancer from benign prostatic disease: A prospective multicenter clinical trial. *JAMA* 279 (19): 1542–1547.

27 Holmstrom, B., Johansson, M., Bergh, A. et al. (2009). Prostate specific antigen for early detection of prostate cancer: Longitudinal study. *BMJ* 339: b3537.

28 Eastham, J.A., Riedel, E., Scardino, P.T. et al. (2003). Variation of serum prostate-specific antigen levels: An evaluation of year-to-year fluctuations. *JAMA* 289 (20): 2695–2700.

29 Thompson, I.M., Pauler, D.K., Goodman, P.J. et al. (2004). Prevalence of prostate cancer among men with a prostate-specific antigen level < or =4.0 ng per milliliter. *N. Engl. J. Med.* 350 (22): 2239–2246.

30 Bryant, R.J., and Lilja, H. (2014). Emerging PSA-based tests to improve screening. *Urol. Clin. North Am.* 41 (2): 267–276.

31 Vickers, A.J., Ulmert, D., Sjoberg, D.D. et al. (2013). Strategy for detection of prostate cancer based on relation between prostate specific antigen at age 40-55 and long term risk of metastasis: Case-control study. *BMJ* 346: f2023.

32 Hessels, D., Klein Gunnewiek, J.M., van Oort, I. et al. (2003). DD3(PCA3)-based molecular urine analysis for the diagnosis of prostate cancer. *Eur. Urol.* 44 (1): 8–15; discussion 6.

33 Loeb, S., Vellekoop, A., Ahmed, H.U. et al. (2013). Systematic review of complications of prostate biopsy. *Eur. Urol.* 64 (6): 876–892.

34 Nam, R.K., Saskin, R., Lee, Y. et al. (2013). Increasing hospital admission rates for urological complications after transrectal ultrasound guided prostate biopsy. *J. Urol.* 189 (1, Suppl.): S12–S17; discussion S7–S8.

35 Murphy, G., Haider, M., Ghai, S., and Sreeharsha, B. (2013). The expanding role of MRI in prostate cancer. *Am. J. Roentgenol.* 201 (6): 1229–1238.

36 Moore, C.M., Robertson, N.L., Arsanious, N. et al. (2013). Image-guided prostate biopsy using magnetic resonance imaging-derived targets: A systematic review. *Eur. Urol.* 63 (1): 125–140.

37 Ahmed, H.U., Pendse, D., Illing, R. et al. (2007). Will focal therapy become a standard of care for men with localized prostate cancer? *Nat. Clin. Pract. Oncol.* 4 (11): 632–642.

38 Ahmed, H.U. et al. (2017). Diagnostic accuracy of multi-parametric MRI and TRUS biopsy in prostate cancer (PROMIS): a paired validating confirmatory study. *Lancet* 389: 815–822, doi:10.1016/S0140-6736(16)32401-1.

39 Kasivisvanathan, V., Rannikko, S., Borghi, M. et al. (2018). MRI-Targeted or Standard Biopsy for Prostate-Cancer Diagnosis. *New Engl J Med*, doi:10.1056/NEJMoa1801993.

40 National Institute for Health and Care Excellence (2014). Prostate cancer: Diagnosis and management. *Clinical Guideline [CG175]*. London: NICE.

41 Klotz, L., Zhang, L., Lam, A. et al. (2010). Clinical results of long-term follow-up of a large, active surveillance cohort with localized prostate cancer. *J. Clin. Oncol.* 28 (1): 126–131.

42 Drazer, M.W., Huo, D., Schonberg, M.A. et al. (2011). Population-based patterns and predictors of prostate-specific antigen screening among older men in the United States. *J. Clin. Oncol.* 29 (13): 1736–1743.

43 Sima, C.S., Panageas, K.S., and Schrag, D. (2010). Cancer screening among patients with advanced cancer. *JAMA* 304 (14): 1584–1591.

44 Gulati, R., Gore, J.L., and Etzioni, R. (2013). Comparative effectiveness of alternative prostate-specific antigen–based prostate cancer screening strategies: Model estimates of potential benefits and harms. *Ann. Intern. Med.* 158 (3): 145–153.

45 de Carvalho, T.M., Heijnsdijk, E.A., and de Koning, H.J. (2015). Screening for prostate cancer in the US? Reduce the harms and keep the benefit. *Int. J. Cancer* 136 (7): 1600–1607.

46 Heijnsdijk, E.A., Wever, E.M., Auvinen, A. et al. (2012). Quality-of-life effects of prostate-specific antigen screening. *N. Engl. J. Med.* 367 (7): 595–605.

47 Scosyrev, E., Wu, G., Mohile, S., and Messing, E.M. (2012). Prostate-specific antigen screening for prostate cancer and the risk of overt metastatic disease at presentation: Analysis of trends over time. *Cancer* 118 (23): 5768–5776.

48 Etzioni, R., Gulati, R., Tsodikov, A. et al. (2012). The prostate cancer conundrum revisited: Treatment changes and prostate cancer mortality declines. *Cancer* 118 (23): 5955–5963.

49 Vertosick, E.A., Poon, B.Y., and Vickers, A.J. (2014). Relative value of race, family history and prostate specific antigen as indications for early initiation of prostate cancer screening. *J. Urol.* 192 (3): 724–728.

50 Loeb, S., Roehl, K.A., Antenor, J.A. et al. (2006). Baseline prostate-specific antigen compared with median prostate-specific antigen for age group as predictor of prostate cancer risk in men younger than 60 years old. *Urology* 67 (2): 316–320.

51 Roobol, M.J., and Carlsson, S.V. (2013). Risk stratification in prostate cancer screening. *Nature Rev. Urol.* 10 (1): 38–48.

52 Gann, P.H., Hennekens, C.H., and Stampfer, M.J. (1995). A prospective evaluation of plasma prostate-specific antigen for detection of prostatic cancer. *JAMA* 273 (4): 289–294.

53 Carlsson, S., Assel, M., Sjoberg, D. et al. (2014). Influence of blood prostate specific antigen levels at age 60 on benefits and harms of prostate cancer screening: Population based cohort study. *BMJ* 348: g2296.

54 Vickers, A., Carlsson, S., Laudone, V., and Lilja, H. (2014). It ain't what you do, it's the way you do it: Five golden rules for transforming prostate-specific antigen screening. *Eur. Urol.* 66 (2): 188–190.

55 Grönberg, H., Adolfsson, J., Aly, M. et al. (2015). Prostate cancer screening in men aged 50–69 years (STHLM3): A prospective population-based diagnostic study. *Lancet Oncol.* 16 (16): 1667–1676.

CHAPTER 14

Colon cancer prevention

John Burn and Harsh Sheth

Institute of Genetic Medicine, International Centre for Life, Newcastle University, UK

SUMMARY BOX

- Genotyping of colorectal cancers (CRCs) for somatic mutations and/or germline variants aids in cancer-specific risk prediction.
- Primary prevention strategies include lifestyle modifications.
- Aspirin use reduces the risk of CRC as well as metastasis and CRC-related mortality, and should be supported as a prophylactic and adjuvant therapy for patients at high risk of developing CRC. Trials are under way to determine the optimal aspirin dose.
- Future work in the field of immunotherapy and colorectal carcinogenesis may provide desperately required insight to develop new, tailored and targeted therapies that would help towards reducing the burden of this disease.

> He is a better physician that keeps diseases off us, than he that cures them being on us; prevention is so much better than healing because it saves the labour of being sick.
>
> *Thomas Adams, 1618*

Colorectal cancer (CRC) is one of the most frequent cancers in the developed world, with an incidence of 160 000 cases diagnosed in the USA every year and 41 804 cases diagnosed in the UK in 2015 [1,2]. Among all cancer types, CRC is the leading cause of cancer-related mortality in developed countries for both males and females, which led to an estimated loss of productivity costs due to premature mortality of €6 billion in Europe in 2008 [3,4], thus posing a significant economic burden to the health-care industry and to society at large.

The striking contrast between rates in the developed world and those seen in rural, low-income populations emphasizes the central role of lifestyle. Factors implicated include obesity, lack of exercise, lack of sun exposure and its associated vitamin D generation, heavy meat consumption, especially red meat, lack of dietary fruit and vegetables, and reduced transit times associated with a lack of fibre (Table 14.1) [5]. Indigestible carbohydrates, also known as fermentable fibre or resistant starch, avoid digestion in the upper intestine by being inaccessible or

---

Cancer Prevention and Screening: Concepts, Principles and Controversies, First Edition.
Edited by Rosalind A. Eeles, Christine D. Berg, and Jeffrey S. Tobias.

Table 14.1 Association between environment and lifestyle risk factors and colorectal cancer risk.

Environment and lifestyle factors	Relative risk	95% confidence intervals
Inflammatory bowel disease	2.93	1.79–4.81
Body mass index[1]	1.10	1.08–1.12
Cigarette smoking[2]	1.06	1.03–1.08
Fruit intake[3]	0.85	0.75–0.96
Physical activity[4]	0.88	0.86–0.91
Red meat intake[5]	1.13	1.09–1.16
Vegetables intake[6]	0.86	0.78–0.94

[1] Risk associated with 8 kg/m^2 increase in body mass index.
[2] Risk associated with 5 pack-years.
[3] Risk associated with 3 servings/day.
[4] Risk associated with 2 standard deviations increase.
[5] Risk associated with 5 servings/week.
[6] Risk associated with 5 servings/day.

crystalline, and are fermented by gut bacteria into anti-neoplastic short-chain fatty acids, especially butyrate. While formal randomized trials of dietary modification have been disappointing [6], few dispute the importance of the combined beneficial effects of taking regular exercise, preferably outdoors, avoidance of obesity, and having a diet rich in fresh fruit and vegetables and a focus on white meat and fish as sources of animal protein. It is also clear that the majority of the Western population struggle to react positively to such advice, and prevention must also rely on interventions.

The accessibility of the colon to examination and removal of pre-cancerous polyps and early cancers is a proven approach to avoiding death from a large proportion of colorectal cancers (CRC). Systematic endoscopy, based either on an age cut-off or evidence of occult blood loss, is the mainstay of the public health response and is dealt with in Chapter 15. There has been a long-term interest in targeted strategies based on offering regular surveillance and/or prophylactic surgery, approaches which have been given added impetus by the genomic revolution, which allows molecular testing of asymptomatic individuals and selection of those at highest risk. A second focus has been on possible chemo-preventive agents suitable for long-term use. Attention has focused on the anti-inflammatory agents, especially aspirin and the selective COX2 inhibitors, though there is also continued interest in the use of DFMO (eflornithine), which suppresses polyamine production by inhibition of ornithine decarboxy-lase. In this chapter we will review the latest achievements in genetic targeting and provide an overview of the benefits of anti-inflammatories, ending with the results from the Cancer Prevention Programme (CaPP), which is exploring the beneficial effects of aspirin in the context of a high-risk population with mismatch repair gene defects.

Genetic architecture of colorectal cancer

A small number of monogenic syndromes account for around 3–5% of CRC. Traditionally, the remainder are divided into 'familial' and 'sporadic'. This is a false dichotomy, as some of the familial cases are simply coincidental occurrence, while many of the isolated cases have a genetic predisposition, usually triggered by a combination of environmental and chance or stochastic factors. Twin studies which compare concordance (both affected) in monozygotic or identical twins compared to dizygotic or fraternal twins suggest around 30% heritability. Rather than being seen as a separate slice of the pie chart, this fraction should be thought of as being a fraction of the ingredients used to make a cake representing the whole population. Each individual slice then can be shown to contain a mixture of genetic and environmental causes, which will vary in amount. Those with an affected first-degree relative will be more likely on average to have a bigger genetic contribution, reflected in an even greater chance of a further relative being affected.

Mutations and genetic variants

The identified genetic risk factors lie between the two extremes: rare high-penetrance mutations, which increase the risk for hereditary syndromes, and common genetic variants that confer individually small effects (Figure 14.1) [7]. To date, 14 genes implicated in CRC syndromes have been identified (Table 14.2), starting with the discovery of the *adenomatous polyposis coli* (*APC*) gene in familial adenomatous polyposis (FAP) patients. Subsequently, human homologues of the DNA mismatch repair (MMR) genes (*MLH1, MSH2, MSH6,* and *PMS2*) were identified through positional cloning, and were originally studied in bacteria and yeast extensively [8]. These genes were implicated in Lynch syndrome patients. Additionally, mutations in genes *STK11, BMPR1A, SMAD4,* and *PTEN* predispose to a high frequency of hamartomas in the gut with malignant potential.

Mutations in the 5′ or 3′ ends of the *APC* gene can result in a less profuse polyposis syndrome called attenuated FAP (AFAP), where patients have an average lifetime cancer risk of around 70% and delayed age of onset (mean 56 years); pathogenic variants in the *MUTYH* gene have been identified as genetic drivers of an adenomatous polyposis syndrome. Mutations in both copies of the *MUTYH* gene lead to a recessive form of adenomatous polyposis known as *MUTYH*-associated polyposis (MAP), where patients have an average lifetime cancer risk of 80%, and most European cases involve one or both of two common alleles. Germline mutations in the proofreading domains of two DNA polymerases (POLE and POLD1) lead to acquisition of a large number of somatically acquired mutations

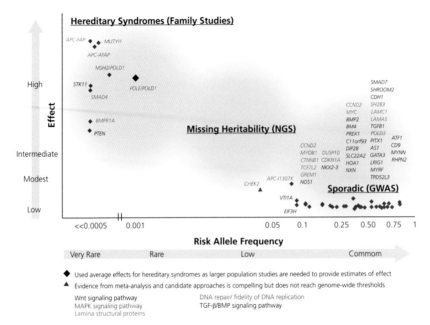

Figure 14.1 Effect size of the association between known risk alleles and colorectal cancer. Minor allele frequency of the variant shown based on the ethnicity in which the locus was discovered, except for variants with a recessive effect (*MUTYH*), for which frequency for homozygous rare genotype is shown. BMP, bone morphogenic protein; CRC, colorectal cancer; GWAS, genome-wide association study; MAPK, mitogen-activated protein kinase; TGFβ, transforming growth factor β. Source: Peters et al. 2015 [7]. Reproduced with permission of BMJ Publishing Group.

(hypermutated tumours) and are known as polymerase proofreading associated polyposis. The latest addition to the polyposis list involves a rare endonuclease gene, *NTHL1,* leading to the proposed acronym NAP.

Familial colorectal cancer type X (FCCTX) is a misleading term coined to describe the presumed missing autosomal dominant forms of nonpolyposis colon cancer. Traditionally the term 'familial' referred to recessive disorders, while the letter 'X' implied a gene on the X chromosome. In practice, linkage studies have failed to identify the presumed dominant traits, leading to the conclusion that we have found most if not all of the monogenic forms of the disease [7].

Family-based linkage studies have been successful in identifying high-penetrance mutations, but have limited statistical power to identify common genetic variants (such as single-nucleotide polymorphisms or SNPs) with weaker effects, as argued by Risch and Merikangas [9]. Given their higher prevalence in the population, low-penetrance mutations and variants can contribute to the overall disease heritability. With the advent of high-throughput genotyping platforms that can genotype up to a million SNPs, several genome-wide association studies (GWAS) have been carried out to identify variants associated with sporadic CRC

Table 14.2 Genes with predisposing mutations in familial colorectal cancer syndromes.

Gene	Hereditary syndrome	Age of onset (years)	Pathway/biological function*
APC	FAP, AFAP	34–43	Wnt signalling pathway
MUTYH	MAP	48–56	Base excision repair
hMLH1, hMSH2, hMSH6, hPMS2, EPCAM	Lynch syndrome	44–56	Mismatch repair
PTEN	Cowden syndrome (includes BRR syndrome)	<50 (BRR paediatric onset)	Negative regulator of metabolic signalling
STK11	PJS	65	Tumour suppressor
GREM1, 15q13 locus	HMPS	48	TGFβ/BMP signalling pathway
BMPR1A	HMPS, juvenile polyposis syndrome	48, 42	TGFβ/BMP signalling pathway
MADH4/ SMAD4	Juvenile polyposis syndrome	42	TGFβ/BMP signalling pathway
POLE, POLD1	Oligopolyposis or polymerase proofreading associated polyposis	23–80	DNA repair

*Many of these pathways interact at multiple levels and are not necessarily independent from each other in biological mechanisms.

AFAP, attenuated familial adenomatous polyposis; BMP, bone morphogenic protein; BRR, Bannayan-Ruvalcaba-Riley syndrome; FAP, familial adenomatous polyposis; HMPS, hereditary mixed polyposis syndrome; MAP, MUTYH-associated polyposis; PJS, Peutz-Jeghers syndrome; TGFβ, transforming growth factor β.

Source: Adapted from Peters et al. 2015 [7]. Reproduced with permission of BMJ Publishing Group Ltd.

risk. To date, GWAS studies have identified over 40 independent loci, with minor allele frequency ranging from 4% to 9% and odds ratio (OR) per risk allele ranging between 1.04 and 1.56. Although most of the commonly associated SNPs with CRC risk are present in the intergenic region, many kilobases (kb) away from the nearest gene, their proximity to the candidate genes has implicated many known CRC carcinogenesis-related genes and pathways. Additionally, GWAS studies have identified SNPs in regions that do not harbour any known candidate genes (e.g. *CDKN1A, EIF3H, TPD52L3, ITIH2, LAMA5,* and *LAMC1*) and SNPs with weak effects in genes linked to hereditary syndromes. It is important to note that while it is tempting to link the most likely candidate gene with the newly identified

SNPs from GWAS studies, functional studies for most of the SNPs have not been carried out, and hence the putative candidate gene list may likely change in the future as more data become available. In saying so, functional studies have been carried out for only a handful of SNPs.

Identification of genetic factors behind high-penetrance syndromes has led to more effective disease surveillance, diagnosis, and management for patients and their families. In contrast, even though the common variants are associated with weaker effects, these variants collectively could enable more accurate risk prediction for an individual in the population, and may modify the risk of CRC in individuals with hereditary syndromes [7]. More recently, subclassification and typing of sporadic CRCs are being carried out based on the gene expression profile of tumours. An international consortium has defined a subclassification system by pooling data from 18 CRC datasets comprising a total of 4151 patients; four major consensus molecular subtypes (CMS) were identified, each with a unique gene expression signature and distinguishing figures [10]. From the entire dataset, 14% of the tumours showed signature for CMS1 (microsatellite instability immune), where tumours were hyper-mutated, microsatellite unstable, hyper-methylated, and had increased expression of genes associated with a diffused immune infiltrate and immune evasion pathways; 37% of the tumours showed signature for CMS2 (canonical), where tumours were marked by Wnt and MYC signalling activation; 13% of the tumours showed signature for CMS3 (metabolic), where tumours had metabolic dysregulation; and 23% of the tumours showed expression for CMS4 (mesenchymal), where tumours had TGFβ activation, stromal invasion, and angiogenesis (Table 14.3) [10].

Table 14.3 Consensus molecular subtypes of colorectal cancer based on gene expression profiling.

CMS 1 MSI Immune	CMS 2 Canonical	CMS 3 Metabolic	CMS 4 Mesenchymal
14%	37%	13%	23%
MSI, CIMP high, hypermutation	SCNA high	Mixed MSI status, SCNA low, CIMP low	SCNA high
BRAF mutations		KRAS mutations	
Immune infiltration and activation	WNT and MYC activation	Metabolic deregulation	Stromal infiltration, TGF-β activation, angiogenesis
Worse survival after relapse			Worse relapse-free and overall survival

CIMP, CpG island methylator phenotype; CMS, consensus molecular subtypes; MSI, microsatellite instability, SCNA, somatic copy number alterations.
Source: Adapted from Guinney et al. 2015 [10]. Reproduced with permission of Nature Publishing Group.

Consensus molecular subtype classification

The CMS1 tumour profile is normally seen in Lynch syndrome cancers with hyper-mutation and increased activation of immune-related pathways, embracing what was previously called the mutator or DNA mismatch repair pathway [2,11]. The CMS2 pattern, previously known as the chromosomal instability (CIN) or 'suppressor' pathway, is the pathway followed by cancers resulting from FAP due to loss of function in the *APC* gene.

CMS1: Lynch syndrome and the DNA mismatch repair defect pathway

MMR pathway defects are observed in approximately 15–20% of sporadic CRCs where the tumours are characterized by high mutation rates, 100 to 1000 fold more common in comparison to normal cells, mainly affecting microsatellite sequences [11,12]. This is caused by the inactivation of MMR genes that are required for base-mismatch repair post-DNA replication (Figure 14.2). In total, there are seven MMR genes that encode functional proteins to carry out mismatch repair: *hMLH1*, *hMLH3*, *hMSH2*, *hMSH3*, *hMSH6*, *hPMS1*, and *hPMS2* [2,11,13]. In sporadic tumours, epigenetic inactivation of *hMLH1* due to methylation and, less frequently, mutation in *hMSH6* are observed [14]. In contrast, germline mutation in *hMLH1* and *hMSH2* genes leads to the hereditary form of CRC, formerly known as hereditary nonpolyposis colorectal cancer (HNPCC), and now renamed Lynch syndrome, which accounts for 2–4% of all CRC cases [15,16]. In both sporadic and hereditary tumours with MMR deficiency, mutations in the mononucleotide or dinucleotide repeat sequences in the functional regions of the tumour suppressor genes such as *TGFβR2*, *BAX*, and *IGF2R* and epigenetic silencing of a number of normally functioning genes are observed [2,11].

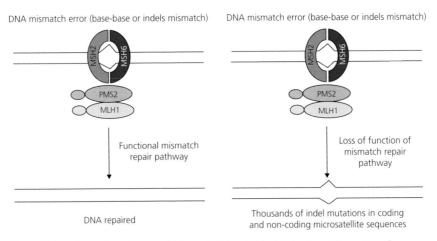

Figure 14.2 Colorectal carcinogenesis through defect in the DNA mismatch repair pathway.

CMS2: FAP and the chromosomal instability pathway

CIN is the most common type of genomic instability observed in 80–85% of tumours; it is assumed to follow the Fearon and Vogelstein model of carcinogenesis [11,17]. The linear model proposed that specific genetic events were correlated with the evolving tissue morphology (Figure 14.3). In cancers caused due to CIN, rare inactivating mutations in genes involved in chromosome stability during replication are observed [2,18]. This leads to physical loss of a wild-type copy of tumour suppressor genes such as *APC*, *P53*, and *SMAD4* and gain of function of oncogenes such as *KRAS* [2,11]. Furthermore, CIN tumours contain a high frequency of allelic imbalance, most commonly on chromosomes 5q, 8p, 17p, and 18q [2,11].

Prevention strategies for colorectal cancer

Currently, two main prevention strategies are being advised: lifestyle modifications that affect risk factors for CRC in the general population, and surveillance and early detection of pre-neoplastic or neoplastic lesions in the colon, in population cohorts containing average to high-risk individuals, mainly because of age, hereditary CRC syndromes, or inflammatory bowel disease (IBD) [19]. Evidence of their application for reducing incidence and CRC-related mortality stems from randomized controlled trials or guidelines from scientific bodies.

Lifestyle modifications and aspirin use

Over the last two decades, long-term use of aspirin and other nonsteroidal anti-inflammatory drugs (NSAIDs) has been shown to reduce CRC risk in epidemiological studies and randomized controlled trials [20]. Aspirin is widely prescribed for its anti-platelet and anti-inflammatory effects; however, in 1988, the first epidemiological evidence for reduced risk of CRC by 42% and 51% in males and females, respectively, who were taking aspirin was observed in a population-based case-control study [21]. In 2011, results from the randomized controlled trial CAPP2 in Lynch syndrome carriers showed that patients taking 600 mg/day aspirin for at least two years had up to a 60% reduction in risk for CRC compared to the placebo group, with the effect apparent after four years of follow-up (hazard ratio [HR] 0.41, 95% confidence interval [CI] 0.19–0.86, p=0.02; incidence rate ratio [IRR] 0.37, 95% CI 0.18–0.78, p=0.008) [22]. While the risk reduction was shown with 600 mg/day aspirin use, this dose cannot be prescribed to the general population, as it is associated with higher gastrointestinal toxicity, thus rendering it unattractive for chemoprevention. In 2013, a follow-up observational study of a randomized controlled trial, the Women's Health Study, showed a reduction in CRC by 20% in the group taking 100 mg alternate day aspirin compared to the placebo group, with the effect commencing 10 years after randomization (HR 0.80, 95% CI 0.67–0.76, p=0.021) [23]. Thus, the chemopreventive effect of aspirin is observed at the now traditional anti-platelet dose, albeit taking longer to achieve the chemopreventive benefit.

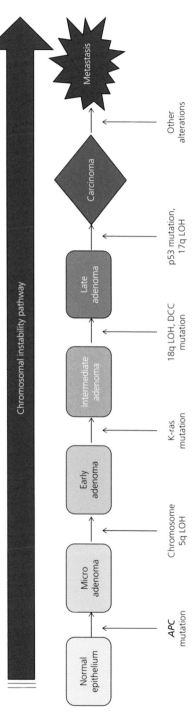

Figure 14.3 Colorectal carcinogenesis through the chromosomal instability pathway.

As colorectal adenomas are the precursors to most CRCs, the chemopreventive effect of aspirin is likely to be observed in the adenomas as they form during the neoplastic transformation of healthy cells to cancer cells. Two randomized controlled trials in patients of European and Japanese ethnicity with FAP showed no significant reduction in the polyp count, but showed reduction in the mean polyp size in patients randomized to aspirin compared to placebo [24,25]. Further meta-analysis of four randomized controlled trials that evaluated secondary prevention of sporadic colorectal adenomas with aspirin showed 17% and 28% risk reduction for developing adenomas (pooled RR 0.83, 95% CI 0.72–0.96, p=0.012) and advanced lesions (pooled RR 0.72, 95% CI 0.57–0.90, p=0.005), respectively [26]. In addition to the evidence from controlled trials, meta-analysis of five observational studies, of which two focused on CRC, showed a 31% reduction in risk of distant metastasis with regular aspirin use (pooled odds ratio [OR] 0.69, 95% CI 0.57–0.83, p<0.0001), but no risk reduction was observed for cancers with regional spread (pooled OR 0.98, 95% CI 0.88–1.09, p=0.71) [20]. Furthermore, regular aspirin use has been associated with a 74% reduction in the risk of later metastasis in patients with CRC without metastasis at the time of initial diagnosis (HR 0.26, 95% CI 0.11–0.57, p=0.0008) and further risk reduction by 87% of later metastasis in patients still on treatment at the time of diagnosis (HR 0.13, 95% CI 0.03–0.56, p=0.007) [27]. Lastly, aspirin use has been associated with a 50% reduction in the risk of death due to cancer in patients with adenocarcinoma without metastasis at initial diagnosis (HR 0.50, 95% CI 0.34–0.74, p=0.0006) [28]. Thus there is convincing evidence for aspirin to be prescribed for prophylaxis and adjuvant therapy in patients at high risk of CRC. The biological mechanism of action and personalized chemoprevention with aspirin are discussed below.

Personalized chemoprevention with aspirin

As colorectal carcinogenesis takes places through a series of complex biological pathways, each with germline variants and somatic mutations that affect cancer susceptibility, it can be hypothesized that these genetic variants modulate aspirin's chemopreventive efficacy. Indeed, this has been shown to be the case through evidence from case-control studies and randomized controlled trials in both general and genetically predisposed populations.

Biological mechanism of aspirin

Several biological pathways have been proposed as the source of aspirin's chemopreventive effect, and the common mechanisms across these pathways include induction of apoptosis, anti-proliferative activity, autophagy, and inhibition of angiogenesis and metastasis. The primary target of aspirin is cyclooxygenase-1 (COX1) enzyme, where it inhibits its enzymatic activity by blocking the access to the catalytic site, which in turn provides an anti-platelet effect [29]. Experimental evidence suggests that cancer patients exhibit increased platelet activation, which in turn aids in tumour metastasis by protecting cells from immune surveillance and helps in attaching tumour cells to the endothelial lining [30]. Thus the reduced risk of metastasis observed in trials [27] could be due to the inhibition of the COX1 enzyme.

An isoform of the COX1 enzyme, COX2, is induced in response to pro-inflammatory and cell division stimuli in monocytes and epithelial cells. Its activity has been shown to be modified by aspirin in a dose-dependent manner [31,32] to produce lipoxins that are involved in resolution of inflammatory reactions, rather than prostaglandin E2 that can cause resistance to apoptosis, cell migration, and angiogenesis [33,34]. Thus modification of the COX2 enzyme activity by aspirin leads to an anti-inflammatory response, which has shown to be beneficial in reducing CRC risk in individuals with overexpression of COX2 in CRC tumours [35].

In addition to the COX-dependent pathway, there is growing evidence of the chemopreventive effects of aspirin through COX-independent pathways. To date, the only COX-independent target known to interact with aspirin is IκB kinase (IKK). *In vivo* and *in vitro* studies have shown that aspirin and salicylic acid, a primary metabolite of aspirin, inhibit IKK, which prevents activation of NF-κB, thereby reducing inflammatory and angiogenic responses [36]. However, another study showed activation and nuclear translocation of NF-κB in CRC cell lines induced by aspirin, followed by apoptosis [37]. The study also showed that this effect was specific to the cells of colonic origin only, thus suggesting a tissue-specific effect of aspirin on NF-κB signalling [37,38]. Other chemopreventive mechanisms mentioned in the literature include inhibitory effects on endothelial cells' ability to undergo angiogenesis [39]; nuclear caspase-dependent cleavage of Sp1, Sp3, and Sp4 specificity protein transcription factors induced by aspirin [40]; decrease in the ATPase and selective inhibition of DNA cleavage activity of topoisomerase IIα enzyme by salicylic acid [41]; inhibition of 6-phosphofructo-1-kinase activity by aspirin and salicylic acid [42]; and activation of polyamine catabolism by increasing expression and activity of spermidine N-acetyltransferase in colonic mucosa by aspirin [43]. Currently, no clear biological mechanism of aspirin's chemopreventive effect has been elucidated, but it has become an active area of research.

Germline variants

Several SNPs have been identified in genes involved in aspirin metabolism or aspirin's mode of action that modulate its chemopreventive efficacy. For example, SNPs rs1105879 and rs2070959 in the *UGT1A6* gene, which is involved in aspirin metabolism, have been shown to have gene x environment interaction, whereby carriers of the SNP variant allele using aspirin had a 34% risk reduction in adenoma formation compared to individuals with a wild-type genotype [44]. A GWAS-based meta-analysis of 10 case-control and cohort studies as part of the GECCO consortium identified SNP rs2965667 near the *MGST1* gene, which showed a significant gene x environment interaction, whereby a 34% risk reduction for CRC was observed among aspirin and/or NSAID users with a wild-type genotype, but an 89% increase in risk in individuals with the variant allele [45]. SNPs in other genes, such as *ODC1, IL16,* and *COX2,* have been identified as modulating aspirin's efficacy. Despite evidence for genetic variants being one of the sources of aspirin's variable efficacy, the relative effect on the risk of CRC or colorectal adenoma (CRA) has been modest, and hence requires further studies to identify key genetic markers, which can be used in clinics to make an informed decision about the risk–benefit ratio for an individual. Furthermore, studies need to be conducted to identify genetic variants that can predict the risk of adverse reactions from taking aspirin. No SNP marker has been identified to date for aspirin that can explain a major proportion of its chemopreventive effect variation. It is likely that the variation in the chemopreventive effect may largely be through somatic mutations that drive cancer development and progression.

Somatic mutations and gene expression

One of the first lines of evidence of the effect of gene expression on aspirin's efficacy was shown in 2007, when Chan et al. [35], using data from the Nurses' Health Study (NHS) and the Health Professional Follow-up Study (HPFS), showed that the risk of developing CRC was reduced by 36% in regular aspirin users who had tumours with overexpression of the COX2 enzyme (RR 0.64, 95% CI 0.52–0.78), but not in individuals with tumours containing weak or absent COX2 expression (RR 0.96, 95% CI 0.73–1.26). Prostaglandins synthesized by COX2 are metabolized by the hydroxyprostaglandin dehydrogenase 15-(nicotinamide adenine dinucleotide) (15-PGDH, HPGD) enzyme, thus HPGD functions as a metabolic antagonist of COX2 [46]. It has been shown that regular aspirin use is associated with a 51% risk reduction in CRCs that are surrounded by colonic mucosa with high HPGD mRNA expression (HR 0.49, 95% CI 0.34–0.71, p=0.0002), but not in cancers surrounded with mucosa having low HPGD expression (HR 0.90, 95% CI 0.63–1.27, p=0.53) compared to nonusers [47].

Research on somatic mutations in CRCs showed that activating mutations in the *PIK3CA* gene that occur in two hotspots (exon 9 and 20) are present in approximately 15–20% of CRCs [48]. The phosphatidylinositol 3-kinase (PI3K) signalling pathway has shown to be involved in colorectal carcinogenesis. PIK3CA is a downstream mediator of COX2, and mutations in PIK3CA lead to increased prostaglandin E2 synthesis and inhibition of apoptosis in colon cancer cells. Improvement in CRC-specific survival by 82% among post-diagnosis regular aspirin users with mutated *PIK3CA* CRC (HR 0.18, 95% CI 0.06–0.61, p<0.001), but not in patients with wild-type *PIK3CA* cancer (HR 0.96, 95% CI 0.69–1.32, p=0.76), has been observed in the NHS and HPFS study cohorts [49].

More recently, research has focused on immune system modulation for improved pre- and post-diagnostic chemoprevention and survival, with a spotlight on cell surface human leukocyte antigens (HLA) that regulate immune recognition. It has been shown that an improved overall survival benefit of 47% is associated with post-cancer diagnosis regular aspirin use (RR 0.53, 95% CI 0.38–0.74, p<0.001) in tumours expressing HLA class I antigen, whereas no benefit is observed in tumours not expressing HLA class I antigen (RR 1.03, 95% CI 0.66–1.61, p = 0.91) [50]. Together, these somatic mutations and gene expression profiles can serve as predictive biomarkers for the efficacy of prophylactic and adjuvant aspirin therapy in CRCs.

Prescribing aspirin to the general and high-risk populations

Aspirin is routinely prescribed as a prophylactic drug for cardiovascular diseases (CVD) and, with rising evidence for its chemopreventive effect for CRC, it is likely to be prescribed as a prophylactic or adjuvant drug for treating CRCs. However, the major issue that needs to be addressed is bleeding risk. A review by Cuzick et al. [51] looked into the risks and benefits of prophylactic use of aspirin in the general population, and observed a delayed chemopreventive effect of aspirin by three years from the start of the treatment. The review also mentioned increase in haemorrhagic strokes and gastrointestinal bleeds in aspirin users by 32–36% and 30–70%, respectively, but the authors estimate a relative reduction of around 9% and 7% in the number of men and women, respectively, with cancer, myocardial infarction, or stroke event over a 15-year period if they have been taking aspirin for 10 years [51]. Furthermore, they also calculated that 61–80% of the overall benefit would be accounted for by the decrease in the cancer risk, especially reduction in the CRC risk, which alone would account for 30–60%. Based on the evidence of risk and benefit of using aspirin, the authors concluded that prophylactic use of 75–325 mg/day aspirin for a minimum of five years would have a favourable risk–benefit ratio [51].

A recent analysis of the CAPP2 trial data, which consisted of patients who were genetically predisposed to Lynch syndrome, showed that there was approximately a 2.5-fold increase in the risk of developing CRC in overweight (body mass index [BMI] 25–29.9 kg/m^2) or obese (BMI >29.9 kg/m^2) individuals compared to under- and normal-weight individuals (HR 2.41, 95% CI 1.22–4.85) [52]. Overall, there was a 7% increase in risk of developing CRC for each 1 kg/m^2 increase in BMI. In the subgroup analysis, the authors observed that the obesity-related excess risk of CRC was confined only to the placebo (HR 2.75, 95% CI 1.12–6.79, p = 0.03), whereas the risk was nullified in the aspirin group [52]. This effect was not supported by analysis of self-reported aspirin use in the large Colon Cancer Family Registry [53]. If the effect is real, the disparity may reflect the 600 mg/day dose used in the CAPP2 trial.

Dose and duration

In the largest randomized controlled trial in Lynch syndrome carrier patients, the protective effect of 600 mg/day aspirin treatment was apparent five years after randomization [22]. In contrast, a long-term follow-up of the only other aspirin randomized trial with cancer as an end-point, the Women's Health Study, showed an 18%

reduction in gastrointestinal cancers, with the effect commencing 10 years post-randomization in people who were randomized to 100 mg alternate day aspirin [23]. Therefore, risk reduction for CRCs is observed in both low-dose and high-dose aspirin users. Furthermore, there is evidence that long-term regular use of aspirin is necessary to achieve chemopreventive benefit, where the incidence is reduced after three years and mortality is reduced after five years [51,54]. While risk reduction is observed for low-dose aspirin users, the benefit of taking a higher dose is not clear.

Since aspirin is an anti-platelet agent, bleeding risk is its most important side effect. There is a relative increase in risk of haemorrhagic strokes by 32–36% and extracranial (mostly gastrointestinal) bleeds by 30–70% from baseline with low- or standard-dose aspirin treatment [51]. There is a sharp increase in gastrointestinal bleeding risk beyond the age of 70 years, however, the bleeding risk is low in individuals below the age of 70 years. Data from the Nurses' Health Study shows that the risk of gastrointestinal bleeding increases with increase in dose and duration of aspirin use [51,55]. Hence it is imperative to carry out a study that will measure the risk–benefit profile of prescribing low-dose or high-dose aspirin treatment in individuals at risk of CRC. The CaPP3 trial, which was launched in 2014, is a randomized trial in Lynch syndrome carriers, where they will be randomized to either 100 mg/day, 300 mg/day, or 600 mg/day aspirin for two years and Lynch syndrome cancer incidence and bleeding rates compared during the 5–10-year follow-up period [56].

Recommendations and considerations

No group, professional society, or national body recommends regular aspirin use for cancer prevention in general or for specific cancers [57–59], except for the international consensus on CRC chemoprevention in the general population [51], and consideration by the American Gastroenterological Association in Lynch syndrome patients based on the data from CAPP2 and Women Health's Study trial data [60]. In 2015, the American Cancer Society recommended against the use of aspirin for CRC prevention in the general population, which is in concordance with the recommendations by the US Preventive Services Task Force (USPSTF) in 2007 [61].

However, in 2015, the USPSTF published findings of cancer prevention, especially CRC, in the population eligible for primary prevention of CVD by assessing the net benefit and harm of regular aspirin use [62]. Based on 10 CVD primary prevention trials, no significant all cancer–related mortality risk reduction was observed in aspirin users compared to nonusers over 3.6–10.1 years (RR 0.96, 95% CI 0.87–1.06). Similarly, based on the data from six trials, no significant all cancer incidence risk reduction was observed in aspirin users compared to nonusers (RR 0.98, 95% CI 0.93–1.04). However, when analysed for CRC-specific incidence in pooled analysis of three trials, a risk reduction of 40% was observed 10–19 years after aspirin initiation (RR 0.60, 95% CI 0.47–0.76). Lastly, when analysed for CRC-specific mortality in pooled analysis of four trials, a 33%

reduction in long-term (0–20+ years) CRC-specific mortality risk was observed (RR 0.67, 95% CI 0.52–0.86). While the findings from both USPSTF [62] and Cuzick et al. [51] suggest a benefit of regular aspirin use in CRC prevention and CRC-specific mortality, the two reviews should be compared with caution, as Cuzick et al. did not report on the overall estimate for total cancers, and USPSTF did not present estimates for individual cancers other than CRC, since other cancers are not frequently reported. Furthermore, relative risk for incidence and mortality differs between the two reviews, in part because Cuzick et al. focused on daily aspirin use and included observational studies, but excluded Women's Health Study and Physicians Health Study data, where aspirin was prescribed on alternate days. The authors suggest using USPSTF's systematic review data on CVD [63] and bleeding harms [64] to determine an overall benefit–harm profile in a CVD primary prevention population.

Future work and novel therapies

Long-term follow-up from trials could provide information on the cancer-specific and overall effects of aspirin on the size and timing of chemopreventive benefits, dose–response relationship, effect of dose, and duration and differences of chemopreventive effects across various subgroups based on sex, age, and genetic make-up. Furthermore, the Non-Vascular outcomes on Aspirin (NoVA) Collaboration is currently collating data from previous and ongoing trials, with the aim of providing comprehensive data on the short-term and long-term effects of aspirin [65]. Lastly, data from observational studies and trials focused on subgroups defined by genetic make-up (germline variants, somatic mutations, and gene expression profile) and lifestyle factors, like the ones mentioned previously, could provide biomarkers that may be useful in stratifying patients who are more likely to benefit from aspirin use.

More recently, a keen interest has been fuelled in the emerging area of immunotherapy and development of anti-cancer vaccines for nonviral cancers such as CRC. Sporadic and hereditary tumours with microsatellite instability (MSI-H) phenotype develop numerous insertion or deletion mutations at well-defined, predictable microsatellite loci, located within approximately 12 000 genes in the human genome [66]. These mutations may lead to a shift in the reading frame and thus generate novel carboxyl-terminated frameshift peptides (FSPs). These FSPs were hypothesized to generate immunological response and provide an anti-cancer effect. In 2008, Schwitalle et al. [66] detected an FSP-specific T-cell response in the peripheral blood from patients with MSI-H CRC and healthy Lynch syndrome mutation carriers, but not from patients with microsatellite stable (MSS) CRC or healthy donors [66]. A vaccine containing FSPs found in approximately 98.5% of MSI-H tumours has been developed and is currently being trialled in patients with mutations in DNA MMR defect, with the aim of generating an immune reaction against malignant cells producing FSPs and thus providing an anti-cancer effect [67].

Further mechanisms of immune evasion by tumour cells are being studied presently in human cell lines and mouse models. A study in a mouse model with a competent immune system and melanoma with Braf[V600E] mutation requires the production of prostaglandin E2 to suppress immunity and fuel tumour-promoting inflammation [68]. Genetic ablation of COX enzymes in Braf[V600E] mouse melanoma cells, Nras[G12D] melanoma, breast, or CRC cells renders them susceptible to immune influence and promotes a shift towards anti-cancer immune pathways [68]. This COX-dependent inflammatory signature is conserved in human cutaneous melanoma biopsies, thus suggesting COX activity as a driver for immune suppression or evasion. In another pathway related to antigen presentation, truncating mutations in the microsatellites of the β-2-microglobulin (*B2M*) gene have been identified in approximately 30% of CRCs and are suggested as the primary mechanism to impair the HLA class I antigen presentation system [69]. Protein expression of B2M in 408 CRCs found that complete loss of B2M expression is more common in MMR-deficient tumours compared to MMR-proficient tumours (19.4% vs 7.1%, $p < 0.001$) [69]. Loss of B2M expression predicted rare local recurrence ($p = 0.03$), absence of distant metastasis ($p = 0.048$, sensitivity 100%), and an overall trend towards favourable survival ($p = 0.12$) in MMR-deficient tumours only. Therefore, patients with MMR-deficient CRC tumours and B2M expression loss have a favourable prognosis.

Immunological approaches to prevention will be informed by advances in the immunotherapy of existing cancers. Therapies that interfere with T-cell checkpoints, particularly the PD-1/PD-L1 axis, have given positive outcomes for a range of malignancies [70,71]. The proposed hypothesis for the mechanism is boosting of T-cell reactivity against 'neo-antigens', which act as epitopes for T cells and are formed as a consequence of tumour-specific mutations [70]. Based on this hypothesis, Le et al. [72] carried out a Phase 2 study that evaluated the activity of PD-1 blockade (pembrolizumab) in 41 patients: 11 patients with MMR-deficient CRC, 21 patients with MMR-proficient CRC, and 9 patients with MMR-deficient cancers other than CRC. Strikingly, 40% of the MMR-deficient CRC patients and 71% of the MMR-deficient non-CRC patients reached an objective immune-related clinical response, whereas none of the patients with MMR-proficient CRC responded [72]. Furthermore, MMR-deficient CRC patients had significantly longer progression-free survival ($p < 0.001$) as well as overall survival ($p = 0.03$).

Conclusion

Genotyping of CRCs for somatic mutations and/or germline variants aids in cancer-specific risk prediction in patients with a family history of CRC and the general population. Primary prevention strategies, including lifestyle modifications and aspirin use, have been shown to reduce the risk of CRC, but cannot replace secondary prevention strategies. Regular aspirin use has been shown to reduce incidence, metastasis, and CRC-related mortality through randomized trials and observational studies, and should be supported as a prophylactic and adjuvant therapy for patients at high risk of developing CRC. Future work in the field of immunotherapy and colorectal carcinogenesis may provide desperately required insight to develop new, tailored and targeted therapies that would help towards reducing the burden of this disease.

References

1   Cancer Reserch UK (2015). *Cancer incidence and mortality in the UK for the 10 most common cancers*. London: Cancer Research UK.

2   Markowitz, S.D., and Bertagnolli, M.M. (2009). Molecular basis of colorectal cancer. *N. Engl. J. Med.* 361 (25): 2449–2460.

3   Hanly, P., Soerjomataram, I., and Sharp, L. (2015). Measuring the societal burden of cancer: The cost of lost productivity due to premature cancer-related mortality in Europe. *Int. J. Cancer* 136 (4): E136–E145.

4   Siegel, R., Naishadham, D., and Jemal, A. (2012). Cancer statistics, 2012. *CA Cancer J. Clin.* 62 (1): 10–29.

5   Johnson, C.M., Wei, C., Ensor, J.E. et al. (2013). Meta-analyses of colorectal cancer risk factors. *Cancer Causes Control* 24 (6): 1207–1222.

6   Mathers, J.C., Movahedi, M., Macrae, F. et al. (2012). Long-term effect of resistant starch on cancer risk in carriers of hereditary colorectal cancer: An analysis from the CAPP2 randomised controlled trial. *Lancet Oncol.* 13 (12): 1242–1249.

7   Peters, U., Bien, S., and Zubair, N. (2015). Genetic architecture of colorectal cancer. *Gut* 64 (10): 1623–1636.

8   Wheeler, J.M.D., Bodmer, W.F., and Mortensen, N.J.M. (2000). DNA mismatch repair genes and colorectal cancer. *Gut* 47 (1): 148–153.

9   Risch, N., and Merikangas, K. (1996). The future of genetic studies of complex human diseases. *Science* 273 (5281): 1516–1517.

10 Guinney, J., Dienstmann, R., Wang, X. et al. (2015). The consensus molecular subtypes of colorectal cancer. *Nature Med.* 21 (11): 1350–1356.

11 Moran, A., Ortega, P., de Juan, C. et al. (2010). Differential colorectal carcinogenesis: Molecular basis and clinical relevance. *World J. Gastrointestin Oncol.* 2 (3): 151–158.

12 Pawlik, T.M., Raut, C.P., and Rodriguez-Bigas, M.A. (2004). Colorectal carcinogenesis: MSI-H versus MSI-L. *Dis. Markers* 20 (4–5): 199–206.

13 Hoeijmakers, J.H. (2001). Genome maintenance mechanisms for preventing cancer. *Nature* 411 (6835): 366–374.

14 Imai, K., and Yamamoto, H. (2008). Carcinogenesis and microsatellite instability: The inter-relationship between genetics and epigenetics. *Carcinogenesis* 29 (4): 673–680.

15 Bronner, C.E., Baker, S.M., Morrison, P.T. et al. (1994). Mutation in the DNA mismatch repair gene homologue hMLH1 is associated with hereditary non-polyposis colon cancer. *Nature* 368 (6468): 258–261.

16 Fishel, R., Lescoe, M.K., Rao, M.R. et al. (1993). The human mutator gene homolog MSH2 and its association with hereditary nonpolyposis colon cancer. *Cell* 75 (5): 1027–1038.

17 Fearon, E.R., and Vogelstein, B. (1990). A genetic model for colorectal tumorigenesis. *Cell* 61 (5): 759–767.

18 Barber, T.D., McManus, K., Yuen, K.W. et al. (2008). Chromatid cohesion defects may underlie chromosome instability in human colorectal cancers. *Proc. Nat. Acad. Sci. U.S.A.* 105 (9): 3443–3448.

19 Roncucci, L., and Mariani, F. (2015). Prevention of colorectal cancer: How many tools do we have in our basket? *Eur. J Intern. Med.* 26 (10): 752–756.

20 Algra, A.M., and Rothwell, P.M. (2012). Effects of regular aspirin on long-term cancer incidence and metastasis: A systematic comparison of evidence from observational studies versus randomised trials. *Lancet Oncol.* 13 (5): 518–527.

21 Kune, G.A., Kune, S., and Watson, L.F. (1988). Colorectal cancer risk, chronic illnesses, operations, and medications: Case control results from the Melbourne Colorectal Cancer Study. *Cancer Res.* 48 (15): 4399–4404.

22 Burn, J., Gerdes, A.M., Macrae, F. et al. (2011). Long-term effect of aspirin on cancer risk in carriers of hereditary colorectal cancer: An analysis from the CAPP2 randomised controlled trial. *Lancet* 378 (9809): 2081–2087.

23 Cook, N.R., Lee, I.M., Zhang, S.M. et al. (2013). Alternate-day, low-dose aspirin and cancer risk: Long-term observational follow-up of a randomized trial. *Ann. Intern. Med.* 159 (2): 77–85.

24 Ishikawa, H., Wakabayashi, K., Suzuki, S. et al. (2013). Preventive effects of low-dose aspirin on colorectal adenoma growth in patients with familial adenomatous polyposis: Double-blind, randomized clinical trial. *Cancer Med.* 2 (1): 50–56.

25 Burn, J., Bishop, D.T., Chapman, P.D. et al. (2011). A randomized placebo-controlled prevention trial of aspirin and/or resistant starch in young people with familial adenomatous polyposis. *Cancer Prevent. Res.* 4 (5): 655–665.

26 Cole, B.F., Logan, R.F., Halabi, S. et al. (2009). Aspirin for the chemoprevention of colorectal adenomas: Meta-analysis of the randomized trials. *J. Nat. Cancer Inst.* 101 (4): 256–266.

27 Rothwell, P.M., Wilson, M., Price, J.F. et al. (2012). Effect of daily aspirin on risk of cancer metastasis: A study of incident cancers during randomised controlled trials. *Lancet* 379 (9826): 1591–1601.

28 Rothwell, P.M., Price, J.F., Fowkes, F.G.R. et al. (2012). Short-term effects of daily aspirin on cancer incidence, mortality, and non-vascular death: Analysis of the time course of risks and benefits in 51 randomised controlled trials. *Lancet* 379 (9826): 1602–1612.

29 Picot, D., Loll, P.J., and Garavito, R.M. (1994). The X-ray crystal structure of the membrane protein prostaglandin H2 synthase-1. *Nature* 367 (6460): 243–249.

30 Gay, L.J., and Felding-Habermann, B. (2011). Contribution of platelets to tumour metastasis. *Nature Rev. Cancer* 11 (2): 123–134.

31 Dovizio, M., Bruno, A., Tacconelli, S., and Patrignani, P. (2013). Mode of action of aspirin as a chemopreventive agent. In: *Prospects for Chemoprevention of Colorectal Neoplasia* (A.T. Chan and E. Detering, ed.), 39–65. Berlin: Springer.

32 Sharma, N.P., Dong, L., Yuan, C. et al. (2010). Asymmetric acetylation of the cyclooxygenase-2 homodimer by aspirin and its effects on the oxygenation of arachidonic, eicosapentaenoic, and docosahexaenoic acids. *Mol. Pharmacol.* 77 (6): 979–986.

33 Alfonso, L., Ai, G., Spitale, R.C., and Bhat, G.J. (2014). Molecular targets of aspirin and cancer prevention. *Br. J. Cancer* 111 (1): 61–67.

34 Ferrandez, A., Piazuelo, E., and Castells, A. (2012). Aspirin and the prevention of colorectal cancer. *Best Pract. Res. Clin. Gastroenterol.* 26 (2): 185–195.

35 Chan, A.T., Ogino, S., and Fuchs, C.S. (2007). Aspirin and the risk of colorectal cancer in relation to the expression of COX-2. *N. Engl. J. Med.* 356 (21): 2131–2142.

36 McCarty, M.F., and Block, K.I. (2006). Preadministration of high-dose salicylates, suppressors of NF-kappaB activation, may increase the chemosensitivity of many cancers: An example of proapoptotic signal modulation therapy. *Integr. Cancer Ther.* 5 (3): 252–268.

37 Stark, L.A., Din, F.V., Zwacka, R.M., and Dunlop, M.G. (2001). Aspirin-induced activation of the NF-kappaB signaling pathway: A novel mechanism for aspirin-mediated apoptosis in colon cancer cells. *FASEB J.* 15 (7): 1273–1275.

38 Din, F.V., Dunlop, M.G., and Stark, L.A. (2004). Evidence for colorectal cancer cell specificity of aspirin effects on NF kappa B signalling and apoptosis. *Br. J. Cancer* 91 (2): 381–388.

39 Borthwick, G.M., Johnson, A.S., Partington, M. et al. (2006). Therapeutic levels of aspirin and salicylate directly inhibit a model of angiogenesis through a Cox-independent mechanism. *FASEB J.* 20 (12): 2009–2016.

40 Pathi, S., Jutooru, I., Chadalapaka, G. et al. (2012). Aspirin inhibits colon cancer cell and tumor growth and downregulates specificity protein (Sp) transcription factors. *PLoS One* 7 (10): e48208.

41 Bau, J.T., Kang, Z., Austin, C.A., and Kurz, E.U. (2014). Salicylate, a catalytic inhibitor of topoisomerase II, inhibits DNA cleavage and is selective for the alpha isoform. *Mol. Pharmacol.* 85 (2): 198–207.

42 Spitz, G.A., Furtado, C.M., Sola-Penna, M., and Zancan, P. (2009). Acetylsalicylic acid and salicylic acid decrease tumor cell viability and glucose metabolism modulating 6-phosphofructo-1-kinase structure and activity. *Biochem. Pharmacol.* 77 (1): 46–53.

43 Martínez, M.E., O'Brien, T.G., Fultz, K.E. et al. (2003). Pronounced reduction in adenoma recurrence associated with aspirin use and a polymorphism in the ornithine decarboxylase gene. *Proc. Nat. Acad. Sci. U.S.A.* 100 (13): 7859–7864.

44 Chan, A.T., Tranah, G.J., Giovannucci, E.L. et al. (2005). Genetic variants in the UGT1A6 enzyme, aspirin use, and the risk of colorectal adenoma. *J. Nat. Cancer Inst.* 97 (6): 457–460.

45 Nan, H., Hutter, C.M., Lin, Y. et al. (2015). Association of aspirin and nsaid use with risk of colorectal cancer according to genetic variants. *JAMA* 313 (11): 1133–1142.

46 Yan, M., Rerko, R.M., Platzer, P. et al. (2004). 15-Hydroxyprostaglandin dehydrogenase, a COX-2 oncogene antagonist, is a TGF-beta-induced suppressor of human gastrointestinal cancers. *Proc. Nat. Acad. Sci. U.S.A.* 101 (50): 17468–17473.

47 Fink, S.P., Yamauchi, M., Nishihara, R. et al. (2014). Aspirin and the risk of colorectal cancer in relation to the expression of 15-hydroxyprostaglandin dehydrogenase (HPGD). *Sci. Transl. Med.* 6 (233): 233re2.

48 Samuels, Y., Wang, Z., Bardelli, A. et al. (2004). High frequency of mutations of the PIK3CA gene in human cancers. *Science* 304 (5670): 554.

49 Liao, X., Lochhead, P., Nishihara, R. et al. (2012). Aspirin use, tumor PIK3CA mutation, and colorectal-cancer survival. *N. Engl. J. Med.* 367 (17): 1596–1606.

50 Reimers, M.S., Bastiaannet, E., Langley, R.E. et al. (2014). Expression of HLA class I antigen, aspirin use, and survival after a diagnosis of colon cancer. *JAMA Intern. Med.* 174 (5): 732–739.

51 Cuzick, J., Thorat, M.A., Bosetti, C. et al. (2014). Estimates of benefits and harms of prophylactic use of aspirin in the general population. *Ann. Oncol.* 26 (1): 47–57.

52 Movahedi, M., Bishop, D.T., Macrae, F. et al. (2015). Obesity, aspirin, and risk of colorectal cancer in carriers of hereditary colorectal cancer: A prospective investigation in the CAPP2 study. *J. Clin. Oncol.* 33 (31): 3591–3597.

53 Ait Ouakrim, D., Dashti, S.G., Chau, R. et al. (2015). Aspirin, ibuprofen, and the risk of colorectal cancer in Lynch syndrome. *J. Nat. Cancer Inst.* 107 (9): djv170.

54 Friis, S., Riis, A.H., Erichsen, R. et al. (2015). Low-dose aspirin or nonsteroidal anti-inflammatory drug use and colorectal cancer risk: A population-based, case-control study. *Ann. Intern. Med.* 163 (5): 347–355.

55 Huang, E.S., Strate, L.L., Ho, W.W. et al. (2011). Long term use of aspirin and the risk of gastrointestinal bleeding. *Am. J. Med.* 124 (5): 426–433.

56 CaPP3 Study (2018) CaPP3 Cancer Prevention Programme. www.capp3.org (accessed 3 January 2018).

57 Spechler, S.J., Sharma, P., Souza, R.F. et al. (2011). American Gastroenterological Association medical position statement on the management of Barrett's esophagus. *Gastroenterology* 140 (3): 1084–1091.

58 Allum, W.H., Blazeby, J.M., Griffin, S.M. et al. (2011). Guidelines for the management of oesophageal and gastric cancer. *Gut* 60 (11): 1449–1472.

59 Gray, J., Mao, J.T., Szabo, E. et al. Lung cancer chemoprevention: ACCP evidence-based clinical practice guidelines (2nd edition). *Chest* 132 (3, Suppl.): 56S–68S.

60 Giardiello, F.M., Allen, J.I., Axilbund, J.E. et al. (2014). Guidelines on genetic evaluation and management of Lynch syndrome: A consensus statement by the US Multi-Society Task Force on Colorectal Cancer. *Gastroenterology* 147: 502–26.

61 U.S. Preventive Services Task Force (2007). Routine aspirin or nonsteroidal anti-inflammatory drugs for the primary prevention of colorectal cancer: U.S. Preventive Services Task Force recommendation statement. *Ann. Intern. Med.* 146 (5): 361–364.

62 Chubak, J., Whitlock, E.P., Williams, S.B. et al. (2016). Aspirin for the prevention of cancer incidence and mortality: Systematic evidence reviews for the U.S. Preventive Services Task Force. *Ann. Intern. Med.* 164 (12): 814–825.

63 Guirguis-Blake, J.M., Evans, C.V., Senger, C.A. et al. (2016). Aspirin for the primary prevention of cardiovascular events: A systematic evidence review for the U.S. Preventive Services Task Force. *Ann. Intern. Med.* 164 (12): 804–813.

64 Whitlock, E.P., Burda, B.U., Williams, S. et al. (2016). Bleeding risks with aspirin use for primary prevention in adults: A systematic evidenvce review for the U.S. Preventive Services Task Force. *Ann. Intern. Med.* 164 (12): 826–835.

65 Henderson, N., and Smith, T. (2013). Aspirin for the next generation. *ecancermedicalscience* 7: 300.

66 Schwitalle, Y., Kloor, M., Eiermann, S. et al. (2008). Immune response against frameshift-induced neopeptides in HNPCC patients and healthy HNPCC mutation carriers. *Gastroenterology* 134 (4): 988–997.

67 Micoryx-Studie (n.d.). Informationen zur Micoryx-Impfstudie für Patienten mit Dickdarmkrebs. www.micoryx.de (accessed 3 January 2018).

68 Zelenay, S., van der Veen, A.G., Bottcher, J.P. et al. (2015). Cyclooxygenase-dependent tumor growth through evasion of immunity. *Cell* 162 (6): 1257–1270.

69 Koelzer, V.H., Baker, K., Kassahn, D. et al. (2012). Prognostic impact of beta-2-microglobulin expression in colorectal cancers stratified by mismatch repair status. *J. Clin. Pathol.* 65 (11): 996–1002.

70 Kelderman, S., Schumacher, T.N., and Kvistborg, P. (2015). Mismatch repair-deficient cancers are targets for anti-PD-1 therapy. *Cancer Cell* 28 (1): 11–13.

71 Topalian, S.L., Hodi, F.S., Brahmer, J.R. et al. (2012). Safety, activity, and immune correlates of anti–PD-1 antibody in cancer. *N. Engl. J. Med.* 366 (26): 2443–2454.

72 Le, D.T., Uram, J.N., Wang, H. et al. (2015). PD-1 blockade in tumors with mismatch-repair deficiency. *N. Engl. J. Med.* 372 (26): 2509–2520.

CHAPTER 15

Colon cancer screening

David F. Ransohoff

Division of Gastroenterology and Hepatology, Department of Medicine; Department of Epidemiology, University of North Carolina, Chapel Hill, NC, USA

SUMMARY BOX

- Screening for colorectal cancer (CRC) has been shown in multiple randomized clinical trials (RCTs) to lower CRC incidence and mortality.

- The early RCTs showed that programmes of guaiac faecal occult blood testing (gFOBT) were successful, even though one annual gFOBT was not highly sensitive.

- Faecal immunochemical testing has demonstrated far superior sensitivity of 70% for invasive cancer, and is now preferred over guaiac-based testing.

- Sigmoidoscopy examines only the left colon, but has been shown in four RCTs to lower CRC mortality from left-colon lesions by 60%.

- Colonoscopy examines the entire colon and enables removal of lesions during the procedure. RCTs are being conducted to quantitatively document its benefits.

- Quality of a screening programme, whether done at the practice level or at the national system level, is an important determinant of outcome. Quality metrics, such as a colonoscopist's adenoma detection rate or a practice's or system's rate of appropriate follow-up of screening findings, are only now being understood and measured.

- While many guidelines for CRC screening have been produced, the quality of guideline-making varies. In general, the US Preventive Services Task Force guidelines have been judged high quality by the National Academy of Medicine in the USA.

This chapter describes key issues in colorectal cancer (CRC) screening and discusses the status of each, as well as challenges and opportunities for the future. The evolution of CRC screening over the last 25 years has been dramatic. In the early 1990s there was no convincing evidence that CRC screening reduced cancer mortality, and guidelines were generally silent about screening. Now multiple randomized controlled clinical trials (RCTs) have shown efficacy, and a variety of CRC screening strategies are being recommended and implemented in countries throughout the world. The reduction of cancer-specific mortality is larger for CRC

Cancer Prevention and Screening: Concepts, Principles and Controversies, First Edition.
Edited by Rosalind A. Eeles, Christine D. Berg, and Jeffrey S. Tobias.
© 2019 John Wiley & Sons, Inc. Published 2019 by John Wiley & Sons, Inc.

screening than for other major cancers like breast, prostate, lung, or ovary. Similar to cervix cancer screening, CRC screening can identify and then remove pre-neoplastic lesions, so it can also lower invasive cancer incidence.

With this background, key questions have evolved from 'Does CRC screening work?' to 'How much can it be made to work?' How can efficacy be improved by considering not just individual tests, but also the systems by which screening is implemented: the testing selected, follow-up of positive results, adherence to repeated testing in a programme over time, and issues of 'quality' at every step? As screening is implemented, the volume and efficient utilization of post-polypectomy surveillance will need to be managed.

Rationale for CRC screening

Overview of evidence

The basis for implementing CRC screening is evidence of efficacy from RCTs, initially assessing for guaiac-based faecal occult blood testing (FOBT). Three RCTs in the 1990s showed a 13–16% reduction in CRC mortality [1–3], and RCTs of sigmoidoscopy published in the 2010s showed a reduction in CRC mortality of about 60% for lesions within the reach of the scope [4–7]. This strong RCT evidence has been considered the 'proof of principle' that benefit accrues from finding early CRC and precancerous lesions, including certain kinds of 'high-risk' adenomas, based on the belief that, biologically, CRC arises from a generally orderly progression from precancerous adenoma to early and then to late-stage cancer.

Targets of screening

Even if RCTs of screening show reduced CRC mortality, there is uncertainty about exactly how that mortality reduction is achieved and what should be the 'targets' of screening. Early-stage CRCs are important targets (Stages I and II, and even many Stage III cases that can be 'cured'), as are the large (over 1 or 2 cm) adenomas thought to be immediate precursors of CRC. However, there is substantial uncertainty about 'where to draw the line' regarding which adenomas should be targets, given that about 50% of persons over age 50 will be found to have at least one adenoma, even if many are quite small, under 5 mm. The vast majority of adenomas, then, will never grow into cancer. Unknown is whether most cancers grow slowly from precursors, over decades, with average 'dwell times' from adenoma incidence to CRC diagnosis of an average of 17–25 years, as suggested in mathematical models [8,9], or whether a substantial portion of cancers grow very quickly from small lesions. It is clear that, for many other cancers, a broad spectrum of growth rates exists, with some growing very slowly and others rapidly, as happens for cancers of the breast, prostate, and lung. An unresolved issue biologically for CRC is whether the long 'average' dwell time is composed of distinct groups of slow-growing and fast-growing lesions, because in that case screening programmes would have to be adjusted to detect the fast-growing (and thus the most dangerous) lesions, through shorter screening intervals if early detection affected the outcome of highly aggressive lesions. The issue of 'which targets' is particularly important for indirect tests like FOBT that are less sensitive for earlier lesions than endoscopy.

Sorting out answers to these questions in the existing literature can be like looking through fog, because so many nonbiological factors affect what lesions can be observed, such as poor preparation for the procedure, limited inspection, and sometimes simple ignorance of knowing what to look for, as has been highlighted by the only recent recognition that serrated lesions in the right colon are both clinically important and hard to detect because of their flat shape and bland coloration. Much of the frustration in trying to understand 'what targets' results from the difficulties these problems cause in studying natural history.

Role of endoscopy versus indirect tests

Colonoscopy, as a test that directly examines the colon, will always have an important role in any programme of CRC screening, because it provides the intervention – detection and removal of targets – that improves outcome. An indirect test such as a stool or blood test can, at most, delay colonoscopy, perhaps forever, if a negative test result correctly indicates the absence of important lesions.

Stool blood testing

Guaiac-based FOBT: RCT evidence of efficacy

Guaiac-based faecal occult blood testing (gFOBT) was the first CRC screening test shown in an RCT to reduce CRC mortality. Involving over a quarter of a million subjects over two decades, three classic RCTs showed a roughly 15% CRC mortality reduction [1–3]. While gFOBT sensitivity for CRC – either at one application of a test or in a programme of repeated testing over time – could not be directly assessed in those studies, a later practice-based study showed sensitivity to be only 13% at one application [10]. On the one hand, then, gFOBT worked fairly well, because it did improve CRC outcome in spite of the low application sensitivity. On the other hand, there seemed to be room for improvement if a stool test more sensitive than gFOBT could be developed.

Faecal immunochemical testing: An improved stool test

Substantial improvement in stool blood testing is now provided by development of the faecal immunochemical test (FIT), which measures human haemoglobin and is approximately 70% sensitive for CRC at a specificity of roughly 95%, similar to gFOBT [11]. FIT avoids the false-positive results from diet that constituted a problem for gFOBT. False-positive results can occur because of biological bleeding, like from angiodysplasia or haemorrhoids. And FIT can be falsely negative to the extent that CRCs or important precursors do not bleed. Its sensitivity for large (1 cm) adenomas or sessile serrated polyps is only about 24% [12]. While this sensitivity is higher than that of gFOBT, it is still low in absolute terms, leaving unclear how much FIT's low sensitivity for important CRC precursors compromises its overall ability to lower CRC mortality in a programme of repeated testing. The answer to that question depends on how fast various lesions grow and on the impact of repeated testing in a programme of screening. These questions may be answered in RCTs involving FIT now under way in the USA (the Veterans Administration's [VA] CONFIRM trial) and in Europe [13].

FIT and guidelines

Programmes of FIT testing are recommended as 'acceptable' by the US Preventive Services Task Force (USPSTF), just as are programmes of colonoscopy and sigmoidoscopy screening [9, 14, 15]. The rationale for 'equal status' or no preference among different testing programmes is discussed later in the section on guidelines.

Challenges for the future
Clinical use

Because FIT has a variable cut-off for positivity, it may be possible to adjust its performance for use in different screening settings, particularly when a defined population is being considered for screening, as is routinely done in Europe and in many health maintenance organizations (HMO) in the USA. Thus the 'constraints and expectations' of screening programmes may specifically be adjusted for, for example when a country [16] has limited colonoscopy resources, via adjusting the overall test positivity rate by changing the FIT cut-off to suit the resources available [17].

Technical issues

Because various FITs being developed utilize different reagents and technical features, practical details are being addressed, such as how to measure haemoglobin amount and concentration in relation to stool volume, along with details of the sampling device and buffer solution, so that reliable comparisons can be provided among different assays [18]. An additional practical problem is understanding the stability of analytes in different ambient temperatures.

FIT sensitivity in a programme of testing repeatedly over time

While FIT's 70% sensitivity for CRC at one application is already quite high, its 'programme sensitivity' – the sensitivity to detect CRC and other lesions when applied repeatedly over time – may be even higher. Increased programme sensitivity would occur if a subsequent test result were 'independent' of the result at a prior application. However, if, biologically, some lesions simply do not bleed, perhaps like right-sided serrated lesions that are not vascular, then a subsequent FIT result would not be independent, and repeated testing in a programme would not lead to higher cumulative sensitivity. Ongoing RCTs may help address this issue.

Sigmoidoscopy

Although sigmoidoscopy examines just half the colon endoscopically, it has been considered to be a recommended stand-alone screening test, both in the USA and in Europe. It is easier to perform than colonoscopy, in terms of bowel preparation, risk, and training, and there is no need for sedation. It achieves a large degree of CRC mortality reduction, at least for the left colon, where more than half of all CRCs are located.

Evidence of efficacy from RCTs

RCT evidence shows that sigmoidoscopy reduces CRC mortality by roughly 60% for lesions within reach of the scope in per-protocol analysis [4–7]. As might be expected, sigmoidoscopy has minimal impact for lesions on the right; any impact in the right colon is due to colonoscopy that may be provoked by finding a lesion in the left colon that prompts colonoscopic detection and removal of that lesion or another elsewhere in the colon.

International variability in the practice of sigmoidoscopy

A fascinating feature of sigmoidoscopy is how dramatically routine practice varies between countries. In the USA, where historically sigmoidoscopy has been performed by primary care physicians, lesions discovered are not removed and often not even biopsied, but rather are left intact until colonoscopy is performed by a gastroenterologist. In a major RCT conducted in practice settings in the USA, roughly 20% of persons screened had some 'lesion' leading to referral for colonoscopy [6]. The lesions included not only adenomas but also non-neoplastic hyperplastic polyps, as well as normal mucosa that, had the histology been known, would have incurred no work-up. In striking contrast, the custom in the UK is for lesions found at screening sigmoidoscopy to be routinely resected at the screening exam, with follow-up colonoscopy done only for persons with large (over 1 cm), histologically advanced, or multiple (three or more) adenomas. In the UK sigmoidoscopy RCT, then, only 5% of participants were referred for colonoscopy work-up [4]. Such differences in custom and referral rate have a substantial impact on cost, effort, and the outcome of screening programmes.

Sigmoidoscopy and guidelines

As for FIT, programmes of sigmoidoscopy, either alone or in combination with FIT, are recommended without preference by the USPSTF.

Challenges for the future: Tailoring screening to risk

In programmes that 'tailor' testing strategies to specific features of risk – like prevalence and location of CRC and advanced adenomas by age and gender – sigmoidoscopy might be particularly useful for persons, for example younger women, who may have a low likelihood of proximal advanced lesions [19].

Colonoscopy

Colonoscopy provides a method that decreases CRC mortality and incidence, by detecting and removing early CRC or advanced or large adenomas and serrated lesions that may soon evolve into CRC. Colonoscopy may be used either as a primary screening test or in follow-up to a positive result of an indirect test like FIT.

How effective could colonoscopy be in assuring low future CRC risk?

Since colonoscopy is the method by which other indirect tests work – by finding and removing early invasive cancers or precancers, or by prompting surgical resection of later-stage lesions – it is worth considering how good colonoscopy could be, meaning how long-lasting could 'protection' be from a single high-quality colonoscopy.

Even though the question may sound simple, it is surprisingly difficult to answer, for two reasons. First, what quality actually is – that is, what features of quality affect outcome – is only recently being understood. Second, learning outcome is difficult in any follow-up study if persons are not left 'undisturbed' so that an important outcome (like CRC or very large adenoma) can develop. Both problems make it difficult to determine the length of protection from a single high-quality exam.

A colonoscopy exam could provide protection in two different ways, depending on whether the colonoscopy result is negative or positive.

A negative exam cannot directly lower CRC risk, but it may predict low future CRC risk

For persons with no neoplastic lesions found at a high-quality examination, how long does this indication of low CRC risk or CRC mortality last? Ten years? Twenty? A lifetime? If, in practice, a high-quality negative exam signifies 'very low future risk' and can take someone out of the screening cycle for 20 years, then a substantial portion of persons – perhaps half or more – might be handled relatively simply in programmes of screening. While CRC risk is related to features like family history, gender, weight, and smoking status, the 'negative' state of the colon – if the examination is high quality – may provide strong prediction of low future risk. A case-control study from Germany showing a low long-term risk of CRC after a negative colonoscopy [20] led to the suggestion that a single negative colonoscopy at age 60, or perhaps two examinations at age 50 and 70, if performed by a 'high detecting colonoscopist', might provide sufficient screening [21]. This kind of approach is clearly worth aggressively considering.

A positive exam may, when lesions are cleared, directly reduce future CRC risk

Second, for persons with a positive colonoscopy whose neoplasms are removed, CRC incidence or mortality could be reduced in the future, as has been shown for example in RCTs of sigmoidoscopy screening. Unclear, however, is how completely the clock can be set back. Is risk set back to that of a person who has never had a neoplasm? Or is that person's risk still increased even if their colon is now 'cleared'? Future risk likely depends on details of a person's history of neoplasms (size, histology, number), along with features like family history, gender, weight, smoking, and so on. In this context, it is still worth trying to learn how much of the reduction may accrue from a high-quality examination.

The logistics of doing studies to answer these questions are daunting, but two European settings may provide at least partial answers. The UK RCT of sigmoidoscopy is following persons who had their left colon cleared and then received no follow-up (no colonoscopy work-up, and no post-polypectomy colonoscopic surveillance), among persons with up to two adenomas under 1 cm [4]. It would be informative to learn whether persons with two 5–10 mm adenomas removed had the same – or higher – CRC outcomes compared to persons with no adenomas. In addition, an RCT of colonoscopy in Europe may provide useful information [22]. Key features for each study include having an unperturbed follow-up period so that outcomes can develop, as well as methods to assess the quality of individual endoscopists, in order to ascertain the long-term outcome of a high-quality endoscopic procedure, both in prediction and in protection.

Can the magnitude of colonoscopy protection be inferred from data from sigmoidoscopy RCTs?

Because RCT evidence is not yet available to directly demonstrate the efficacy of colonoscopy screening, RCT evidence about sigmoidoscopy may provide some insight. One could argue that the 60% reduction of CRC mortality for endoscopy on the left would be an optimistic estimate of reduction on the right, which is more difficult to reach endoscopically and more difficult to prepare, and because right-sided lesions are harder to find because they can be flat and with less distinctive colour. Ongoing RCTs of colonoscopy, including the USA's CONFIRM trial and Europe's NordiCC trial [22], may help address these questions.

Can the magnitude of colonoscopy protection be inferred from non-RCT studies?

The main source of estimates of colonoscopy protection includes studies that are not RCTs and that, lacking a direct comparison group, use historical controls or other methods to calculate expected outcomes for comparison. Not only is the lack of a direct and concurrent comparison group a problem, but also it can be unclear what the intervention was. To the extent that subjects in such studies may have had multiple colonoscopies done over time (e.g. including post-polypectomy surveillance), it can be difficult to know at the individual patient level how many colonoscopies were done and to relate that intensity to outcome. While such studies overall strongly suggest protection stemming from colonoscopy, both the magnitude of protection – and the intensity of the intervention responsible for protection – are not nearly as clear as they would be in an RCT.

The National Polyp Study initially reported a 76–90% reduction in CRC incidence [23] and, later, a 53% reduction in CRC mortality [24] in persons who had had a colonoscopy, including multiple colonoscopies over time. Other non-RCT studies show protection as well, but also lack important detail (detail that is admittedly very difficult to assess) about the overall intensity of intervention in individual subjects [25, 26]. Of particular interest for such longitudinal studies would be to try to determine how much protection comes from an initial examination compared to subsequent surveillance.

Colonoscopy quality: Very variable and very significant

It is only recently being appreciated that colonoscopy quality varies widely and how it depends on features like bowel preparation and on operator-based features like thoroughness of inspection and completeness of removal of lesions. While initial efforts to assess quality focused on the relation of caecal intubation rate and withdrawal time to numbers of lesions detected, recent reports have begun to relate important outcomes, like CRC mortality and incidence, to the adenoma detection rate (ADR) of individual practitioners. A report of over 300 000 colonoscopies done by 136 gastroenterologists in an HMO showed that ADRs from 7.4% to 52.5% were associated with a roughly 60% lower risk of fatal CRC for practitioners in the highest quintile of ADR compared to the lowest [27, 28].

While these data show that outcome is dramatically related to ADR, it is not clear whether ADR – and increasing ADR – is the 'cause' that would improve outcome. For example, ADR might be a surrogate marker for another feature of quality that is causal, like better detection of large lesions or flat lesions, or better resection. Correctly determining cause is critical, because efforts to improve the incorrect metric (for example, simply increasing ADR by finding tiny adenomas that may be unimportant) may not improve outcome and may be wasteful.

Measuring and improving components of quality are being addressed particularly intensely in Europe, where countries are responsible for managing entire systems of health care [29–31].

Challenges for the future

Important questions about the possible role of colonoscopy include:
- What is the length of 'predictive effect' (if colonoscopy is negative) and 'protective effect' (if positive) of a single high-quality colonoscopy?
- For persons with a high-quality negative exam, is the long-term risk of CRC low enough that they can be taken out of the screening system for 15 or 20 years?
- Can available data and modelling indicate how much CRC reduction is contributed by the initial colonoscopy versus a subsequent colonoscopy?
- Can methods to reduce cost be adopted in the USA, like doing procedures unsedated, as is done in parts of Europe? Does lack of sedation compromise quality, such as thoroughness of inspection?
- To what extent can nonphysicians perform high-quality colonoscopy?

Post-polypectomy surveillance

Surveillance is the practice of more aggressive (more aggressive than for persons with average risk) follow-up of persons thought to have an increased risk of developing future CRC. 'High-risk' polyps – composed of 'advanced adenomas' including ones over 1 cm, multiple (three or more, though this number is under reconsideration), and with advanced histology (e.g. villous or tubulovillous) – are thought to indicate, after being cleared from a colon, higher future risk of CRC in the rest of the colon.

The volume of post-polypectomy colonoscopic surveillance will grow in the next decade as CRC screening is increasingly implemented. When colonoscopy is done, either as the primary screening test or when provoked by an indirect screening test, adenomas will be discovered, since about 50% of persons over age 50 have an adenoma if one looks hard enough for very small ones. These findings will incur decisions about surveillance. Further contributing to increased detection is the use of high-definition colonoscopes and the increasing focus on ADRs as a quality metric. All these forces will tend to place screened persons in a high-risk group thought to require intensive surveillance.

Surveillance guidelines have varied over time and have at times been overaggressive

Surveillance guidelines have varied dramatically and have, at times, reflected an overestimate of the seriousness of finding polyps. In the early 1990s, the CRC risk of 'polyp-formers' – almost anyone with any adenomatous polyp – was thought to be so high that every three-year or even every one-year post-polypectomy surveillance was commonly recommended. It was in this era that the National Polyp Study (NPS) RCT was designed to test the hypothesis that a CRC difference would occur in persons having one-year post-polypectomy follow-up compared to three years. The 1993 NPS RCT report of almost no cancers (a total of three) in either group [23] was both welcome news and a shocking indicator of how off-target the expectations had been.

Another surprise, showing that at least some kinds of adenomas indicate no increased future risk of CRC, came from a UK cohort study in which persons with recto-sigmoid adenomas removed at sigmoidoscopy were followed 13 years for development of CRC anywhere in the colon. A subgroup of persons with one or two small (under 1 cm) adenomas was shown, unexpectedly, to have average risk of CRC – that is, the same risk (actually it was a little lower) as persons considered average risk – for lesions anywhere in the colon [32]. Because risk was so low, even though these persons had had adenomas, such persons could be recommended to have no surveillance more aggressive than regular screening. (A group was also identified with high risk, including persons with over 1 cm adenomas and multiple adenomas, that is three or more.)

Based on these data, the first two published polyp guidelines recommended that persons with one or two low-risk adenomas (under 1 cm) may not need any surveillance at all after polypectomy, but rather merely routine screening [33–35]. In the following decades, however, surveillance recommendations became more aggressive for this low-risk group, even in the absence of clear evidence that natural history was more ominous [35].

Last, physicians tend to recommend aggressive surveillance even for persons in the low-risk group, in both the USA and Europe [35,36]. At the same time, there is evidence that some persons in higher-risk groups do not receive aggressive enough surveillance, so problems in clinician behaviour exist at both ends of the risk spectrum.

Challenges for the future

Several forces operate to make post-polypectomy surveillance – and oversurveillance – a pressing problem to be managed:

- As programmes of screening are implemented, planners will need to consider the downstream effort and cost of surveillance, how to frame guidelines, and how to incentivize physicians not to be overly aggressive.
- In an era when better scopes and increased focus on ADRs lead to finding more and more adenomas and to classifying people into a high-risk group (if simply because of more than three adenomas, even if they are tiny), it would be useful to know how much 'upstaging' can be accounted for as an artefact of improved diagnostic technology. Perhaps the criteria for a low-risk group should be adjusted to include persons who now might be considered high risk because of more than three tiny adenomas, since these lesions never would have been discovered before and we do not have empirical evidence about the natural history of such persons. Research about post-polypectomy surveillance in Europe (EPoS) [37] or the USA should consider how to adjust for this problem of upstaging.

Screening guidelines

Guidelines have consequences for practice by influencing physicians, payers, and overall expectations. While virtually all guidelines claim to be evidence based, enormous variation can occur. In the mid-2000s, over 250 guideline-making organizations had created over 2500 guidelines, many of which disagreed on the same topic. Guideline-making is complicated and labour intensive, when done in the detailed, prespecified, quantitative, explicit manner developed by the USPSTF, and there is almost no review process or method to judge guidelines' trustworthiness or quality. In this setting, the US Congress asked the National Academy of Sciences' Institute of Medicine (IOM; now the National Academy of Medicine) to write a report describing how to judge the trustworthiness of guidelines. The IOM report used two CRC-screening guidelines, both written in 2008, to illustrate differences in the output and in the process and quality of guideline-making [38].

Different recommendations

The USPSTF 2008 CRC guidelines had concluded that 'any of several strategies is acceptable', including programmes of FOBT/FIT screening, sigmoidoscopy alone, colonoscopy and so on [14]. In contrast, the MSTF/ACS (Multisociety Task Force, comprised of US gastrointestinal (GI) subspecialty societies and the American College of Radiology, along with the American Cancer Society) said that 'structural exams were preferred' because 'prevention is better than early detection' [39], a statement widely interpreted as saying that colonoscopy was preferred compared to programmes of FIT testing or other strategies.

These differences were dramatic to both the GI and primary care communities. The phrase 'prevention is better than early detection' – which favoured colonoscopy – became a popular message, including in advertisements by GI professional societies.

Different processes

The differing recommendations were products of different processes, and those processes had different degrees of quality. The USPSTF – as one of the organizations that developed the field of evidence-based medicine – uses explicit, prespecified, and transparent methods to quantitatively project outcomes of benefit versus harm for individual patients. The reason that different strategies (like FIT and colonoscopy) have been recommended as acceptable and without preference is that the USPSTF has found, in its quantitative assessment of outcomes, that programmes of screening using a less sensitive test (like FOBT) applied more frequently over time can be as effective, and sometimes even more effective, than a more sensitive test (like colonoscopy) applied less frequently over time. This seemingly counter-intuitive result can occur when the dwell times of lesions that cause death are short, because those lesions would be missed by a more sensitive test applied less frequently [40].

The MSTF/ACS did no quantitative projection of outcome. Rather, it based its choices on new rules of thumb that were developed during the process of guideline-making, including whether a test had a sensitivity for CRC of 50% at one point in time, and on whether the test was a 'structural exam', because of the idea that prevention is better than early detection.

The IOM report used the MSTF/ACS guidelines as an example of a lesser-quality process, because of the lack of quantitative, explicit consideration of outcomes as well as other reasons [38].

The USPSTF CRC screening guidelines, updated in 2016, now consider acceptable seven different screening strategies (colonoscopy, sigmoidoscopy plus annual FIT, annual FIT alone, CT colonograpy, stool FIT-DNA, guaiac-based FOBT, and sigmoidoscopy without a stool-based test) [15] that doctors and patients may select from, using results of models projecting outcomes that patients and doctors may consider in 'shared decision-making' [9]. In the process of developing its 2016 recommendations, the USPSTF 'now acknowledges, appropriately, the many … "moving parts" that affect the clinical outcomes of screening programs in practice [including how] … colonoscopy quality may vary widely as may the performance and accuracy of imaging procedures and stool-based screening tests' [41]. Within this context, the task force 'appears to believe that the most important of these moving parts is the likelihood that the patient will actually undergo screening with a test that has been deemed "acceptable"' [41].

Challenges for the future

Creating guidelines and judging their quality provide a fascinating challenge for the field of medicine. In the USA, where professional organizations' goals include both to promote 'best care' of patients and also to promote their professional members' economic interests, conflicts can occur that must be appropriately managed, as suggested by the National Academy of Medicine [38]. The USPSTF needs to clarify its currently evolving standards for where the bar is that must be cleared to make a testing strategy 'acceptable' [41]. The situation in Europe is less fraught, because there are fewer groups making guidelines, and the economic conflicts of medical professionals may be less strong.

References

1 Mandel, J.S., Bond, J.H., Church, T.R. et al. (1993). Reducing mortality from colorectal cancer by screening for fecal occult blood. Minnesota Colon Cancer Control Study. *N. Engl. J. Med.* 328 (19): 1365–1371.

2 Hardcastle, J.D., and Justin, T.A. (1996). Screening high-risk groups for colorectal neoplasia. *Am. J. Gastroenterol.* 91: 850–852.

3 Kronborg, O., Fenger, C., Olsen, J. et al. (1996). Randomised study of screening for colorectal cancer with faecal-occult-blood test. *Lancet* 348 (9040): 1467–1471.

4 Atkin, W.S., Edwards, R., Kralj-Hans, I. et al. (2010). Once-only flexible sigmoidoscopy screening in prevention of colorectal cancer: A multicentre randomised controlled trial. *Lancet* 375 (9726): 1624–1633.

5 Segnan, N., Armaroli, P., Bonelli, L. et al. (2011). Once-only sigmoidoscopy in colorectal cancer screening: Follow-up findings of the Italian Randomized Controlled Trial – SCORE. *J. Natl Cancer Inst.* 103 (17): 1310–1322.

6 Schoen, R.E., Pinsky, P.F., Weissfeld, J.L. et al. (2012). Colorectal-cancer incidence and mortality with screening flexible sigmoidoscopy. *N. Engl. J. Med.* 366 (25): 2345–2357.

7 Holme, O., Loberg, M., Kalager, M. et al. (2014). Effect of flexible sigmoidoscopy screening on colorectal cancer incidence and mortality: A randomized clinical trial. *JAMA* 312 (6): 606–615.

8 van Ballegooijen, M., Rutter, C.M., Knudsen, A.B. et al. (2011). Clarifying differences in natural history between models of screening: The case of colorectal cancer. *Med. Decis. Making* 31 (4): 540–549.

9 Knudsen, A.B., Zauber, A.G., Rutter, C.M. et al. (2016). Estimation of benefits, burden, and harms of colorectal cancer screening strategies: Modeling study for the US Preventive Services Task Force. *JAMA* 315 (23): 2595–2609.

10 Imperiale, T.F., Ransohoff, D.F., Itzkowitz, S.H. et al. (2004). Fecal DNA versus fecal occult blood for colorectal-cancer screening in an average-risk population. *N. Engl. J. Med.* 351 (26): 2704–2714.

11 Lee, J.K., Liles, E.G., Bent, S. et al. Accuracy of fecal immunochemical tests for colorectal cancer: Systematic review and meta-analysis. *Ann. Intern. Med.* 160 (3): 171.

12 Imperiale, T.F., Ransohoff, D.F., Itzkowitz, S.H. et al. (2014). Multitarget stool DNA testing for colorectal-cancer screening. *N. Engl. J. Med.* 370 (14): 1287–1297.

13 Quintero, E., Castells, A., Bujanda, L. et al. (2012). Colonoscopy versus fecal immuno-chemical testing in colorectal-cancer screening. *N. Engl. J. Med.* 366 (8): 697–706.

14 U.S. Preventive Services Task Force (2008). Screening for colorectal cancer: U.S. Preventive Services Task Force recommendation statement. *Ann. Intern. Med.* 149 (9): 627–637.

15 U.S. Preventive Services Task Force; Bibbins-Domingo, K., Grossman, D.C., Curry, S.J. et al. (2016). Screening for colorectal cancer: US Preventive Services Task Force recommendation statement. *JAMA* 315 (23): 2564–2575.

16 Wilschut, J.A., Habbema, J.D., van Leerdam, M.E. et al. (2011). Fecal occult blood testing when colonoscopy capacity is limited. *J. Natl Cancer Inst.* 103 (23): 1741–1751.

17 Young, G.P., Symonds, E.L., Allison, J.E. et al. (2015). Advances in fecal occult blood tests: The FIT revolution. *Dig. Dis. Sci.* 60 (3): 609–622.

18 Fraser, C.G., Allison, J.E., Halloran, S.P., and Young, G.P.; Expert Working Group on Fecal Immunochemical Tests for Hemoglobin CCSCWEO (2012). A proposal to standardize reporting units for fecal immunochemical tests for hemoglobin. *J. Natl Cancer Inst.* 104 (11): 810–814.

19 Imperiale, T.F., Monahan, P.O., Stump, T.E. et al. (2015). Derivation and validation of a scoring system to stratify risk for advanced colorectal neoplasia in asymptomatic adults: A cross-sectional study. *Ann. Intern. Med.* 163 (5): 339–346.

20 Brenner, H., Chang-Claude, J., Seiler, C.M., and Hoffmeister, M. (2011). Long-term risk of colorectal cancer after negative colonoscopy. *J. Clin. Oncol.* 29 (28): 3761–3767.

21 Rex, D.K. (2015). Colonoscopy: The current king of the hill in the USA. *Dig. Dis. Sci.* 60 (3): 639–646.

22 Kaminski, M.F., Bretthauer, M., Zauber, A.G. et al. (2012). The NordICC Study: Rationale and design of a randomized trial on colonoscopy screening for colorectal cancer. *Endoscopy* 44 (7): 695–702.

23 Winawer, S.J., Zauber, A.G., Ho, M.N. et al. (1993). Prevention of colorectal cancer by colonoscopic polypectomy. The National Polyp Study Workgroup. *N. Engl. J. Med.* 329 (27): 1977–1981.

24 Zauber, A.G., Winawer, S.J., O'Brien, M.J. et al. (2012). Colonoscopic polypectomy and long-term prevention of colorectal-cancer deaths. *N. Engl. J. Med.* 366 (8): 687–696.

25 Nishihara, R., Wu, K., Lochhead, P. et al. (2013). Long-term colorectal-cancer incidence and mortality after lower endoscopy. *N. Engl. J. Med.* 369 (12): 1095–1105.

26 Loberg, M., Kalager, M., Holme, O. et al. (2014). Long-term colorectal-cancer mortality after adenoma removal. *N. Engl. J. Med.* 371 (9): 799–807.

27 Corley, D.A., Jensen, C.D., Marks, A.R. et al. (2014). Adenoma detection rate and risk of colorectal cancer and death. *N. Engl. J. Med.* 370 (14): 1298–1306.

28 Meester, R.G., Doubeni, C.A., Lansdorp-Vogelaar, I. et al. (2015). Variation in adenoma detection rate and the lifetime benefits and cost of colorectal cancer screening: A micro-simulation model. *JAMA* 313 (23): 2349–2358.

29 Gupta, S., Anderson, J., Bhandari, P. et al. (2011). Development and validation of a novel method for assessing competency in polypectomy: Direct observation of polypectomy skills. *Gastrointest. Endosc.* 73 (6): 1232–1239.

30 Bourikas, L.A., Tsiamoulos, Z.P., Haycock, A. et al. (2013). How we can measure quality in colonoscopy? *World J. Gastrointest. Endosc.* 5 (10): 468–475.

31 Kaminski, M.F., Anderson, J., Valori, R. et al. (2015). Leadership training to improve adenoma detection rate in screening colonoscopy: A randomised trial. *Gut* 65 (4): 616–624.

32 Atkin, W.S., Morson, B.C., and Cuzick, J. (1992). Long-term risk of colorectal cancer after excision of rectosigmoid adenomas. *N. Engl. J. Med.* 326 (10): 658–662.

33 Winawer, S.J., Fletcher, R.H., Miller, L. et al. (1997). Colorectal cancer screening: Clinical guidelines and rationale. *Gastroenterology* 112 (2): 594–642.

34 Bond, J.H. (2000). Polyp guideline: Diagnosis, treatment, and surveillance for patients with colorectal polyps. Practice Parameters Committee of the American College of Gastroenterology. *Am. J. Gastroenterol.* 95 (11): 3053–3063.

35 Ransohoff, D.F., Yankaskas, B., Gizlice, Z., and Gangarosa, L. (2011). Recommendations for post-polypectomy surveillance in community practice. *Dig. Dis. Sci.* 56 (9): 2623–2630.

36 van Heijningen, E.M., Lansdorp-Vogelaar, I., Steyerberg, E.W. et al. (2015). Adherence to surveillance guidelines after removal of colorectal adenomas: A large, community-based study. *Gut* 64 (10): 1584–1592.

37 UiO Institute of Health and Safety (2014). EPoS (European Polyp Surveillance). http://www.med.uio.no/helsam/english/research/projects/epos/ (accessed 3 January 2018).

38 Graham, R., Mancher, M., Wolman, D.M. et al., ed. (2011). *Clinical Practice Guidelines We Can Trust*. Washington, DC: Institute of Medicine/National Academies Press.

39 Levin, B., Lieberman, D.A., McFarland, B. et al. (2008). Screening and surveillance for the early detection of colorectal cancer and adenomatous polyps, 2008: A joint guideline from the American Cancer Society, the US Multi-Society Task Force on Colorectal Cancer, and the American College of Radiology. *CA Cancer J. Clin.* 58 (3): 130–160.

40 Pignone, M., Russell, L., and Wagner, J. (2005). *Economic models of colorectal cancer screening in average-risk adults: Workshop summary.* http://www.nap.edu/catalog/11228.html. Washington, DC: National Academies Press.

41 Ransohoff, D.F., and Sox, H.C. (2016). Clinical practice guidelines for colorectal cancer screening: New recommendations and new challenges. *JAMA* 315 (23): 2529–2531.

CHAPTER 16

Lung cancer prevention

Jonathan M. Samet

Colorado School of Public Health, Aurora, USA

SUMMARY BOX

- Lung cancer, the leading cause of cancer death in the USA, is largely preventable.
- Tobacco smoking, the main driver of the lung cancer epidemic, can be reduced through comprehensive tobacco control programmes.
- Environmental agents causing lung cancer include air pollution, indoor radon, and various occupational exposures. Exposures can be reduced through a variety of regulatory and policy actions.
- Chemoprevention has not proved to be efficacious for lung cancer.
- Globally, the multinational tobacco companies are seeking to maintain and expand their markets. The World Health Organization's Framework Convention on Tobacco Control (FCTC) is a global public health treaty directed at ending the epidemic of tobacco use.

Lung cancer, now the leading cause of cancer death in the USA and worldwide, was quite uncommon a century ago. The rapid increase in its occurrence reflects powerful environmental causal factors, and indicates the potential for prevention by mitigating these agents. The course of the lung cancer epidemic has been largely driven by the strongest of these causal factors, the twentieth-century epidemic of cigarette smoking, which began about 20 years before the rise of lung cancer (Figure 16.1). Other environmental contributors to the epidemic, some widespread and ubiquitous, include outdoor air pollution and indoor radon, and workplace exposures that place certain worker groups at particularly high risk, such as underground uranium miners and asbestos workers. While genetic factors contributing to lung cancer risk have been vigorously sought, findings of the genome-wide association studies (GWAS) and other studies to date have not identified loci that contribute substantially to lung cancer risk [1]. Thus, prevention of lung cancer occurrence is grounded in mitigating its environmental causes,

---

Cancer Prevention and Screening: Concepts, Principles and Controversies, First Edition.
Edited by Rosalind A. Eeles, Christine D. Berg, and Jeffrey S. Tobias.
© 2019 John Wiley & Sons, Inc. Published 2019 by John Wiley & Sons, Inc.

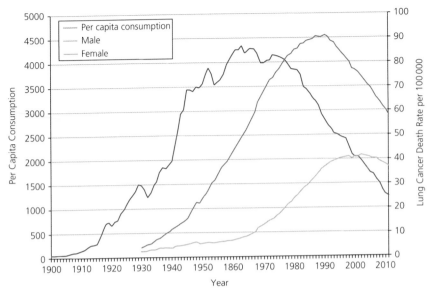

Figure 16.1 Per capita cigarette consumption and age-standardized death rates from lung cancer, US males and females, 1900–2011.
Per capita consumption data for ages 18 and above.
Death rates per 100 000 and age-standardized to the year 2000 US population.

particularly cigarette smoking. Chemoprevention, considered promising decades ago, has yet to be found efficacious [2].

These two approaches, identifying and mitigating risk factors and chemoprevention, are termed primary prevention; that is, the goal is to prevent the occurrence of disease. Secondary prevention – that is, screening – has the objective of identifying disease at a sufficiently early stage so that intervention will improve the long-run natural history and prevent death from the disease. For lung cancer, the National Lung Cancer Screening Trial (NLST) in the USA has shown screening to be efficacious [3]. Screening for lung cancer is covered in Chapter 17.

The lung's function and structure underlie the causation of lung cancer by environmental agents. The lung is the site of gas exchange, a purpose reflected by its myriad airways and the large surface area of the alveoli, equivalent to that of a tennis court. Typically, an adult inhales 10 000 litres of air daily, so that doses of harmful carcinogens delivered to the lung can be substantial, even if present in low concentrations in inhaled air. Inhaled gases and particles deposit across the lung's myriad airways and the large alveolar surface, potentially exposing the epithelial cells lining the surfaces to carcinogens and other toxic agents. While the respiratory tract has elegant defence systems to handle inhaled agents that are harmful, these defences may be overwhelmed at high doses, as with cigarette smoking and some occupational exposures. For sustained exposures, such as radon and air pollution, risk mounts cumulatively as exposure is sustained. In considering prevention of lung cancer, consideration also needs to be given to how exposure to inhaled carcinogens and other damaging agents occurs. For inhaled agents, exposure is the product of the pollutant concentration with the time spent at the concentration; for example, 10 hours spent breathing air with a particle concentration of 100 mcg/m^3 results in an exposure of 1000 mcg/m^3-hour, and hence a potential inhaled dose of 1 mg of particulate matter. Exposures are accrued across the day in multiple venues, referred to as microenvironments, having particular profiles of contaminants in their air. For example, for an adult, relevant microenvironments might be the home, the workplace, the outdoors, transportation environments, and various public places. The exposures accrued across these locations drive the doses of contaminants delivered to the lung and the associated risk for diseases, including lung cancer.

Inhaled agents likely cause lung cancer through specific, for example mutations, and nonspecific mechanisms, for instance inflammation. Combustion-generated pollution mixtures may contain polycyclic aromatic hydrocarbons, such as the known carcinogen benzo(a)pyrene, and tobacco smoke contains 70 agents classified as carcinogenic by the International Agency for Research on Cancer (IARC) [4,5]. Ionizing radiation, whether from X-ray or the internal emitters, such as radon decay products, damages DNA. Many inhaled pollutants also cause inflammation through oxidative and other mechanisms, potentially adding to lung cancer risk through this mechanism. There has been interest in preventing lung cancer by chemoprevention with agents that interfere with these mechanisms. For example, some putative chemoprevention agents, such as beta-carotene, were hypothesized as acting through anti-inflammatory mechanisms.

This chapter addresses the prevention of lung cancer, both by primary prevention through reduction of exposure to risk factors and by use of chemopreventive agents in people at high risk. It covers major causal agents for lung cancer and the strategies used to control them. While chemopreventive agents have not yet been proven effective, in spite of trials involving promising agents, the topic remains of interest because there are still high-risk groups [2]. The chapter begins by covering the occurrence and the burden of avoidable lung cancer.

The occurrence of lung cancer

Figure 16.1 charts the lung cancer epidemic in the USA over the 80 years from 1930 to 2010. Among males, the overall age-adjusted rate peaked in 1990 and has steadily declined since; for females, decline is now beginning. However, the number of new cases has risen steadily, now reaching an estimated 221 200 in 2015, and the annual deaths from lung cancer currently number 158 040 [6]. Over recent decades, incidence rates in males have declined most steeply in younger

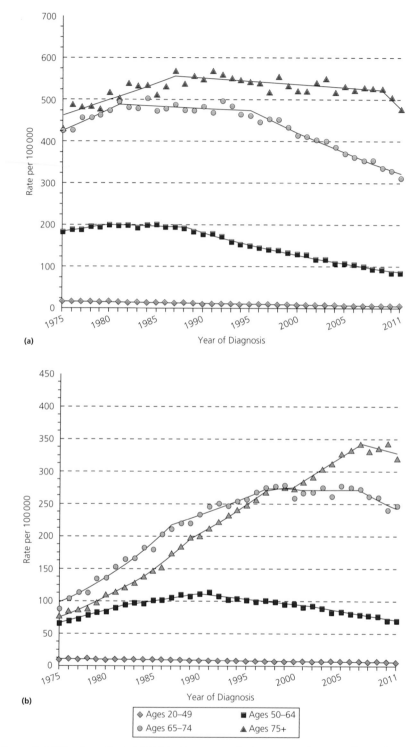

(a)

(b)

◆ Ages 20–49	■ Ages 50–64
● Ages 65–74	▲ Ages 75+

Figure 16.2 Title: Age-adjusted SEER incidence rates for lung cancer, by age at diagnosis, (a) males and (b) females, 1975–2011. Incidence rates per 100 000 and age-adjusted to the year 2000 US population, from the Surveillance, Epidemiology, and End Results Program (SEER) 9 registries (Atlanta, Connecticut, Detroit, Hawaii, Iowa, New Mexico, San Francisco-Oakland, Seattle-Puget Sound, and Utah). Note scale change on y-axis.

Table 16.1 Age-adjusted SEER incidence and US mortality rates* for lung cancer by race/ethnicity and sex, 2007–2011.

Race/ethnicity	Males		Females	
	Incidence[†]	Mortality[‡]	Incidence[†]	Mortality[‡]
All races	72.2	61.6	51.1	38.5
White	72.4	61.4	53.8	39.8
White Hispanic[#]	41.0	31.9	26.3	14.6
White Non-Hispanic[#]	77.0	63.9	58.1	42.1
Black	93.0	75.7	51.2	36.5
Asian/Pacific Islander	49.4	34.7	28.1	18.4
American Indian/Alaska Native	49.5	41.0	34.7	26.1
Hispanic[#]	39.6	30.5	25.5	14.0

*Rates per 100 000 and age-adjusted to year 2000 US population.
[†]Incidence data from the Surveillance, Epidemiology, and End Results Program (SEER) 18 registries (Alaska Native Tumor Registry, Atlanta, Connecticut, Detroit, Greater California, Greater Georgia, Hawaii, Iowa, Kentucky, Los Angeles, Louisiana, New Jersey, New Mexico, Rural Georgia, San Francisco-Oakland, San Jose-Monterey, Seattle-Puget Sound, and Utah).
[‡]Mortality data from the US Mortality Files, National Center for Health Statistics, CDC.
[#]Hispanic and Non-Hispanic are not mutually exclusive from whites, blacks, Asian/Pacific Islanders, and American Indians/Alaska Natives.

males, reflecting smoking patterns in more recent birth cohorts (Figure 16.2). Rates are also declining over time in younger women. Incidence and mortality rates vary widely by racial/ethnic group in the USA (Table 16.1), highlighting the need to target those groups at highest risk. For still unexplained reasons, African American males have the highest rates, even though cigarette smoking is more prevalent in non-Hispanic white males, with the second highest rates. The low rates among male and female Hispanics and Asian/Pacific Island females reflect smoking patterns.

Worldwide, lung cancer occurrence varies greatly (Figure 16.3) [7]. Uniformly, rates are higher in males compared with females. At present, the more developed regions have higher rates, reflecting historical patterns of tobacco use. Of the less-developed regions, much of Africa has very low incidence and mortality rates, as does Central America. Historically, smoking has been infrequent in these regions, and cigarette smokers tend to smoke only small numbers of cigarettes. The variation of lung cancer occurrence across the various regions of the world identifies differing priorities for tobacco control: to promote smoking cessation where rates are already high and to limit initiation where rates are low.

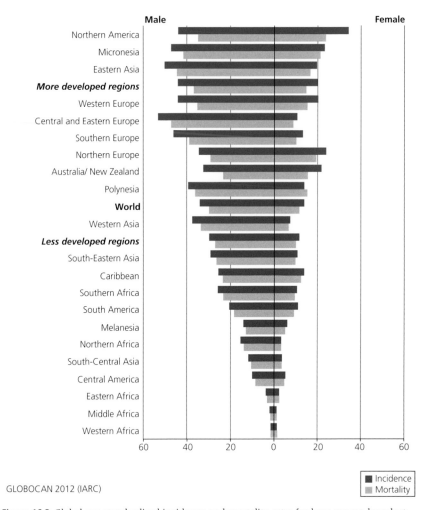

Figure 16.3 Global age-standardized incidence and mortality rates for lung cancer, by select regions of the world, 2012.

The causes of lung cancer and opportunities for prevention

Tobacco smoking
Tobacco smoking and lung cancer risk

By the 1950s, epidemiological and other evidence supported the conclusion that smoking was a cause of lung cancer, a conclusion reached with definitive support (for men) in the landmark 1964 report of the US Surgeon General on smoking and health [8]. By then, case-control and cohort studies had provided evidence of a very strong association of smoking with lung cancer risk; temporal patterns of lung cancer occurrence were consistent with a causal role of smoking (Figure 16.1); and tobacco smoke was known to contain carcinogens [8]. At the time of the report, smoking was associated with an approximately 10-fold increased risk of lung cancer in men, but a much lower relative risk in women, reflecting historical patterns of smoking. The evidence was soon conclusive for women as well, and epidemiological studies, spanning 1959–2010, show that the relative risk of lung cancer mortality for current smoking has risen sharply in women, reaching 12.7 during 1982–1988 from 2.7 in 1959–1965. and more recently (2000–2010) reaching 25.7, equal to that in men, at 25.0 for the period 2000–2010 [9,10]. The relative risk for lung cancer, compared with that in continuing smokers, drops progressively, but even 20 years after successful cessation, the risk remains above that for those who never smoked. Smoking is causally linked with all major histological types of lung cancer, and the shift to a predominance of adenocarcinoma over the last four decades is thought to be consequent to changes in cigarettes and how they are smoked [5]. Given the high relative risk for lung cancer in cigarette smokers and the scope of past cigarette smoking, much of the burden of lung cancer in most countries, including the USA, comes from cigarette smoking. Thus, tobacco smoking, particularly cigarette smoking, is a critical target for lung cancer prevention.

Tobacco control

Tobacco control has had a lengthy evolution that has been closely linked to the increasing evidence on the health effects of active and passive smoking and on what tobacco control modalities have been effective [5,11,12]. Historically, the initial findings on lung cancer and smoking were followed by efforts to educate the public about the risks of smoking, with the expectation that smokers would stop smoking. Since then, we have learned that tobacco control requires far more complex approaches that acknowledge the hierarchy of factors determining the use of tobacco and the interplay of these factors across the life course, as health is damaged by smoking from conception on. At each age, the emphasis of tobacco control shifts, moving from ending maternal smoking during pregnancy and secondhand smoke (SHS) exposure during childhood, to preventing initiation, and then to promoting successful cessation. Additionally, tobacco control efforts need to be dynamic in time, changing as the tobacco industry attempts to counter any tobacco control measures. For lung cancer, both cessation and prevention of initiation are needed: cessation is requisite to most quickly reduce the current lung cancer burden, while reduction of initiation is critical for the long run.

Figure 16.4 provides a hierarchical model that is useful for framing tobacco control and for providing a rationale for implementing a package of measures to limit tobacco use [13]. At the lowest level, emerging evidence shows that genetic factors figure in determining susceptibility to addiction and risk for disease in smokers. Intermediate levels are also relevant: the roles of family and peers in initiation are well established. The broader neighbourhood, municipal and state, and national levels are also critical in establishing both positive and negative pressures for tobacco use and in setting the critical 'cultural norm' around smoking.

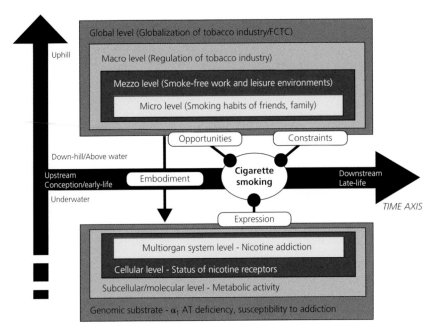

Figure 16.4 Hierarchical model for tobacco control across the life course.

The cultural norms may be that smoking is acceptable, as in present-day China, where cigarettes have well-established roles in social interactions; or unacceptable, as in much of the USA and many other high-income countries today, where workplaces and public places are largely smoke free. Advertising bans, pack warnings, and taxation rates – potentially determined at multiple governmental levels – also affect the environment for smoking and tobacco control. The global level is ever more relevant, as the tobacco industry has consolidated into a limited number of multinational companies, including Philip Morris International, British American Tobacco, Japan Tobacco International, and Imperial Tobacco/Altadis [14]. The largest producer is China National Tobacco Corporation, a state monopoly that manufactures more than 90% of cigarettes consumed by China's 300 million smokers, and hence China faces a unique constellation of issues in addressing its massive tobacco epidemic [15].

The industry has a critical role, as the 'root cause' of the tobacco epidemic. Considered in the classic epidemiological triangle of agent, vector, and host, the tobacco industry is the vector that conveys tobacco to people, the host. It also contributes to setting the environment by advertising and promoting its addicting product, attempting to alter the regulatory and policy landscape, and even by attempting to affect the environment around smoking by paying for placement of smoking in movies. For decades, the industry used diverse tactics to undermine the scientific evidence linking active and passive smoking to the causation of disease [16]. Notably, the industry is adaptive and changes strategies in a dynamic way to target by host characteristics (age, gender, and race) and to counter emerging efforts at tobacco control. The need to address the industry broadly is reflected in control measures that directly address its activities, including regulation, litigation, and the World Health Organization's (WHO) Framework Convention on Tobacco Control (FCTC) [17].

Over time, approaches to tobacco control have evolved such that they incorporate a package of interventions [5]. This evolution reflects the expanding understanding of the impact of various tobacco control strategies. For example, the finding that passive smoking caused lung cancer in never smokers motivated the implementation of smoking bans in public places and workplaces, and initiated a change in social norms around smoking that moved smoking from being viewed as acceptable to unacceptable. As noted by Surgeon General Koop in the preface to his 1986 report, 'The right of smokers to smoke ends where their behavior affects the health and well-being of others' [18]. Approaches to smoking cessation became more effective when nicotine was identified as addicting, nicotine replacement therapy and other pharmacological approaches were introduced, and stronger behavioural approaches were devised. Research and experience also documented the need to raise taxes, to use aggressive counter-marketing to denormalize smoking, and to protect children from the reach of the tobacco industry. Increasing price through higher taxes is a particularly efficient strategy, as implementation is at no cost and for the short run revenues to governments do not fall, even if smoking decreases [5,19]. Most importantly, evidence from decades of research shows that a multicomponent strategy is needed that targets nonsmokers to keep them from smoking, and that encourages and supports smokers to quit. Experience in New York City, for example, shows that an aggressive, multifaceted programme can have a rapid impact. Following implementation of a smoking ban, tax increases, hard-hitting anti-smoking campaigns, and an active cessation programme, smoking prevalence fell by 11% from 2002 to 2003, a reduction of approximately 140 000 smokers during this period [20].

Many nations have implemented tobacco control programmes. Most importantly, there is now the FCTC, ratified and in force for most nations of the world, although not for the USA. Many universal elements of national tobacco control policy are core elements of the FCTC, including a comprehensive ban on tobacco advertising, promotion, and sponsorship; a ban on misleading descriptors such as 'light'; and a mandate to place rotating warnings that cover at least 30% of tobacco packaging and encouragement for even larger, graphic warnings. The FCTC also urges countries to implement smoke-free workplace laws, address tobacco smuggling, and increase tobacco taxes. The FCTC has now been in place for than 10 years and progress is slowly being made in implementing its components [21].

Building on the FCTC process, the WHO released its first 'Report on Control of the Tobacco Epidemic', entitled 'MPOWER', in 2008 [22]. MPOWER is a comprehensive tobacco control strategy intended to provide a programmatic counterpart to the FCTC. It includes six key tobacco control measures: Monitoring the epidemic; Protecting nonsmokers from exposure to SHS; Offering help to cease tobacco use; Warning smokers of the health effects of smoking with strong, effective health warnings; Enforcing advertising bans; and Raising the price of tobacco products. The WHO is tracking implementation of MPOWER and coverage of the world's population by its provisions. To date, its reach is still limited, although increasing coverage of the global population by its elements can be anticipated [23].

Air pollution
Outdoor air pollution

Outdoor air can be contaminated by many respiratory carcinogens, coming from vehicles, industrial sources, power generation, fuel combustion for space heating and cooking, and refuse burning [24]. Thus, the carcinogens in outdoor air primarily come from the combustion of various carbon-based fuels; carcinogens generated by combustion, such as polycyclic aromatic hydrocarbons; and components of the combusted materials, such as metals: arsenic, nickel, and chromium. Depending on the pollution source mix, the constituents of 'air pollution' will vary by locale and over time.

Air pollution exposure is ubiquitous in the world's cities and an increasing problem in many mega-cities [25]. A now substantial body of evidence links outdoor air pollution to lung cancer and possibly other cancers [26]. The evidence includes studies of the components of the air pollution mixture and their biological activity, including extensive data on the mutagenicity of atmospheric particles; animal bioassays; and epidemiological studies of cancer risk in relation to long-term air pollution exposure. The epidemiological evidence comes from ecological studies, case-control studies, and cohort studies. The most recent and conclusive evidence comes from long-term and large cohort studies, including the Harvard Six Cities Study, the American Cancer Society's Cancer Prevention Study II, and the ESCAPE project, a pooling of European cohorts using a standard protocol for exposure estimation. Hamra et al. [27] carried out a meta-analysis of 18 studies, finding a significantly increased risk of lung cancer associated with exposure to fine particulate matter ($PM_{2.5}$) (risk ratio [RR] 1.09, 95% confidence interval [CI] 1.04–1.14) per 10 micrograms per cubic meter increase [27]. By smoking status, the increase was statistically significant in never smokers and greatest for former smokers.

Based on the evidence available, the International Agency for Research on Cancer (IARC) has now classified outdoor air pollution, and particulate matter specifically, as carcinogenic for humans; that is, Group 1 carcinogens [26]. Ambient air pollution is genotoxic and mutagenic, and the exposure–risk relationship likely has no threshold. While IARC does not quantify the risks associated with carcinogens, the meta-analysis by Hamra et al. [27] was a component of the evidence evaluation. The Global Burden of Disease estimates 223 000 lung cancer deaths worldwide in 2010 from air pollution [28]. The conclusion that air pollution causes lung cancer has critical regulatory and public health implications. Given that the anticipated risk would extend to lower levels of exposure, control strategies cannot eliminate risk, and some acceptable target level of risk needs to be determined.

The IARC classification of outdoor air pollution has significant policy implications, strengthening the rationale for air pollution control, particularly in low- and middle-income countries where pollution is worsening. Prevention of some of the burden of lung cancer caused by air pollution is possible through general air pollution control measures, though all risk cannot be eliminated. Additionally, critical sources of airborne carcinogens might be targeted, such as coke oven refineries and highly polluting diesel vehicles.

Biomass fuel burning

An estimated 2.4 billion people are exposed to smoke from biomass fuel combustion for the purposes of cooking and space heating [29]. Various fuels are used, including twigs and animal dung, charcoal, wood, and coal, and the smoke may be unvented, resulting in very high concentrations. While there are carcinogens in the smoke, IARC classified biomass smoke as a Group 2A (probable) carcinogen, while designating smoke from coal combustion as Group 1 [30]. As a combustion product of various carbon-containing fuel stocks, biomass fuel smoke has components that are specific carcinogens, as well as components that could nonspecifically contribute to carcinogenesis [30]. A meta-analysis of 14 case-control studies reported in 2015 estimated the lung cancer risk associated with biomass smoke exposure from cooking and/or heating as an odds ratio of 1.17 (95% CI 1.01–1.37) overall, and 1.15 (95% CI 0.97–1.37) for cooking only [29].

Exposure to biomass smoke can be reduced and numerous initiatives are under way worldwide to do so [31,32]. These include substitution of lower-emission stoves and use of cleaner fuels. The enormity of the problem is a logistical and financial challenge, but one that is finally being addressed on the global scale.

Ionizing radiation
Ionizing radiation and lung cancer risk

Together, mechanistic considerations and findings of epidemiological studies show that lung cancer is causally associated with exposure to ionizing radiation. Two types of radiation, classified by rate of energy transfer to tissues, cause lung cancer: high–linear energy transfer (high-LET) radiation (e.g. radon) and low-LET radiation (e.g. X-rays and gamma rays). The decay products of radon are the principal source of human exposure to high-LET radiation; radon is ubiquitous in indoor air, and underground miners may have high exposures from naturally occurring radon released from radium-containing ore. For low-LET radiation, medical imaging has now become the principal source of exposure for the population generally, while some occupations also result in exposures. The radioactive decay products of radon – that is, radon progeny – release alpha particles; while radon is a gas, the progeny are particulate and, when deposited in the respiratory tract, the alpha particles that they release penetrate to the basal cells in the epithelium and damage DNA. Low-LET radiation also produces ionization in tissues. For both types of radiation, the epidemiological evidence initially came primarily from cohorts exposed at levels substantially greater than those experienced by the general population, and risk assessment methods were used to estimate risks to the general population.

Radon is an inert gas produced naturally from radium in the decay series of uranium. Two of the radon progeny emit alpha particles that can, consequent to high energy and mass, cause damage to the DNA of cells of the respiratory epithelium. Epidemiological studies of underground miners of uranium and other ores have established exposure to radon daughters as a cause of lung cancer [33]. In the underground miners exposed to radon in past centuries, very high lung cancer risks were observed, even in never smokers; in the miners in more contemporary workplaces, the observed risks have been much less, as exposure concentrations have been better controlled, but studies still show clear evidence of continuing cancer risk. Risk models based on the studies of underground miners show that risk increases with cumulative exposure to radon; declines with increasing time since exposure occurred; and also drops with increasing age. Cigarette smoking and radon decay products synergistically influence lung cancer risk, for example, in a manner that is greater than simply adding the risks of each together. For this reason, the bulk of the lung cancer burden caused by radon exposure in the general population is concentrated within cigarette smokers [33,34].

Radon control

Radon is of broader societal interest, because it is a ubiquitous air pollutant that enters buildings from the underlying soil, where it is generated by naturally occurring precursors in the uranium decay chain. As an inert component of soil gas, radon diffuses into homes through basements and cracks in foundations; indoor levels thus depend on the radon concentration in the soil gas and the rate of exchange of indoor air with outdoor air, which lowers the radon concentration. Radon in water and radium in gypsum wallboard are also potential sources.

On average, indoor exposures to radon for the general population are much less than for occupational groups such as uranium miners, although some homes have been documented as having concentrations as high as those in underground uranium mines. Case-control studies of indoor radon exposure have documented that residential exposure to radon in indoor air is significantly associated with increased risk for lung cancer [33,34]. Additionally, because of the mechanism by which radon progeny cause lung cancer, any exposure is anticipated to have some risk, because the high energy of the alpha particles damaging the respiratory epithelium is invariant with the radon concentration. The risk models used by the US Environmental Protection Agency indicate that approximately 15 000–20 000 lung cancer deaths per year in the USA are caused by radon, making radon the second leading cause of lung cancer. The Global Burden of Disease attributes 99 000 lung cancer deaths globally to radon in 2010 [28].

Radon mitigation strategies for existing homes involve measurement of radon and mitigation if levels exceed a guideline value. Radon concentration in air can be measured relatively inexpensively with passive devices that can measure concentrations over time spans ranging from a few days up to a year, in order to gain an assessment of the long-term concentration that is relevant to lung cancer risk. If the concentration exceeds the recommended limit, then mitigation by a specialist is recommended, which might involve sealing of openings into a home or use of a pump to exhaust air with high radon concentration from a basement. In the USA, the Environmental Protection Agency has a guideline value of 4 pico-curies per litre [35], while the WHO recommends a reference level of 100 Bq/m³ (about 3 pico-curies per litre) to minimize health hazards due to indoor radon exposure [36].

Radon has also been a powerful occupational carcinogen, although at present underground uranium mining is quite limited in the USA and most mining globally is now open pit, where radon concentrations are quickly diluted rather than building up as with underground mines. Consequently, regulations provide limits for exposure for underground miners; in the USA, the Mine Safety and Health Administration (MSHA) sets the standard [37], while globally the International Commission on Radiological Protection provides guidance values [38]. Because the lung cancer risk caused by radon progeny follows a linear no-threshold relationship, meeting existing occupational standards cannot eliminate increased risk for miners.

Low-LET radiation: X-rays and gamma-rays

Earlier epidemiological data relating low-LET radiation to lung cancer stem from three principal populations: the atomic bomb survivors in Japan, patients with diseases such as ankylosing spondylitis or tuberculosis who received multiple radiation treatments, and occupational groups in professions exposed to radiation [39]. The single, high-dose exposure of the atomic bomb survivors was associated with significant lung cancer risk. Regardless of age at the time of the blast, the excess of lung cancer occurred when the survivors reached the older ages when cancer usually occurs [40]. Quantitative risk models are available that describe how risk rises with radiation dose.

Over the last several decades, medical radiation has replaced radon as the leading contributor to the population's radiation exposure [41]. In general, a substantial proportion of the US population is now exposed to ionizing radiation from medical diagnostics, particularly from computed tomography (CT) scans. The exposure is of sufficient magnitude to be of concern as a cause of increased population risk for cancer. In the USA, the Food and Drug Administration (FDA) regulates exposure from radiation-emitting electronic products, including medical devices [42].

Occupational factors
Occupational exposures and lung cancer risk

Lung cancer has been found to be associated causally with many workplace exposures, including radon, asbestos, arsenic, chromium, silica, coke oven fumes, and nickel. Historically, exposures to some of these agents were at high concentrations by current workplace standards, large numbers of workers were exposed, and there were numerous cases of occupational lung cancer. In high-income countries, occupational exposures to lung carcinogens have been estimated by case-control studies to account for 5–10% of lung cancer cases [43,44], although in high-income countries the burden of occupational lung cancer is likely falling, as the high exposures that harmed past cohorts of workers have been abated and much manufacturing has shifted to lower-income countries.

Occupational lung cancer can be potentially prevented through the combination of careful surveillance and stringent regulation. Unfortunately, by the time that excess cases have been identified in a group of workers, a large number of people may have been exposed and be at risk. For example, epidemiological studies did not link asbestos to lung cancer until Doll's study in the 1950s, approximately a half-century after asbestos use became widespread [45,46]. Control of these carcinogens has been driven by the epidemiological and other evidence on their risks, although delayed in some notable examples by industries that attempted to deflect culpability, such the asbestos industry. In the USA, relevant regulations are promulgated by a variety of agencies, depending on the agent and the context. Occupational carcinogens would generally fall under the Occupational Safety and Health Administration (OSHA). For radiation, exposures are regulated by various agencies, depending on the radiation source and the context of exposure: MSHA, the Department of Energy (DOE), the Department of Transportation (DOT), FDA, the Nuclear Regulatory Commission (NRC), and the Environmental Protection Agency (EPA). Globally, the International Labor Organization (ILO) adopts over 40 conventions, recommendations, and codes of practice that cover fundamental principles of occupational safety and health, as well as protection against specific risks such as radiation and asbestos, and protection in specific branches of activity including mining and agriculture [47]. These ILO standards on occupational safety and health are not legally binding, but they do provide guidelines for governments, employers, and workers to establish sound prevention, reporting, and inspection practices at the workplace. Cigarette smoking also potentiates the effect of some of the known occupational lung carcinogens, including asbestos and radon [4], such that tobacco control will also contribute to a reduction of occupational lung cancer.

Chemoprevention of lung cancer

Chemoprevention is another possible strategy to prevent lung cancer. The possibility of chemoprevention draws plausibility from early animal experiments on changes in the respiratory epithelium associated with vitamin A deficiency, and epidemiological observations showing lower lung cancer risk for those with higher consumption of fruits and vegetables [48]. Beta-carotene was a promising early agent tested in clinical trials; it was hypothesized to protect against oxidative injury to DNA and was considered to be without harmful effects itself [49]. However, clinical trials provided the surprising finding that the administration of beta-carotene was associated with an increased risk of lung cancer among smokers [20]. Other micronutrients, including vitamins E and A and selenium, are not recommended. Retinoids, another class of promising agents, have not shown efficacy. Various pharmaceutical agents are under consideration as chemopreventive agents [2].

The burden of avoidable lung cancer

The Global Burden of Disease project has estimated the lung cancer deaths attributable to the various risk factors for the USA and globally between 1990 and 2010 (Tables 16.2 and 16.3). For the USA, the burden from smoking currently accounts for approximately 75% of deaths in both men and women; the rise in attributable deaths among women reflects the increasing prevalence of smoking and the rising relative risk for lung cancer among smoking women in the last three decades. Two forms of air pollution, ambient air pollution and indoor radon, both account for approximately 10 000 lung cancer deaths. The radon estimate by the Global Burden of Disease project is less than that by the EPA because of differing methodology and assumptions. Fortunately, the burden of lung cancer from occupational agents has declined in the USA. While the evidence on diet and lung cancer risk is much less certain than for other risk factors, the Global Burden project does provide an estimate, indicating another potential strategy for reducing lung cancer: dietary modification.

Globally, the burden of avoidable lung cancer continues to rise as the epidemic continues. While the worldwide burden is enormous, there is great opportunity

Table 16.2 Lung cancer deaths attributable to risk factors, USA, 1990 and 2010.

Risk factors	Attributable deaths			
	Male		Female	
	1990	2010	1990	2010
Smoking (including exposure to SHS)	83 343	81 583	45 262	59 832
Diet low in fruits	14 510	15 137	7635	10 601
Ambient PM pollution	8473	5661	5012	4373
Occupational carcinogens	3978	2961	1050	777
Residential radon*	N/A	5578	N/A	4293
Total	110 304	110 920	58 959	79 876

*Data on residential radon available from 2005 onwards.
N/A, not available; PM, particulate matter; SHS, secondhand smoke.
Source: Institute for Health Metrics and Evaluations. Global Burden of Disease 2010 [28].

Table 16.3 Lung cancer deaths attributable to specific risk factors, by global, developed, and developing regions, 2010.

Risk factors	Attributable deaths		
	Global	Developed Region	Developing Region
Smoking (including exposure to SHS)	956 517	523 230	442 287
Diet low in fruits	257 802	88 413	169 389
Ambient PM pollution	222 944	45 799	177 145
Household air pollution	124 926	5188	119 739
Occupational carcinogens	95 271	22 734	72 537
Residential radon*	98 992	41 458	57 534
Total	1 756 452	726 822	1 038 631

*Data on residential radon available from 2005 onwards.
Total may not sum due to rounding.
N/A, not available; PM, particulate matter; SHS, secondhand smoke.
Source: Institute for Health Metrics and Evaluations. Global Burden of Disease 2010 [28].

for prevention (Table 16.3). One avoidable causal agent – tobacco smoke – is the predominant contributor, and a global tobacco control movement has been launched through the FCTC. Many nations, including the USA, have made great progress. In some countries, such as Panama, the prevalence of smoking is below 10% and discussion is under way concerning the 'end game' for tobacco. Known occupational carcinogens can also be controlled, although the circumstances of industries in low- and middle-income countries may limit effective regulation. Control of outdoor air pollution and biomass smoke, which together affect the entire world population, represents a formidable challenge. Attention is increasingly focused on mitigation of exposure to biomass smoke, primarily to lower the burden of respiratory illness in children. Reduction of lung cancer should follow. Outdoor air pollution is of concern because of rising exposures for billions of people in Asia and the complexities of control.

Conclusion

A global epidemic of lung cancer began with the start of the twentieth century; it continues today. Fortunately, the most critical drivers of the epidemic have been identified; unfortunately, understanding of causation has proved to be only the starting point for the complex task of mitigating avoidable exposures. The epidemic of tobacco-caused lung cancer persists more than a half-century after cigarette smoking was identified as a predominant cause. Control of the enormous burden of avoidable morbidity and premature mortality from lung cancer requires ongoing multisectoral and international activities, involving education, synergistic policies, regulation, and litigation.

References

1 Marshall, A.L., and Christiani, D.C. (2013). Genetic susceptibility to lung cancer: Light at the end of the tunnel? *Carcinogenesis* 34 (3): 487–502.

2 Szabo, E., Mao, J.T., Lam, S. et al. (2013). Chemoprevention of lung cancer: Diagnosis and management of lung cancer, 3rd ed. American College of Chest Physicians evidence-based clinical practice guidelines. *Chest* 143 (5, Suppl.): e40S–60S.

3 National Lung Screening Trial Research Team; Aberle, D.R., Adams, A.M., Berg, C.D. et al. (2011). Reduced lung-cancer mortality with low-dose computed tomographic screening. *N. Engl. J. Med.* 365 (5): 395–409.

4 International Agency for Research on Cancer (2004). Tobacco smoke and involuntary smoking. *IARC Monographs on the Evaluation of Carcinogenic Risks to Humans*, vol. 83. Lyon: IARC.

5 U.S. Department of Health and Human Services (2014). *The health consequences of smoking – 50 years of progress: A report of the Surgeon General.* Atlanta, GA: U.S. Department of Health and Human Services, Centers for Disease Control and Prevention, National Center for Chronic Disease Prevention and Health Promotion, Office on Smoking and Health.

6 American Cancer Society (2015). Cancer facts and figures 2015. Atlanta, GA: American Cancer Society.

7 Ferlay, J., Soerjomataram, I., Ervik, M. et al. (2013). GLOBOCAN 2012 v1.0, Cancer Incidence and Mortality Worldwide: IARC CancerBase No. 11. http://globocan.iarc.fr (accessed 20 February 2015).

8 U.S. Department of Health Education and Welfare (1964). *Smoking and health. Report of the Advisory Committee to the Surgeon General. DHEW Publication No. [PHS] 1103.* Washington, DC: U.S. Government Printing Office.

9 Thun, M.J., Carter, B.D., Feskanich, D. et al. (2013). 50-year trends in smoking-related mortality in the United States. *N. Engl. J. Med.* 368 (4): 351–364.

10 National Cancer Institute (1997). Changes in cigarette-related disease risks and their implication for prevention and control. Monograph 8 (NIH Publication No. 97-4213). Bethesda, MD: U.S. Government Printing Office.

11 U.S. Department of Health and Human Services (2000). *Reducing tobacco use: A report of the Surgeon General.* Atlanta, GA: U.S. Department of Health and Human Services, Centers for Disease Control and Prevention, National Center for Chronic Disease Prevention and Health Promotion, Office on Smoking and Health.

12 Wipfli, H., and Samet, J.M. (2009). Global economic and health benefits of tobacco control: Part 2. *Clin. Pharmacol. Ther.* 86 (3): 272–280.

13 Samet, J.M., and Wipfli, H.L. (2013). Ending the tobacco epidemic: From the genetic to the global level. In: *Structural Approaches in Public Health* (ed. M. Sommer and R. Parker), 231–243. New York: Routledge.

14 Eriksen, M., Mackay, J., and Ross, H. (2012). *The Tobacco Atlas*, 4ed. Atlanta, GA: American Cancer Society/World Lung Foundation.

15 Yang, G., Wang, Y., Wu, Y. et al. (2015). The road to effective tobacco control in China. *Lancet* 385 (9972): 1019–1028.

16 Proctor, R. (2012). *Golden Holocaust: Origins of the Cigarette Catastrophe and the Case for Abolition.* Berkeley, CA: University of California Press.

17 World Health Organization (n.d.). WHO Framework Convention on Tobacco Control (FCTC). http://www.who.int/fctc/en/index.html (accessed 19 March 2015).

18 U.S. Department of Health and Human Services (1986). *The health consequences of involuntary smoking: A report of the Surgeon General. DHHS Publication No. (CDC) 87-8398.* Washington, DC: U.S. Department of Health and Human Services, Public Health Service, Office on Smoking and Health.

19 World Bank (1999). *Curbing the epidemic: Governments and the economics of tobacco control.* Washington, DC: International Bank for Reconstruction and Development.

20 Frieden, T.R., Mostashari, F., Kerker, B.D. et al. (2005). Adult tobacco use levels after intensive tobacco control measures: New York City, 2002–2003. *Am. J. Public Health* 95 (6): 1016–1023.

21 Beaglehole, R., Bonita, R., Yach, D. et al. (2015). A tobacco-free world: A call to action to phase out the sale of tobacco products by 2040. *Lancet* 385 (9972): 1011–1018.

22 World Health Organization (2008). *WHO report on the global tobacco epidemic, 2008: The MPOWER package.* Geneva: WHO.

23 World Health Organization (2013). *WHO report on the global tobacco epidemic, 2013: Enforcing bans on tobacco advertising, promotion and sponsorship.* Geneva: WHO.

24 Straif, K., Cohen, A., Samet, J.M., ed. (2013). Air pollution and cancer. IARC Scientific Publication No. 161. Geneva: IARC.

25 Krzyzanowski, M., Apte, J.S., Bonjour, S.P. et al. (2014). Air pollution in the mega-cities. *Curr. Envir. Health Rpt.* 1: 185–191.

26 Loomis, D., Grosse, Y., Lauby-Secretan, B. et al. (2013). The carcinogenicity of outdoor air pollution. *Lancet Oncol.* 14 (13): 1262–1263.

27 Hamra, G.B., Guha, N., Cohen, A. et al. (2014). Outdoor particulate matter exposure and lung cancer: A systematic review and meta-analysis. *Environ. Health Perspect.* 122 (9): 906–911.

28 Institute for Health Metrics and Evaluation (2015). Global Burden of Disease Cause Patterns 2015. https://vizhub.healthdata.org/gbd-compare/patterns (accessed 3 January 2018).

29 Bruce, N., Dherani, M., Liu, R. et al. (2015). Does household use of biomass fuel cause lung cancer? A systematic review and evaluation of the evidence for the GBD 2010 study. *Thorax* 70 (5): 433–441.

30 International Agency for Research on Cancer (2010). Household use of solid fuels and high-temperature frying. *IARC Monographs on the Evaluation of Carcinogenic Risks to Humans,* vol. 95. Lyon: IARC.

31 Smith, K.R., Frumkin, H., Balakrishnan, K. et al. (2013). Energy and human health. *Annu. Rev. Public Health* 34: 159–188.

32 Wilkinson, P., Smith, K.R., Davies, M. et al. (2009). Public health benefits of strategies to reduce greenhouse-gas emissions: Household energy. *Lancet* 374 (9705): 1917–1929.

33 National Research Council, Committee on Health Risks of Exposure to Radon (1999). *Health effects of exposure to radon: BEIR VI.* Washington, DC: National Academy Press.

34 United Nations Scientific Committee on the Effects of Atomic Radiation (2006). *Effects of ionizing radiation: Vol. II – Report to the General Assembly, with Scientific Annexes C, D, and E.* Vienna: United Nations.

35 U.S. Environmental Protection Agency (2012). *A citizen's guide to radon: The guide to protecting yourself and your family from radon.* Washington, DC: U.S. Environmental Protection Agency.

36 World Health Organization (2009). *WHO handbook on indoor radon: A public health perspective.* Geneva: WHO.

37 Mine Safety and Health Administration (1986). *30 CFR Part 57: Safety and health standards – underground metal and nonmetal mines.* Washington, DC: Department of Labor.

38 International Commission on Radiation Protection (1997). General principles for the radiation protection of workers. *Ann. ICRP* 27 (1).

39 National Research Council (2006). *Health risks from exposure to low levels of ionizing radiation: BEIR VII Phase 2*. Washington, DC: National Academy of Sciences.

40 Ozasa, K., Shimizu, Y., Suyama, A. et al. (2012). Studies of the mortality of atomic bomb survivors, Report 14, 1950–2003: An overview of cancer and noncancer diseases. *Radiat. Res.* 177 (3): 229–243.

41 National Council on Radiation Protection and Measurements (2009). *Ionizing radiation exposure of the population of the United States: Recommendations of the National Council on Radiation Protection and Measurements*. Bethesda, MD: National Council on Radiation Protection and Measurements.

42 U.S. Food and Drug Administration (n.d.). Electronic Product Radiation Control Program. http://www.fda.gov/Radiation-EmittingProducts/ElectronicProductRadiationControlProgram/default.htm (accessed 23 March 2015).

43 Siemiatycki, J. (1991). *Risk Factors for Cancer in the Workplace*. Boston, MA: CRC Press.

44 Vineis, P., and Simonato, L. (1991). Proportion of lung and bladder cancers in males resulting from occupation: A systematic approach. *Arch. Environ. Health* 46 (1): 6–15.

45 Becklake, M.R. (1976). Asbestos-related diseases of the lung and other organs: Their epidemiology and implications for clinical practice. *Am. Rev. Resp. Dis.* 114 (1): 187–227.

46 Doll, R. (1955). Mortality from lung cancer in asbestos workers. *Br. J. Indus. Med.* 12: 81–86.

47 International Labor Organization (n.d.). International labour standards on occupational safety and health. http://www.ilo.org/global/standards/subjects-covered-by-international-labour-standards/occupational-safety-and-health/lang--en/index.htm (accessed 23 March 2015).

48 World Cancer Research Fund, American Institute for Cancer Research (1997). *Food, nutrition, and the prevention of cancer: A global perspective*. Washington, DC: American Institute for Cancer Research.

49 Peto, R., Doll, R., Buckley, J.D., and Sporn, M.B. (1981). Can dietary beta-carotene materially reduce human cancer rates? *Nature* 290: 201–208.

CHAPTER 17

Lung cancer screening

Christine D. Berg[1], Kwun M. Fong[2], and Henry M. Marshall[2]

[1] Division of Cancer Epidemiology and Genetics, National Cancer Institute, Bethesda, Maryland, USA
[2] University of Queensland Thoracic Research Centre, and Department of Thoracic Medicine,
The Prince Charles Hospital, Brisbane, Australia

SUMMARY BOX

- The US National Lung Screening Trial provided definitive evidence that lung cancer screening with low-dose helical computerized tomography in a high-risk cohort can lower lung cancer–specific mortality by 20%.

- Achieving this reduction comes with several defined consequences: a high rate of false positives, overdiagnosis, and radiation risks.

- Smoking cessation rates decline in participants in screening trials, with higher quit rates in those with abnormal scans. All screening programmes should offer smoking cessation interventions.

- Many major medical groups in North America and Europe recommend screening high-risk groups. The US Preventive Services Task Force and Medicare have recommended screening, which should facilitate insurance coverage.

- The implementation of screening is complex and best practices are emerging, such as through protocols developed by the American College of Radiology.

Screening of high-risk individuals for lung cancer has been shown to reduce lung cancer mortality. The US National Lung Screening Trial (NLST) compared low-dose helical computerized tomography (LDCT) to chest X-ray [1]. The results documented a 20% decrease in lung cancer–specific mortality as a consequence of LDCT screening, with a beneficial effect on overall mortality as well.

However, implementation of lung cancer screening will be a serious challenge. As worldwide lung cancer is the leading cause of cancer death, with 1.6 million deaths in 2013, high-quality implementation of screening may improve these grim lung cancer mortality statistics [2].

Cancer Prevention and Screening: Concepts, Principles and Controversies, First Edition.
Edited by Rosalind A. Eeles, Christine D. Berg, and Jeffrey S. Tobias.
© 2019 John Wiley & Sons, Inc. Published 2019 by John Wiley & Sons, Inc.

Screening for lung cancer: Early approaches

Trials of lung cancer screening with chest X-ray (CXR) have been uniformly disappointing and demonstrated that CXR screening does not reduce lung cancer mortality. The four early randomized trials, including one study in Czechoslovakia and three US National Cancer Institute (NCI)–sponsored trials, which incorporated sputum cytology, demonstrated no effect on lung cancer–specific mortality [3, 4]. As these four studies were small and felt to be inconclusive, the Prostate, Lung, Colorectal and Ovarian Cancer screening trial (PLCO) studied the effect of CXR (postero-anterior only) screening (three rounds for nonsmokers and four rounds for current or former smokers) compared with no screening on lung cancer mortality. The trial enrolled 154 901 individuals, 10% of whom were current smokers and 41.5% former smokers. The result unfortunately confirmed that this approach did not affect lung cancer mortality [5].

With the advent of LDCT, several groups undertook screening of at-risk individuals in observational cohort studies in the USA and Japan [3, 4]. CT appeared to be three to four times more sensitive than CXR in the Early Lung Cancer Action Project (ELCAP) study, and the majority of tumors were Stage I. A serious downside also emerged, that of a very high positivity rate for nodules suspicious for lung cancer, most of which were false positive. Single-arm studies have many well-known limitations such as lead-time bias, length bias, and overdiagnosis bias, and are therefore not considered definitive proof of efficacy.

Randomized controlled trials

National Lung Screening Trial

The US-based National Lung Screening Trial was designed as a randomized trial to test the effect of LDCT screening on lung cancer mortality [1]. The entry criteria were set to bring a high-risk group into the study: current or former smokers ages 55–74, 30 pack-years of smoking (product of packs smoked daily and years of smoking), or if former smokers those having quit within 15 years. The trial compared three rounds of screening at 12-month intervals of LDCT to postero-anterior CXR. Accrual was rapid and 53 454 individuals were enrolled. Overall, the trial participants were younger, of higher educational status, and more likely to be former smokers than those who also matched the NLST entry criteria in the US population, leading to concerns about generalizability [6]. Screening with LDCT was shown to result in a 20% decrease in lung cancer–specific mortality in the study cohort. A subset of the PLCO that matched the NLST was compared, and there was no evidence that there was any lung cancer mortality reduction with CXR when compared with community care [5]. Fewer late-stage cancers were found in NLST rounds two and three; this reflected a true stage shift consistent with the lung cancer mortality reduction. Overall mortality was also lowered. However, when lung cancer deaths were removed, this difference was no longer statistically significant.

The NLST had incidental findings in 7.5% of all LDCT scans, but it did not appear that the detection of these findings had any effect on overall mortality.

A concern in all screening is a phenomenon called overdiagnosis, which in this context is generally defined as the detection of lung cancers (primarily indolent ones) that will not be clinically significant during a person's lifetime. An estimate of overdiagnosis within the NLST has been done [7]. Using follow-up data extended from that in the primary manuscript, a total of 1089 lung cancers occurred in the LDCT arm compared with 969 in the CXR arm; that is, 120 additional lung cancer cases detected in the LDCT arm. Two estimates of the highest range for overdiagnosis were calculated: 18.5% of the cases detected during screening and 11% of the cases overall. Longer follow-up would be helpful to determine the extent of continued catch-up in cases in the CXR arm. The Cancer Intervention and Surveillance Modeling Network (CISNET) calculated overdiagnosis rates, and with annual screening from 55 to 80 estimated a rate of 4% [8]. It should be noted that a study of women's reaction to the concept of overdiagnosis in breast cancer screening indicated that they were pleased to be informed, but that they considered the issue more important for treatment decisions, and that it would not alter their planned cancer screening [9].

Subset analyses within the NLST

Retrospective subset analyses, while imperfect, are useful, providing some information about potential variations in effectiveness in subgroups. Analysis of performance within the NLST was conducted by age, gender, and smoking status [10]. This analysis was conducted on extended follow-up compared to the primary paper, such that the mortality reduction was diluted from 20% to 16%. The mortality risk ratios by age, under 65 and 65 or over, were 0.82 and 0.87; gender, males and females, 0.92 and 0.73; and by smoking status, current versus former, 0.81 and 0.91. Lung cancer incidence rates were similar between men and women within each trial arm. Analyses across different histologies revealed mortality risk ratios of 0.75 for adenocarcinoma, 0.90 for small cell carcinoma, and 1.23 for squamous cell carcinoma. A separate report provided more detail comparing the Medicare-eligible versus under-65 populations [11]. Only 25% of the NLST population was 65 and over. The false-positive rate (FPR) was higher, 27.7% versus 22.0%, and prevalence and positive predictive value (PPV) were higher in the over-65 cohort (PPV 4.9% versus 3.0%). A concern in the elderly is the comorbid conditions that decrease the ability to have surgery and increase its risks. While those in NLST were a healthy volunteer cohort, detection of Stage I disease was as common in the over 65 group compared to those under 65, and rates of resection of Stage I were 93.0% versus 96.9%. Ninety-day postsurgical mortality rates were 1.0% and 1.8%, respectively.

The European Randomized Controlled Trials (RCT)

Seven European RCTs (collectively titled EUCT [12]) have randomized 36 000 participants to LDCT screening or usual care (no screening), and are in various stages of completion (Table 17.1). The Nederlands-Leuvens

Table 17.1 Summary of European randomized low-dose computed tomography (LDCT) lung cancer screening trials.

Study	DANTE, Italy [13]	DLCST, Denmark [14, 15]	NELSON, Netherlands and Belgium [16–19]	ITALUNG, Italy [20]	MILD, Italy [21]	LUSI, Germany [22, 23]	UKLS (pilot study), UK [24, 25]
Design and Recruitment							
Eligibility age range	60–74 (men only)	50–70	50–74	55–69	49–75	50–69	50–75, 5% risk of developing lung cancer in 5 years*
Smoking history	Current or former smokers >20 PY, quit <10yr	Current or former smokers >20 PY, quit <10yr	Current or former smokers >15 PY, quit <10yr	Current or former smokers >20 PY, quit <10yr	Current or former smokers >20 PY, quit <10yr	Current or former smokers >15 PY, quit <10yr	
Years of recruitment	2001–2006	2004–2006	2003–2006	2004–2006	2005–2011	2007–2011	2011–2013
Recruitment method	Via media and general practitioners	Via media	Population sample	Via general practitioners	Via media	Population sample	Randomized population sample
Planned years of follow-up from randomization	4	10	10	7	10	NR	10
Completion/expected completion year	2010	2016	2015	2014 onwards	Ongoing	Ongoing	2018
Reported results	Eight-year results reported 2015	Five-year results reported 2012	Three-year results reported 2013	Four-year results reported 2013	Five-year results reported 2012	Three-year results reported 2015	First-year results reported 2013 (abstract)
Control group	Usual care (no intervention)†	Usual care (no intervention)	Usual care (no intervention)	Usual care (no intervention)	Usual care (no intervention)	Usual care (no intervention)	Usual care (no intervention)

Screening schedule (years)	1, 2, 3, 4, 5	1, 2, 3, 4, 5	1, 2, 4, 6.5	1, 2, 3, 4	Annual or biennial for 10 years		1, 2, 3, 4, 5	1
LDCT arm, n	1264	2052	7915	1613	1190 annual	1186 biennial	2029	2000
Control arm, n	1186	2052	7907	1593	1723		2023	2000
Baseline Scan Result Nodule Categories‡								
Positive	Smooth NCN ≥10mm, spiculated NCN ≥6mm; GGO >10mm§	>15mm or with suspicious morphology	Solid >500mm³, pleural based >10mm, or VDT <400days	Solid ≥5mm, nonsolid ≥10mm	>250mm³		>10mm or VDT ≤400days	>500mm³, pleural based >10mm, or VDT <400days
Indeterminate	Smooth NCN <10mm, spiculated NCN <6mm, or lesion not clearly benign; GGO <10mm	5–15mm	50–500mm³, pleural based 5–10mm, nonsolid ≥8mm, or VDT 400–600 days	NA	60–250mm³ (~5–8mm diameter)		5–10mm or VDT 400–600 days	15–500mm³, pleural based <10mm, or VDT >400days
Negative	≤5mm smooth or calcified NCN	<5mm or benign characteristics	<50mm³ or VDT >600days	Solid <5mm, nonsolid <10mm	<6 0mm³		<5mm or VDT >600days	<15mm³, pleural based ≤3mm
Incidence Scan Result Nodule Categories‡								
Positive	New >5mm or any growth**; GGO >10mm	Any new or growth** VDT <400days	New >500mm³, pleural based >10mm, or growth** plus VDT <400days	New >3mm or any growth**	New >250mm³ or growth**		>10mm or VDT ≤400days	NA

Continued

Table 17.1 Continued

Study	DANTE, Italy [13]	DLCST, Denmark [14, 15]	NELSON, Netherlands and Belgium [16–19]	ITALUNG, Italy [20]	MILD, Italy [21]	LUSI, Germany [22, 23]	UKLS (pilot study), UK [24, 25]
Indeterminate	No new, no growth, or existing solid NCN 5–10 mm	Growth but VDT 400–600 days	New 50–500 mm³, pleural based 5—10 mm, nonsolid ≥8 mm, or growth plus VDT 400–600 days	New ≤3 mm	New 0–250 mm³	5–10 mm or VDT 400–600 days	NA
Negative	No new, no growth, or existing solid NCN <5 mm	No new, no growth, or VDT >600 days	No new or new <50 mm³, no growth, or VDT >600 days	No new or no growth	No new and no growth	<5 mm or VDT >600 days	NA
Participant Characteristics (LDCT Arm)							
Age at randomization, years, median	64	57	59	60.7	57 and 58	NR (50.3% were in the age group 50–54)	NR
Males, %	100	55.9	84	64	68	50.1	NR
Current smokers at randomization, %	56	75.3	55.6	65.7	68††	50.2	NR
Pack years smoking at randomization	47	36.4	42	42.9	39	NR	NR

Total patients with cancers diagnosed (screen detected and interval)	104##	69 cancers in 68 patients	NR	40	34	25	62	NR
Cancer diagnosis rate per 100 000 person-years follow-up	NR	NR	NR	NR	620	457	674	NR

2D, two-dimensional measurement (on axial view); 3D, three-dimensional (volumetric) measurement; CXR, chest radiograph; GGO, ground-glass (nonsolid) nodule; NA, not applicable; NCN, noncalcified (solid) nodule; NR not recorded; PY, Pack-years (cigarettes per day/20 x duration of smoking in years); VDT, volume doubling time (days).

DANTE, Detection and Screening of Early Lung Cancer by Novel Imaging Technology and Molecular Assays. Milan, Bergamo, Catania, Italy.

DLCST, Danish Randomized Lung Cancer CT Screening Trial. Copenhagen, Denmark.

ITALUNG, Italian CT Trial. Florence, Pisa, Pistoia, Italy.

LUSI, Lung Cancer Screening Intervention Trial. Heidelberg, Germany.

MILD, Multicentric Italian Lung Detection Trial. Milan, Italy.

NELSON, Nederlands-Leuvens Longkanker Screenings Onderzoek (Dutch–Belgian Lung Cancer Screening Trial). Groningen, Utrecht, Haarlem, Netherlands; Leuven, Belgium.

UKLS, UK Lung Cancer Screening Trial. Liverpool, Cambridge, UK.

*Using the Liverpool Lung Project risk model [23].

†All participants received plain chest radiograph and sputum cytology at baseline.

‡Positive scan indicates nodule requires clinical work-up; indeterminate scan indicates nodule requires interval radiological assessment within 12 months.

§DANTE work-up protocol is not rigid, and may be adjusted on the basis of personal preferences, experience, and availability of facilities.

**Growth was defined as volume change ≥25% and VDT estimate (DLCST, NELSON, MILD); diameter increase ≥1 mm or increasing solid component of nonsolid nodule (ITALUNG); VDT estimate (LUSI, UKLS).

††Control group contained 90% current smokers, a statistically significant difference.

‡‡Includes four patients with two synchronous primary tumours and eight patients with metachronous second primaries.

Longkanker Screenings (NELSON) trial has 80% power to show a lung cancer mortality reduction of at least 25% 10 years after randomization. In addition, the EUCT plan to combine their data once a minimum of 170 300 person-years follow-up is reached in the control arm. This should achieve 90% power to demonstrate a lung cancer mortality reduction of at least 25% depending on lung cancer risk, compliance, and contamination rates [12].

The EUCT differ from the NLST in several respects:

- *Eligibility*. EUCT eligibility criteria are based on age and smoking history, apart from the UK Lung Cancer Screening Trial (UKLS), which is driven by predicted five-year lung cancer risk. EUCT recruited participants between age 49 and 75, with a median age probably in the late 50s. This population is likely to be slightly younger than NLST (median age 60 years), but to have higher proportions of males and current smokers.

- *Recruitment*. Four EUCT trials recruited volunteers through media releases and/or primary care providers, whereas NELSON, the Lung Cancer Screening Intervention Trial (LUSI), and UKLS used population-based samples. However, healthy volunteer bias is still possible; for example, NELSON and UKLS reported that participants were less likely to be current smokers than eligible nonparticipants or the general population, which could affect generalizability [19, 25].

- *Nonscreened control groups*. Unlike NLST, EUCT randomized LDCT screening against no screening, with the exception that all Detection and Screening of Early Lung Cancer by Novel Imaging Technology and Molecular Assays (DANTE) participants received chest radiography and sputum cytology at baseline.

- *Volumetric assessment of nodules*. In general, EUCT utilize three-dimensional (3D) volumetric analysis rather than two-dimensional (2D) caliper measurement for solid parenchymal nodule assessment. Volumetry is likely to be more accurate and reproducible than manual 2D measurement, and hence a more sensitive tool for detecting growth. However, due to software limitations, ground-glass (nonsolid) lesions and nodules attached to pleura or other structures still require manual measurement.

- *Definition of positive scans*. This is discussed in the following section on false-positive examinations.

- *Varied incidence scan intervals*. Most clinical guidelines, supported by Cancer Intervention and Surveillance Modeling Network (CISNET) microsimulation modelling, recommend annual LDCT screening. However, extended incidence scan intervals may offer improved cost-effectiveness or be clinically appropriate for lower-risk participants. NELSON and the Multicentric Italian Lung Detection Trial (MILD) have specifically addressed the question of optimal screening interval, incorporating 2- and 2.5-year intervals in NELSON (for all screenees) and random allocation to annual versus biennial screens in MILD.

False-positive examinations: A serious challenge

Across nearly every trial, over 90% of all positive screening scans are falsely positive [24]; that is, they show indeterminate nodules which ultimately are not diagnosed as cancerous. Unfortunately, the number of positive scans can be large (up to 51% in some studies [24]), representing a significant false-positive burden on participants in screening programmes and health providers alike, and a potential barrier to screening implementation [26].

Nodule measurement, definition of positive scan, and nodule management

There is no consensus definition of a 'positive' scan result or required length of follow-up before a positive screening examination can be declared false positive. Consequently, definitions may vary across studies. NLST, using 2D calipers (maximum diameter), considered scans positive if any nodule ≥4 mm was detected (recall for interval CT examination if size 4–10 mm, or clinical work-up for those >10 mm), whereas NELSON, using 3D volumetry, considered scans positive if a nodule >500 mm^3 (~9.8 mm diameter) was detected (requiring pulmonologist referral for work-up) and indeterminate if a nodule 50–500 mm^3 was detected (requiring recall scan to assess volume doubling time [VDT]) [1, 18]. Accordingly, 39.1% of participants in the NLST LDCT arm had at least one positive scan [1]. The rate of positive scans was 24.2% across all three screening rounds and 96.4% of these were false positive [1]. In NELSON, the rate of positive and indeterminate scans was 2.0% and 10.8%, respectively, across all three screening rounds [18], a substantially lower result than NLST. Even so, 59.4% of the positive scan results were false positive. Thus, 3D volumetric assessment of size could reduce the FPR, although NELSON mortality data are awaited.

I-ELCAP and NLST retrospectively assessed how changing the nodule size threshold for positivity could have an impact on screening accuracy and diagnostic delay. I-ELCAP, the largest nonrandomized screening trial, evaluated 21 136 baseline scans between 2006 and 2010 [27]. The working definition of positivity was any nodule >5 mm diameter (the average of length and width measured on the same slice); 16% of baseline scans were positive and 119 cancers were diagnosed. Nodules <9 mm accounted for 75.3% of positive scans. NLST evaluated 75 126 scans of which 26 309 were baseline scans [28]. The working definition of positivity was any nodule ≥4 mm maximal diameter. At baseline, 27.3% of scans were positive, 263 cancers were diagnosed, and nodules <9 mm accounted for 70.6% of positive scans. Both analyses found that increasing the nodule size threshold reduced the number of positive scans, need for work-up, FPR, and number of invasive procedures for false-positive scans; however, this was at the cost of reduced sensitivity and delayed diagnostic work-up for a proportion of participants with lung cancer.

These illustrative data have been criticized for not accounting for other known risk variables such as nodule attenuation [29], and it is worth reflecting that the largest nodule on a scan may not always harbour cancer. For example, among the 102 Pan-Canadian Early Detection of Lung Cancer (PanCan) participants with lung cancer, cancer was diagnosed from the largest nodule in 82 participants, in the second largest in 16, in the third largest in 1, in the fourth largest in 2, and in the fifth largest in 1 [30]. The PanCan investigators therefore developed a multi-variable cancer risk prediction model for nodules detected on baseline scan [30]. Variables in the full model ('2a') included age, sex, family history, emphysema, nodule size, attenuation, location, and count. A parsimonious model ('1a') included sex, nodule size, and location. In a validation set (1090 participants; 5021 nodules; 42 lung cancers; median follow-up 8.6 years), discrimination appeared excellent; full model ROC (receiver operative characteristic) AUC = 0.970, parsimonious model = 0.960. When applied to the subset of nodules ≤10 mm diameter, discrimination was still very good (AUC 0.938 and 0.907, respectively). A more comprehensive risk assessment such as the PanCan model could easily be incorporated into reporting software, but has yet to be proven prospectively.

Radiologists vary considerably when detecting and reporting nodules. The mean individual FPR of 112 NLST radiologists was 28.7%, but ranged from 3.8 to 69.0% [31]. In an attempt to reduce reporting heterogeneity, an expert commit-tee, convened by the American College of Radiology, developed the Lung-RADS nodule classification system [32]. Lung-RADS uses an average axial length and width measured on the same slice and incorporates the PanCan nodule risk model for suspicious nodules (Category 4B). When applied retrospectively to NLST data (26 455 baseline scans and 48 671 incidence scans), Lung-RADS 1.0 substantially reduced FPR (12.8% versus 26.6% at baseline and 5.3% versus 21.8% at incidence scans, respectively). However, the trade-off for improved specificity was reduced sensitivity compared to NLST criteria: 84.9% versus 93.5% at baseline, and 78.6% versus 93.8% for incidence scans [33]. This trade-off was also seen in the NLST trial itself: radiologists with below-median FPR (1-specificity) had aggregate lower sensitivity for lung cancer than those above median FPR (91.9% versus 96.5%) [31].

Radiation risk

Unlike many other kinds of screening, screening involving ionizing radiation such as LDCT (and mammography) has a risk of radiation carcinogenesis. The screen-ing risk must be balanced against the benefit of mortality reduction. The estimated whole-body effective dose from an LDCT administered in the NLST was 1.4 mil-lisievert (mSv) [34]. An estimate of radiation-induced cancers in an individual screened at 55, 56, and 57 years with the NLST LDCT technique is 1–3 lung cancer deaths per 10 000, and breast cancers induced is 0.3 per 10 000. This compares with 30 lung cancer deaths prevented per 10 000 screened three times (Berrington de Gonzalez, personal communication). CISNET incorporated risk of lung cancer death into its models and, with a lifetime of annual screens, it estimated that 0.8% of lung cancer deaths (24 per 100 000 persons) would be related to radiation exposure [8]. In never smokers the calculation is different. The lifetime risk from three rounds of LDCT screening for a nonsmoking 40-year-old woman would be 3/10 000 lung cancer deaths and 5/10 000 breast cancers compared with 0.36/10 000 lung cancer deaths averted [34]. In persons who are candidates for screening, prudence dictates that radiation exposure be kept to the lowest possible dose for good image quality, and that follow-up imaging be optimized to limit further exposures.

Recommendations for screening

On review of lung cancer screening study results, the US Preventive Services Task Force (USPSTF) recommended it at a Grade B level [35]. The USPSTF recommendations that achieve an A or a B level indicate high or moderate certainty that the net benefits are moderate to substantial. Under the terms of the Affordable Care Act (ACA), many insurance companies offering plans that are ACA compliant must offer preventive and screening interventions without a deductible that obtain a USPSTF A or B recommendation [36]. The recommendations followed the NLST criteria, but extended the age for screening to cover 55–80 years. The USPSTF utilized an evidence review from the Pacific Northwest Evidence-based Practice Center, Oregon Health & Science University, and also modelling from CISNET [8, 37].

The evidence review included the NLST and the published European trials discussed earlier. While concluding that lung cancer screening lowered lung cancer mortality, the known drawbacks of high FPR, overdiagnosis potential, radiation risk, psychosocial consequences, effect on smoking behaviour, and incidental findings were acknowledged.

The CISNET lung group used five independent models developed by their members to estimate the long-term harms and benefit of screening if applied to a US cohort born in 1950 [8]. They used individual-level data from the NLST and the PLCO, so as to have information on a cohort that had no screening. The most efficient scenario, defined as the greatest mortality reduction for the number of screens, was annual screening from ages 55–80. This is reasonable, as lung cancer incidence increases with age, but in the very elderly comorbid conditions increase the risk of invasive procedures. CISNET did note that increasing quit time to 25 years also was efficient, since enhanced lung cancer risk persists after cessation. The Centers for Medicare & Medicaid Services (CMS) released a final decision memo in 2015 recommending annual screening with LDCT for Medicare beneficiaries who meet NLST criteria, but with an upper age limit of 77 [38]. The coverage includes a counselling and shared decision-making visit with a written order for the procedure. Requirements also included radiologist credentials, image acquisition standards, and participation in a CMS registry. Other major medical groups in the USA, Canada, and France have evaluated lung cancer screening and issued recommendations [39–41].

Risk-based models to better select screening populations

A screening programme for the approximately 7 million individuals in the USA who met the NLST eligibility criteria, estimated by proportions from the 2010 National Health Interview Survey in the 2007–2008 SEER dataset, would detect approximately 27% of lung cancers [42]. If this age range were expanded to 55–79, 32.9% of lung cancers would be detected. In this 2007–2008 SEER data, 19% of lung cancers were in the 80+ population, currently not recommended by CMS or the USPSTF for screening due to comorbidities and decreased life expectancy. Clearly, many lung cancers occur in the US population outside of the NLST criteria.

Also, even within the NLST there is a broad variation of risk of death from lung cancer. In an analysis of lung cancer death, the lowest-risk quintile had no discernible benefit from screening, albeit the power was low [43]. Therefore, more efficient screening strategies may use different criteria than the NLST, excluding those at lower risk while including those outside NLST criteria who are at identifiable high risk.

Several risk prediction models exist, as reviewed by Tammemagi [44]. The $PLCO_{m2012}$ model is the best validated and compares favourably with NLST and USPSTF selection criteria when applied to smokers in the PLCO intervention (chest radiograph) arm (Table 17.2) [45, 46]. The $PLCO_{m2012}$ model has been developed utilizing data from the PLCO control group. Selected risk factors included age, race, ethnicity, education, body mass index, self-reported chronic obstructive pulmonary disease, personal and family history of lung cancer, and smoking variables. To compare $PLCO_{m2012}$ with the USPSTF criteria, a risk threshold of 1.5% over six years was chosen, as below this threshold there was no reliable evidence of screening benefit and much higher numbers needed to screen. Comparing this risk model threshold to the USPSTF criteria in the PLCO CXR arm demonstrates that the $PLCO_{m2012}$ risk model approach is more efficient. Fewer individuals would need to be screened (8.8%) and 12.4% more lung cancers would be detected.

More complex approaches requiring medical assessment may also make screening more efficient. Chronic obstructive pulmonary disease and emphysema are well-known risk factors for lung cancer. Adding pulmonary function test results to an earlier $PLCO_{m2011}$ model improved performance [3]. Biomarkers in blood, sputum, bronchial washings, and nasal swabs are all being explored, both to bring individuals into screening and to assist with management of the indeterminate pulmonary nodule.

Table 17.2 Selection criteria for lung cancer screening: Comparison of PLCO$_{m2012}$, NLST, and USPSTF.

	PLCO$_{m2012}$ vs NLST [45]		PLCO$_{m2012}$ vs USPSTF [46]	
	PLCO$_{m2012}$	NLST	PLCO$_{m2012}$	USPSTF
Selection criteria	>1.3455%[§§]	Age 55–74, current/former smoker (quit within the past 15 years) ≥30 PY	≥1.51%[‡‡]	Age 55–80, current/former smoker (quit within the past 15 years) ≥30 PY
Validation cohort	14 144 PLCO trial screening arm smokers	14 144 PLCO trial screening arm smokers who met NLST inclusion criteria	37 327 PLCO trial screening arm smokers	37 327 PLCO trial screening arm smokers who met USPSTF inclusion criteria
Sensitivity, % (95% CI)	83.0	71.1[***]	80.1 (76.8–83.0)	71.2 (67.6–74.6)[§§]
Specificity, % (95% CI)	62.9	62.7[†††]	66.2 (65.7–66.7)	62.7 (62.2–63.1)[§§]
Positive predictive value, % (95% CI)	4.0	3.4[‡‡‡]	4.2 (3.9–4.6)	3.4 (3.1–3.7)[§§]

CI, confidence interval; NLST, National Lung Screening Trial; PLCO, Prostate, Lung, Colorectal and Ovarian Cancer screening trial; PY, pack-years smoking history; USPSTF, US Preventive Services Task Force.

§§Estimated. lung cancer risk over six years.

***p<0.001.

†††p=0.54.

‡‡‡p=0.01.

Selection of high-risk individuals may reduce false-positive rate

The lung cancer mortality model mentioned earlier in NLST participants demonstrated a significant decreasing trend in the ratio of false-positive results per screening-prevented lung cancer death, when categorized according to quintile of risk (e.g. 1648:1 in the lowest-risk quintile compared to 65:1 in the highest-risk quintile). Although the number of false-positive scans was reasonably equally distributed across all quintiles, screening-prevented lung cancer deaths were not, such that the 60% of participants at highest risk for lung cancer death accounted for 64% of false-positive results, but 88% of the screening-prevented lung cancer deaths. Thus, restricting screening to individuals at highest risk could reduce the false-positive burden, but at the cost of missing some lung cancers [43].

Screening in never smokers

The risk of lung cancer in never smokers is low. It rises with age and appears to be equivalent in males and females [47]. Risk factors include genetics, radon exposure, occupational exposure, cooking techniques, and, most importantly, second-hand smoke exposure. The PLCO had a large population of never smokers. To assess whether or not risk factors could be quantified to determine whether or not a never smoker had a risk high enough to merit screening, a modified $PLCO_{all2014}$ model similar to the $PLCO_{m2012}$ model already discussed was developed and tested [46]. No group was identified that met the risk cut-off of 1.5%. The conclusion was that screening was not currently recommended in most never smokers. An ongoing RCT of LDCT in Japan in 50–64-year-olds with under 30 pack-years of smoking, including nonsmokers, will provide useful information [48]. However, given the known increased risk of lung cancer in Japanese never smokers, there would be concerns about generalizability. Additionally, radiation risk in never smokers also cautions against screening.

Cost-effectiveness

Lung cancer screening with LDCT is costly, and also large numbers of individuals must be screened to achieve mortality reductions at the population level. Many groups have been reluctant to embark on screening programmes because of this concern. Initial efforts to estimate cost-effectiveness depended on extrapolations of benefit from nonrandomized estimates of benefit [49]. A preliminary analysis from PanCan provocatively suggested that screening would be cost neutral, as more early-stage disease would be discovered which could be treated surgically, without the substantive expenses of systemic therapy needed in late-stage disease [50].

The cost-effectiveness analysis from the NLST utilized data from medical record abstraction, covering in exhaustive detail medical interventions delivered as a consequence of screening [51]. As compared with no screening, screening with low-dose CT cost an additional $1631 per person and provided an additional 0.0316 life-years and 0.0201 quality-adjusted life-years (QALY) per person. The corresponding incremental cost-effectiveness ratios were $52 000 per life-year gained and $81 000 per QALY gained, but they varied widely by underlying risk group. A narrower selection of higher-risk individuals for screening, more streamlined evaluation protocols, and potential reductions in screening frequency for lower-risk participants could reduce these costs. Health systems have varying thresholds for cost-effectiveness for the implementation of medical interventions, but these numbers serve as a reasonable starting point for discussion.

Critical interface with smoking cessation programmes

Many authorities have been concerned that lung cancer screening could be seen as an excuse to continue smoking. Others see screening as a 'teachable moment' for smoking cessation. In the randomized Danish Lung Screening Trial, smoking cessation rates depended on LDCT result, with 12% quitting if the scan was negative and 18% quitting with a positive result [52]. Current smokers in the Lung Screening Study portion of the NLST were evaluated for smoking cessation and results also analysed by findings on LDCT [53]. Those with normal scans did show a decline in smoking prevalence that continued for the seven years of assessment (38.2% quit rate). Those with abnormal scans had higher cessation rates; the more abnormal the scan, the higher the rate (43.3% quit: suspicious for lung cancer, new or changed). All lung cancer screening programmes should incorporate proven smoking cessation strategies.

Implementation of screening programmes

Lung cancer screening programmes can learn from successful cancer screening efforts in other malignancies. Screening is a complex endeavour involving public health officials, health-care providers, and the public. As cigarette smoking in countries such as the USA continues primarily in lower socio-economic and medically underserved communities, the challenges are multiplied. An effective mechanism for determining whom to screen is important, and outreach to this group can be through simple questionnaire-based risk tools via self-report. As risk models incorporate more variables such as pulmonary function tests or biomarkers, the process becomes more medically intensive and more costly for enrolment, but may provide better effectiveness through screening better-defined, higher-risk groups.

The actual screening in radiology departments will require the close cooperation of radiologists and medical physicists, to ensure that image acquisition protocols provide optimal image quality at the lowest reasonable radiation exposure. Given the high positivity rate of initial screens, it is important that a process for evaluation of abnormal screens be in place to maximize cancer case yield at early stages, while minimizing the number of diagnostic images and, importantly, the number of biopsies for benign disease. In the USA, CMS has set out standards for lung cancer screening that address all of these issues and require reporting of performance to a central registry. This central registry may serve as a valuable resource to improve screening practice.

The American College of Radiology (ACR) has developed a process for accreditation of lung cancer screening programmes within its existing computerized tomography accreditation program [32], where Lung-RADS will be used and machine parameters and image acquisition parameters are codified. This ACR Lung Cancer Screening Registry has been approved by CMS.

Continued research into improvements in the screening process and novel screening technologies will be critical. Developments in dose reduction technology are important. Computer-aided detection (CAD) and diagnosis are eagerly awaited [3].

Conclusion

Screening appears to have potential to reduce mortality from lung cancer. While the NLST documented a highly promising 20% reduction in lung cancer mortality from screening, the many challenges include overall costs, patient recruitment, optimal image acquisition with low radiation exposure, and developing efficient paradigms to evaluate positive screens. At the same time, we need to find ways of minimizing the work-up burden, which increases radiation risk and the risk from biopsies for benign disease. Evaluation of programme effectiveness is critical to ensure that more early-stage cancers are being detected and the burden from advanced disease minimized. While the USPSTF and CMS recommendations for screening are an excellent start, there are substantial numbers of lung cancers that occur in the population in those who do not meet those risk criteria. Finding more efficient approaches such as risk-based algorithms like the $PLCO_{m2012}$ will be helpful.

There is no substitute for effective tobacco control policies that prevent nonsmokers from starting and support smokers to stop. Effective measures include bans on tobacco advertising, increases in tobacco taxes, and smoke-free workplaces. Screening should be a stop-gap measure until these and other strong anti-smoking measures bring to an end the tragedy of smoking-related lung cancer.

References

1 National Lung Screening Trial Research Team (2011). Reduced lung-cancer mortality with low-dose computed tomographic screening. *N. Engl. J. Med.* 365: 395–409.

2 GBD 2013 Mortality and Causes of Death Collaborators (2015). Global, regional, and national age-sex specific all-cause and cause-specific mortality for 240 causes of death, 1990–2013: A systematic analysis for the Global Burden of Disease Study 2013. *Lancet* 385: 117–171.

3 Tammemagi, M.C., and Lam, S. (2014). Screening for lung cancer using low dose computed tomography. *BMJ* 348: g2253.

4 Marshall, H.M., Bowman, R.V., Yang, I.A. et al. (2013). Screening for lung cancer with low-dose computed tomography: A review of current status. *J. Thoracic. Dis.* 5 (Suppl. 5): S524–S539.

5 Oken, M.M., Hocking, W.G., Kvale, P.A. et al. (2011). Screening by chest radiograph and lung cancer mortality: The Prostate, Lung, Colorectal, and Ovarian (PLCO) randomized trial. *JAMA* 306: 1865–1873.

6 National Lung Screening Trial Research Team; Aberle, D.R., Adams, A.M., Berg, C.D. et al. (2010). Baseline characteristics of participants in the randomized national lung screening trial. *J. Natl Cancer Inst.* 102: 1771–1779.

7 Patz, E.F., Pinsky, P., Gatsonis, C.G. et al. (2014). Overdiagnosis in low-dose computed tomography screening for lung cancer. *JAMA Intern. Med.* 174: 269–274.

8 De Koning, H.J., Meza, R., Plevritis, S.K. et al. (2014). Benefits and harms of computed tomography lung cancer screening strategies: A comparative modeling study for the U.S. Preventive Services Task Force. *Ann. Int. Med.* 160: 311–320.

9 Waller, J., Douglas, E., Whitaker, K.L., and Wardle, J. (2013). Women's responses to information about overdiagnosis in the UK breast cancer screening programme: A qualitative study. *BMJ Open* 3: e002703.

10 Pinsky, P.F., Church, T.R., Izmirlian, G. et al. (2013). The National Lung Screening Trial: Results stratified by demographics, smoking history, and lung cancer histology. *Cancer* 119: 3976–3973.

11 Pinsky, P.F., Gierada, D.S., Hocking, W. et al. (2014). National Lung Screening Trial findings by age: Medicare-eligible versus under-65 population. *Ann. Intern. Med.* 161: 627–633.

12 Field, J.K., van Klaveren, R., Pedersen, J.H. et al. (2013). European randomized lung cancer screening trials: Post NLST. *J. Surg. Oncol.* 108: 280–286.

13 Infante, M., Cavuto, S., Lutman, F.R. et al. (2015). Long-term follow-up results of the DANTE trial, a randomized study of lung cancer screening with spiral computed tomography. *Am. J. Respir. Crit. Care Med.* 191: 1166–1175.

14 Saghir, Z., Dirksen, A., Ashraf, H. et al. (2012). CT screening for lung cancer brings forward early disease. The randomised Danish Lung Cancer Screening Trial: Status after five annual screening rounds with low-dose CT. *Thorax* 67: 296–301.

15 Rasmussen, J.F., Siersma, V., Pedersen, J.H. et al. (2014). Healthcare costs in the Danish randomised controlled lung cancer CT-screening trial: A registry study. *Lung Cancer* 83: 347–355.

16 van Iersel, C.A., de Koning, H.J., Draisma, G. et al. (2007). Risk-based selection from the general population in a screening trial: Selection criteria, recruitment and power for the Dutch-Belgian randomised lung cancer multi-slice CT screening trial (NELSON). *Int. J. Cancer* 120: 868–874.

17 van Klaveren, R.J., Oudkerk, M., Prokop, M. et al. (2009).Management of lung nodules detected by volume CT scanning. *N. Engl. J. Med.* 361: 2221–2229.

18 Horeweg, N., van der Aalst, C.M., Vliegenthart, R. et al. (2013). Volumetric computed tomography screening for lung cancer: Three rounds of the NELSON trial. *Eur. Respir. J.* 42: 1659–1667.

19 Yousaf-Khan, U., Horeweg, N., van der Aalst, H. et al. (2015). Baseline characteristics and mortality outcomes of NELSON control group participants and eligible non-responders. *J. Thorac. Oncol.* 10: 747–753.

20 Lopes Pegna, A., Picozzi, G., Falaschi, F. et al. (2013). Four-year results of low-dose CT screening and nodule management in the ITALUNG trial. *J. Thorac. Oncol.* 8: 866–875.

21 Pastorino, U., Rossi, M., Rosato, V. et al. (2012). Annual or biennial CT screening versus observation in heavy smokers: 5-year results of the MILD trial. *Eur. J. Cancer Prev.* 21: 308–315.

22 Becker, N., Motsch, E., Gross, M.L. et al. (2012). Randomized study on early detection of lung cancer with MSCT in Germany: Study design and results of the first screening round. *J. Cancer Res. Clin. Oncol.* 138: 1475–1486.

23 Becker, N., Motsch, E., Gross, M.-L. et al. (2015). Randomised study on early detection of lung cancer with MSCT in Germany: Results of the first 3 years of follow-up after randomisation. *J. Thorac. Oncol.* 10: 890–896.

24 Field, J.K., Devaraj, A., Baldwin, D.R. et al. (2013). P1.20-004 UK Lung Cancer Screening Trial (UKLS): Baseline data. *J. Thorac. Oncol.* 8: S685.

25 McRonald, F.E., Yadegarfar, G., Baldwin, D.R. et al. (2014). The UK Lung Screen (UKLS): Demographic profile of first 88,897 approaches provides recommendations for population screening. *Cancer Prev. Res.* 7: 362–371.

26 Woolf, S.H., Harris, R.P., and Campos-Outcalt, D. (2014). Low-dose computed tomography screening for lung cancer: How strong is the evidence? *JAMA Intern. Med.* 174: 2019–2022.

27 Henschke, C.H.I., Yip, R., Yankelevitz, D.F. et al. (2013). Definition of a positive test result in computed tomography screening for lung cancer: A cohort study. *Ann Intern Med* 158: 246–252.

28 Gierada, D.S., Pinsky, P., Nath, H. et al. (2014). Projected outcomes using different nodule sizes to define a positive CT lung cancer screening examination. *J. Natl Cancer Inst.* 106: dju284.

29 Lam, S., McWilliams, A., Mayo, J., and Tammemagi, M. (2013). Computed tomography screening for lung cancer: What is a positive screen? *Ann. Intern. Med.* 158: 289–290.

30 McWilliams, A., Tammemagi, M.C., Mayo, J.R. et al. (2013). Probability of cancer in pulmonary nodules detected on first screening CT. *N. Engl. J. Med.* 369: 910–919.

31 Pinsky, P.F., Gierada, D.S., Nath, P.H. et al. (2013). National lung screening trial: Variability in nodule detection rates in chest CT studies. *Radiology* 268: 865–873.

32 American College of Radiology (n.d.) ACR-STR Practice Guideline for the Performance and Reporting of Lung Cancer Screening Thoracic Computed Tomography. http://www.acr.org/~/media/ACR/Documents/PGTS/guidelines/LungScreening.pdf (accessed 14 July 2015).

33 Pinsky, P.F., Gierada, D.S., Black, W. et al. (2015). Performance of Lung-RADS in the National Lung Screening Trial. *Ann. Intern. Med.* 162: 485–491.

34 Berrington de Gonzalez, A., Kim, K.P., and Berg, C.D. (2008). Low-dose lung computed tomography screening before age 55: Estimates of the mortality reduction required to outweigh the radiation-induced cancer risk. *J. Med. Screen* 15: 153–158.

35 Moyer, V.A. (2014). Screening for lung cancer: U.S. Preventive Services Task Force recommendation statement. *Ann. Int. Med.* 160: 330–338.

36 Kaiser Family Foundation (2015). *Preventive services covered by private health plans under the Affordable Care Act.* http://kff.org/health-reform/fact-sheet/preventive-services-covered-by-private-health-plans/ (accessed 14 July 2015).

37 Humphrey, L., Deffebach, M., Pappas, M. et al. (2013). Screening for lung cancer: Systematic review to update the U.S. Preventive Services Task Force recommendation. *Evidence Syntheses*, No. 105. Rockville, MD: Agency for Healthcare Research and Quality. http://www.ncbi.nlm.nih.gov/sites/books/NBK154610/ (accessed 14 July 2015).

38 Centers for Medicare and Medicaid Services (2015). *Decision memo for screening for lung cancer with low dose computed tomography (LDCT) (CAG-00439N)*. http://www.cms.gov/medicare-coverage-database/details/nca-decision-memo.aspx?NCAId=274 (accessed 14 July 2015).

39 Centers for Disease Control (n.d.). Lung cancer screening guidelines and recommendations. http://www.cdc.gov/cancer/lung/pdf/guidelines.pdf (accessed 14 July 2015).

40 Roberts, H., Walker-Dilks, C., Sivjee, K. et al. (2013). Screening high-risk populations for lung cancer. *J. Thorac. Oncol.* 8: 1232–1237.

41 Courand, S., Cortot, A.B., Greiller, L. et al. (2013). From randomized trials to the clinic: Is it time to implement individual lung-cancer screening in clinical practice? A multidisciplinary statement from French experts on behalf of the French intergroup (IFCT) and the group d'Oncologie de langue francaise (GOLF). *Ann. Oncol.* 24: 586–597.

42 Pinsky, P.F., and Berg, C.D. (2012). Applying the National Lung Screening Trial eligibility criteria to the US population: What percent of the population and of incident lung cancers would be covered. *J. Med. Screen* 19: 154–156.

43 Kovalchik, S.A., Tammemagi, M., Berg, C.D. et al. (2013). Targeting of low-dose CT screening according to the risk of lung-cancer death. *N. Engl. J. Med.* 369: 245–254.

44 Tammemagi, M.C. (2015). Application of risk prediction models to lung cancer screening: A review. *J. Thorac. Imaging* 30: 88–100.

45 Tammemägi, M.C., Katki, H.A., Hocking, W.G. et al. (2013). Selection criteria for lung-cancer screening. *N. Engl. J. Med.* 368: 728–736.

46 Tammemagi, M.C., Church, T.R., Hocking, W.G. et al. (2014). Evaluation of the lung cancer risks at which to screen ever- and never-smokers: Screening rules applied to the PLCO and NLST cohorts. *PLoS Med.* 11: e10001764.

47 Thun, M.J., Hannan, L.M., Adams-Campbell, L.L. et al. (2008). Lung cancer occurrence in never-smokers: An analysis of 13 cohorts and 22 cancer registry studies. *PLoS Med.* 5: e185.

48 Sagawa, M., Nakayama, T., Tanaka, M. et al. (2012). A randomized controlled trial on the efficacy of thoracic CT screening for lung cancer in non-smokers and smokers of <30 pack-years aged 50–64 years (JECS study): Research design. *Jpn J. Clin. Oncol.* 42: 1219–1221.

49 McMahon, P.M., Kong, C.Y., Bouzan, C. et al. Cost-effectiveness of computed tomography screening for lung cancer in the United States. *J. Thorac. Oncol.* 6: 1841–1848.

50 Cressman, S., Lam, S., Tammemagi, M.C. et al. Resource utilization and costs during the initial years of lung cancer screening with computed tomography in Canada. *J. Thorac. Oncol.* 9: 1449–1458.

51 Black, W.C., Gareen, I.F., Soneji, S.S. et al. (2014). Cost-effectiveness of CT screening in the National Lung Screening Trial. *N. Engl. J. Med.* 371: 1793–1802.

52 Ashraf, H., Saghir, Z., Dirksen, A. et al. (2014). Smoking habits in the randomized Danish Lung Cancer Screening Trial with low-dose CT: Final results after a 5-year screening programme. *Thorax* 69: 574–579.

53 Tammemagi, M.C., Berg, C.D., Riley, T.L. et al. (2014). Impact of lung cancer screening results on smoking cessation. *J. Natl Cancer Inst.* 106: dju084.

CHAPTER 18

Mesothelioma: Screening in the modern age

Joanna Sesti, Sabina Musovic, Jessica S. Donington, and Harvey I. Pass

Department of Cardiothoracic Surgery, NYU School of Medicine, New York, USA

SUMMARY BOX

- Malignant mesothelioma is a rare cancer, which accounts for 0.10% of cancer deaths annually in the USA, with six-month, one-year, and five-year overall survival (OS) of 55%, 33%, and 5%, respectively.

- Asbestos exposure has been linked to the development of malignant pleural mesothelioma.

- Despite the widespread use of chest X-ray and computed tomography, there are no data to support their use in early-stage malignant mesothelioma screening.

- Studies suggest that the use of biomarkers such as SMRP, osteopontin, fibulin-3, and ILK may be useful screening tests, but require further prospective validation.

- Novel approaches like the SOMamer assay, breath testing, and microRNA analysis may become useful adjuncts in screening.

- A prospective, screening study looking at the use of HMGB1, SMRP, fibulin-3, and osteopontin will be performed along with serial computerized tomography every six months for three years in asbestos-exposed workers in order to validate their use as screening tools.

Role of screening

Malignant pleural mesothelioma (MPM) is a relatively rare cancer arising from mesothelium, a protective lining that covers many of the internal organs of the body. The three main histological subtypes of mesothelioma are epithelioid, sarcomatoid, and biphasic, which combines epithelioid and sarcomatoid features. Most cases of mesothelioma arise from the pleural mesothelium, and of those

Cancer Prevention and Screening: Concepts, Principles and Controversies, First Edition.
Edited by Rosalind A. Eeles, Christine D. Berg, and Jeffrey S. Tobias.
© 2019 John Wiley & Sons, Inc. Published 2019 by John Wiley & Sons, Inc.

cases, approximately 60–70% are associated with asbestos exposure [1]. Analysis from the Surveillance Epidemiology and End Results (SEER) database revealed around 2500–3000 malignant pleural mesothelioma (MPM) cases per year, of which, most were in older, white males. Contrary to trends in other nations, where the incidence of pleural mesothelioma has yet to reach a peak, in the USA the incidence has been downtrending since 2005 [1]. Nevertheless, it is estimated that there will be approximately 30 000 new cases among females and around 50 000 among males for 2008–2054 [1].

While relatively rare, MPM accounts for 0.10% of cancer deaths annually in the USA, with six-month, one-year, and five-year overall survival (OS) of 55%, 33%, and 5%, respectively [2]. Using the IASLC (International Association for the Study of Lung Cancer) Mesothelioma Staging Database in an analysis of 2141 patients having surgery for mesothelioma, Pass et al. [3] found that advanced-stage, nonepithelial histology, male gender, age over 50 years, palliative surgery rather than curative intent surgery, the lack of adjuvant therapy, and elevated platelet and white blood cell counts were the most significant factors for poor prognosis. The clinical course of MPM usually involves substantial pain and respiratory symptoms. Most patients are currently diagnosed at a clinically advanced stage when cure is difficult, which makes early detection imperative.

Designing a clinically useful screening test for a rare disease like MPM requires that:
- The disease occurs with reasonable frequency within the population for which screening is recommended.
- The disease must result in substantial morbidity and mortality.
- The screening test must have reasonable specificity and sensitivity.
- The screening test should be noninvasive or only minimally invasive, and have low morbidity.
- One or more effective therapeutic interventions must exist for the early-stage cancer, with improved outcomes in comparison to the prognosis for patients whose disease is diagnosed at a more advanced stage.

In light of the ability to identify high-risk individuals, the substantial morbidity and mortality associated with MPM, and the improved OS associated with earlier-stage disease and surgical intervention, as well as the high economic burden ($200 billion in compensation is estimated over the next 35–40 years [4]) resulting from MPM, it would seem reasonable to develop a screening tool for high-risk groups. The best long-term survival results for MPM are achieved with multidisciplinary strategies, including maximal cytoreductive operations for patients with early-stage disease treated either with neo- or adjuvant chemotherapy. Such interventions can yield median survivals in excess of two years in selected studies. What remains to be proven is whether stage shifting by screening would define more patients who would fulfil criteria for maximal cytoreduction and thus improve their prognosis.

Identifying the at-risk population

Asbestos has been implicated in the development of MPM since Wagner's cohort report in 1960 [5]. Conventional wisdom dictates that a minimum 10-year interval from first asbestos exposure to diagnosis is required before a case of MPM can be attributed to asbestos, but the usual interval is 20–50 years. At-risk professions include pipefitters, boilermakers, maintenance workers, machinists, electricians, and sheet metal workers [6]. Although the risk of asbestos exposure in the USA has significantly decreased since 1972, when federal regulations were instituted to limit asbestos exposure, it remains a significant risk, as 1.3 million workers in the construction industry as well as building and equipment maintenance are estimated to be exposed [7]. The lifetime risk for MPM in an asbestos-exposed worker is around 10% [8]. In addition to individuals with direct occupational exposure, other means for contact with fibres include passive or low-level exposure from deterioration of buildings or offices that contain asbestos, environmental exposure such as the first responders to the terrorist attack on the World Trade Center on 11 September 2001, and direct and constant contact with others who are exposed to asbestos, such as family members [2, 9–11]. No direct relationship has been found between smoking and development of MPM [12].

Moreover, recent discoveries point to cohorts of patients with a familial propensity for mesothelioma. Two unrelated US families have been reported with a high incidence of mesothelioma despite only minimal potential exposure to asbestos, and it was noted that two members in one of these families developed uveal melanoma (UVM); one of them died of the disease and the other was treated at an early stage and cured, but subsequently developed mesothelioma [13, 14]. In each family member who had developed mesothelioma, UVM, or other cancers, *BAP1*, a member of the ubiquitin C-terminal hydrolases (UCH) subfamily of deubiquitylating enzymes (DUBs), was mutated. Family members who did not carry *BAP1* mutations did not develop these tumours. Germline *BAP1* mutations seem to cause a new cancer syndrome characterized by mesothelioma and UVM [15], and the monitoring of patients for mesothelioma who have a germline *BAP1* mutation may be another indication for screening in the future.

Screening methodologies

Since 1973, the US Occupational Safety and Health Administration (OSHA) has mandated screening of individuals with occupations that involve asbestos exposure. Employers must provide annual medical and work histories, with special emphasis directed to respiratory, cardiac, and gastrointestinal (GI) symptoms; completion of the respiratory disease questionnaire; physical exam including chest X-ray and pulmonary function tests, including forced vital capacity (FVC) and forced expiratory volume in one second (FEV1); and any laboratory or other test necessitated by sound medical practice [16]. Although data supporting the efficacy of this strategy are lacking, it highlights the need to develop better screening methodologies.

The role of chest X-ray

The first attempt at defining the role of chest X-ray in the screening for MPM dates back to 1972 in the UK. Over 2400 individuals with known asbestos exposure underwent standard chest X-rays. The overall incidence of asbestos-related abnormalities was 3–16%, yet no cases of MPM were detected [17]. Several screening studies were performed in Finland by the Finnish Institute of Occupation Health (FIOH). One in particular, which was carried out in 1990–1992 as part of the Asbestos Program of the FIOH, enrolled 18 943 workers under 70 years of age who had worked at least 10 years in construction, 1 year in a shipyard, or in the manufacture of asbestos products. The mean age was 53 years; 95% were employed in construction, 2% in shipyards, and 3% in the asbestos industry [17]. A positive screening result was defined as (1) a radiographic finding clearly indicating lung fibrosis (International Labour Organization [ILO] category 1/1); (2) a radiographic finding indicating mild lung fibrosis (ILO category 1/0) with unilateral or bilateral pleural plaques; (3) marked abnormalities of the visceral pleura (marked adhesions with or without pleural thickening); or (4) bilateral pleural plaques. Positive radiographs were found in 4133 (22%), who were then sent for further investigation and found not to have asbestosis (a chronic inflammatory and fibrotic medical condition affecting the pulmonary parenchyma associated with asbestos exposure) [17]. Yet another Finnish study used the FIOH database to investigate the associations between certain specific X-ray changes and malignancy risk. The study followed 1376 patients through the Finnish Cancer Registry who had been diagnosed with either asbestosis or benign pleural disease. The incidence of MPM was 32-fold higher and 5.5-fold higher in the asbestosis population and benign pleural disease cohorts compared to the general population. Although a direct correlation between X-ray findings and malignancy could not be made, it reinforced the notion of increased risk of malignancy with certain X-ray findings; specifically, the presence of fibrosis was a stronger predictor of MPM than plaques [18].

The largest systematic examination by chest X-ray for an asbestos-exposed cohort was the Beta-Carotene and Retinol Efficacy Trial (CARET). This was a multicentre, randomized, double-blinded, placebo-controlled trial from the USA. Its initial intent was to study the efficacy of daily pharmacological doses of vitamin A and beta-carotene in preventing lung cancer among heavy smokers and asbestos workers, who had baseline chest radiographs. Although the trial was terminated early after preliminary analysis suggested an increased risk of lung cancer, it provided investigators with the opportunity to identify radiographic findings in patients with asbestos exposure (4060) as well as monitor the development of mesothelioma. Observed radiographic changes in the asbestos cohort included benign pleural disease, defined as thickening or fibrotic plaques on pleural surfaces of the lung bilaterally; and/or asbestosis, defined as diffuse lung scarring [19, 20]. The cumulative risk of developing MPM and lung cancer during the 12–19-year follow-up was 0.9% and 6.9%, respectively [21]. Specific radiographic abnormalities or ILO readings that could predict the presence of MPM were not identified. Despite the widespread use of chest X-ray in the screening of asbestos-exposed workers, there are no data to support its usefulness in early-stage diagnosis of MPM. The CARET serum archive represents a valuable resource for blood-based biomarker discovery for the diagnosis or preclinical screening for MPM.

The role of computed tomography

Many of the studies of computed tomography (CT) in the asbestos-exposed population were performed with an interest in early detection of lung cancer more than MPM. A study of asbestos-exposed, smoking individuals in Helsinki was the first large-scale screening study evaluating CT. In this study, 602 workers with asbestos-related occupational disease were screened using helical CT and chest radiography [22]. Of those screened, 601 had bilateral pleural plaques, and 85 had asbestosis. A total of 111 patients were found to have non-calcified nodules more than 0.5 cm in diameter and 66 were referred for further examination based on the degree of suspicion that nodules were malignant. They found five lung cancers and one peritoneal mesothelioma [22]. A second Finnish study by the FIOH screened 633 individuals with heavy asbestos exposure from 2003–2004 using chest X-ray and/or high-resolution chest CT. Five lung cancers and one pleural mesothelioma were found [23]. Overall, these two studies did not conclude that CT was an acceptable method for early detection of mesothelioma.

Another European study from Italy enrolled 1045 volunteers in a surveillance programme for asbestos-exposed workers and former workers to determine if there was a screening role for low-dose helical CT (LHCT) [24]. Abnormalities were classified as pleural thickening/plaque, pleural effusion, parenchymal focal opacity, endobronchial lesion, fibrosis/scar, bone/soft-tissue lesion, cardiac abnormality, emphysema/chronic obstructive bronchopneumonopathy, or other. LDCT identified pleural abnormalities in 880 (70%) patients, of which 10 (0.96%) were diagnosed with a thoracic malignancy (9 lung cancers and 1 thymic carcinoid) [24].

In North America, a screening study performed in collaboration with the Occupational Health Clinics for Ontario Workers recruited 516 patients with a remote asbestos exposure history (at least 20 years prior). This study was the first to scrupulously characterize plaque abnormalities based on their presence, extent, location, and shape. Serial CTs were then obtained of the target area. Overall, six lung cancers, two MPMs, and two peritoneal mesotheliomas were detected. Unfortunately, both MPM patients died soon after diagnosis, and so the conclusion was that despite their meticulous characterization of plaque abnormalities, serial LDCT did not lead to early diagnosis of MPM [25]. While a recent meta-analysis by Ollier et al. [26] regarding the use of chest CT in asbestos-exposed individuals concluded that CT scan screening was effective in detecting asymptomatic lung cancer, its role in MPM screening is unsupported.

The current consensus is that neither chest X-ray nor CT is able to have an impact on early detection of MPM and thus affect survival. While in the USA OSHA continues to mandate annual chest X-rays in asbestos-exposed workers, other organizations like the British Thoracic Society Standards of Care Committee and the French Speaking Society for Chest Medicine (SPLF) no longer recommend it [27, 28]. Moreover, OSHA does not recommend the use of CT in its guidelines.

The role of circulating biomarkers

The early diagnosis of MPM proves challenging not only on a radiographic level, but also on a cytological and pathological level. To that effect, organizations such as the International Mesothelioma Interest Group (IMIG) and the British Thoracic Society recommend a multidisciplinary approach to the diagnosis of MPM, including cytological, pathological, and radiographic evaluation [29, 30]. Over the last several years, the role of biomarkers in distinguishing MPM from benign mesothelial reactions, other carcinomas, and other benign pleural pathologies has been investigated. At the infancy of biomarker research, most studies have attempted to identify proteins or genes responsible for secreted extracellular proteins from mesotheliomas, and adapt them to serum analysis, including mesothelin, osteopontin, and fibulin-3.

Circulating biomarker studies for distinguishing MPM from controls

High-mobility group protein B1 (HMGB-1)

One of the first issues regarding the use of circulating biomarkers for the possible early detection of mesothelioma is the choice of subjects to screen, as detailed earlier. Certainly, asbestos exposure is correlated with mesothelioma, but in the majority of cases the asbestos exposure is detailed in a patient's history without correlation with imaging studies or specifically an ILO score. A biomarker which first stratifies patients as to their exposure to fibres would help in the selection of patients for further longitudinal follow-up with blood samples, and in fact a profile of biomarkers for the evolution of mesothelioma may indeed be different from one that simply identifies asbestos exposure. Yang et al. [31, 32] reported that transformed mesothelial cells are 'addicted' to the damage-associated molecular pattern (DAMP) protein HMGB1, and that MPM cells actively secrete HMGB1, which is required for MPM growth and invasion. The secretion of HMGB1 by MPM cells suggested that HMGB1 might be a serological biomarker for MPM. Thirty MPM patients were found to have significantly higher serum and plasma levels of HMGB1 compared to healthy individuals. Moreover, HMGB1 levels in serum and plasma were comparable. Since many MPM patients are exposed to asbestos, it is unknown whether the sustained high levels of HMGB1 are linked solely to asbestos exposure, to MPM, or both, or whether the levels of HMGB1 in asbestos-exposed individuals may further increase on MPM development. Other investigators have validated these findings [33, 34], and HMGB1 deserves validation in prospective trials as either a marker of asbestos exposure and/or MPM.

Hyaluronic acid

Hyaluronic acid (HA) was the first circulating biomarker to be explored for the early detection of MPM [35]. Several studies showed that serum HA levels were elevated in patients with MPM [35–39]. In addition, further work revealed a significant difference in the levels of HA in healthy volunteers versus those with malignant tumours other than MPM [40, 41]. Nevertheless, HA has been found to have a limited role as a marker for early diagnosis of MPM due to its prevalence in late-stage disease [36, 42]; and elevation in other pathologies such as hepatic fibrosis, inflammatory joint disease, and pleural metastases of various carcinomas [43, 44].

CA-125

Serum CA-125 is a well-known tumour marker that can be elevated in the serum of patients with various malignancies, most notably ovarian cancer. A few small-scale studies have investigated its role in the diagnosis of MPM. In 2007, Creaney et al. [45] collected serum CA-125 levels in 117 patients at the time of diagnosis, 33 healthy asbestos-exposed individuals, 53 with asbestos-related lung or pleural disease, and 30 with benign pleural effusions. They found that despite the fact that 117 (42%) patients with MPM had elevated CA-125 levels, 50% of individuals with benign effusions and 10% with asbestos exposure also had elevated levels. This confirmed the lack of diagnostic specificity of CA-125 in the setting of MPM diagnosis [45].

Soluble mesothelin-related protein

The mesothelin gene (*MSLN*) encodes a precursor protein that is cleaved into megakaryocyte potentiating factor and mesothelin, and an enzyme-linked immunosorbent assay (ELISA) was developed which measured soluble mesothelin-related protein (SMRP). SMRP was first identified as a useful marker in the diagnosis of MPM in 2003. The study by Robinson et al. [46] included 44 patients with confirmed MPM; 68 matched controls, of which 40 had been exposed to asbestos; and 160 patients with other inflammatory or malignant lung and pleural diseases. Their results showed a sensitivity of 85% (37/44) for MPM and a specificity of 100% (38/38) versus other pleural disease. In addition, they found that SMRP was elevated in only 1 out of 30 lung cancers, 0 out of 28 non-asbestos-exposed individuals, and 7 out of 40 asbestos-exposed patients without cancer [46]. Several studies have attempted to determine the optimal SMRP level to achieve an appropriate sensitivity and specificity as a screening study (Table 18.1). The largest North American SMRP study assessed serum levels in 90 MPM patients, 170 lung cancer patients, 66 age- and tobacco-matched asbestos-exposed individuals, along with 45 malignant pleural effusions, 30 benign effusions, and

Table 18.1 Studies investigating the diagnostic accuracy of SRMP in malignant pleural mesothelioma.

	SMRP Cut-off Level (nmol/mL)	Sensitvity	Specificity	AUC
Robinson et al. [70]	1.6	83%	95%	–
Scherpereel et al. [71]	0.93	80%	82.6%	0.872
Pass et al. [47]	1.9	60%	89%	0.81
Rodriguez-Portal et al. [72]	0.55	72%	72%	0.75
Hollovoet et al. [73]	2.0	64%	95%	0.871

AUC, area under curve; SRMP, soluble mesothelin-related protein.

20 nonmesothelial malignant effusions [47]. They noted that SMRP levels correlated with histology (epithelioid and biphasic higher than sarcomatoid), stage (Stage II: 2.09 ± 0.41, > Stage I: 10.61 ± 3.89, p=0.03), and sample source (pleural higher than serum). The association between SMRP level and disease progression was highlighted by Grigoriu et al. [48]. They found that SMRP levels increased in patients with disease progression despite treatment, while those with treatment response had a temporary (six-month) decrease and then return to baseline. It has been suggested that SMRP should be used in combination with a baseline CT, then followed at defined intervals over time, with patients demonstrating rising levels progressing to more invasive testing [21]. Despite numerous published reports (of possible diagnostic utility), the routine use of SMRP in the diagnosis of MPM has not been fully adopted. It is used extensively in Australia, but only sparingly in the USA, where it is measured in a reference laboratory. A recent meta-analysis was conducted by Hoolevoet et al. [49]. They concluded that at 95% specificity, SMRP displayed a sensitivity of 32%. Therefore, in a patient suspected to have MPM, an elevated serum SMRP would present a strong incentive to pursue further diagnostic steps, but due to its poor sensitivity its role in early diagnosis of MPM is limited.

Megakaryocyte-potentiating factor

Megakaryocyte-potentiating factor (MPF) is a protein made from posttranslational modification of mesothelin. While some studies have suggested that MPF has adequate sensitivity and specificity as a MPM biomarker, others have shown the opposite. A Japanese team showed that 51 out of 56 patients (91%) had elevated MPF levels compared with healthy controls [50]. Shiomi et al. [51] developed an ELISA system to detect levels of N-ERC/mesothelin, and found that levels in MPM patients were on average higher than healthy controls. However, when comparing osteopontin, MPF, and serum mesothelin as MPM markers, MPF had a sensitivity of only 34% at a specificity of 95%. So while the data are somewhat conflicting, it is evident that MPF does not demonstrate a clear advantage over SMRP for the early detection of MPM [52].

Osteopontin

Osteopontin (OPN) is a regulatory protein secreted from malignant cells, and is an important intermediate in the tumour microenvironment. The use of OPN as a biomarker in MPM was initially investigated by Pass et al. [53], using serum OPN levels of age-matched asbestos-exposed, non-asbestos-exposed, and MPM patients. Serum OPN levels were noted to be significantly higher in the MPM group versus the asbestos-exposed group (133 ± 10 ng/mL and 30 ± 3 ng/mL, $p < 0.001$). At a cut-off value of 48.3 ng/mL, serum OPN had a sensitivity of 77.6% and a specificity of 85.5%. Serum OPN levels were also noted to be higher depending on the length of asbestos exposure (greater if over 10 years) and the presence of asbestos-related radiographic findings (plaques or fibrosis). Not all projects have been as optimistic regarding OPN. Grigoriu et al. [54] measured serum OPN levels in 43 individuals with pleural effusions secondary to non-mesothelioma-related malignancies, 33 with benign pleural asbestos-related lesions, 96 with MPM, and 112 asbestos-exposed healthy subjects. They concluded that while OPN was higher in MPM patients compared to healthy asbestos-exposed subjects, it was unable to distinguish between MPM and pleural metastatic carcinoma or benign pleural effusions in asbestos-exposed patients [54]. Since serum OPN is susceptible to degradation secondary to its central thrombin cleavage site, differences in laboratory handling could explain the differing conclusions previously mentioned. Measuring plasma OPN may negate the latter issues, and in some studies has been promising when analysing asbestos-exposed and MPM patient samples [55–57].

Fibulin-3

Fibulin-3 is a highly conserved member of the extracellular glycoprotein fibulin family. After genomic comparison of normal peritoneum and matched mesotheliomas revealed elevated levels of EFEMP1 whose gene product is fibulin-3, plasma levels were investigated in a number of cohorts [58]. Fibulin-3 plasma levels were measured in 92 MPM patients, 136 healthy asbestos-exposed individuals, 93 patients with nonmesothelioma effusions, and 43 healthy controls. Fibulin-3 levels in the pleural effusions were also investigated from 74 MPM patients, 39 with benign effusions, and 54 with nonmesothelioma effusions. The study was conducted in independent discovery and validation cohorts from New York and Detroit. It found that plasma fibulin-3 levels did not vary according to age, sex, duration of asbestos exposure, or degree of radiographic changes. Nevertheless, levels were higher in patients with MPM compared to asbestos-exposed persons (105 ± 7 ng/mL vs 14 ± 1 ng/mL in the Detroit cohort and 113 ± 8 ng/mL vs 24 ± 1 ng/mL in the New York cohort, $p < 0.001$). When data from both groups were combined, at a cut-off value of 52.8 ng/mL, the sensitivity and specificity were 96.7% and 95.5%, respectively, for MPM versus nonmesothelioma. In addition, the ability of fibulin-3 to distinguish between nonmesothelioma and early-stage disease was even more striking; a cut-off value of 46.0 ng/mL provided a sensitivity and specificity of 100% and 94.1%, respectively [58]. A blinded validation trial using plasma from asbestos-exposed individuals as well as from MPM patients accumulated at the Princess Margaret Cancer Center in Toronto, Canada was then performed, which revealed an area under the curve of 0.87 for plasma specimens from 96 asbestos-exposed versus 48 MPM patients. This compares favourably to previous work on biomarkers such as mesothelin (area under curve [AUC] 0.72–0.93) [49].

Integrin-linked Kinase

It is thought that chronic inflammation is one of the key pathophysiological mechanisms in the development of MPM. Integrin-linked kinase (ILK), an intracellular serine/threonine kinase, has been implicated in chronic inflammatory processes, and high levels have been associated with ovarian cancer as well as MPM [59]. Watzka et al. [59] hypothesized that ILK may be useful as an MPM diagnostic biomarker. Their group assessed levels of ILK using an ELISA on serum samples from 46 MPM patients, 98 nonmesothelioma patients with other malignancies, and 23 with benign chest pathology. They found ILK levels to be significantly higher in MPM patients compared to patients with nonmesothelioma malignancies or benign pulmonary pathologies (8.89 ng/mL, 0.66 ng/mL, and 0.78 ng/mL, respectively). At a cut-off level of 2.48 ng/mL, ILK had a diagnostic sensitivity of 80% and a specificity of 95% for distinction between MPM and other diseases [59]. In a subsequent study, serum ILK concentrations were found to vary significantly based on stage (stages I+II: 6.7 ± 7.8 ng/mL, stages III+IV: 13.7 ± 15.9 ng/mL, p =0.02) [60].

SOMAmer

SomaLogic has developed a proteomic assay (SOMAscan™) that solves width, depth, and scale problems encountered by other proteomic platforms such as LCMS and ELISA-based assays. The assay is a highly multiplexed, sensitive, quantitative, and reproducible affinity-based proteomic tool for discovering previously undetected biomarkers of disease, prognosis, therapeutic response, and physiological changes. The SOMAscan assay currently measures 1129 protein analytes from 65 mcL of plasma and offers a wide dynamic range, quantifying proteins that span over 8 logs in abundance (from femtomolar to micromolar), with low limits of detection (40 fM median LOD) and good reproducibility (5.1% median %CV).

The SOMAscan proteomic assay is enabled by protein-capture SOMAmer (Slow Off-rate Modified Aptamer) reagents. SOMAmer reagents are constructed with chemically modified nucleotides that greatly expand the physicochemical diversity of the large randomized nucleic acid libraries from which the SOMAmer reagents are selected [61]. The SOMAscan assay measures native proteins in complex matrices by transforming each individual protein concentration into a corresponding SOMAmer concentration, which is then quantified by standard DNA techniques such as microarrays or quantitative polymerase chain reaction (PCR). The assay takes advantage of SOMAmers' dual nature as both protein affinity-binding reagents with defined three-dimensional structures, and unique nucleotide sequences recognizable by specific DNA hybridization probes.

The SomaLogic proteomic assay was recently used in a multicentre, case-control study of 117 MPM cases and 142 asbestos-exposed control individuals [62]. Using univariate and multivariate approaches, 64 candidate protein biomarkers were identified, from which a 13-marker random forest classifier was used. This panel demonstrated an AUC of 0.99 ± 0.01 in training, 0.98 ± 0.04 in independent blinded verification, and 0.95 ± 0.04 in blinded validation studies. Sensitivity and specificity in blinded verification were 90% and 95%, respectively [62]. Future studies defining the role of this panel for the early detection of mesothelioma in a screening trial of asbestos-exposed individuals are being planned.

Micro-RNAs

MicroRNAs (miRNAs) are small (approx. 22 nt) noncoding RNA molecules that play a central role in the regulation of gene expression. In patients with cancer, miRNAs can function as tumor suppressors or oncogenes [63]. In addition, some studies have demonstrated that certain neoplasms have characteristic miRNA fingerprints in human peripheral blood samples [64]. This has led some investigators to look at miRNAs as potential diagnostic biomarkers for MPM. Weber et al. [65] used oligonucleotide microarrays to identify miRNA levels in peripheral blood samples of patients with MPM and healthy, asbestos-exposed controls. They identified miR-103 as a potential biomarker for early detection of MPM. Real-time PCR was then used for validation of miR-103 in 23 MPM patients, 17 asbestos-exposed patients, and 25 controls. At a cut-off level of 0.621, miR-103 had a sensitivity and specificity of 83% and 71%, respectively, for MPM versus asbestos-exposed patients. Other miRNAs have been identified at other laboratories, including miR-625p and miR-29c [66]. In fact, there is some evidence to suggest that miR-29c may be linked to prognosis in MPM [67]. Kirschner et al. [66] found that miR-29c* and miR-92a, as well as 15 novel miRNAs, were elevated in plasma samples from MPM patients compared to healthy controls; miR-625-3p was also present in significantly higher concentration in plasma/serum from MPM patients, and was able to discriminate between cases and controls, in both the original and the independent series of patients. As with other biomarkers, the inconsistency of results for microRNAs in the blood which could be used for early detection is a function of small numbers of cases, as well as differences in what the cases are compared to; that is, normal healthy individuals or individuals with known asbestos exposure.

Breath-testing

Breathomics is a noninvasive tool that uses highly sensitive probes to detect breath-volatile organic compounds (BVOCs) in exhaled breath, and it is hypothesized that patients with different malignancies have specific and reproducible patterns of BVOCs, almost like a fingerprint. Chapman et al. [68] analysed breath samples from 20 MPM patients, 18 acute respiratory distress syndrome (ARD) patients, and 42 healthy controls. A 'smell print' was derived from 10 MPM subjects, which was able to distinguish 10 independent MPM patients from controls with an accuracy of 95%. In fact, MPM, ARDs, and control subjects were correctly identified in 88% of cases. A simultaneous study by Dragonieri et al. [69] looked at 13 histology-confirmed MPM patients, 13 asbestos-exposed patients, and 13 healthy subjects. Breathprints distinguished MPM from asbestos-exposed controls with a sensitivity and specificity of 92.5% and 85.7%, respectively. There is certainly promise in this technology, and it could become a useful tool for the diagnosis of asbestos-related diseases; however, large, prospective, case-control studies are still needed.

Conclusion

Although MPM is a rare disease, its impact in terms of morbidity and mortality is substantial. With early detection and treatment, survival can be improved. The identification of economical, easily administered, and highly specific and sensitive screening tests has been fraught with adversity. Large-scale radiological screening studies with plain chest X-ray and chest CT have proven ineffective. The trend towards research on biomarkers that can be sampled in patient serum, plasma, or pleural effusions is encouraging, but limited by small cohorts and inconsistent results. A comparison of different biomarkers is presented in Table 18.2. Nevertheless, despite early promise, no one biomarker has proven to have sufficient specificity and sensitivity in a prospective trial to be adapted to public use. It is possible that screening for MPM in the asbestos-exposed population will be a multimodal approach, consisting of imaging, combination biomarker assays, and breathomics; however, prospective randomized trials looking at multimodal screening methods are needed. Such a trial will be commenced through a collaboration of the National Cancer Institute Early Detection Research Network and the Government of Chile, in which a cohort of workers exposed to asbestos products will be studied prospectively for the development of mesothelioma. Longitudinal blood sampling for HMGB1, SMRP, fibulin-3, and osteopontin will be performed along with serial computerized tomography every six months for three years. Only SMRP will be used as an 'actionable' biomarker, depending on its absolute level and change over time. A valuable reference set of plasma and serum from this study will be made available to the research community for future discovery and validation of asbestos/MPM–associated markers.

Table 18.2 Specificity and sensitivity of different biomarkers.

Biomarkers	Cut-off Level (nmol/mL)	Sensitivity	Specificity
SMRP [70]	1.6	83%	95%
Osteopontin [47]	48.3	77.6%	85.5%
MPF [52]	–	34%	95%
Fibulin-3 [47] (nonmesothelioma vs all-stage disease)	52.8	96.7%	95.5%
Fibulin-3 [47] (nonmesothelioma vs early-stage disease)	46.0	100%	94.1%
ILK [47]	2.48	80%	95%

ILK, interleukin-linked kinase; MPF, megakaryocyte-potentiating factor; SMRP, soluble mesothelin-related protein.

References

1 Price, B., and Ware, A. (2009). Time trend of mesothelioma incidence in the United States and projection of future cases: An update based on SEER data for 1973 through 2005. *Crit. Rev. Toxicol.* 39 (7): 576–588.

2 Helland, A., Solberg, S., and Brustugun, O.T. (2012). Incidence and survival of malignant pleural mesothelioma in Norway: A population-based study of 1686 cases. *J. Thorac. Oncol.* 7(12): 1858–1861.

3 Pass, H.I., Giroux, D., Kennedy, C. et al. (2014). Supplementary prognostic variables for pleural mesothelioma: A report from the IASLC staging committee. *J. Thorac. Oncol.* 9 (6): 856–864.

4 Carroll, S., Hensler, D.R., Abrahamse A. et al. (2002). Asbestos litigation costs and compensation: An interim report. Report No. DB-397-ICJ. Santa Monica, CA: Rand Corporation.

5 Wagner, J.C., Sleggs, C.A., and Marchand, P. (1960). Diffuse pleural mesothelioma and asbestos exposure in the North Western Cape Province. *Br. J. Ind. Med.* 17: 260–271.

6 Roggli, V.L., Sharma, A., Butnor, K.J. et al. (2002). Malignant mesothelioma and occupational exposure to asbestos: A clinicopathological correlation of 1445 cases. *Ultrastruct. Pathol.* 26 (2): 55–65.

7 U.S. Department of Labor (2003). Asbestos: OSHA standards. https://www.osha.gov/SLTC/asbestos/standards.html (accessed 3 January 2018).

8 Selikoff, I.J., Hammond, E.C., and Seidman, H. (1980). Latency of asbestos disease among insulation workers in the United States and Canada. *Cancer* 46 (12): 2736–2740.

9 National Academy of Sciences (1984). *Asbestiform Fibers: Non-Occupational Health Risks.* Washington, DC: National Academies Press.

10 Lange, J.H. (2003). Cough and bronchial responsiveness in firefighters at the World Trade Center site. *N. Engl. J. Med.* 348 (1): 76–77.

11 Lioy, P.J., Weisel, C.P., Millette, J.R. et al. (2002). Characterization of the dust/smoke aerosol that settled east of the World Trade Center (WTC) in lower Manhattan after the collapse of the WTC 11 September 2001. *Environ. Health Perspect.* 110 (7): 703–714.

12 Muscat, J.E., and Wynder, E.L. (1991). Cigarette smoking, asbestos exposure, and malignant mesothelioma. *Cancer Res.* 51 (9): 2263–2267.

13 Carbone, M., Yang, H., Pass, H.I. et al. (2013). BAP1 and cancer. *Nat. Rev. Cancer* 13 (3): 153–159.

14 Testa, J.R., Cheung, M., Pei, J. et al. (2011). Germline BAP1 mutations predispose to malignant mesothelioma. *Nat. Genet.* 43 (10): 1022–1025.

15 Carbone, M., Ferris, L.K., Baumann, F. et al. (2012). BAP1 cancer syndrome: Malignant mesothelioma, uveal and cutaneous melanoma, and MBAITs. *J. Transl. Med.* 10: 179.

16 US Department of Labor (1994). OSHA Regulations (Standards – 29 CFR). https://www.osha.gov/pls/oshaweb/owadisp.show_document?p_table=STANDARDS&p_id=10003 (accessed 3 January 2018).

17 Harries, P.G., Mackenzie, F.A.F., Sheers, G. et al. (1972). Radiological survey of men exposed to asbestos in naval dockyards. *Br. J. Ind. Med.* 29 (3): 274–279.

18 Karjalainen, A., Pukkala, E., Kauppinen, T., and Partanen, T. (1999). Incidence of cancer among Finnish patients with asbestos-related pulmonary or pleural fibrosis. *Cancer Causes Control* 10 (1): 51–57.

19 Barnhart, S., Keogh, J., Cullen, M.R. et al. (1997). The CARET asbestos-exposed cohort: Baseline characteristics and comparison to other asbestos-exposed cohorts. *Am. J. Ind. Med.* 32 (6): 573–581.

20 Omenn, G.S., Goodman, G., Thornquist, M. et al. (1994). The beta-carotene and retinol efficacy trial (CARET) for chemoprevention of lung cancer in high risk populations: Smokers and asbestos-exposed workers. *Cancer Res.* 54 (7, Suppl.): 2038s–2043s.

21 Pass, H.I., and Carbone, M. (2009). Current status of screening for malignant pleural mesothelioma. *Semin. Thorac. Cardiovasc. Surg.* 21 (2): 97–104.

22 Tiitola, M., Kivasaari, L., Huuskonen, M.S. et al. (2002). Computed tomography screening for lung cancer in asbestos-exposed workers. *Lung Cancer* 35 (1): 17–22.

23 Vierikko, T., Järvenpää, R., Autti, T. et al. (2007). Chest CT screening of asbestos-exposed workers: Lung lesions and incidental findings. *Eur. Respir. J.* 29 (1): 78–84.

24 Fasola, G., Belvedere, O., Aita, M. et al. (2007). Low-dose computed tomography screening for lung cancer and pleural mesothelioma in an asbestos-exposed population: Baseline results of a prospective, nonrandomized feasibility trial – an Alpe-adria Thoracic Oncology Multidisciplinary Group Study (ATOM 002). *Oncologist* 12 (10): 1215–1224.

25 Egedahl, R.D., Olsen, G.W., Coppock, E. et al. (1989). An historical prospective mortality study of the Sarnia Division of Dow Chemical Canada Inc., Sarnia, Ontario (1950–1984). *Can. J. Public Health* 80 (6): 441–446.

26 Ollier, M., Chamoux, A., Naughton, G. et al. (2014). Chest CT scan screening for lung cancer in asbestos occupational exposure: A systematic review and meta-analysis. *Chest* 145 (6): 1339–1346.

27 Robinson, M., and Wiggins, J. (2002). Statement on malignant mesothelioma in the UK. *Thorax* 57 (2): 187.

28 Scherpereel, A.; French Speaking Society for Chest Medicine Experts (2007). Guidelines of the French Speaking Society for Chest Medicine for management of malignant pleural mesothelioma. *Respir. Med.* 101 (6): 1265–1276.

29 British Thoracic Society Standards of Care Committee (2007). BTS statement on malignant mesothelioma in the UK, 2007. *Thorax* 62 (Suppl. 2): ii1–ii19.

30 Husain, A.N., Colby, T.V., Ordóñez, N.G. et al. (2009). Guidelines for pathologic diagnosis of malignant mesothelioma: A consensus statement from the International Mesothelioma Interest Group. *Arch. Pathol. Lab. Med.* 133 (8): 1317–1331.

31 Jube, S., Rivera, Z.S., Bianchi, M.E. et al. (2012). Cancer cell secretion of the DAMP protein HMGB1 supports progression in malignant mesothelioma. *Cancer Res.* 72 (13): 3290–3301.

32 Yang, H., Rivera, Z., Jube, S. et al. (2010). Programmed necrosis induced by asbestos in human mesothelial cells causes high-mobility group box 1 protein release and resultant inflammation. *Proc. Natl Acad. Sci. U.S.A.* 107 (28): 12611–12616.

33 Tabata, C., Kanemura, S., Tabata, R. et al. (2013). Serum HMGB1 as a diagnostic marker for malignant peritoneal mesothelioma. *J. Clin. Gastroenterol.* 47 (8): 684–688.

34 Tabata, C., Shibata, E., Tabata, R. et al. (2013). Serum HMGB1 as a prognostic marker for malignant pleural mesothelioma. *BMC Cancer* 13: 205.

35 Chiu, B., Churg, A., Tengblad, A. et al. (1984). Analysis of hyaluronic acid in the diagnosis of malignant mesothelioma. *Cancer* 54 (10): 2195–2199.

36 Frebourg, T., Lerebours, G., Delpech, B. et al. (1987). Serum hyaluronate in malignant pleural mesothelioma. *Cancer* 59 (12): 2104–2107.

37 Pettersson, T., Fröseth, B., Riska, H., and Klockars, M. (1988). Concentration of hyaluronic acid in pleural fluid as a diagnostic aid for malignant mesothelioma. *Chest* 94 (5): 1037–1039.

38 Roboz, J., Greaves, J., Silides D. et al. (1985). Hyaluronic acid content of effusions as a diagnostic aid for malignant mesothelioma. *Cancer Res.* 45 (4): 1850–1854.

39 Fuhrman, C., Duche, J.C., Chouaid, C. et al. (2000). Use of tumor markers for differential diagnosis of mesothelioma and secondary pleural malignancies. *Clin. Biochem.* 33 (5): 405–410.

40 Pluygers, E., Baldewyns, P., Minette, P. et al. (1992). Biomarker assessments in asbestos-exposed workers as indicators for selective prevention of mesothelioma or bronchogenic carcinoma: Rationale and practical implementations. *Eur. J. Cancer Prev.* 1 (2): 129–138.

41 Thylen, A., Wallin, J., and Martensson, G. (1999). Hyaluronan in serum as an indicator of progressive disease in hyaluronan-producing malignant mesothelioma. *Cancer* 86 (10): 2000–2005.

42 Hedman, M., Arnberg, H., Wernlund, J. et al. (2003). Tissue polypeptide antigen (TPA), hyaluronan and CA 125 as serum markers in malignant mesothelioma. *Anticancer Res.* 23 (1B): 531–536.

43 Atagi, S., Ogawara, M., Kawahara, M. et al. (1997). Utility of hyaluronic acid in pleural fluid for differential diagnosis of pleural effusions: Likelihood ratios for malignant mesothelioma. *Jpn J. Clin. Oncol.* 27 (5): 293–297.

44 Soderblom, T., Pettersson, T., Nyberg, P. et al. (1999). High pleural fluid hyaluronan concentrations in rheumatoid arthritis. *Eur. Respir. J.* 13 (3): 519–522.

45 Creaney, J., van Bruggen, I., Hof, M. et al. (2007). Combined CA125 and mesothelin levels for the diagnosis of malignant mesothelioma. *Chest* 132 (4): 1239–1246.

46 Robinson, B.W., Creaney, J., Lake, R. et al. (2003). Mesothelin-family proteins and diagnosis of mesothelioma. *Lancet* 362 (9396): 1612–1616.

47 Pass, H.I., Wali, A., Tang, N. et al. (2008). Soluble mesothelin-related peptide level elevation in mesothelioma serum and pleural effusions. *Ann. Thorac. Surg.* 85 (1): 265–272.

48 Grigoriu, B.D., Chahine, B., Vachani, A. et al. (2009). Kinetics of soluble mesothelin in patients with malignant pleural mesothelioma during treatment. *Am. J. Respir. Crit. Care Med.* 179 (10): 950–954.

49 Hollevoet, K., Reitsma, J.B., Creaney, J. et al. (2012). Serum mesothelin for diagnosing malignant pleural mesothelioma: An individual patient data meta-analysis. *J. Clin. Oncol.* 30 (13): 1541–1549.

50 Onda, M., Nagata, S., Ho, M. et al. (2006). Megakaryocyte potentiation factor cleaved from mesothelin precursor is a useful tumor marker in the serum of patients with mesothelioma. *Clin. Cancer Res.* 12 (14, Part 1): 4225–4231.

51 Shiomi, K., Miyamoto, H., Segawa, T. et al. (2006). Novel ELISA system for detection of N-ERC/mesothelin in the sera of mesothelioma patients. *Cancer Sci.* 97 (9): 928–932.

52 Creaney, J., Yeoman, D., Demelker, Y. et al. (2008). Comparison of osteopontin, megakaryocyte potentiating factor, and mesothelin proteins as markers in the serum of patients with malignant mesothelioma. *J. Thorac. Oncol.* 3 (8): 851–857.

53 Pass, H.I., Goparaju, C., Espin-Garcia, O. et al. (2016). Plasma biomarker enrichment of clinical prognostic indices in malignant pleural mesothelioma. *J. Thorac. Oncol.* 11 (6): 900–909.

54 Grigoriu, B.D., Scherpereel, A., Devos, P. et al. (2007)(. Utility of osteopontin and serum mesothelin in malignant pleural mesothelioma diagnosis and prognosis assessment. *Clin. Cancer Res.* 13 (10): 2928–2935.

55 Creaney, J., Yeoman, D., Musk, A.W. et al. (2011). Plasma versus serum levels of osteopontin and mesothelin in patients with malignant mesothelioma: Which is best? *Lung Cancer* 74 (1): 55–60.

56 Hu, Z.D., Liu, X.F., Liu, X.C. et al. (2014). Diagnostic accuracy of osteopontin for malignant pleural mesothelioma: A systematic review and meta-analysis. *Clin. Chim. Acta* 433: 44–48.

57 Joseph, S., Harrington, R., Walter, D. et al. (2012). Plasma osteopontin velocity differentiates lung cancers from controls in a CT screening population. *Cancer Biomark.* 12 (4): 177–184.

58 Pass, H.I., Levin, S.M., Harbut, M.R. et al. (2012). Fibulin-3 as a blood and effusion biomarker for pleural mesothelioma. *N. Engl. J. Med.* 367 (15): 1417–1427.

59 Watzka, S.B., Posch, F., Pass, H.I. et al. (2011). Detection of integrin-linked kinase in the serum of patients with malignant pleural mesothelioma. *J. Thorac. Cardiovasc. Surg.* 142 (2): 384–389.

60 Watzka, S.B., Posch, F., Pass, H.I. et al. (2013). Serum concentration of integrin-linked kinase in malignant pleural mesothelioma and after asbestos exposure. *Eur. J. Cardiothorac. Surg.* 43 (5): 940–945.

61 Gold, L., Ayers, D., Bertino, J. et al. (2010). Aptamer-based multiplexed proteomic technology for biomarker discovery. *PLoS One* 5 (12): e15004.

62 Ostroff, R.M., Mehan, M.R., Stewart, A. et al. (2012). Early detection of malignant pleural mesothelioma in asbestos-exposed individuals with a noninvasive proteomics-based surveillance tool. *PLoS One* 7 (10): e46091.

63 Kent, O.A., and Mendell, J.T. (2006). A small piece in the cancer puzzle: MicroRNAs as tumor suppressors and oncogenes. *Oncogene* 25 (46): 6188–6196.

64 Hausler, S.F., Keller, A., Chandran, P.A. et al. (2010). Whole blood-derived miRNA profiles as potential new tools for ovarian cancer screening. *Br. J. Cancer* 103 (5): 693–700.

65 Weber, D.G., Johnen, G., Bryk, O. et al. (2012). Identification of miRNA-103 in the cellular fraction of human peripheral blood as a potential biomarker for malignant mesothelioma: A pilot study. *PLoS One* 7 (1): e30221.

66 Kirschner, M.B., Cheng, Y.Y., Badrian, B. et al. (2012). Increased circulating miR-625-3p: A potential biomarker for patients with malignant pleural mesothelioma. *J. Thorac. Oncol.* 7 (7): 1184–1191.

67 Pass, H.I., Goparaju, C., Ivanov, S. et al. (2010). hsa-miR-29c* is linked to the prognosis of malignant pleural mesothelioma. *Cancer Res.* 70 (5): 1916–1924.

68 Chapman, E.A., Thomas, P.S., Stone, E. et al. (2012). A breath test for malignant mesothelioma using an electronic nose. *Eur. Respir. J.* 40 (2): 448–454.

69 Dragonieri, S., van der Schee, M.P., Massaro, T. et al. (2012). An electronic nose distinguishes exhaled breath of patients with Malignant Pleural Mesothelioma from controls. *Lung Cancer* 75 (3): 326–331.

70 Robinson, B.W., Creaney, J., Lake, R. et al. (2005). Soluble mesothelin-related protein: A blood test for mesothelioma. *Lung Cancer* 49 (Suppl. 1): S109–S111.

71 Scherpereel, A., Grigoriu, B., Conti, M. et al. (2006). Soluble mesothelin-related peptides in the diagnosis of malignant pleural mesothelioma. *Am. J. Respir. Crit. Care Med.* 173 (10): 1155–1160.

72 Rodriguez Portal, J.A., Becerra, E.R., Rodríguez, D.R. et al. (2009). Serum levels of soluble mesothelin-related peptides in malignant and nonmalignant asbestos-related pleural disease: Relation with past asbestos exposure. *Cancer Epidemiol. Biomarkers Prev.* 18 (2): 646–650.

73 Hollevoet, K., Nackaerts, K., Thimpont, J. et al. (2010). Diagnostic performance of soluble mesothelin and megakaryocyte potentiating factor in mesothelioma. *Am. J. Respir. Crit. Care Med.* 181 (6): 620–625.

CHAPTER 19

Skin cancer prevention and screening

Mark Elwood[1] and Terry Slevin[2]

[1] *School of Population Health, University of Auckland, New Zealand*
[2] *Cancer Council of Western Australia, Perth, Australia*

SUMMARY BOX

- Skin cancer is the commonest cancer in fair-skinned people.
- It is predominantly caused by ultraviolet (UV) light, solar or artificial.
- Squamous cell and basal cell cancers are a major health-care cost; melanoma is a major cause of death.
- Melanoma incidence is beginning to decrease in countries with active population-level prevention programmes.
- Sunscreens are effective if properly used. UV solaria are banned in many countries. Modest UV exposure is needed to optimize vitamin D levels.
- Screening for melanoma has never been tested in a randomized trial, but is supported by other studies.
- Screening is often done without organization, quality control, or evaluation.
- Overdiagnosis of thin melanomas is recognized.
- Diagnosis and monitoring of high-risk patients may use dermoscopy, photography, and computer systems.

Skin cancer is generally divided into two categories: cutaneous malignant melanoma (CMM, melanoma); and keratinocyte or nonmelanoma skin cancers (NMSC), the most common of which are basal cell carcinoma (BCC) and squamous cell carcinoma (SCC). Melanoma is generally considered the most dangerous, if far less common, form of skin cancer. This chapter will focus primarily on issues related to melanoma. Many but not all factors relating to the causation,

---

Cancer Prevention and Screening: Concepts, Principles and Controversies, First Edition.
Edited by Rosalind A. Eeles, Christine D. Berg, and Jeffrey S. Tobias.
© 2019 John Wiley & Sons, Inc. Published 2019 by John Wiley & Sons, Inc.

prevention of, and screening for melanoma also relate to NMSCs. When these categories are combined, skin cancers are the most common cancers diagnosed in humans.

Causes of skin cancer

Excessive ultraviolet radiation (UVR) from the sun is the primary modifiable risk factor for melanoma and other skin cancers [1, 2]. Other established risk factors are UVR from artificial sources such as the use of solaria [3]. The greater quantum of the exposure and the earlier in life the first use of sunbeds, the greater the skin cancer risk.

Skin type, hair colour, and eye colour are important recognized risk factors. Broadly, the lighter the colour of a person's skin, hair, and eyes, the greater the risk of melanoma. Risk is roughly double for those with lighter skin colours (types I and II on the Fitzpatrick skin type [4]) compared to those with dark skin. Those with heavily freckled skin have double the skin cancer risk compared to those who do not have lots of freckles. Compared to people with dark or black hair, risk is almost three times greater for those with red or red/blonde hair, double for blondes, and one and a half times higher for those with light brown hair. A similar risk increase (46%) is linked to those with blue/green/grey eyes compared to those with brown eyes [5].

Other risk factors include people with many nevi (sometimes also called moles), which are benign precursor lesions to melanoma. As with many cancers, people with a family history of melanoma are at substantially greater risk, as are people with previous skin cancers.

UVR exposure levels early in life, such as the first 10 years, influence to a major degree the lifetime potential risk of skin cancer, while exposure in later years of life appears to determine the extent to which that potential is realized [6]. The pattern of exposure also influences risk, with intermittent intensive exposure, more typical of that experienced by a modern office worker, being more strongly connected to risk of BCC and melanoma, while more continuous exposure, more linked to outdoor workers' exposure patterns, being more likely to increase SCC risk [6, 7].

Incidence

Figure 19.1 shows international comparisons of melanoma incidence and mortality rates (age standardized rates (ASR), both males and females combined) across major areas of the world. It shows the highest rates in populations in the more economically advantaged nations, particularly those with predominantly pale-skinned populations. Australia and New Zealand have clearly the highest ASRs of around 35 per 100 000, and the highest mortality rates, particularly in men.

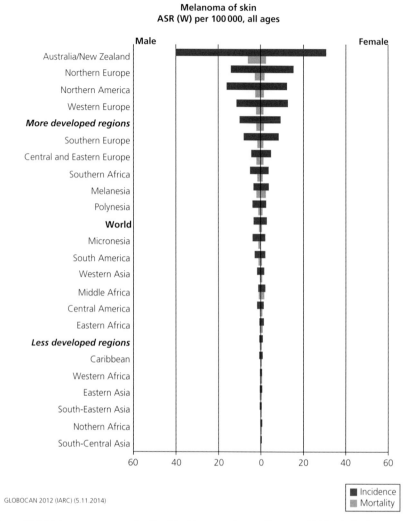

Figure 19.1 Melanoma age-standardized incidence and mortality rates (ASRs) in both sexes combined. Source: International Agency for Research on Cancer. Public domain.

Northern Europe, North America, and Western Europe are also highly ranked, with ASRs of around 12–20 per 100 000 [8]. Some caution should be applied, however, as these are also the countries with the best cancer data capture. Pale-skinned populations living closer to the equator report higher rates, but the relatively high incidence rates in Scandinavian countries may be linked to greater access to artificial sources of UVR, as well as cheaper access to holidays in sunny destinations and associated sun exposure [9].

Changes in incidence trends internationally: Are prevention efforts working?

Many studies have reported steady and in some cases more dramatic increases in melanoma rates in a range of countries [10, 11]. Erdmann et al. [11] report that while melanoma incidence in 39 countries for which there is good data has been increasing for the past 50 years, there is evidence of that increase 'levelling off', particularly in the younger cohorts in countries that have been more active and early in promoting skin cancer prevention, such as Australia, New Zealand, Canada, and the USA [10]. Other countries with a less active focus on skin cancer prevention, or later to adopt prevention initiatives, such as Slovenia, Denmark, Belarus, the UK, and Sweden, show no similar trend.

Supporting the notion that there may be evidence of efforts to prevent skin cancer contributing to reduced disease incidence is the reduction in the number of keratinous (NMSC) cancer excisions in younger age groups in Australia between 2000 and 2011 [12].

The question has been raised that any reduction in melanoma in countries like Australia may be an artefact of an increase in inward migration of subpopulations with more heavily pigmented skin, lowering the skin cancer risk profile of the whole population [13]. Other researchers challenge whether the migration effect is of sufficient volume to account for the measured incidence reduction effect. Despite evidence of progress, Leiter et al. [14] suggest that incidence rates in Europe may increase to 40–50 per 100 000 over the next decades.

Questions have been posed regarding the genuine benefit of any incidence reduction achieved. Some evidence suggests that the fall in incidence has been mainly in thin lesions, which some researchers argue may be the less aggressive form of melanoma, unlikely to proceed to metastatic disease; thus the incidence reduction may have little influence on melanoma-related mortality. This issue of overdiagnosis is discussed later in this chapter.

Cost of skin cancer

Increasingly, the prospect of investing in programmes or initiatives to achieve disease prevention is insufficient to attract the interest of governments and policymakers. Public health efforts need to be couched in terms of economic benefits or cost savings. As a result, more effort is being put into assessing the cost burden of diseases. Skin cancer broadly is recognized as one of the most expensive cancers, if not the most expensive, in higher-income countries when the cost of managing NMSC and melanoma is combined.

The annual cost of treating skin cancer in the USA is estimated at $8.1 billion (of which $4.8 billion is for NMSC) [15], and the cost of treating NMSC in Australia for 2015 was put at AUS$703 million [16]. Costs in other countries were captured in a review paper [17], which estimated the expenditure on skin cancer treatment in 2008 in the UK at £112 million; in Denmark at €33.3 million, of which 59% was from melanoma and accounted for 0.2% of the Danish health budget; R$109 million in Brazil (capturing public and private health service costs); and in Canada CAN$66.1 million (made up of CAN$36.5 million for NMSCs and CAN$29.6 million for melanoma). All estimates are likely to be underestimates; none includes the cost of removal of benign lesions thought to be suspicious. These figures can be considered the minimum baseline for assessing the cost of excessive UV exposure in these populations.

With the clear and substantial burden of disease linked to skin cancer established and some indication of prevention efforts proving beneficial, where might any modest skin cancer public health investment best be made?

Controversies in prevention

As has been heralded in the tobacco control sphere for many decades, the importance of a 'comprehensive approach' to skin cancer prevention is paramount. Put another way, no single sandbag ever stopped a flood.

When assessed in isolation, evidence remains thin for individual skin cancer prevention programmes proving effective [18]. This is likely to be linked to the complex and variant drivers for individual risk behaviours and UVR exposure, including the significant number of quite different behaviours that are likely to influence skin cancer risk.

Prevention options are broadly focused on reduced UVR exposure. There remains a variety of individual behaviours likely to achieve or influence that objective. The choice of hats, sun-protective clothing or swimwear, sunglasses, the use of sunscreen, choices about timing of UVR exposure (during high- or low-UVR periods of the day and year), and the use of shade are all influenced by a range of factors, from personal knowledge, attitudes, and beliefs, to the built and natural environment, societal norms, and much more.

For this reason, the application of a wide range of strategies to promote skin cancer prevention becomes necessary before any realistic expectation of cancer risk reduction can be made. Iannacone and Green [19] capture the range of components and interventions that might be reasonably placed, in combination, to influence UVR exposure in a population. The emphasis on high-profile mass media social marketing and advertising campaigns is understandable, but ignores the importance of a range of policy initiatives, school and workplace programmes, and efforts to influence the environment to maximize availability of shade in outdoor workplaces and recreation facilities. Glanz et al. concluded in 2004 [20]: 'The ideal intervention strategies to reduce UVR exposure are coordinated, sustained, community-wide approaches that combine education, mass media, and environmental and structural change.'

This summary remains a relevant and succinct expression of the 'comprehensive approach' towards skin cancer prevention that is needed to achieve success, as it sees beyond the clear limitations of individual programmes. Action in workplaces, schools, childcare facilities, communities, health-care settings, and sporting settings, alongside education and mass media efforts, investment in influencing policies, the built environment, and tax structures to favour affordable sun protection, are all essential ingredients to make progress.

The prospect of meaningfully delineating the impact of these various individual strategies on a population is minimal. There is no evidence that any one component is the single most influential one.

Linked to the theme of assessing the most important aspects of effective prevention programmes is the challenge around the accurate measurement of skin cancer prevention behaviours. Measuring trends in the use of sunscreen, clothing choice, hat wearing (and if worn, what type of hat), use and adequacy of use of sunscreen, use and adequacy of shade, total quantum of UVR exposure (be it deliberate tanning behaviour or incidental exposure associated with preferred outdoor activities), the influence of weather and other factors, all add to the issues to be tackled. A range of sun protection behaviours in Australia has been monitored in the National Sun Survey, with data collection in the summers of 2003/2004, 2006/2007 and 2010/2011, in an effort to track trends in relevant behaviours [21]. The findings generally support the hypothesis that there has been a progressive improvement in sun protection behaviours. However, the capture of many quite different key behaviours and even factors like the variance in weather patterns make unequivocal conclusions difficult; for example, during the final summer reported there was an unusually long period of heavy rainfall over a substantial part of the Australian east coast, influencing behaviour and data collection.

Accepting that there is a considerable level of complexity in the task, it is worth examining individual key issues in skin cancer prevention.

Does sunscreen make things better or worse?

Sunscreens were originally designed to avoid erythema (sunburn) and have increasingly been recommended as a tool for skin cancer prevention. The International Agency for Research on Cancer (IARC) released a monograph in 2001 recommending the daily use of sunscreen rated SPF15 or better in high-UVR environments, while warning against the use of sunscreen to allow extended UVR exposure [22]. Since that time, a randomized study conducted in Nambour, Australia has shown that when sunscreen (SPF15+ was used in the trial) is used regularly, it is effective in reducing melanoma [23]. Some support for the benefit of sunscreen in melanoma prevention was found also in a case-control study in the USA [24]. More evidence of the preventive benefit (or otherwise) of sunscreen use in melanoma would be welcome.

Sunscreen is seen as a useful skin cancer prevention tool, but caution should be applied. A substantial body of evidence indicates that most users apply an insufficient quantity to achieve the protection level claimed on the label, and that broadspectrum (protecting against UVA and UVB) sunscreen with an SPF rating of 30 or better should be used. The safety of sunscreen remains under scrutiny, with concerns about adverse effects of long-term use being raised regularly. The current evidence suggests that sunscreen remains a safe product to use. Improved formulation of the protective efficacy and cosmetic acceptability of sunscreen is an ongoing process that is to be encouraged. The dominant view is that sunscreen should be considered a useful but not sole strategy for skin cancer prevention [25].

Banning solariums and sunbeds

Brazil was the first country in the world to ban commercial solarium operations, in 2009. Australia followed suit, with most jurisdictions applying a ban as of 2015 after progressive tightening of regulations relating to their commercial use over a period of more than 10 years, and a concerted advocacy effort by a range of groups [26]. The increasing body of evidence linking solarium use with skin cancer has heightened calls for, and in more jurisdictions implementation of, bans on allowing solarium use for people under the age of 18 years [27].

Vitamin D

It is impossible to address skin cancer prevention without considering the development of a body of research examining the benefits of vitamin D and the harms linked to its paucity. Vitamin D deficiency is unquestionably linked to compromised bone health, and while levels of evidence vary, is considered to be associated with a wide range of other adverse health effects [28]. Serum levels of 25-OHD have been used as a measure of adequacy for vitamin D. While some dietary sources of vitamin D are available, it is broadly viewed that exposure to UVR is the most common and effective source of vitamin D for the majority of the world's population. There remains active debate about where cut-points for deficiency and sufficiency might be drawn. The Institutes of Medicine (IOM) 2011 report recommended deficiency be defined as 25-OHD less than 30 nmol/L (12 ng/mL) and adequacy as 50–125 nmol/L (20–50 ng/mL), with the range of 30–50 nmol/L being defined as 'insufficient' – a range indicating some health risk to some but not all individuals. The report advises: 'Use of higher than appropriate cut-points for serum 25-OHD levels would be expected to artificially increase the estimates of the prevalence of vitamin D deficiency' [29].

The level of UVR exposure – in combination with dietary and other factors – to establish and maintain optimum levels of Vitamin D will obviously vary across the world, being influenced by variables such as geography, season, age, skin type, and more. However, in higher-UVR locations the importance of minimizing UVR exposure during high-UVR times of the day and of the year remain a health priority, with a view to skin cancer prevention. A challenge in seeking to strike this balance is to avoid extreme interpretation of public health advice, driving consumers excessively in one direction or the other.

Conclusions on prevention

On balance, skin cancer is largely but not entirely preventable with reduced exposure to UVR, particularly among high-risk populations living in or spending time in high-UVR environments. Claiming proven efficacy for skin cancer prevention efforts may be slightly premature. The time line linking prevention efforts with sun exposure behaviour change, leading to population-level UVR exposure reductions and subsequent skin cancer incidence reductions, is likely to be a minimum of three or more decades. The available evidence at present suggests encouraging progress, being sufficient to support a continued effort among communities where prevention efforts have commenced. It also offers guidance and encouragement in populations where little progress on this issue has been made that investment in prevention may be highly beneficial.

Population screening for melanoma

The scientific and policy issues around screening for melanoma are epitomized in the US Surgeon General's 2014 report on skin cancer prevention [18], which notes: 'despite the insufficient evidence supporting screening in the general population, an estimated 87% of Americans believe that skin cancer screening is recommended'.

The key question is [30]: 'Does screening in asymptomatic persons with whole body examination by a primary care clinician or by self-examination reduce morbidity and mortality from skin cancer?' This question distinguishes screening from case-finding by assessment of those who seek advice for a suspicious lesion, and also from surveillance of selected high-risk groups, such as those with prior melanoma, a strong family history, or multiple dysplastic naevi. While the question relates to skin cancer, the real target is melanoma, as other skin cancers are generally very successfully treated after a routine clinical diagnosis and cause little mortality; but any detection programme for melanoma will result in assessments for other skin lesions as well.

The absence of randomized trials

The normal evidence-based approach to population-based screening for cancer relies on having randomized trial evidence for the main benefit, a reduction in mortality. Indeed, often randomized trial evidence of benefit is stated to be *required* to justify publicly funded programmes. Thus, for breast and colorectal cancer screening, most discussion is around the interpretation of the considerable number of randomized trials available; and even so, opinions on the interpretation and implementation of such evidence may still vary considerably. However, the most well-established screening programme for cancer, for uterine cervical cancer, does not rely on randomized trial evidence, as Pap smear screening was developed in the 1940s, whereas large-scale, long-term, population-based randomized trials are a more recent development.

The challenge with screening for melanoma is that there is no randomized trial evidence, because no trial has been done, and a trial may never be done. It has been attempted. In Queensland, Australia, with one of the highest incidence rates of melanoma in the world, it was proposed to randomize small communities with an aggregate population of around 280 000 over age 30 into intervention and control groups, and to offer free whole-body skin examinations by primary care practitioners over a three-year period, backed up by publicity and community interventions to encourage screening [31, 32]. The trial was designed to reach 40% uptake of screening in the intervention communities, giving sufficient power to detect a 20% reduction in mortality, on the appropriate 'offer to screen' comparison. However, while the research funding was obtained after the usual peer-review processes, the service delivery funding depended on administrative decisions and was not obtained [33]. A pilot phase was completed, with 18 communities randomized. The intervention group showed a successful increase in screening, increases in the detection rate of melanoma, and a lower proportion of deeply invasive lesions compared to Queensland general statistics; estimated specificity was 86% [34]. Assessment of screening in Queensland depends on a case-control study, described later in this chapter. In Germany, a randomized trial was proposed, but rejected by the administrative body in favour of a programme with nonrandomized comparisons, also described later [35].

Recommendations of major groups

The usual approach to authoritative recommendations and guidelines is dominated by the conventional evidence-based paradigm, and therefore breaks down in the absence of randomized trial evidence. For example, in the USA multidisciplinary groups emphasizing reliance on empirical evidence do not recommend screening, although they do not clearly recommend against it; thus the US Preventive Services Task Force and the National Cancer Institute state that the evidence is insufficient to assess benefits and harms [36], while the American Academy of Dermatology recommends self-examination – 'persons should examine their skin for signs of skin cancer' – and the American Cancer Society recommends skin examination as part of the 'cancer related check-up' (along with examination of the thyroid, testicles, ovaries, lymph nodes, and oral cavity). In other countries, similar variations often exist.

Case-control studies

Following the evidence-based paradigm, the next most reliable study designs are cohort and case-control studies, involving individuals selected and studied carefully. There are no such cohort studies with defined control groups for melanoma.

There are case-control studies, the first published over 20 years ago [37]. In Connecticut, USA, 650 newly diagnosed melanoma patients were compared with control subjects from the general population, using a personal interview on whether the individuals had previously conducted 'a careful, deliberate, and purposeful examination of the skin' – skin self-examination (SSE). The melanoma patients were then followed for five years to identify 'lethal' melanoma; that is, subjects who died or developed advanced disease with distant metastases. Thus, the question tested is whether practising self-examination reduces the risk of lethal melanoma. It did: the risk was reduced by 63%, and the effect was significant, although only 15% of all subjects had carried out SSE. Case-control studies of cancer screening are notoriously difficult to interpret, and there are some curious features of these results: for example, part of the benefit was because doing SSE was associated with a lower incidence of total melanoma [38], whereas an unchanged or higher incidence would be expected.

A large population-based case-control study in Queensland, Australia compared previous screening histories in over 3700 patients with newly diagnosed melanomas and in population-based controls, using detailed interviews. The study showed that previous participation in skin examinations by a physician resulted in a significant 14% reduction in the incidence of invasive melanoma over 0.75 mm deep, and a 40% reduction in lesions over 3 mm; this change in depth distribution was projected to lead to a 26% decrease in mortality over five years [39]. Also, there was a significant 38% higher risk of being diagnosed with a thin invasive melanoma (<0.75 mm), which represents the combination of true earlier diagnosis and overdiagnosis. The investigators concluded that 'these results suggest that screening would reduce melanoma mortality', but the study does not extend to assessing mortality directly.

Population-based comparisons

For other evidence, we have population-based comparisons. One small example is that there was great concern in the 1980s about a possible cluster of melanoma at the Lawrence Livermore National Laboratory in California, USA, mainly around possible nuclear exposures. While no such association was shown in subsequent investigations, the concern led to an extensive programme of education, promotion of self-examination, and provision of physician skin screening in the employees. Over the period 1984–1996, no deaths from melanoma occurred, while 3.4 would have been expected; and the incidence rate of more deeply invasive melanomas, over 0.75 mm, was reduced compared to previous experience [40].

Switzerland has the highest melanoma incidence in Europe, and early detection by self-examination and skin examinations by health professionals has been funded since the 1990s, with the proportion of the population having a skin examination by a health professional reaching 38% in women and 33% of men by 2007. Analysis of melanoma incidence trends in one region of southern Switzerland showed no change in all-age mortality; there were increases in incidence to 2003, with some decreases thereafter. The increases were restricted to melanoma in the thin and intermediate categories (less than 2 mm), and to superficial spreading melanoma [41]. The investigators concluded that an opportunistic screening strategy does not change the incidence of thick melanomas or the overall mortality. However, this study has no defined comparison group and the information on participation in screening is limited.

The German SCREEN programme

Most attention recently has concentrated on the SCREEN project in Germany (Skin Cancer Research to provide Evidence for Effectiveness of Screening in Northern Germany) [35, 42]. The government of Schleswig-Holstein provided funding for a standardized whole-body examination by a primary care physician over a 12-month period (2003–2004) for all citizens aged over 20 with statutory health insurance. Physicians had to complete an eight-hour training programme and were paid for each examination performed. Subjects could choose to be screened by a dermatologist, and 23% did so. Of 1.88 million eligible citizens, over 360 000 participated, 19%. Of those screened, 26% were considered at increased risk or had a suspicious lesion, and 9% had a personal or first-degree relative history of melanoma, showing some self-selection of higher-risk individuals. Over 3000 malignancies were detected, including 585 melanomas. In an early analysis, mortality trends were compared over the decade 2000–2009, showing a decrease of 48% in the screening area, contrasting with increases of 2–32% in four adjacent regions, and 10% in all of Germany excluding the screening area [42]. But this choice of time period was questionable: much of the decrease seems too soon to attribute to screening, and many melanoma deaths after 2003–2004 would have resulted from melanoma diagnosed prior to that period. The decline over 2000–2009 was virtually the same in men (47%) and in women (49%), although participation in screening was much higher in women (27% compared with 10%). However, in melanoma diagnosed in people who had participated, the proportions were not as different (56% in women, 46% in men). Furthermore, the year 2000, the starting point of the trend analysis, showed a peak, with higher rates than in the previous decade in men, but not for women. Thus, the investigators' conclusion that this shows 'strong evidence, but not absolute proof' of screening reducing mortality is questionable. Nevertheless, the programme was successful in policy terms, leading to a nationwide programme in Germany from 2008 offering screening to individuals 35 years and over [43]. Later evaluations show that the mortality rates in the screening area returned to preprogramme levels, and no decrease in national rates was shown, thus there is no clear evidence for the success of this programme [44, 45].

Other studies assessing depth distribution

A considerable number of other studies also show that patients using self-examination or participating in physician examination tend to be diagnosed with thinner melanomas, but these studies do not involve carefully documented population-based controls, and are more open to selection and recall biases. For example, in US studies, thinner melanomas were associated with both physician screening and self-examination [46, 47], and also with more regular medical care indicated by insurance coverage [48]. Individually these studies are weak, but together they do provide supportive evidence of benefits.

Overdiagnosis and indolent lesions

Overdiagnosis is a problem with all cancer diagnosis and cancer screening, and is probably most severe with prostate cancer [49, 50]. Overdiagnosis in melanoma screening is shown by increases in the incidence of thin melanomas, with no decrease in the incidence of thick lesions, or in mortality; this pattern has been shown in several countries over the last 30 years (e.g. [51, 52]). Melanoma provided one of the first clear examples of overdiagnosis, related to increasing awareness and case-finding rather than screening: an analysis in one region in Australia demonstrated a rapid rise in total incidence and in the incidence of in situ and thin invasive melanomas, and a reduction in the proportion, but no reduction in the absolute incidence rate, of thicker melanomas [53]. Often the misleading impression of benefit is given by assessing the proportional distribution by depth, rather than the population-based rates. The Queensland case-control study gave one of the quantitative estimates of overdiagnosis, showing a 38% excess rate of very thin melanoma associated with previous physician skin examination [39]. A change in approach including the use of the term 'indolent lesion of epithelial origin' – IDLE – has been proposed [50]. Factors contributing to overdiagnosis include increased public concern about common skin lesions, greater clinical surveillance, a higher number of biopsies, partially for medico-legal reasons, changes in pathology classifications and 'diagnostic drift', and the added impetus of screening – 'error amplification by population screening' [54, 55].

Selective screening and risk-prediction models

It is often recommended that screening be restricted or concentrated on subjects at increased risk. With very greatly increased risk, this becomes clinical surveillance of reasonably small numbers of identified high-risk subjects, such as those with prior melanoma, multiple dysplastic naevi, or familial disease, which will not be dealt with here.

The more general question of targeting screening to subjects at higher risk than normal is more complex. Many discussions look only at the likely performance of screening in the high-risk subjects. On general principles, if the same screening procedure is applied to a higher-risk group, sensitivity and specificity may be the same, but the yield in cases diagnosed, the predictive value of a positive test, and the overall benefit–risk and cost-effectiveness should be considerably increased. Targeting screening by simple factors such as age and sex is appropriate, and is of course used for every other medical intervention. Many studies have pointed to the concentration of the risk of deeply invasive, poor-prognosis melanoma in men over age 50, whereas the first responders to many screening and educational programmes tend to be younger women.

More detailed selective screening is a two-step process, the first step being the identification of the defined 'higher-risk' group. This is in itself a screening process, with false positives and false negatives; it may be expensive, and like all screening processes has the potential to create anxiety and generate clinical workload. Many models of selective screening incorporate a risk model based on risk factors for melanoma, such as skin type, sunburn history, or naevi. However, the discriminatory power of such models may be modest. Two systematic reviews of risk-prediction models for melanoma included 25 and 28 models respectively [15, 56]. While there are many models using a large number of risk factors, and most giving reasonable and generally similar levels of discrimination, few studies have had validation in independent populations or have demonstrated applications in clinical and public health practice. A US model is regarded as the most clinically useful in one review [57], while the other review notes that only two models, one in the USA and the other developed in Italy and tested in Brazil, have been validated in separate populations; both showed good discrimination [58, 59].

Improving the management of patients presenting

In melanoma, issues of screening are closely related to those of the appropriate management of presenting signs and symptoms in primary care. While a comprehensive review of this large topic is inappropriate here, a few recent advances are worth noting.

The traditional approach uses the history and clinical examination, not assisted by any special technology. Many schemes have been suggested to assist practitioners in distinguishing suspicious skin lesions for which referral to a specialist and/or biopsy is appropriate. In the UK, the emphasis has been on referral to a specialist, whereas for example in Australia and New Zealand, general practitioners often carry out their own biopsies. Of the simple clinical rules, the seven-point checklist developed by MacKie and colleagues in Glasgow in the 1980s [60] has been widely used. It was modified in 1989, and the revised 'Weighted 7PCL' recommended for use in primary care in the UK by the National Institute for Health and Clinical Excellence (NICE). A substantial primary care assessment study concluded that score performed well, although a change in the cut-off was recommended. With the recommended cut-off of 4, there was a sensitivity of 92% from melanoma and specificity of 53% [61]; using a single item, an irregular border, also gave good results. In North America the ABCDE system, a five-point checklist [62], was developed primarily for awareness programmes aimed at the general public; its elements are Asymmetry, Border (irregular), Colour (variety or change), Diameter (larger than 6 mm), and Evolving (any change). A comparison of the ABCDE and the seven-point rules in Australia showed that two features of the seven-point scale, a change in size and a change in colour, are the most useful discriminators between benign lesions and melanoma [63].

Many technical aids to discriminate between benign and malignant lesions have been developed [64]. All of these understandably have been developed in secondary care, where large numbers of patients are available for intensive investigation. Many of these methods are only applicable for small groups of patients, seen as referrals or as high-risk subjects under surveillance, although they may often be suggested as screening methods. Such methods include total body photography, to which can be added computer image capture allowing external review and surveillance, and extra imaging of selected lesions with dermoscopy. Such methods are marketed to physicians and to the general public in many countries, but trials and follow-up studies are very limited [64]. There are many more complex methods at various stages of development, including confocal scanning microscopy, infrared spectroscopy, Raman spectroscopy, and thermographic imaging [64]. Multispectral imaging is used in the MelaFind device, approved by the Food and Drug Administration (FDA) in the USA [65, 66].

In relation to screening, only techniques simple and inexpensive enough for widespread use in primary care are relevant. Two methods have been evaluated thoroughly in primary care: dermoscopy and spectrophotometry.

Dermoscopy is the use of a hand-held magnifying device which is placed directly on the lesion, often with a smear of oil to improve clarity. As with clinical examination, its value depends on the physician's interpretation, but the process shows more detail and can give both improved sensitivity and specificity (that is, correctly identifying innocent lesions which need no further action) when used by dermatologists who have considerable experience [67]. A European study in primary care showed increases in sensitivity, with no change in specificity [68]. Dermoscopy can incorporate a digital camera and so facilitates teledermatology, with the images being sent to an expert dermatologist located anywhere, and the digital images can be stored and compared at a later dermoscopic examination, allowing 'digital monitoring'. In Australasian primary care, training courses in dermoscopy have been popular, either as a one-day clinical course, or using textbooks and image banks in self-administered programmes. Then the practitioner can use dermoscopy, including sending images for expert assessment, and offer follow-up and reassessment as an alternative to immediate biopsy or referral. The primary focus of this approach is to reduce biopsies and referrals, while maintaining the existing high level of suspicion for melanoma diagnosis. In a trial in Australian primary care, 63 practitioners completed online training, and assessed subsequent patients first by conventional clinical assessment, with the results and management plan then recorded, and then reassessed them at the same visit, adding digital dermoscopy [69]. Of those lesions recommended for biopsy or referral on the basis of clinical examination alone, the majority (64%) were recognized as benign and not excised or referred, being managed by immediate reassurance or short-term follow-up with reassurance after showing no change. Both physicians and patients were very satisfied with this process; this combined approach suggests that many referrals and excisions of skin lesions presenting in primary care in Australia could be avoided.

Employing multispectral imaging, the 'MoleMate' system uses a hand-held Spectrophotometric Intracutaneous Analysis (SIAcopy) scanner and a scoring algorithm based on UK primary care experience. The spectrophotometry images have been shown to be predictive of melanoma in experimental and secondary care applications. In a randomized trial in England, patients aged over 18 with a suspicious pigmented lesion which 'could not immediately be diagnosed as benign and about which the patient could not be reassured' were randomized to receive either a standard examination using clinical history and unassisted visual inspection, or the standard examination with SIAcopy assessment, by general practitioners with a short training in the technique [70]. The primary outcome was the proportion of referred lesions that specialist experts decided were 'appropriate referrals', justifying referral or biopsy. In contrast to the dermoscopy trial described, this trial showed no improvement in appropriate referrals; indeed, with the SIAcopy a higher proportion of lesions were referred, and agreement with the final diagnosis was lower. Despite this, the clinicians were confident that the system improved their practice, and patients were more satisfied with the enhanced consultation; the authors note that 'the novel technology provided false reassurance'.

Conclusions on screening

The situation is still uncertain [71]. The question of the value of screening for melanoma is made complex by the lack of randomized trial evidence. Perhaps no definitive trial will ever be done. Thus, concluding that 'screening cannot be supported because of a lack of randomized trial evidence' avoids the issue rather than dealing with it. The existing evidence, based on case-control and population-based comparisons supplemented by clinical studies, modelling, and cost–benefit assessments, has to be used even though it is limited. Overall, this evidence is consistent with a beneficial effect of screening by skin examination, either as self-examination or by a doctor. In many countries, the current situation is very unsatisfactory, as screening is widely practised and supported, indeed expected, by much of the population, but because it is not 'officially' supported or funded, there is little or no monitoring or quality control, so gaining further knowledge is inhibited. Selective, high-risk, or opportunistic screening is widely done, without a strong evidence base. In countries where melanoma is a major problem, the advantages of supporting skin screening and doing it well should outweigh the hazards of inaction.

References

1 International Agency for Research on Cancer (2012). Solar and ultraviolet radiation. *IARC Monographs on the Evaluation of Carcinogenic Risks to Humans*, vol. 100D. Lyon: IARC.

2 International Agency for Research on Cancer (2004). Solar and ultraviolet radiation. *IARC Monographs on the Evaluation of Carcinogenic Risks to Humans*, vol. 55. Lyon, France: International Agency for Research on Cancer; 2004.

3 El Ghissassi, F., Baan, R., Straif, K. et al. (2009). A review of human carcinogens – Part D: Radiation. *Lancet Oncol.* 10 (8): 751–752.

4 Fitzpatrick, T.B. (1975). Soleil et peau. *J. Med. Esthet.* 2: 33–34.

5 Olsen, C.M., Carroll, H.J., and Whiteman, D.C. (2010). Estimating the attributable fraction for cancer: A meta-analysis of nevi and melanoma. *Cancer Prev. Res.* 3 (2): 233–245.

6 Armstrong, B.K. (2004). How sun exposure causes skin cancer: An epidemiological perspective. In: *Prevention of Skin Cancer* (ed. D.J. Hill, J.M. Elwood, and D.R. English), 89–116. Dordrecht: Kluwer.

7 Elwood, J.M., Gallagher, R.P., Hill, G.B., and Pearson, J.C.G. (1985). Cutaneous melanoma in relation to intermittent and constant sun exposure: The Western Canada Melanoma Study. *Int. J. Cancer* 35: 427–443.

 8 Ferlay, J., Soerjomataram, I., Ervik, M. et al. (2012). *GLOBOCAN 2012 v1.0, Cancer incidence and mortality worldwide: IARC CancerBase No. 11*. Lyon: IARX. http://globocan.iarc.fr/Default. aspx (accessed 3 January 2018).

 9 Bentham, G., and Aase, A. (1996). Incidence of malignant melanoma of the skin in Norway, 1955–1989: Associations with solar ultraviolet radiation, income and holidays abroad. *Int. J. Epidemiol.* 25 (6): 1132–1138.

10 Jemal, A., Saraiya, M., Patel, P. et al. (2011). Recent trends in cutaneous melanoma incidence and death rates in the United States, 1992–2006. *J. Am. Acad. Dermatol.* 65 (5, Suppl. 1): S17–S25.

11 Erdmann, F., Lortet-Tieulent, J., Schuz, J. et al. (2013). International trends in the incidence of malignant melanoma 1953–2008: Are recent generations at higher or lower risk? *Int. J. Cancer* 132 (2): 385–400.

12 Olsen, C.M., Williams, P.F., and Whiteman, D.C. (2014). Turning the tide? Changes in treatment rates for keratinocyte cancers in Australia 2000 through 2011. *J. Am. Acad. Dermatol.* 71 (1): 21–26.

13 Czarnecki, D. (2014). The incidence of melanoma is increasing in the susceptible young Australian population. *Acta Derm. Venereol.* 94 (5): 539–541.

14 Leiter, U., Eigentler, T., and Garbe, C. (2014). Epidemiology of skin cancer. *Adv. Exp. Med. Biol.* 810: 120–140.

15 Usher-Smith, J.A., Emery, J., Kassianos, A.P., and Walter, F.M. (2014). Risk prediction models for melanoma: A systematic review. *Cancer Epidemiol. Biomarkers Prev.* 23 (8): 1450–1463.

16 Fransen, M., Karahalios, A., Sharma, N. et al. Non-melanoma skin cancer in Australia. *Med. J. Aust.* 197 (10): 565–568.

17 Gordon, L.G., and Rowell, D. (2015). Health system costs of skin cancer and cost-effectiveness of skin cancer prevention and screening: A systematic review. *Eur. J. Cancer Prev.* 24 (2): 141–149

18 U.S. Department of Health and Human Services (2014). *The Surgeon General's call to action to prevent skin cancer*. Washington, DC: Office of the Surgeon General.

19 Iannacone, M.R., and Green, A.C. (2014). Towards skin cancer prevention and early detection: Evolution of skin cancer awareness campaigns in Australia. *Melanoma Manag.* 1 (1): 75–84.

20 Glanz, K., Saraiya, M., and Briss, P. (2004). Impact of intervention strategies to reduce UVR exposure. In: *Prevention of Skin Cancer* (ed. D. Hill, J.M. Elwood, and D.R. English), 259–293. Dordrecht: Kluwer.

21 Volkov, A., Dobbinson, S., Wakefield, M., and Slevin, T. (2013). Seven-year trends in sun protection and sunburn among Australian adolescents and adults. *Aust. N. Z. J. Public Health* 37 (1): 63–69.

22 International Agency for Research on Cancer (2001). Sunscreens. *IARC Handbooks of Cancer Prevention*. Lyon: IARC.

23 Green, A.C., Williams, G.M., Logan, V., an Strutton, G.M. (2011). Reduced melanoma after regular sunscreen use: Randomized trial follow-up. *J. Clin. Oncol.* 29 (3): 257–263.

24 Lazovich, D., Vogel, R.I., Berwick, M. et al. (2011). Melanoma risk in relation to use of sunscreen or other sun protection methods. *Cancer Epidemiol. Biomarkers Prev.* 20 (12): 2583–2593.

25 Mancebo, S.E., Hu, J.Y., and Wang, S.Q. (2014). Sunscreens: A review of health benefits, regulations, and controversies. *Dermatol. Clin.* 32 (3): 427–438.

26 Sinclair, C.A., Makin, J.K., Tang, A. et al. (2014). The role of public health advocacy in achieving an outright ban on commercial tanning beds in Australia. *Am. J. Public Health* 104 (2): e7–e9.

27 Dore, J.F., and Chignol, M.C. (2012). Tanning salons and skin cancer. *Photochem. Photobiol. Sci.* 11 (1): 30–37.

28 Autier, P., Boniol, M., Pizot, C., and Mullie, P. (2014). Vitamin D status and ill health: A systematic review. *Lancet Diabetes Endocrinol.* 2 (1): 76–89.

29 Ross, C.A., Taylor, C.L., Aktine, A.L., and el Valle, H.B., ed.; Committee to review dietary reference intakes for vitamin D and calcium FaNBIoM (2011). *Dietary reference intakes for calcium and vitamin D*. Washington DC: National Academies Press.

30 Wolff, T., Tai, E., and Miller, T. (2009). Screening for skin cancer: An update of the evidence for the U.S. Preventive Services Task Force. *Ann. Intern. Med.* 150 (3): 194–198.

31 Aitken, J., and Elwood, M. (2004). Population screening for melanoma: Current evidence and a population-based randomised trial. In: *Textbook of Melanoma* (ed. J.F. Thompson, D.L. Morton, and B.B.R. Kroon), 100–114. London: Martin Dunitz.

32 Aitken, J.F., Elwood, J.M., Lowe, J.B. et al. (2002). A randomised trial of population screening for melanoma. *J. Med. Screen* 9 (1): 33–37.

33 Elwood, M., Aitken, J.F., and English, D.R. (2003). Prevention and screening. In: *Cutaneous Melanoma*, 4e (ed. C.M. Balch, A.N. Houghton, A.J. Sober, and S. Soong), 93–120. St Louis, MO: Quality Medical Publishing.

34 Aitken, J.F., Janda, M., Elwood, M. et al. (2006). Clinical outcomes from skin screening clinics within a community-based melanoma screening program. *J. Am. Acad. Dermatol.* 54 (1): 105–114.

35 Breitbart, E.W., Waldmann, A., Nolte, S. et al. (2012). Systematic skin cancer screening in Northern Germany. *J. Am. Acad. Dermatol.* 66 (2): 201–211.

36 Collins, M.K., Secrest, A.M., and Ferris, L.K. (2014). Screening for melanoma. *Melanoma Res.* 24 (5): 428–436.

37 Berwick, M., Begg, C.B., Fine, J.A. et al. (1996). Screening for cutaneous melanoma by skin self-examination. *J. Natl Cancer Inst.* 88 (1): 17–23.

38 Elwood, J.M. (1996). Skin self-examination and melanoma. *J. Natl Cancer Inst.* 88 (1): 3–5.

39 Aitken, J.F., Elwood, J.M., Baade, P.D. et al. (2010). Clinical whole-body skin examination reduces the incidence of thick melanomas. *Int. J. Cancer* 126 (2): 450–458.

40 Schneider, J.S., Moore, D.H., and Mendelsohn, M.L. (2007). Screening program reduced melanoma mortality at the Lawrence Livermore National Laboratory, 1984 to 1996. *J. Am. Acad. Dermatol.* 58 (5): 741–749.

41 Bordoni, A., Leoni-Parvex, S., Peverelli, S. et al. (2013). Opportunistic screening strategy for cutaneous melanoma does not change the incidence of nodular and thick lesions nor reduce mortality: A population-based descriptive study in the European region with the highest incidence. *Melanoma Res.* 23 (5): 402–407.

42 Katalinic, A., Waldmann, A., Weinstock, M.A. et al. (2012). Does skin cancer screening save lives? An observational study comparing trends in melanoma mortality in regions with and without screening. *Cancer* 118 (21): 5395–5402.

43 Geller, A.C., Greinert, R., Sinclair, C. et al. (2010). A nationwide population-based skin cancer screening in Germany: Proceedings of the first meeting of the International Task Force on Skin Cancer Screening and Prevention (September 24–25, 2009). *Cancer Epidemiol.* 34 (3): 355–358.

44 Stang, A., Garbe, C., Autier, P., and Jockel, K.H. (2016). The many unanswered questions related to the German skin cancer screening programme. *Eur. J. Cancer* 64: 83–88.

45 Boniol, M., Autier, P., and Gandini, S. (2015). Melanoma mortality following skin cancer screening in Germany. *BMJ Open* 5 (9): e008158.

46 Swetter, S.M., Pollitt, R.A., Johnson, T.M. et al. (2012). Behavioral determinants of successful early melanoma detection: Role of self and physician skin examination. *Cancer* 118 (15): 3725–3734.

47 Pollitt, R.A., Geller, A.C., Brooks, D.R. et al. (2009). Efficacy of skin self-examination practices for early melanoma detection. *Cancer Epidemiol. Biomarkers Prev.* 18 (11): 3018–3023.

48 Pollitt, R.A., Clarke, C.A., Shema, S.J., and Swetter, S.M. (2008). California Medicaid enrollment and melanoma stage at diagnosis: A population-based study. *Am. J. Prev. Med.* 35 (1): 7–13.

49 Black, W.C. (2000). Overdiagnosis: An underrecognized cause of confusion and harm in cancer screening. *J. Natl Cancer Inst.* 92 (16): 1280–1282.

50 Esserman, L.J., Thompson, I.M., Reid, B. et al. (2014). Addressing overdiagnosis and over-treatment in cancer: A prescription for change. *Lancet Oncol.* 15 (6): e234–e242.

51 Forsea, A.M., del Marmol, V., de Vries, E. et al. (2012). Melanoma incidence and mortality in Europe: New estimates, persistent disparities. *Br. J. Dermatol.* 167 (5): 1124–1130.

52 Geller, A.C., Clapp, R.W., Sober, A.J. et al. (2013). Melanoma epidemic: An analysis of six decades of data from the Connecticut Tumor Registry. *J. Clin. Oncol.* 31 (33): 4172–4178.

53 Burton, R.C., Coates, M.S., Hersey, P. et al. (1993). An analysis of a melanoma epidemic. *Int. J. Cancer* 55: 765–770.

54 Norgaard, C., Glud, M., and Gniadecki, R. (2011). Are all melanomas dangerous? *Acta Derm. Venereol.* 91 (5): 499–503.

55 Shuster, S. (2009). Malignant melanoma: How error amplification by screening creates spurious disease. *Br. J. Dermatol.* 161 (5): 977–979.

56 Vuong, K., McGeechan, K., Armstrong, B.K., and Cust, A.E. (2014). Risk prediction models for incident primary cutaneous melanoma: A systematic review. *JAMA Dermatol.* 150 (4): 434–444.

57 Fears, T.R., Guerry, D., Pfeiffer, R.M. et al. (2006). Identifying individuals at high risk of melanoma: A practical predictor of absolute risk. *J. Clin. Oncol.* 24 (22): 3590–3596.

58 Williams, L.H., Shors, A.R., Barlow, W.E. et al. Identifying persons at highest risk of melanoma using self-assessed risk factors. *J. Clin. Exp. Dermatol. Res.* 2 (6): 1000129.

59 Fortes, C., Mastroeni, S., Bakos, L. et al. (2010). Identifying individuals at high risk of mela-noma: A simple tool. *Eur. J. Cancer Prev.* 19 (5): 393–400.

60 MacKie, R.M. (1990). Clinical recognition of early invasive malignant melanoma: Looking for changes in size, shape, and colour is successful. *BMJ* 301: 1005–1006.

61 Walter, F.M., Prevost, A.T., Vasconcelos, J. et al. (2013). Using the 7-point checklist as a diagnostic aid for pigmented skin lesions in general practice: A diagnostic validation study. *Br. J. Gen. Pract.* 63 (610): e345–e353.

62 Friedman, R.J., Rigel, D.S., and Kopf, A.W. (1985). Early detection of malignant melanoma: The role of physician examination and self-examination of the skin. *CA Cancer J. Clin.* 35: 130–151.

63 Liu, W., Hill, D., Gibbs, A.F. et al.(2005). What features do patients notice that help to dis-tinguish between benign pigmented lesions and melanomas? The ABCD(E) rule versus the seven-point checklist. *Melanoma Res.* 15 (6): 549–554.

64 Higgins, H.W., Lee, K.C., and Leffell, D.J. (2014). Point of care cutaneous imaging technol-ogy in melanoma screening and mole mapping. *F1000Prime Rep.* 6: 34.

65 Monheit, G., Cognetta, A.B., Ferris, L. et al. (2011). The performance of MelaFind: A prospective multicenter study. *Arch. Dermatol.* 147 (2): 188–194.

66 Hauschild, A., Chen, S.C., Weichenthal, M. et al. (2014). To excise or not: Impact of MelaFind on German dermatologists' decisions to biopsy atypical lesions. *J. Dtsch Dermatol. Ges.* 12 (7): 606–614.

67 Vestergaard, M.E., Macaskill, P., Holt, P.E., and Menzies, S.W. (2008). Dermoscopy com-pared with naked eye examination for the diagnosis of primary melanoma: A meta-analysis of studies performed in a clinical setting. *Br. J. Dermatol.* 159 (3): 669–676.

68 Argenziano, G., Puig, S., Zalaudek, I. et al. (2006). Dermoscopy improves accuracy of pri-mary care physicians to triage lesions suggestive of skin cancer. *J. Clin. Oncol.* 24 (12): 1877–1882.

69 Menzies, S.W., Emery, J., Staples, M. et al. (2009). Impact of dermoscopy and short-term sequential digital dermoscopy imaging for the management of pigmented lesions in primary care: A sequential intervention trial. *Br. J. Dermatol.* 161 (6): 1270–1277.

70 Walter, F.M., Morris, H.C., Humphrys, E. et al. (2012). Effect of adding a diagnostic aid to best practice to manage suspicious pigmented lesions in primary care: Randomised controlled trial. *BMJ* 345: e4110.

71 Wernli, K.J., Henrikson, N.B., Morrison, C.C. et al. (2016). Screening for skin cancer in adults: Updated evidence report and systematic review for the US Preventive Services Task Force. *JAMA* 316 (4): 436–447.

CHAPTER 20

Screening and prevention of oral cancer

Apurva Garg, Pankaj Chaturvedi, and Rajiv Sarin

Tata Memorial Hospital, Mumbai, India

SUMMARY BOX

- Oral cancer is the sixth most common cancer in the world, with high incidence in countries with a high rate of tobacco usage, especially smokeless tobacco.

- Tobacco, alcohol, areca nut, and human papilloma virus are the most important causative factors in the development of oral cancer.

- Identification of high-risk cases based on tobacco habits and premalignant oral lesions, their screening and effective management, is the most cost-effective means of primary and secondary prevention of oral cancer.

- Primary care physicians, health workers, and mouth self-examination play a very important part in screening of the oral cavity.

- A variety of screening methods are available, ranging from older methods of exfoliative cytology and Lugol's iodine to newer methods using nanoparticles, narrow-band imaging, and lab-on-a-chip.

- Numerous drugs, natural agents, and nutritional supplements have been studied for their role in chemoprevention, but there is insufficient evidence to recommend their use.

Oral cancers are almost always squamous carcinomas [1] and refer to cancers of the oral or anterior two-thirds tongue, gingivo-buccal complex (GBC), floor of mouth, hard palate, and lips. Oral cancer is the sixth most common cancer in the world, with more than 300 000 new cases and 145 000 deaths annually [2]. It is more common in developing countries where tobacco chewing is very prevalent, and is the most common cancer in males in South Asia and parts of South-East Asia. Its incidence is also increasing in Germany, Denmark, Scotland, and central and eastern France. In the Indian subcontinent and some other counties where tobacco chewing is very common, the predominant site of cancer in the oral cavity is the gingivo-buccal complex (GBC). In Europe, the USA, and other regions

Cancer Prevention and Screening: Concepts, Principles and Controversies, First Edition.
Edited by Rosalind A. Eeles, Christine D. Berg, and Jeffrey S. Tobias.
© 2019 John Wiley & Sons, Inc. Published 2019 by John Wiley & Sons, Inc.

where tobacco abuse is primarily in the form of cigarette smoking with or without alcohol, the tongue is the most common site of oral cancer.

The estimated five-year survival of oral cancer patients is about 81% for localized, 42% for regional, and 17% for distant metastatic disease [3]. The mortality rate is higher in developing countries due to late-stage presentation and limited access to multidisciplinary treatment [1]. Oral squamous cell carcinomas (OSCCs) are generally preceded by premalignant lesions. These premalignant lesions may be very distinct, like the white patch of leukoplakia, the red patch of erythroplakia, and oral submucous fibrosis (OSMF). The long latent period of malignant transformation, the reversible nature of some premalignant lesions, and the high cure rates of early-stage oral cancer are the basis for primary and secondary prevention [4].

Screening

Screening is the process of evaluating an asymptomatic person to determine if he or she is 'likely' or 'unlikely' to have a potentially malignant or malignant lesion [5]. The oral cavity being easily visible and accessible, it is amenable to screening by self-examination, or examination by doctors or health workers [6]. Oral cancers are ideally suited for screening. A cluster randomized trial done in Kerala, India involving 191 873 individuals showed 34% reduction in oral cancer mortality in high-risk individuals with tobacco use and/or alcohol consumption after three rounds of screening and nine years of follow-up [6]. After four rounds of screening and fifteen years of follow-up there was a 38% reduction in incidence and an 81% decrease in oral cancer mortality, which was statistically significant [7]. Targeted screening of individuals using tobacco with or without alcohol is the most cost-effective way. A Cochrane review in 2013 recommends oral cancer screening of high-risk individuals, which will lead to improvement of survival and stage shift across the whole population [8]. The American Dental Association recommends that visual and tactile screening in high-risk individuals may result in detection of cancer in the early stages. There is insufficient evidence to show the benefit of screening asymptomatic individuals without habits [5]. Recommendations regarding screening for oral cancer by various agencies are summarized in Table 20.1.

Role of primary care clinicians and health workers in screening

Primary care clinicians play a very important role in screening high-risk cases who are either tobacco users or have oral premalignant lesions. The sensitivity of clinical oral examination varies from 50% to 99% and specificity from 90% to 98% [9]. Visual examination is the gold standard for detecting early epithelial changes.

Table 20.1 Guidelines for oral cancer screening.

Agency	Recommendations
American Cancer Society [9]	Oral examination should be part of routine health check-ups after the age of 20. High-risk individuals should be screened annually.
American Dental Association [5]	Screening is recommended in high-risk individuals. No benefit of screening in asymptomatic individuals.
U.S. Preventive Services Task Force [10]	Evidence is insufficient to support screening in asymptomatic individuals.
UK National Health Service [11]	Screening programmes among high-risk individuals is the most cost-effective option for screening Screening not recommended in asymptomatic individuals.
Canadian Task Force [12]	Insufficient evidence for or against screening for oral cancer. Annual examination for high-risk individuals.

After an accurate history regarding high-risk behaviour such as use of tobacco and alcohol, a systematic visual and tactile oral cavity examination should be performed. A systematic oral examination can be performed within two minutes with a very basic set-up and can be done equally well in the field or community setting. It is important to evaluate and document orodental health and any premalignant lesion such as submucous fibrosis, leukoplakia, erythroplakia, and so on, and to biopsy if indicated. Health workers should take relevant history and perform oral examination for any restriction in mouth opening or any mucosal changes in the form of ulceration, bleeding, or changes in colour, texture, or mobility [13]. Cases with any suspicious findings should be referred to the clinician for re-evaluation and biopsy if warranted.

Leukoplakic lesions have a higher probability of malignant transformation if they are present in females, occur in the absence of addiction, are larger (>200 mm^2), or in specific sites such as the ventral surface of the tongue, soft palate, and retro-molar trigone [4].

Role of mouth self-examination.

Mouth self-examination (MSE) is a simple but systematic self-examination method performed using a mirror under good illumination. The quality and utility of MSE will depend on the information and training provided by the clinicians or health workers and the use of teaching aids. During MSE, a person should look for any suspicious lesions like white or red patches, ulcers, bleeding, restricted mouth opening, or burning, and report to physicians or screening clinics if any suspicious features are noted. A demonstration project for MSE was conducted in

Kerala, India involving 22 000 individuals. Compliance with MSE was observed in 36% participants. Of the 247 individuals who reported to clinics, 34% had oral precancerous lesions and 3% were diagnosed with cancer [14]. Another study from Kerala evaluated the role of MSE in 57 704 high-risk individuals [15]. Concordance between the findings of MSE and health workers was 77%, and between health workers and clinicians it was 100%. The sensitivity and specificity of MSE were 18% and 99.9%, respectively. MSE detected 42.9% of nonhealing ulcers, 66.7% of red patches, but only 12.7% of white patches. It created over 80% awareness about oral cancer and its risk factors, but the 32% compliance rate was poor and similar to a previous study [14]. A recent Cochrane review [9] shows that the sensitivity of MSE is low (18–33%), but its specificity is high in some studies (54–100%). Considering the lack of better methods which can be applied widely, MSE is recommended for individuals with high-risk behaviour.

Tests for screening (see Table 20.2)

Exfoliative cytology

Exfoliative cytology is the study and interpretation of epithelial cells from the oral mucosa that flake off naturally or artificially with the help of a brush or spatula. It helps in guiding the sites for scalpel biopsy and in monitoring the different regions within a larger lesion [16]. A multicentre study has shown that in 5% of the clinically benign lesions, malignancy was found after biopsy was taken from areas with abnormal exfoliative cytology [17, 18]. The OralCDx® brush biopsy is an oral transepithelial 'biopsy' system using computer-assisted brushing, and helps in identifying dysplasia in areas which are clinically not suspicious [16, 17]. Although

Table 20.2 Sensitivity and specificity of various screening tests for oral cancer.

Test	Sensitivity (%)	Specificity (%)
Exfoliative cytology	52–100	29–100
Toulidine blue	78–100	31–100
Lugol's iodine	87.5	84.2
Chemiluminescence	77	70
Microendoscopy	98	92
Elastic scattering spectroscopy	72	75
Optical coherence tomography	80–98	80–98
Narrow-band imaging	87–96	94–98
Salivary biomarkers	71	75

it has high false-positive rates and overestimates dysplastic lesions, the specimen obtained can be used for further evaluation, including tumour markers and molecular and DNA analysis [16].

Toluidine blue

This is a vital dye which is used to stain abnormal cells and nucleic acids. Surgeons have used it to demarcate epithelial lesions before excision. There is some evidence that toluidine blue (TB) can stain premalignant lesions. Various studies have reported the sensitivity of this technique as from 78% to 100% and specificity from 31% to 100% [16]. Its main disadvantage is that while it stains all areas with malignancy, only 40–70% of dysplastic areas are stained. Gray et al. [19] have shown that toluidine blue is not suitable as a primary method for screening due to the high false-positive rate and low rate in detecting dysplasia [20]. Toluidine blue staining of lesions has been correlated with loss of hetrozygosity (LOH) at 3p, 17p for carcinoma, and with LOH at 9p for dysplasia [21, 22].

Lugol's iodine

Iodine in solution reacts with the cytoplasmic glycogen to produce a colour change. The degree of colour change is directly proportional to the glycogen content of the cell, which is inversely proportional to the keratinization. On staining with Lugol's iodine, the normal cells take a brown or mahogany colour and the dysplastic mucosa does not stain and appears pale. Petruzzi et al. [23] have reviewed the use of Lugol's iodine in oral cancer diagnosis. Almost all studies with Lugol's iodine in oral potentially malignant lesions (OPMLs) or cancers have been done in tertiary centres. It is useful in mapping the suspicious areas for biopsy and to determine the extent of the margin of resection. The sensitivity of this technique is 87.5% and its specificity is 84.2%. There are little data on the utility of this method in a healthy population or in the community setting. Lugol's iodine staining cannot detect subepithelial spread or invasion, and its use is limited to nonkeratinized lesions.

Light-based detection systems

Tissue reflectance was previously used as a method to differentiate between malignant and benign lesions of the cervix. This technique is now also available for similar use in oral lesions [20]. It is based on the principle that the metabolic changes that occur during carcinogenesis cause distinct changes in absorption and refraction on exposure to different types of light [16].

Chemiluminescence

Vizilite® is a well-known system where the subject rinses the mouth with acetic acid and the oral cavity is illuminated with a chemiluminent light stick [17]. It has sensitivity of 100%, but specificity of only 0–14.2%, with a low positive predictive value. To improve its specificity, a combination of this technique with toluidine blue (Vizilite® plus) has been proposed. However, robust scientific evidence to support its use is lacking [16, 24]. Microlux/DL® is another method using an autoclavable, battery-powered light-emitting diode with a light guide, which produces a diffuse light. The sensitivity and specificity of this technique are 77% and 70%, respectively [16].

Tissue fluorescence imaging

The VELscope® system (Visually Enhanced Lesion Scope), by applying direct fluorescence (400–430 nm), detects the loss of fluorescence in malignant and premalignant lesions [16]. The normal mucosa appears pale green, but the abnormal mucosa appears dark in colour [20]. The sensitivity of this system is 97–100% and specificity is 94–100%. It is helpful in deciding the margins of resection, but its efficacy has not been proven when used in a low-risk population [16]. The IDENTAFI 3000 system is a combination of confocal microscopy, fibreoptics, and fluorescence. It is more accessible than VELscope as it is smaller. It has sensitivity and specificity of 82% and 87%, respectively, in differentiating malignant and nonmalignant lesions [21, 25].

Tissue fluorescence spectroscopy

This consists of an optical fibre that produces excitations of different wavelengths. The data are received by a spectroscope, recorded on a computer, and analysed by special software, thereby reducing subjective interpretation of the results. It is useful in differentiating malignant and nonmalignant lesions, but cannot differentiate between types of lesions, as the optical fibre can sample only a small area at a time [16, 26].

Microendoscopy

This technique is useful for in vivo histopathological assessment. It has a camera attached to a microendoscope with 150X magnification. On comparison with frozen and paraffin section, it has sensitivity and specificity of 98% and 92%, respectively [27, 28].

Elastic scattering spectroscopy

This system generates a wavelength which shows properties within the tissues, like proteins, lipids, nucleus, and other organelles. It has sensitivity of 72% and specificity of 75% in differentiating malignant and nonmalignant lesions. It can also be used to assess the depth of invasion in the mandible and to differentiate types of skin lesions [27].

Optical coherence tomography

Optical coherence tomography uses infrared and records reflectance from the tissue to reconstruct the micro-anatomical architecture. Studies have shown that it co-relates with the histopathological findings, with sensitivity and specificity ranging between 80% and 98%. It can be used to identify skin lesions and to estimate the margin of resection in basal cell carcinoma (BCC) [27].

Narrow-band imaging

This technique uses a narrow-band spectrum filter to identify superficial capillaries and neoangiogenesis in abnormal tissues by enhanced contrast. Abnormal vessels appear as brown dots and dilatations. It is helpful in identifying premalignant and malignant lesions. Various studies report its sensitivity, specificity, positive predictive value, negative predictive value, and accuracy in the range of 87–96%, 94–98%, 73–96%, 97–98%, and 92–97%, respectively [27, 29]. This technique can help in assessment of the primary or recurrent tumour and margins [29]. Narrow-band imaging is not widely used, however, due to the learning curve and lack of robust evidence of its clinical utility [27, 29].

Biopsy

While biopsy is the gold standard, it is an invasive procedure with associated discomfort and also some interpretative issues. For extensive lesions the biopsy should be taken from the most representative area. Incisional biopsy should be of sufficient depth and size, and include the area of the advancing margin of the tumour. Some studies have shown the advantage of punch biopsy over scalpel biopsy in terms of fewer artefacts [30]. Several others have described high inter- and intra-observer variability in diagnosing dysplasia, with concordance of only 56%, and limited reproducibility could lead to more aggressive treatment [17, 30, 31].

Biomarkers, microscopy, and other methods

Various biomarkers, microscopy, and other techniques have been developed and evaluated for diagnosing or characterizing oral premalignant lesions and cancers. A general description is provided here, but the findings of specific studies are beyond the scope of this chapter.

Salivary biomarkers

Several studies have evaluated the role of salivary biomarkers for screening and diagnosis of OPML and oral cancer. Most commonly studied salivary markers are Cyfra 21-1, CA 19-9, CA 125, carcinoembryonic antigen (CEA), and tissue polypeptide-specific antigen (TPS). The presence of Cystain SA-I deletion in saliva is a marker of oral tumours. The sensitivity, specificity, negative, and positive predictive value of significant increase (400%) in salivary concentrations of Cyfra 21-1, TPS, and CA 125 are 71%, 75%, 71%, and 75%, respectively [17]. Levels of IL-8 and Il-1β are also elevated in oral cancer patients [32].

Serum biomarkers

Increased levels of plasma micro RNA mir-31 and circulatory vascular endothelial growth factor (VEGF) in serum are markers of OSCC. Autoantibody against p53 is detected in 25% of patients with head and neck squamous cell carcinoma (HNSCC). OSCC is associated with increased levels of C16 and C24 and a decrease in C18-ceramide [32].

DNA analysis

DNA image cytometry determines the malignant potential of cells by measuring ploidy status. Combined cytogenetic and morphological analysis of oral brush samples is helpful in detecting premalignant cells [17]. Samples are assessed for loss of heterozygosity at 3p14 and 9p21, p53 protein expression, chromosomal polysomy, and so on [4]. In a study with 25 patients, allelic imbalance was present in 40% of patients with leukoplakia as compared to controls, giving it sensitivity and positive predictive value of 78% and 100%, respectively [17, 33].

Spectral cytopathology

In this technique, the biochemical composition of exfoliated cells is evaluated by infrared micro-spectral measurement, which is followed by multivariate analysis. The spectral patterns produced are specific to the disease [17].

Multispectral digital microscope

This takes images in narrow-band reflectance, fluorescence, and orthogonal polarized reflectance modes. It helps in differentiation between malignant and nonmalignant lesions [17].

Spectroscopy

Raman spectroscopy, named after its discoverer, Sir C.V. Raman, is a biophysical technique based on inelastic scattering of light emitted from a diode laser. It is able to identify between normal mucosa, premalignant lesions, and malignant lesions [34].

Lab-on-a-chip

This represents the miniaturization of lab analytical procedures on a single chip. It involves microfluidics, which is the chemistry equivalent of silicon chips. The lab-on-a-chip analyses cell membrane proteins that are uniquely expressed on malignant or dysplastic cells [20].

Nano-particles

This is an emerging technology where gold nano-particles are conjugated to anti- epidermal growth factor receptor (EGFR) antibodies. These contrast agents have the potential to extend the ability of vital reflectance microscopies for in vivo molecular imaging. They can potentially enable combined screening and detection [35].

Prevention of oral cancer

Tobacco, alcohol, and betel quid are the most significant risk factors for oral cancer. Countries in the Indian subcontinent, Taiwan, and some South-East Asian and African countries have a high incidence of oral cancer due to the widespread use of smokeless tobacco. In these regions, the most common site of oral cancer is gingivo-buccal, followed by the oral tongue. Prevention is the most cost-effective strategy for long-term control of cancer. A national cancer programme can help policymakers make the best use of available resources for the benefit of the population [1]. Awareness, screening programmes, and enabling legislation for tobacco control and early detection of OPML and oral cancer form the best way of preventing oral cancer morbidity and mortality. The precancerous changes are reversed after cessation over a period of time. Important known carcinogens for oral cancer and their associated risks are described here.

Smokeless tobacco, betel quid, and areca nut

Smokeless tobacco and preparation of areca nut are available in various combinations and forms around the world. Areca nut and betel quid are especially prevalent in the Indian subcontinent, parts of South-East Asia, Taiwan, and North and East Africa. In the Indian subcontinent, traditionally the areca nut was eaten in betel leaves prepared with slaked lime and acacia Catechu, with or without tobacco. Lime lowers the pH, thereby increasing the absorption of nicotine. In the last few decades, processed betel quid with areca nut has become widely available as ready-to-eat pouches. These may contain tobacco (Gutka) or may not contain tobacco (Pan Masala). Other forms of betel quid with tobacco are zarda and mawa. According to the Global Adult Tobacco Survey (GATS) 2009, 25.9% of adults in India use smokeless tobacco [36]. Smokeless tobacco has 28 known carcinogens, which include tobacco-specific nitrosamines (most harmful), N-nitrosamino acids, benzopyrenes, volatile N-nitrosamines, nickel, cadmium, and arsenic [37].

A recent meta-analysis and systematic review of 21 case-control studies and 4 cohort studies confirms that smokeless tobacco and betel quid without tobacco are independent risk factors for oral cancers [38]. For smokeless tobacco, in the 14 case-control studies (4553 cases, 8632 controls) under the random effects model, the adjusted main effect summary computed was an odds ratio (OR) of 7.46 (95% confidence interval [CI] 5.86–9.50, p=0.001). The adjusted main effect summary for 4 cohort studies (163 430) was a relative risk (RR) of 5.48 (95% CI 2.56–11.71, p=0.001). For betel quid without tobacco, in the 15 case-control studies (4648 cases; 7847 controls) under the random effects model, the adjusted main effect summary computed was OR 2.82 (95% CI 2.35–3.40, p=0.001). The risk conferred by betel quid without tobacco is presumably due to the areca nut.

Tobacco smoking

Cigarettes are the most common form of smoked tobacco around the world. A meta-analysis reported a pooled RR of 3.43 (95% CI 2.37–4.94) for oral cancer in 12 studies comparing current smokers with never smokers, and a RR of 1.4 (95% CI.99–2.0) in 9 studies comparing former smokers with never smokers [39]. Most studies included in this meta-analysis are from Europe or North America where the predominant form of tobacco use is cigarette smoking. In the Indian subcontinent use of bidi is very common. Bidis are made of sun-dried flaked tobacco rolled in dried tendu or temburni leaf [40]. The cancer risk associated with bidi was examined in a large cohort of 66 277 men in the age range of 30–80 years in Kerala [40]. This study reported that tobacco chewing was associated with increased oral cancer risk (p<0.001), and that the risk increased with greater frequencies (p<0.001) and duration (p<0.001) of use. While an increased risk of oral cancer with alcohol was not found in this study, bidi smoking in men without tobacco chewing was associated with an increased oral cancer risk, with RR 2.6 (95% CI 1.4–4.9). This risk increased with duration and frequency of bidi smoking (p<0.001) and younger age at start of bidi smoking (p=0.007). After smoking cessation, the level of risk for cancer approaches that of a nonsmoker in about 10 years [41].

Alcohol

Alcohol is an important risk factor for oral cancer, as it may potentiate the carcinogenic effects of tobacco with a multiplicative rather than additive effect [42]. A meta-analysis [43] reported a slight increased risk for oral cancer in light drinkers (RR 1.17, 95% CI 1.01–1.35) and a higher risk in heavy drinkers (four or more drinks; RR 4.64, 95% CI 3.78–5.70). Alcohol cessation leads to a 40% decrease in the risk of oral cancer after 20 years or more of cessation as compared to drinkers [41].

Human papilloma virus

The human papilloma virus (HPV) is an important risk factor for oropharyngeal cancers. Association of HPV has been seen in other head and neck cancer sites, and one study reported HPV in 25% of oral cancers, with the majority being HPV-16 followed by HPV-18 [44].

Diet and nutritional factors

In developing countries 20% of cancers are related to dietary factors. A diet rich in fresh fruits and vegetables is protective against oral cancerous and precancerous lesions [1]. Foods protecting against oral cancer include fish, pulses, and buttermilk. Foods protecting against oral precancer are fibres, tomatoes, and those containing vitamin C, iron, copper, zinc, and other micronutrients [41]. Consuming very hot liquids increases the risk of oral cancer [1].

Genetic predisposition

While environmental factors play a major role in the development of oral cancer, a weak inherited susceptibility for oral cancer may be conferred due to specific gene–environment interactions. A family history of HNSCC has an RR of 3.5–3.8 for first-degree relatives. Null genotype or mutation in genes coding for detoxifying enzymes, glutathione S-transferase (GST), and UDP-glucuronyl transferase 1A7 (UGT1A7) are associated with an increased risk of oral cancer. Germline p16 and p53 mutations also predispose to an increased risk for oral cancer. Various cancer syndromes, like Bloom's syndrome, Fanconi's anaemia, and ataxia telengectasia, have a defective DNA repair mechanism and are associated with an increased risk of oral cancer [44]. A study through whole exome sequencing has identified several recurrent and novel somatic genetic alterations in gingivo-buccal cancer, which is the most common type of oral cancer in the Indian subcontinent [45].

Chemoprevention of oral cancer

Chemoprevention is the use of drugs or natural products that can reverse or arrest malignant transformation. Foy et al. [4] have reviewed the role of chemoprevention in oral premalignant lesions. Use of retinoids in a secondary setting produces a clinical and histological response in 64% and 57% cases of OPML, respectively, but may cause hypertriglyceridemia, mucocutaneous effects, and relapse after stoppage. Use of retinoids with N-acetylcysteine or COX-2 inhibitors has not shown any benefit so far. Thiazolidinediones have shown promising results in a Phase IIa study, with a 68% histological response in leukoplakia, and further Phase IIb studies are under way. Numerous dietary agents like green tea polyphenols, curcumin, herbs, fruits, and vegetables have been reported to show promising chemopreventive effects. Curcumin from turmeric has been shown to downregulate nicotine-induced COX-2 and nuclear factor-KappaB (NF-kB) in vitro. Spirulina, black raspberries, vitamin supplements, resveratrol, and lycopene have all been evaluated for their protective role against OPML and OSCC. Attempts at restoring p53 function using a genetically engineered virus have been made using ONYX-015, but the response is short-lived and unpredictable [4]. Erlotinib, an EGFR inhibitor, is being evaluated in a Phase III trial as an oral chemopreventive agent for OPML with LOH. However, for none of these agents is there high-quality scientific evidence of clinical benefit to recommend their use outside clinical trials.

Conclusion

Oral cancer is ideally suited for prevention and early detection, but it continues to be a major health problem in many parts of the world. Screening of high-risk individuals using simple methods is a proven and cost-effective way of reducing morbidity and mortality from oral cancer. Mouth self-examination and physicians have very important roles to play in screening and effective management of this disease. There are various tests available for screening, but a test with high sensitivity, specificity, and cost-effectiveness is still not available. Almost all cases of oral cancer can be prevented by abstaining from tobacco and alcohol. Several natural agents and anti-oxidants have shown promise as chemopreventive agents, and their role in oral cancer prevention needs to be established through large randomized trials with suitable surrogate biomarker end-points. Health campaigns are required to create public health awareness about mouth self-examination, the risks of various forms of tobacco use, the effective management of precancerous lesions, and tobacco cessation programmes for high-risk cases. Governments need to devise strong strategies and legislation for reducing the production, marketing, and use of tobacco products.

References

1 Peterson, P.E. (2009). Oral cancer prevention and control: The approach of the World Health Organization. *Oral Oncol.* 45: 454–460.

2 GLOBOCON 2012 (2013). Estimated cancer incidence, mortality and prevalence worldwide in 2012. http://globocan.iarc.fr/Default.aspx (accessed 20 October 2014).

3 Gloeckler Ries, L.A., Kosary, C.L., Hankey, B.F. et al. (1997). SEER cancer statistics review, 1973–1994. Bethesda, MD: National Cancer Institute.

4 Foy, J.P., Bertolus, C., William, W.N., Jr et al. (2013). Oral premalignancy: The roles of early detection and chemoprevention. *Otolaryngol. Clin. N. Am.* 46: 579–597.

5 Rethman, M.P., Carpenter, W., Cohen, E.E.W. et al. (2010). Evidence-based clinical recommendations regarding screening for oral squamous cell carcinomas. *J. Am. Dental Assoc.* 141 (5): 509–520.

6 Sankarnarayanan, R., Ramdas, K., Thomas, G. et al. (2005). Effect of screening on oral cancer mortality in Kerala, India: A cluster-randomised controlled trial. *Lancet* 365: 1927–1933.

7 Sankarnarayanan, R.. Ramdas, K., Thara, S. et al. (2013). Long term effect of visual screening on oral cancer incidence and mortality in a randomized trial in Kerala, *India. Oral Oncol.* 49: 314–321.

8 Brocklehurst, P., Kujan, O., Glenny, A.M. et al. (2013). Screening programmes for the early detection and prevention of oral cancer. *Cochrane Database Syst. Rev.* 11 (Art. No.: CD004150. doi: 10.1002/14651858.CD004150.pub4.

9 Walsh, T., Liu, J.L.Y., Brocklehurst, P. et al. (2013). Clinical assessment to screen for the detection of oral cavity cancer and potentially malignant disorders in apparently healthy adults. *Cochrane Database Syst. Rev.* 11 (Art. No.: CD010173). doi: 10.1002/14651858. CD010173.pub2.

10 U.S. Preventive Services Task Force (2013). Oral cancer: Screening. https://www. uspreventiveservicestaskforce.org/Page/Document/UpdateSummaryFinal/oral-cancer-screening1 (accessed 3 January 2018).

11 Speight, P.M., and Warnakulasuriya, R. (2010). Evaluation of screening for oral cancer against NSC Criteria. Report produced for the National Screening Committee, May 2010. http://www.screening.nhs.uk/oralcancer (accessed 31 October 2014).

12 Epstein, B., Gorsky, M., Cabay, R.J. et al. (2008). Screening for and diagnosis of oral premalignant lesions and oropharyngeal squamous cell carcinoma: Role of primary care physicians. *Can. Fam. Physician* 54: 870–875.

13 Messadi, D.V., Wilder-Smith, P., and Wolinsky, L. (2009). Improving oral cancer survival: The role of dental providers. *J. Calif. Dent. Assoc.* 37 (11): 789–798.

14 Mathew, B., Sankarnarayan, R., Wesley, R. et al. (1995). Evaluation of mouth self-examination in control of oral cancer. *Br. J. Cancer* 71: 397–399.

15 Elango, K.J., Anandkrishnan, N., Suresh, A. et al. (2011). Mouth self-examination to improve oral cancer awareness and early detection in a high-risk population. *Oral Oncol.* 47 (7): 620–624.

16 Lestón, J.S., and Dios, P.D. (2010). Diagnostic clinical aids in oral cancer. *Oral Oncol.* 46: 418–422.

17 Mehrotra, R., and Gupta, D.K. (2011). Exciting new advances in oral cancer diagnosis: Avenues to early detection. *Head Neck Oncol.* 3: 33.

18 Sciubba, J.J. (1999). Improving detection of precancerous and cancerous oral lesions: Computer-assisted analysis of the oral brush biopsy. *J. Am. Dent. Assoc.* 130: 1445–1457.

19 Gray, M.G.L., Burls, A., and Elley, K. (2000). The clinical effectiveness of toluidine blue dye as an adjunct to oral cancer screening in general dental practice. A West Midlands Development and Evaluation Service Report. Birmingham: University of Birmingham.

20 Lingen, M.W., Kalmar, J.R., Karrison, T. et al. (2008). Critical evaluation of diagnostic aids for the detection of oral cancer. *Oral Oncol.* 44: 10–22.

21 Messadi, D.V. (2013). Diagnostic aids for detection of oral precancerous conditions. *Int. J. Oral Sci.* 5: 59–65.

22 Awan, K.H., Yang, Y.H., Morgan, P.R. et al. (2012). Utility of toluidine blue as a diagnostic adjunct in the detection of potentially malignant disorders of the oral cavity: A clinical and histological assessment. *Oral Dis.* 18 (8): 728–733.

23 Petruzzi, M., Lucchese, A., Baldoni, E. et al. (2010). Use of Lugol's iodine in oral cancer diagnosis: An overview. *Oral Oncol.* 46: 811–813.

24 Epstein, J.B., Silverman, S., Epstein, J.D. et al. (2008). Analysis of oral lesion biopsies identified and evaluated by visual examination, chemiluminescence and toluidine blue. *Oral Oncol.* 44: 538–544.

25 Schwarz, R.A., Gao, W., Redden Weber, C. et al. (2009). Noninvasive evaluation of oral lesions using depth-sensitive optical spectroscopy: Simple device for the direct visualization of oral-cavity tissue fluorescence. *Cancer* 115 (8): 1669–1679.

26 De Veld, D.C., Witjes, M.J., Sterenborg, H.J., and Roodenburg, J.L. (2005). The status of in vivo autofluorescence spectroscopy and imaging for oral oncology. *Oral Oncol.* 41: 117–131.

27 Green, B., Cobb, A.R.M., Brennan, P.A. et al. (2014). Optical diagnostic techniques for use in lesions of the head and neck: Review of the latest developments. *Br. J. Oral Maxillofac. Surg.* 52: 675–680.

28 Upile, T., Jerjes, W., Mahil, J. et al. (2012). Microendoscopy: A clinical reality in intra-operative margin analysis of head and neck lesions. *Head Neck Oncol.* 4: 43.

29 Vu, A.N., and Farah, C.S. (2014). Efficacy of narrow band imaging for detection and surveillance of potentially malignant and malignant lesions in the oral cavity and oropharynx: A systematic review. *Oral Oncol.* 50: 413–420.

30 Meghana, S.M., and Ahmedmujib, B.R. (2007). Surgical artefacts in oral biopsy specimens: Punch biopsy compared to conventional scalpel biopsy. *J. Oral Maxillofac. Pathol.* 11 (1): 11–14.

31 Holmstrup, P., Vedtofte, P., Reibel, J., and Stoltze, K. (2007). Oral premalignant lesions: Is biopsy reliable? *J. Oral Path. Med.* 36: 262–266.

32 Mishra, R. (2012). Biomarkers of oral premalignant epithelial lesions for clinical application. *Oral Oncol.* 48: 578–584.

33 Bremmer, J.F., Graveland, A.P., Brink, A. et al. (2009). Screening for oral precancer with noninvasive genetic cytology. *Cancer Prev. Res.* 2 (2): 128–133.

34 Sahu, A., Deshmukh, A., Ghanate, A.D. et al. (2012). Raman spectroscopy of oral buccal mucosa: A study on age-related physiological changes and tobacco-related pathological changes. *Tech. Cancer Res. Treat.* 11: 529–541.

35 Sokolov, K., Follen, M., Aaron, J. et al. (2003). Real-time vital optical imaging of precancer using anti-epidermal growth factor receptor antibodies conjugated to gold nanoparticles. *Cancer Res.* 63: 1999–2004.

36 Ministry of Health and Family Welfare, Government of India (n.d.) Global Adult Tobacco Survey (GATS). Fact Sheet India: 2009–2010. http://www.who.int/tobacco/surveillance/en_tfi_india_gats_fact_sheet.pdf (accessed 31 October 2014).

37 Brunnemann, K.D., and Hoffmann, D. (1991). Analytical studies on tobacco specific N-nitrosamines in tobacco and tobacco smoke. *Crit. Rev. Toxicol.* 21: 235–240.

38 Gupta, B., and Johnson, N.W. (2014). Systematic review and meta-analysis of association of smokeless tobacco and of betel quid without tobacco with incidence of oral cancer in South Asia and the Pacific. *PLoS One* 9 (11): e113385.

39 Gandini, S., Botteri, E., Iodice, S. et al. (2008). Tobacco smoking and cancer: A meta-analysis. *Int. J. Cancer* 122 (1): 155–164.

40 Jayalekshmi, P.A., Gangadharan, P., Akiba, S. et al. (2011). Oral cavity cancer risk in relation to tobacco chewing and bidi smoking among men in Karunagappally, Kerala, India: Karunagappally cohort study. *Cancer Sci.* 102 (2): 460–467.

41 Marron, M., Boffetta, P., Zhang, Z.F. et al. (2010). Cessation of alcohol drinking, tobacco smoking and the reversal of head and neck cancer risk. *Int. J. Epidemiol.* 39: 182–196.

42 Gupta, P.C., and Ray, C.S. (2009). Epidemiology in head and neck cancers. In: Head and Neck Surgery (ed. C. de Souza, Z. Gil, and D.M. Fliss), 617–647. New Delhi: Jaypee Brothers.

43 Turati, F., Garavello, W., Tramacere, I. et al. (2010). A meta-analysis of alcohol drinking and oral and pharyngeal cancers. Part 2: Results by subsites. *Oral Oncol.* 46 (10): 720–726.

44 Jefferies, S., and Foulkes, W.D. (2001). Genetic mechanisms in squamous cell carcinoma of the head and neck. *Oral Oncol.* 37: 115–126.

45 India Project Team of ICGC (2013). Mutational landscape of gingivobuccal oral squamous cell carcinoma reveals new recurrently-mutated genes and molecular subgroups. *Nat. Comm.* 4: 2873.

CHAPTER 21

Oesophageal cancer

Timothy J. Underwood

Cancer Sciences Unit, Faculty of Medicine, University of Southampton, UK

SUMMARY BOX

- Screening for oesophageal cancer cannot currently be recommended.
- Risk factors for oesophageal cancer are dependent on histological subtype.
- Modifiable factors such as obesity, gastro-oesophageal reflux disease, and smoking are the major risk factors for adenocarcinoma.
- A number of potential genetic factors have been identified.
- The combination of epidemiological and genetic factors with novel, primary care–based oesophageal sampling devices may tailor screening strategies in the future.

The case for cancer prevention and screening in oesophageal cancer is based on the global burden and natural history of the disease, and acceptable strategies to intervene before patients present with locally advanced, incurable tumours.

Global perspective

Oesophageal cancer is important worldwide: 450 000 people were diagnosed with the disease in 2012 [1]. In the first quantification of the global burden of oesophageal cancer subtypes by the International Agency for Research on Cancer, the incidence of squamous cell cancer (SCC) and adenocarcinoma (EAC) was 5.2 per 100 000 and 0.7 per 100 000, respectively [1]. However, these overall data mask wide geographical variations, with 79% of SCC cases being found in South-East and Central Asia, and 46% of EAC cases in North-West Europe, North America, and Oceania. The UK is the world's capital of EAC, with an incidence of 7.2 per 100 000 and 2.5 per 100 000 for men and women, respectively [1]. By contrast, China alone contributes nearly half of the global total of SCC. Oesophageal cancer is more common in men, especially in the case of EAC (male-to-female ratio EAC

4.4; SCC 2.7) [1]. This is most evident in the USA, where of the 100 000 people diagnosed with EAC in 2012, 88% were male [1].

These clear differences in the incidence of the major subtypes of oesophageal cancer, East versus West, developed world versus developing world, and male versus female, mean that strategies aimed at cancer prevention, early diagnosis, and screening will need careful consideration of the population at risk in the local environment.

Fortunately, there are characteristics of both SCC and EAC that make cancer prevention and screening possible, at least in theory. As our understanding of the natural history of oesophageal cancer has developed, we have identified risk factors in genetics, the environment, and individual behaviour that predispose to disease. Both types of oesophageal cancer have recognized premalignant lesions that progress through defined stages towards invasive disease [2]. For clarity, this chapter will focus on EAC as a worked example of the opportunities and controversies in cancer prevention and screening, but the principles described could equally be applied to SCC.

Oesophageal adenocarcinoma

Before considering potentially expensive and harmful cancer prevention and/or screening programmes, the case must be made for the potential benefits at the population level, and perhaps most importantly for the individual at risk. Oesophageal cancer kills people. While over the last 40 years survival from all forms of cancer in the UK has doubled, mortality for EAC has risen by 50% [3]. This is attributable to an unprecedented increase in incidence, and because approximately two-thirds of patients will have incurable disease at the time of diagnosis [4]. Despite substantial incremental improvements in staging, neoadjuvant therapies, and surgery for EAC, five-year survival for all-comers remains below 15% [1, 3–5]. Investment in research in oesophageal cancer lags behind that of other common cancers.

Risk factors

Age
EAC is predominantly a disease of middle age. The median age at diagnosis is between 65 and 70 years in the majority of reported series. Alarmingly, the recent increase in incidence of EAC has coincided with a rise in the number of younger patients (<50) being diagnosed with advanced disease. In the most recent pooled analysis of eight population-based, case-control studies, which included nearly 3000 patients and 5700 controls, 10.5% of cases were observed in patients under 50 years of age, with one-third occurring in the under-60s [6]. This changing demographic has important implications for public health messaging and awareness campaigns.

Sex

EAC is more common in men, for reasons that are yet to be understood.

Gastro-oesophageal reflux disease

The association between gastro-oesophageal reflux disease (GORD), hiatus hernia, and EAC has long been established [7]. GORD is believed to lead to the development of Barrett's oesophagus (BE), the only recognized precursor for EAC. More recent evidence confirms that GORD is strongly associated with EAC at any age, but early-onset EAC (<50 years) has the strongest association with recurrent reflux relative to older age groups [6].

Obesity

High body mass index is associated with EAC at all ages. Central adiposity is believed to have adverse effects on the mechanics of the lower oesophageal sphincter, increasing the likelihood of reflux. Obesity is also independently associated with a higher risk of EAC via mechanisms that probably involve pro-inflammatory and immune modulation. Early-onset EAC is also more strongly associated with obesity than EAC diagnosed at older ages [6].

Lifestyle factors

Smoking, alcohol consumption, and poor diet have all been associated with a higher risk of EAC [8].

Genetic predisposition

Genome-wide association studies have revealed single-nucleotide polymorphisms (SNPs) associated with BE (6p21; within the HLA region, 16q24; close to FOXF1 [9], GDF7, and TBX5 [10]) and EAC (CRTC1, BARX1, and FOXP1 [11]). Interestingly, transcription factors involved in thoracic, diaphragmatic, and oesophageal development or proteins involved in the inflammatory response predominate. These SNPs might influence an individual's tendency towards GORD, but this hypothesis is yet to be tested.

Prevention and screening in EAC

Interventions to improve outcomes for EAC are required across every stage of the disease, but effective therapies for locally advanced and metastatic disease are unlikely to become available in the short term. Potential points of intervention to prevent disease progression can be understood from the natural history of EAC. The oesophagus is lined by a stratified squamous mucosa. The development of EAC requires the establishment of a glandular mucosa, most commonly in the distal oesophagus and at the gastro-oesophageal junction (GOJ). The accepted model for this change describes columnar metaplasia (BE) in response to chronic inflammation after long-term exposure to supra-physiological levels of acid and bile as part of GORD [12–14]. For this to take place, either terminally differentiated squamous cells or, more likely, stem cells in the oesophageal mucosa are reprogrammed to a glandular phenotype. However, recent reports suggest that the architecture of BE closely represents the gastric antrum, raising the possibility that BE is actually derived from the gastric mucosa [15]. This is a controversial area that has been vigorously debated since the first description of a glandular mucosa in the distal oesophagus by Barrett himself, and it has profound implications for the design of novel therapies [16].

No matter what the origin of the columnar metaplasia in the oesophagus is, there is expert consensus that EAC develops as a consequence of progressive cellular dysplasia in BE over time. BE is the only known precursor lesion for EAC [17]. Patients with BE are at risk of developing EAC, but the annual conversion rate is low (0.12–0.5%) [17, 18]. Patients with BE are more likely to die of a cause other than EAC. Medicine is currently unable to accurately identify which patients with BE will progress to cancer, and we rely on surveillance programmes of unproven efficacy. Patients with long-segment BE (>3 cm) and where intestinal metaplasia is present are believed to be at higher risk of progression to cancer. US and UK guidelines are conflicting, but recommend endoscopic screening of high-risk individuals (chronic GORD symptoms and multiple risk factors, with special consideration of family history) in an attempt to identify patients with BE. If BE is detected, then 2–3-yearly surveillance endoscopy with biopsy of visible lesions and quadrantic biopsies taken every 1–2 cm throughout the Barrett's segment is recommended for patients with long-segment Barrett's (>3 cm) [19]. There is some evidence that surveillance of BE correlates with earlier-stage and improved survival from EAC [20, 21], but this is controversial [22, 23], and there are no conclusive randomized controlled trials of benefit. A quadrantic biopsy protocol is designed to provide an adequate 'sample' of the BE segment, with the aim of identifying cellular dysplasia and/or early cancer. However, only a tiny fraction of the BE segment is ever sampled, with the very real possibility that important cellular changes elsewhere will be missed. Intensive biopsy protocols are associated with cancer detection, but they are demanding of the patient and health-care resources [24].

The value of this surveillance strategy is further questioned by a number of findings. First, 90–95% of patients with BE will never develop cancer [18, 25]. Secondly, the majority of cancers observed in large-cohort studies arise soon after the index endoscopy [18]; and, thirdly, advanced EAC has been documented to develop in patients under intense surveillance [26]. This is possibly explained by the rapidity of somatic genomic alterations in BE from patients who progress to cancer, compared with the relative chromosomal stability of BE of 'nonprogressors' [26]. This leads to a relative overdiagnosis of nonprogressive BE, but underdiagnosis of unstable and rapidly progressive BE. It is important to note that the majority of patients with BE, whether they be 'progressors' or 'nonprogressors', are still at large in the general population, unaware that they have the condition.

In this context, it will be important to know whether or not endoscopic surveillance of BE is of benefit at all. The Barrett's Oesophagus Surveillance Study

(BOSS) aims to determine if endoscopic surveillance is beneficial in practice, in which 3400 patients have been randomized (1:1) to receive a standard upper gastrointestinal endoscopy with biopsy every two years for ten years, or endoscopy at need [27, 28]. This study is not due to report for several years.

In the meantime, new strategies for the assessment and treatment of BE are being developed. Understanding and identifying the population at risk are perhaps the most important considerations in EAC. Endoscopic therapies (endoscopic mucosal resection [EMR], radio-frequency ablation [RFA], etc.) can treat BE with a high risk of progression, and they are currently recommended for BE with low-grade or high-grade dysplasia and early cancers [19]. This avoids the necessity for high-risk surgery, but there is little, if any, evidence that endoscopic therapies reduce population mortality from EAC. Given the difficulty associated with identifying progressive and nonprogressive BE, a pragmatic approach to cancer prevention could be to eradicate all visible BE in all patients. However, this would lead to substantial overtreatment and individual harm: RFA is associated with a risk of perforation of 0.02% and stricture formation of 6%, in addition to more minor side effects. Therefore, more targeted strategies are required.

The Cytosponge™ offers considerable promise as a more cost-effective and less invasive device for screening and surveillance. It is a sponge-on-a-string that is contained in a dissolving capsule. It is swallowed to the stomach and then withdrawn up the oesophagus, removing mucosal cells from the GOJ and the entire length of the oesophagus, thus avoiding sampling bias. Coupled with Trefoil Factor 3 (TTF3), an immunohistochemical marker of BE, the Cytosponge has shown early promise for the diagnosis of BE in primary care [29]. Results of the prospective, multicentre, case-control BEST2 study conducted in over 1000 patients show that patients prefer the Cytosponge to endoscopy, with excellent diagnostic accuracy for BE over 3 cm in length (sensitivity 87.2% [95% CI 83.0–90.6%], specificity 92.4% [95% CI 89.5–94.7%]) [30]. TTF3 is only useful to identify patients with BE, and another biomarker or panel of biomarkers will be required to determine patients at risk of disease progression. Using data from the first comprehensive whole-genome sequencing study in EAC, the Cytosponge was combined with mutations in TP53 in a simple, clinically applicable test to define high-grade dysplasia in 86% of known cases with 100% specificity [31]. Together, these findings suggest that the Cytosponge may be able to replace endoscopy for targeted screening and subsequent surveillance of BE, with endoscopy reserved for high-risk cases and therapeutic procedures.

Future perspectives

Current strategies for the prevention of EAC are focused on the understanding, detection, and treatment of BE, but at a population level this alone will have limited impact. More than 90% of cases of EAC arise outside of surveillance programmes and the majority of people with BE will never develop cancer. EAC can be cured if detected at an early stage, but this requires timely referral for diagnosis and treatment from primary care [32]. In turn, people need to understand the risk factors for the disease and be prepared to present themselves to the health-care system. Initiatives such as the UK 'Be Clear on Cancer' campaign show early promise in improving detection rates for oesophageal and gastric cancer. Seeking medical attention for persistent heartburn is the key message of this campaign, with the aim of capturing the majority of patients with EAC who report a long history of GORD. However, it must be remembered that up to 40% of cases occur in people without chronic reflux.

More can be done to address lifestyle factors associated with EAC. EAC is clearly linked with obesity [33], and effective public health programmes that lead to weight reduction could address much of the burden of disease. Unfortunately, Western countries seem to be getting fatter rather than thinner, compounded by the finding that the majority of the adult obese population, at least in Great Britain, do not identify themselves as either 'obese' or even 'very overweight' [34].

We have gained some insight into inherited risk from large-scale genome-wide association studies. So far, a limited number of reports have revealed polymorphisms in loci close to genes involved with oesophageal development to predict risk of EAC and BE, but this is yet to be translated in a meaningful way [35].

Offering patients with proven BE the possibility of chemoprevention is also attractive. Currently only proton-pump inhibitors have been demonstrated to have any association with risk modification, but no randomized controlled trials have been performed. Results of the AspECT study are eagerly awaited and will give insight into the use of aspirin with a proton-pump inhibitor (PPI) for chemoprevention in BE.

A new approach to cancer prevention for EAC has recently been suggested by Vaughan and Fitzgerald [36]. They propose the categorization of individuals into more precise risk groups, each of which can be targeted for further investigation and/or prevention interventions in a manner that is appropriate for their absolute risk of EAC. People flow from the general population, through primary care, and on into secondary and tertiary care providers for more complex interventions, based on combinations of risk factors including heritable characteristics, novel oesophageal sampling devices coupled with biomarker assessment, and endoscopy. The value of a combinatorial model such as this is that it may more precisely target interventions to the individual at risk and limit the underdiagnosis of EAC and overtreatment of BE that currently occur. It is also modifiable over time, and could include novel biomarkers (e.g. blood-based proteomics) as they become available.

Conclusion

Oesophageal cancer represents a significant challenge for prevention and screening. Lifestyle modification with risk factor reduction is likely to deliver the most benefit at a population level, but changes such as weight reduction are hard to achieve. In the case of adenocarcinoma in Western populations, persistent heart-burn is the only recognized symptom for early disease, but the majority of people with heartburn will never develop cancer or Barrett's oesophagus. Screening with endoscopy, the current gold standard for diagnosis, is not feasible in this context. Significant progress is required in both our understanding of the underlying causes of oesophageal cancer and methods for screening and surveillance before a significant reduction in deaths can be achieved.

References

1 Arnold, M., Soerjomataram, I., Ferlay, J., and Forman, D. (2014). Global incidence of oesophageal cancer by histological subtype in 2012. *Gut* 64 (3): 381–387.

2 Lambert, R., Hainaut, P., and Parkin, D.M. (2004). Premalignant lesions of the esophago-gastric mucosa. *Sem. Oncol.* 31 (4): 498–512.

3 Cancer Research UK (2010). Oesophageal cancer incidence statistics. http://www.cancerresearchuk.org/health-professional/cancer-statistics/statistics-by-cancer-type/oesophageal-cancer/incidence (accessed 3 January 2018).

4 National Oesophago-Gastric Cancer Audit (2013). Second annual report: 2013. London: NHS Information Centre.

5 Allum, W.H., Blazeby, J.M., Griffin, S.M. et al. (2011). Guidelines for the management of oesophageal and gastric cancer. *Gut* 60 (11): 1449–1472.

6 Drahos, J., Xiao, Q., Risch, H.A. et al. (2016). Age-specific risk factor profiles of adenocarci-nomas of the esophagus: A pooled analysis from the international BEACON consortium. *Int. J. Cancer* 138 (1): 55–64.

7 Lagergren, J., Bergstrom, R., Lindgren, A., and Nyren, O. (1999). Symptomatic gastroe-sophageal reflux as a risk factor for esophageal adenocarcinoma. *N. Engl. J. Med.* 340 (11): 825–831.

8 Lubin, J.H., Cook, M.B., Pandeya, N. et al. (2012). The importance of exposure rate on odds ratios by cigarette smoking and alcohol consumption for esophageal adenocarcinoma and squamous cell carcinoma in the Barrett's Esophagus and Esophageal Adenocarcinoma Consortium. *Cancer Epidemiol.* 36 (3): 306–316.

9 Su, Z., Gay, L.J., Strange, A. et al. (2012). Common variants at the MHC locus and at chro-mosome 16q24.1 predispose to Barrett's esophagus. *Nat. Genet.* 44 (10): 1131–1136.

10 Palles, C., Chegwidden, L., Li, X. et al. (2015). Polymorphisms near TBX5 and GDF7 are associated with increased risk for Barrett's esophagus. *Gastroenterology* 148 (2): 367–378.

11 Levine, D.M., Ek, W.E., Zhang, R. et al. (2013). A genome-wide association study identifies new susceptibility loci for esophageal adenocarcinoma and Barrett's esophagus. *Nat. Genet.* 45 (12): 1487–1493.

12 Fitzgerald, R.C. (2005). Barrett's oesophagus and oesophageal adenocarcinoma: How does acid interfere with cell proliferation and differentiation? *Gut* 54 (Suppl. 1): i21–i26.

13 Fitzgerald, R.C. (2008). Dissecting out the genetic origins of Barrett's oesophagus. *Gut* 57 (8): 1033–1034.

14 Flejou, J.F. (2005). Barrett's oesophagus: From metaplasia to dysplasia and cancer. *Gut* 54 (Suppl. 1): i6–i12.

15 Lavery, D.L., Nicholson, A.M., Poulsom, R. et al. (2014). The stem cell organisation, and the proliferative and gene expression profile of Barrett's epithelium, replicates pyloric-type gastric glands. *Gut* 63 (12): 1854–1863.

16 Barrett, N.R. (1956). The oesophagus lined by columnar epithelium. *Gastroenterologia* 86 (3): 183–186.

17 di Pietro, M., Alzoubaidi, D., and Fitzgerald, R.C. (2014). Barrett's esophagus and cancer risk: How research advances can impact clinical practice. *Gut Liver* 8 (4): 356–370.

18 Hvid-Jensen, F., Pedersen, L., Drewes, A.M. et al. (2011). Incidence of adenocarcinoma among patients with Barrett's esophagus. *N. Engl. J. Med.* 365 (15): 1375–1383.

19 Fitzgerald, R.C., di Pietro, M., Ragunath, K. et al. (2014). British Society of Gastroenterology guidelines on the diagnosis and management of Barrett's oesophagus. *Gut* 63 (1): 7–42.

20 Streitz, J.M., Jr, Andrews, C.W., Jr, and Ellis, F.H., Jr. (1993). Endoscopic surveillance of Barrett's esophagus: Does it help? *J. Thorac. Cardiovasc. Surg.* 105 (3): 383–387; discussion 7–8.

21 Corley, D.A., Levin, T.R., Habel, L.A. et al. (2002). Surveillance and survival in Barrett's adenocarcinomas: A population-based study. *Gastroenterology* 122 (3): 633–640.

22 Conio, M., Blanchi, S., Lapertosa, G. et al. (2003). Long-term endoscopic surveillance of patients with Barrett's esophagus: Incidence of dysplasia and adenocarcinoma: A prospective study. *Am. J. Gastroenterol.* 98 (9): 1931–1939.

23 Corley, D.A., Mehtani, K., Quesenberry, C. et al. (2013). Impact of endoscopic surveillance on mortality from Barrett's esophagus-associated esophageal adenocarcinomas. *Gastroenterology* 145 (2): 312–319.

24 Reid, B.J., Blount, P.L., Feng, Z., and Levine, D.S. (2000). Optimizing endoscopic biopsy detection of early cancers in Barrett's high-grade dysplasia. *Am. J. Gastroenterol.* 95 (11): 3089–3096.

25 Sikkema, M., de Jonge, P.J., Steyerberg, E.W., and Kuipers, E.J. (2010). Risk of esophageal adenocarcinoma and mortality in patients with Barrett's esophagus: A systematic review and meta-analysis. *Clin. Gastroenterol. Hepatol.* 8 (3): 235–244.

26 Li, X., Galipeau, P.C., Paulson, T.G. et al. (2014). Temporal and spatial evolution of somatic chromosomal alterations: A case-cohort study of Barrett's esophagus. *Cancer Prev. Res.* 7 (1): 114–127.

27 Jankowski, J., and Barr, H. (2006). Improving surveillance for Barrett's oesophagus: AspECT and BOSS trials provide an evidence base. *BMJ* 332 (7556): 1512.

28 Barr, H. (2008). Randomised controlled trial of surveillance and no surveillance for patients with Barrett's oesophagus: BOSS (Barrett's Oesophagus Surveillance Study). http://www.controlled-trials.com/ISRCTN54190466 (accessed 3 January 2018).

29 Kadri, S.R., Lao-Sirieix, P., O'Donovan, M. et al. (2010). Acceptability and accuracy of a non-endoscopic screening test for Barrett's oesophagus in primary care: Cohort study. *BMJ* 341: c4372.

30 Ross-Innes, C., O'Donovan, M., Walker, E.; BEST2 Study Group. (2014). Prospective, multi-centre, case-control study to evaluate a novel Cytosponge™–TFF3 test for diagnosing Barrett's oesophagus. 2014 NCRI Cancer Conference, Liverpool.

31 Weaver, J.M., Ross-Innes, C.S., Shannon, N. et al. (2014). Ordering of mutations in preinvasive disease stages of esophageal carcinogenesis. *Nat. Genet.* 46 (8): 837–843.

32 Shawihdi, M., Thompson, E., Kapoor, N. et al. (2014). Variation in gastroscopy rate in English general practice and outcome for oesophagogastric cancer: Retrospective analysis of Hospital Episode Statistics. *Gut* 63 (2): 250–261.

33 Long, E., and Beales, I.L. (2014). The role of obesity in oesophageal cancer development. *Ther. Adv. Gastroenterol.* 7 (6): 247–268.

34 Johnson, F., Beeken, R.J., Croker, H., and Wardle, J. (2014). Do weight perceptions among obese adults in Great Britain match clinical definitions? Analysis of cross-sectional surveys from 2007 and 2012. *BMJ Open* 4 (11): e005561.

35 Jankowski, J.A., and Satsangi, J. (2013). Barrett's esophagus: Evolutionary insights from genomics. *Gastroenterology* 144 (4): 667–669.

36 Vaughan, T.L., and Fitzgerald, R.C. (2015). Precision prevention of oesophageal adenocarcinoma. *Nature Rev. Gastroenterol. Hepatol.* 12 (4): 243–248.

CHAPTER 22

Hepatocellular carcinoma: Prevention and screening

Aileen Marshall[1] and Tim Meyer[2]

[1]The Royal Free Sheila Sherlock Liver Centre, and UCL Institute of Liver and Digestive Health, Royal Free Hospital, London, UK
[2]Department of Oncology, UCL Medical School, and UCL Cancer Institute, London, UK

SUMMARY BOX

- Liver cancer is the second most common cause of cancer death worldwide, and its incidence is rising in Western populations.

- The major risk factor for HCC is chronic liver disease, which is present in around 80% of patients.

- The most common underlying causes are viral hepatitis, alcohol, and nonalcoholic fatty liver disease.

- For HCC, an at-risk population can be identified, so that screening can be targeted rather than whole population based. The current EASL-EORTC guidelines recommend screening the defined populations of patients with cirrhosis; noncirrhotic hepatitis B carriers with active hepatitis or a family history of HCC; and noncirrhotic patients with chronic hepatitis C and severe fibrosis.

- Ultrasound is regarded as the standard method for surveillance.

Definition and epidemiology

Hepatocellular carcinoma (HCC) is a primary liver cancer thought to arise from hepatocytes. Globally, liver cancer is the second commonest cause of cancer death. Over 780 000 cases occur per year and there were 746 000 deaths from HCC in 2012 [1]. If diagnosed at an early stage, HCC is treatable by liver transplantation, liver resection, or tumour ablation. However, the vast majority of cases are currently diagnosed at an advanced stage, where treatment options are limited and prognosis is poor. Once considered rare in UK and other Western countries, HCC

Cancer Prevention and Screening: Concepts, Principles and Controversies, First Edition.
Edited by Rosalind A. Eeles, Christine D. Berg, and Jeffrey S. Tobias.
© 2019 John Wiley & Sons, Inc. Published 2019 by John Wiley & Sons, Inc.

has been steadily increasing in incidence and now has the highest increase in mortality of all cancers in the UK over the last 10 years, increasing by 44% in males and 50% in females [2].

HCC is an ideal cancer to target for prevention. There is a strong association between chronic liver disease and HCC, and environmental factors play an important part in affecting the risk of HCC.

Liver cirrhosis and HCC

More than 80% of HCCs occur in people with liver cirrhosis. The risk of HCC is associated with the cause of cirrhosis, being highest in those with chronic hepatitis B virus (HBV) or chronic hepatitis C virus (HCV) infection. Cirrhosis can be regarded as a pre-neoplastic field change, predisposing to HCC. Chronic liver diseases share the common features of chronic inflammation, oxidative stress, hepatocyte death and senescence, and activation of pro-fibrogenic pathways. In addition, HBV can integrate into the host genome to disrupt regulation of oncogenes and tumour suppressors. A full understanding of the molecular mechanisms underlying the pathogenesis of HCC in cirrhosis has not yet been reached, but new genomic techniques have provided a better insight. HCC is a heterogeneous cancer, with a number of common mutations, especially in p53 and beta catenin, altered signalling pathways, and epigenetic modifications. This knowledge offers opportunity for HCC prevention in patients with cirrhosis, and in patients who have been successfully treated for HCC and then remain at risk of recurrence or developing a second tumour.

Risk factors for HCC: Specific liver diseases

Hepatitis B virus

Globally, the vast majority of HCCs occur in people chronically infected with HBV. It is estimated that over 2 billion people have been exposed to HBV and 240 million have chronic infection. The risk of acute infection becoming chronic is related to the age of exposure, with approximately 90% of exposed infants developing chronic infection, 30–50% below the age of 6, and 10% if infection occurs as an adult [3]. In sub-Saharan Africa and East Asia, approximately 5–10% of the population is chronically infected with HBV, 2–5% in the Middle East and Indian subcontinent, and 1% in Western countries. The predominant route of transmission in high-prevalence countries is perinatal.

The long-term outcome of chronic HBV infection is variable and a proportion will develop chronic hepatitis leading to cirrhosis. The presence of liver cirrhosis is the most important additional risk factor for HCC in patients with chronic HBV infection, such that the annual risk is estimated between 3% and 8% [4].

Unique among the causes of liver cirrhosis, patients with noncirrhotic chronic HBV infection also have an increased risk of HCC. Increasing age, male gender, high serum HBV DNA >2000 IU/ml [5], high serum hepatitis B surface antigen level >1000 IU/ml [6], and family history of HCC are additional independent risk factors. Risk stratification using these variables might be an important means of targeting prevention to those at highest risk.

Hepatitis C virus

Hepatitis C virus is a blood-borne virus that is predominantly transmitted through unsafe injection practices, such as needle-sharing between people who inject drugs, inadequate sterilization of medical equipment, and transfusion of unscreened blood or blood products. In contrast to HBV, vertical transmission is rare. Acute infection is usually associated with minimal symptoms and the majority of those exposed, approximately 55–85%, will develop chronic infection. It is estimated that 130–150 million individuals worldwide are chronically infected with HCC, particularly in North Africa, Central and East Asia, and Japan [7].

Again, the long-term outcome of chronic HCV infection is variable, and a proportion will develop chronic hepatitis leading to cirrhosis. The annual incidence of HCC in patients with HCV-related cirrhosis is approximately 3–5%, with a much-reduced risk in noncirrhotic chronic HCV.

Hereditary haemochromatosis

Hereditary haemochromatosis (HH) is an autosomal recessive condition associated with iron overload in solid organs, including the liver. If untreated, this may lead to cirrhosis and subsequent increased risk of HCC in approximately 3–4% of patients with cirrhosis per year. More than 90% of HH is caused by homozygosity for a single mutation in the HFE gene, namely a G-to-A missense mutation, leading to the substitution of tyrosine for cysteine at amino acid position 282 (C282Y). Hence, genetic diagnosis is relatively straightforward in patients presenting with iron overload and to screen for the disease in their relatives. However, the disease has incomplete penetrance, with only approximately 30% of homozygotes developing iron overload [8]. Genetic screening of the general population to identify C282Y homozygotes is not recommended.

Aflatoxin

Aflatoxin is produced by the fungus aspergillus in nuts or grains stored in damp conditions. It is particularly a problem in sub-Saharan Africa and East Asia, populations with a high prevalence of HBV. Aflatoxin exposure is linked to specific mutations in the tumour suppressor p53, most commonly an arginine to serine mutation at codon 249, which abrogates p53 function. Aflatoxin acts synergistically with chronic HBV infection; a 73-fold increase is HCC risk is reported with high-level aflatoxin exposure and chronic HBV infection [9].

Risk factors for HCC: General risk factors

Alcohol and smoking

Heavy alcohol consumption is associated with the development of alcohol-related liver disease and cirrhosis. In Western populations with HCC, alcohol-related liver disease is the risk factor in 35% of cases. In a prospective study of patients with alcohol-related cirrhosis aged 40–75 years, the annual incidence was 2.5% [10]. In the absence of liver cirrhosis, it is not known whether alcohol consumption increases the risk of HCC. However, in patients with chronic viral hepatitis, heavy alcohol consumption is a co-factor increasing the risk of HCC two- to threefold compared to nondrinkers [11]. There is a correlation between alcohol consumption and tobacco smoking which is a potential confounder, but after adjusting for alcohol consumption, smoking appears to be an independent risk factor for HCC [12].

Diabetes, obesity, and the metabolic syndrome

The prevalence of obesity and the metabolic syndrome has increased dramatically in Western countries during the last 50 years. Non-alcohol-related fatty liver disease (NAFLD) is regarded as the liver manifestation of the metabolic syndrome. NAFLD encompasses simple hepatic steatosis, to steatohepatitis, fibrosis, and cirrhosis. The risk of HCC in NAFLD is estimated at 2% per year and is becoming a greater proportion of HCC cases. The importance of diabetes is underlined by studies showing a threefold increased risk of HCC in diabetic individuals in populations not stratified for the presence of liver disease [13]. A recent US study found that diabetes and obesity have the largest population attributable fraction for HCC, thus public health measures aimed at tackling these factors could have the greatest impact [14].

Interventions to reduce risk

Prevention of HBV infection

Prevention of HBV-related HCC begins with prevention of HBV infection. Worldwide, the predominant mode of HBV transmission is vertical at the time of delivery. Many countries implement screening of pregnant women to identify HBV carriers. It is recommended to vaccinate infants born to mothers who are chronic HBV carriers, with the addition of hepatitis B immune globulin if the mother has a high serum HBV DNA titre. This prevents infection in 95% of cases.

Many countries have a policy of universal HBV vaccination, although this is not the case in the UK, where only those perceived to be at high risk of HBV infection are offered vaccination. Taiwan, previously a high-prevalence country for HBV and HCC, was one of the first to introduce a policy of universal vaccination in 1984. Initially this was offered to infants of HBV surface antigen–positive mothers, then extended to all infants under 12 months old in 1997. The 20-year follow-up was reported in 2009 [15]; vaccinated cohorts aged 6–19 years old had an HCC rate ratio of 0.31 compared with nonvaccinated cohorts. Incomplete vaccination course and maternal HB surface antigen positivity were associated with HCC development in the vaccinated cohort. As this first cohort reaches the age where HBV-related HCC becomes more common, it remains to be seen whether there will still be a protective effect or if other risk factors will now affect this population.

Treatment of viral hepatitis

Prevention of HCC in patients with chronic viral hepatitis can be considered on three levels: first to prevent progression to cirrhosis; secondly to prevent HCC development in patients with established cirrhosis; and thirdly to prevent recurrence or *de novo* HCC in patients successfully treated for HCC.

The mainstay of therapy for chronic HBV is interferon, usually in a time-limited course, or long-term treatment with nucleo(t)side analogues (NA) that suppress HBV replication. In general, international guidelines recommend treating individuals with significant necro-inflammatory activity measured biochemically or histologically, or high-serum HBV DNA titre. The newer NAs such as entecavir and tenofovir are well tolerated and efficacious to suppress HBV DNA. Regression of liver fibrosis has been reported with long-term use of tenofovir [16].

A meta-analysis of NA treatment demonstrated a reduced risk of HCC in treated versus untreated patients overall (2.8% vs 6.4%) [17]. Within this cohort, the reduction of risk was not apparent in patients with established cirrhosis. However, these patients were commonly treated with the first-generation drugs lamivudine and adefovir, which were less efficacious to suppress HBV DNA and drug resistance developed frequently.

Worldwide, liver resection is often used as primary treatment for HBV-related HCC. There are historical data to suggest a beneficial effect of interferons on HCC recurrence following treatment, but interferons are now rarely used in chronic HBV due to side-effect profile. High viral load is a risk factor for adverse outcome following resection for HCC, and a recent meta-analysis including over 8400 patients found that NA treatment reduced HCC recurrence, and improved disease-free survival and overall survival (risk ratios [RR] 0.69, 0.7, and 0.46, respectively) [18]. Thus, the benefit of anti-viral treatment in patients with hepatitis B reduces both the risk of HCC recurrence and liver disease–related mortality.

There is no vaccine against HCV at present, so prevention of infection is based on public health measures to limit unsafe injection and, in health-care settings at risk, to provide adequate sterilisation and screened blood products.

Treatment of hepatitis C virus is a rapidly developing field. In the past, treatment was based on a combination of pegylated interferon and ribavirin, with the recent addition of the protease inhibitors telaprevir and boceprevir. The side-effect profile and limited efficacy of these drugs in patients with cirrhosis, the group at risk of HCC, meant that many patients were not suitable for treatment. In those cirrhotic patients who could be treated, a meta-analysis indicated an RR for HCC of 0.43 overall, and 0.35 in patients who achieved a sustained viral response [19].

A new generation of direct-acting anti-HCV drugs is now being evaluated in clinical trials and the first few are entering clinical practice. According to the clinical trials, these new drugs are highly efficacious to clear HCV with a better side-effect profile. The major barrier to widespread treatment of all patients with HCV is the cost. As these drugs are used more widely, we should see whether they are effective in reducing HCC risk in patients with cirrhosis. Ultimately, the goal should be early treatment of HCV before the development of cirrhosis.

Lifestyle modification

Theoretically, advice to modify lifestyle and behaviour to reduce weight through diet and exercise, reduce alcohol consumption, and avoid smoking should have beneficial effects on risk of diabetes, metabolic syndrome, alcoholic liver disease, NAFLD, and HCC. Apart from alcohol abstinence in patients with alcohol-related cirrhosis, evidence of reduced HCC risk through lifestyle modification is lacking.

Coffee consumption appears to protect against HCC. A recent meta-analysis reports a relative risk of 0.72 for low coffee consumption and 0.44 for high coffee consumption [20], independent of gender, alcohol consumption, or history of liver disease or hepatitis.

Chemoprevention

An active area of research interest is the use of specific drugs to prevent HCC in patients with cirrhosis. Large-scale epidemiological data indicate a reduced risk of several cancers, including HCC, in patients taking statins, metformin, or aspirin [21–23]. For metformin, a meta-analysis of observational studies showed a 50% reduction in HCC incidence with metformin use. In contrast, there was an increased incidence of HCC with sulphonylurea or insulin, and no evidence of a difference with thiazolidinediones [21]. For statins, a meta-analysis of 10 studies including almost 1.5 million patients found an odds ratio [OR] of 0.63 for HCC incidence in statin users compared to nonusers. The effect was greatest in Asian populations [22]. The American Association of Retired Persons Diet and Health study [23] observed both reduced HCC incidence (RR 0.59) and death from chronic liver disease (RR 0.59) in aspirin users compared to nonusers. No effect on HCC or liver disease mortality was seen with other nonsteroidal inflammatory drugs.

While these data are promising, it should be noted that all these studies are observational and in general populations, not specifically targeted to patients with liver disease. The effect is seen for a number of cancers, and all three drugs are being evaluated in clinical of trials as adjunctive treatment for cancer or to prevent cancer in high-risk patients, including lung, breast, prostate, colon, and oesophagus. A clinical trial of aspirin as secondary prevention of HCC in patients treated with liver resection is also under way.

Screening for HCC

Principles of screening

The objective of screening is to reduce mortality in patients who develop cancer by detecting a tumour at a stage when curative interventions are available. The effectiveness of a screening programme is determined by the incidence of the condition, the sensitivity and specificity of the screening test to detect potentially curable disease, the compliance of the at-risk population, the cost of implementation, and the risks associated with the test.

Effectiveness of treating early disease

Early disease that can be treated with resection, ablation, or transplantation is associated with improved outcome and cure in a proportion of patients. Resection is generally reserved for those with limited disease occurring in a noncirrhotic liver or those with well-compensated liver disease. Transplantation, on the other hand, can be undertaken in patients with cirrhosis, but is limited by organ availability and, in order to achieve parity with benign indications, is confined to those within the so-called Milan Criteria [24]. An intention to treat analysis comparing the outcomes for resection and transplantation in cirrhotic patients reported a five-year survival of 51% and 69%, respectively; however, for patients without significant portal hypertension, the five-year survival for resected patients was 74% [25]. For patients with tumours of 2 cm or less, radiofrequency ablation (RFA) appears to have equivalent survival to surgical resection in uncontrolled studies [26], but randomized trials have been conflicting [27, 28]. Patients who are outside criteria for these potentially curative options may receive palliative therapies, offering median survivals of 20 months for embolization, 11 months for systemic therapy, or 3 months for supportive care. Overall, there is clear evidence that patients with early-stage disease have a better outcome and can be cured. Strategies that can reliably detect early disease in asymptomatic patients therefore have the potential to have an impact on overall mortality from this disease.

Target population

For HCC, an at-risk population can be identified so that screening can be targeted rather than whole population based. Hence, the current EASL-EORTC guidelines recommend screening the following defined populations [29]:

- Patients with cirrhosis. Liver cirrhosis is associated with an annual risk of developing HCC for between 1% and 8%, and cirrhosis is present in more than 80% patients who present with HCC. Since cirrhosis itself is a potentially life-limiting condition, screening is recommended for Child-Pugh stages A and B, and for those with stage C who are awaiting liver transplantation.
- Noncirrhotic HBV carriers with active hepatitis or family history of HCC. Chronic hepatitis B infection is associated with a 223-fold risk of developing

HCC [30], and those who are HBe-antigen positive or high HBV DNA carry the highest risk [31, 32]. Worldwide, HBV infections account for 52.3% of HCC, and 40% are not cirrhotic.

- Noncirrhotic patients with chronic HCV and severe fibrosis F3. In the USA, chronic liver disease from HCV infection is present in 20% of patients presenting with HCC, but the majority also have cirrhosis. However, data from the HALT-C study demonstrated a 4.1% five-year risk of developing HCC in the presence of bridging fibrosis [33]. A sustained viral response may reduce the risk, but does not obviate it [34].

While hepatitis B and C may be detected though surveillance programmes, other risk factors for cirrhosis, such as alcohol and nonalcoholic steatohepatitis (NASH), are more difficult to detect and treat at an early stage and, for this reason, the data from screening programmes performed in one at-risk population may not necessarily be transferable to another.

Screening methodology

Imaging

Ultrasound (US) is regarded as the standard method for surveillance and is endorsed by the EASL guidelines. It is noninvasive, safe, and relatively cheap, but is operator dependent. The reported sensitivity for US ranges from 58% to 89%, with a specificity of more than 90% [35, 36]. A systematic review of 13 studies demonstrated a sensitivity of 94% for US to detect tumours before they were clinically evident, but only 63% for early tumours as defined by the Milan Criteria [37]. A Japanese study, however, reported that under 2% of cases detected by US surveillance exceeded 3 cm [38]. A recently published meta-analysis including 47 trials published between 1990 and 2014 and involving 15 158 patients demonstrated that surveillance was associated with better early-stage detection (OR 2.08) and curative treatment rates (OR 2.24) [39]. Moreover, surveillance was associated with a significantly prolonged survival (OR 1.90). However, the study was limited by lack of sufficient follow-up for survival in some studies, and failure to correct for lead-time bias in others. Neither computed tomography (CT) nor magnetic resonance imaging (MRI) has been formally evaluated for surveillance; both are limited by cost, and CT by the additional risk of increased radiation exposure. These modalities tend to be reserved for those on the transplant waiting list.

Blood-based tests

The most widely investigated blood test for screening is serum alpha-fetoprotein (AFP). AFP has been extensively investigated in patients with HCC and has an established role as a diagnostic and prognostic biomarker. However, AFP can be elevated in patients with hepatitis and negative in patients with confirmed HCC. Overall, AFP has been reported to have sensitivity of 39–65% and specificity of 76–94% [40–42]; both sensitivity and specificity vary depending on the cut-off level chosen and the stage of the disease. At a threshold of 20 ng/mL, the sensitivity has been reported to be 41–64% while the specificity is 82–91% [40, 43]. The positive (PPV) and negative predictive values (NPV) of a screening test are determined by the prevalence of the condition and, at a prevalence of 5%, the PPV is only 25%, using an AFP threshold of 20 ng/mL [41]. Finally, only 10–20% early HCC present with elevated AFP, and for all these reasons, AFP is not recommended for screening in international guidelines [29]. Des-gamma-carboxy prothrombin (DCP) has also been evaluated and, as a single marker, found to lack sensitivity for early detection [44, 45].

Effectiveness of screening

The effectiveness of screening for HCC remains a subject of debate, and robust data from randomized trials are lacking for most patient populations. To date, the only randomized controlled trials conducted have been in Chinese patients with HBV infection. The study by Zhang et al. [46] included around 18 000 subjects aged 35–59 with HBV infection or a history of chronic hepatitis. They were randomized to surveillance: six-monthly US and AFP (cut-off 20 mcg/L) or no surveillance. In the surveillance group there were 86 HCC detected, and in the nonsurveillance group 67 were detected. Moreover, resection was achieved in 46.5% and 7%, respectively, and overall there was a 37% reduction in HCC-related mortality in the surveillance group. However, compliance with the surveillance programme was only 60% and the sensitivity of AFP was only 60%, confirming its limitation as a screening tool. Another study of 5581 male HBsAg carriers aged 30–69 randomly assigned subjects to surveillance with six-monthly AFP and follow-up US for those with an AFP of ≥20 mcg/L, or no surveillance [47]. The overall sensitivity and specificity of the surveillance was 55% and 86%, respectively, but rose to 80.0% and 80.9% in those who complied with all scheduled visits. There was a higher proportion of Stage I cancers detected in the surveillance group compared with the nonsurveillance group: 29.6% versus 6.0%. However, neither the five-year survival nor the mortality rate differed between the two groups, and screening in this case was deemed ineffective. The failure was attributed to inadequate methods of screening, diagnosis, and available treatment, and may not be relevant to other regions offering US as a primary surveillance tool and other curative modalities such as transplantation.

In the non-HBV population, there are no randomized trials and most of the reported studies are subject to significant bias. An Italian study [48] performed a retrospective study of the impact of surveillance US in 649 HCC patients with Child-Pugh class A or B, of which the majority had HCV infection. Patients were separated into two groups: Group 1 had six-monthly US (n = 510) and Group 2 had yearly US (n = 139). In Group 1, HCC was detected at an earlier stage, with 24% having tumours ≤2 cm compared to 5% in Group 2, and median survival was significantly better, at 45 months versus 30 months. When corrected for a calculated lead-time bias of 141 days, the difference between the two groups remained significant. Interestingly, the improvement in survival was not attributable to increased rates of resection or transplantation, which were equivalent between the two groups.

The difference between three- and six-monthly surveillance US has also been evaluated in a European randomized trial involving 1278 patients with histologically confirmed cirrhosis [49]. Focal lesions were detected in 28% of patients, but HCC only confirmed in 9.6%, and focal lesions less than 10 mm were more commonly detected in the three-monthly US group. However, there was no difference in the rate of HCC detection or the prevalence of HCC ≤3 cm between the two groups. Although survival was not the primary end-point of this trial, there was no difference in estimated five-year survival. The potential benefit of US in well-compensated HCV cirrhotic patients has also been investigated using a modelling approach, in which variable rates of access and screening efficiency were considered and lead-time bias taken into account [50]. Assuming existing practices have an access of 57% and diagnostic effectiveness of 42%, screening was determined to reduce five-year mortality by 6% compared to no screening. Optimal screening resulting in the detection of 87% of patients at Barcelona Clinic liver cancer (BCLC) stage 0/A would lead to decrease in five-year mortality of 20%. Modelling has also been used more systematically to assess the impact of lead-time bias [51]. The model was informed by a cohort of 1380 patients, of whom 850 had HCC detected during six-monthly surveillance, 234 during annual surveillance, and 296 after symptomatic presentation. The respective five-year survival among these groups was 32.7%, 25.2%, and 12.2%, respectively, and the lead-time was calculated to be 7.2 months for six-monthly and 4.1 months for annual surveillance. While lead-time was found to be the major determinant for short-term survival up to three years, surveillance was found to be beneficial on longer follow-up.

Cost-effectiveness

The cost-effectiveness of screening for HCC has been assessed using modelling approaches and analysis of retrospective series. The estimates vary widely, since they are influenced by a number of variables or assumptions, including incidence in the screened population, screening interval, screening modality used, and effectiveness of interventions. An Italian study evaluated the cost-effectiveness of a surveillance programme which enrolled 313 patients to six-monthly US and AFP. The incidence of HCC was 4.1% per year, but only 69% were detected at a stage at which potentially curative options could be offered. Compared with a cohort of 104 incidentally detected HCCs, the survival of the screened population was significantly improved, but the overall cost of the surveillance programme per life-year saved was $112 993 [43]. This figure is consistent with a decision analysis model which estimated the cost of screening European patients with

Child-Pugh A cirrhosis at between $48 000 and $284 000 per life-year gained [52]. Another modelling study examined the cost-effectiveness of a range of surveillance modalities, including CT and MRI, and concluded that six-monthly US was the only strategy which came below the threshold of $50 000 per quality-adjusted life-year [53].

Conclusion

HCC is a common cancer and is now the leading cause of increased cancer mortality in Western populations. Most patients are diagnosed with advanced-stage disease with a poor outcome. The populations at risk can be identified, and the key priorities to improve outcome are better surveillance and early diagnosis, as well as preventing HCC development through modification of environmental risk factors (diet, alcohol, smoking, and aflatoxin), HBV vaccination, and specific antiviral therapies. Future studies should focus on chemoprevention of HCC with aspirin, statins, and metformin.

The efficacy of surveillance for HCC remains the subject of debate but, given the data from randomized trials from China, and retrospective and modelling analyses undertaken in Western populations, it is recommended for high-risk patients by international guidelines. It is unlikely that a randomized trial will be undertaken, and the focus for the future will be to define more sensitive and specific methods to detect early disease and improve treatment outcomes for those in whom HCC is detected.

References

1 GLOBOCAN 2012 (2012). Estimated cancer incidence, mortality and prevalence worldwide. Liver cancer fact sheet. http://globocan.iarc.fr/Pages/fact_sheets_cancer.aspx (accessed 4 January 2015).

2 Cancer Research UK (2014). Cancer mortality statistics. http://www.cancerresearchuk.org/health-professional/cancer-statistics/mortality (accessed 3 January 2018).

3 World Health Organization (2014). Hepatitis B. http://www.who.int/mediacentre/factsheets/fs204/en/ (accessed 4 January 2015).

4 Bruix, J., and Sherman, M. (2011). AASLD Practice Guideline: Management of hepatocellular carcinoma: An update. American Association for the Study of Liver Diseases. http://www.aasld.org/sites/default/files/guideline_documents/HCCUpdate2010.pdf (accessed 4 January 2015).

5 Chen, C.F., Lee, W.C., Yang, H.I. et al.; Risk Evaluation of Viral Load Elevation and Associated Liver Disease/Cancer in HBV (REVEAL–HBV) Study Group (2011). Changes in serum levels of HBV DNA and alanine aminotransferase determine risk for hepatocellular carcinoma. *Gastroenterology* 141 (4): 1240–1248.

6 Tseng, T.C., Liu, C.J., Yang, H.C. et al. (202). High levels of hepatitis B surface antigen increase risk of hepatocellular carcinoma in patients with low HBV load. *Gastroenterology* 142 (5): 1140–1149.

7 World Health Organization (2014). Hepatitis C. http://www.who.int/mediacentre/factsheets/fs164/en/ (accessed 4 January 2015).

8 Gurrin, L.C., Osborne, N.J., Constantine, C.C. et al.; HealthIron Study Investigators (2008). The natural history of serum iron indices for HFE C282Y homozygosity associated with hereditary hemochromatosis. *Gastroenterology* 135 (6): 1945–1952.

9 Kew, MC (2013). Aflatoxins as a cause of hepatocellular carcinoma. *J. Gastrointestin. Liver Dis.* 22 (3): 305–310.

10 Mancebo, A., González-Diéguez, M.L., Cadahía, V. et al. (2013). Annual incidence of hepatocellular carcinoma among patients with alcoholic cirrhosis and identification of risk groups. *Clin. Gastroenterol. Hepatol.* 11 (1): 95–101.

11 Lin, C.W., Lin, C.C., Mo, L.R. et al. (2013). Heavy alcohol consumption increases the incidence of hepatocellular carcinoma in hepatitis B virus-related cirrhosis. *J. Hepatol.* 58 (4): 730–735.

12 Koh, W.P., Robien, K., Wang, R. et al. (2011). Smoking as an independent risk factor for hepatocellular carcinoma: The Singapore Chinese Health Study. *Br. J. Cancer* 105 (9): 1430–1435.

13 El-Serag, H.B., and Rudolph, K.L. (2007). Hepatocellular carcinoma: Epidemiology and molecular carcinogenesis. *Gastroenterology* 132 (7): 2557–2576.

14 Welzel, T.M., Graubard, B.I., Quraishi, S. et al. (2013). Population-attributable fractions of risk factors for hepatocellular carcinoma in the United States. *Am. J. Gastroenterol.* 108 (8): 1314–1321.

15 Chang, M.H., You, S.L., Chen, C.J. et al.; Taiwan Hepatoma Study Group (2009). Decreased incidence of hepatocellular carcinoma in hepatitis B vaccinees: A 20-year follow-up study. *J. Natl Cancer Inst.* 101: 1348–1355.

16 Marcellin, P., Gane, E., Buti, M. et al. (2013). Regression of cirrhosis during treatment with tenofovir disoproxil fumarate for chronic hepatitis B: A 5-year open-label follow-up study. *Lancet* 381 (9865): 468–475.

17 Papatheodoridis, G.V., Lampertico, P., Manolakopoulos, S., and Lok, A. (2010). Incidence of hepatocellular carcinoma in chronic hepatitis B patients receiving nucleos(t)ide therapy: A systematic review. *J. Hepatol.* 53: 348–356.

18 Zhou, Y., Zhang, Z., Zhao, Y. et al. (2014). Antiviral therapy decreases recurrence of hepatitis B virus-related hepatocellular carcinoma after curative resection: A meta-analysis. *World J. Surg.* 38 (9): 2395–2402.

19 Singal, A.K., Singh, A., Jaganmohan, S. et al. (2010). Antiviral therapy reduces risk of hepatocellular carcinoma in patients with hepatitis C virus-related cirrhosis. *Clin. Gastroenterol. Hepatol.* 8 (2): 192–199.

20 Bravi, F., Bosetti, C., Tavani, A. et al. (2013). Coffee reduces risk for hepatocellular carcinoma: An updated meta-analysis. *Clin. Gastroenterol. Hepatol.* 11 (11): 1413–1421.

21 Singh, S., Singh, P.P., Singh, A.G. et al. (2013). Anti-diabetic medications and the risk of hepatocellular cancer: A systematic review and meta-analysis. *Am. J. Gastroenterol.* 108 (6): 881–891.

22 Singh, S., Singh, P.P., Singh, A.G. et al. (2013). Statins are associated with a reduced risk of hepatocellular cancer: A systematic review and meta-analysis. *Gastroenterology* 144: 323–332.

23 Sahasrabuddhe, V.V., Gunja, M.Z., Graubard, B.I. et al. (2012). Nonsteroidal anti-inflammatory drug use, chronic liver disease, and hepatocellular carcinoma. *J. Natl Cancer Inst.* 104 (23): 1808–1814.

24 Mazzaferro, V., Regalia, E., Doci, R. et al. (1996). Liver transplantation for the treatment of small hepatocellular carcinomas in patients with cirrhosis. *N. Engl. J. Med.* 334: 693–699.

25 Llovet, J.M., Fuster, J., and Bruix, J. (1999). Intention-to-treat analysis of surgical treatment for early hepatocellular carcinoma: Resection versus transplantation. *Hepatology* 30: 1434–1440.

26 Livraghi, T., Meloni, F., Di, S.M. et al. (2008). Sustained complete response and complications rates after radiofrequency ablation of very early hepatocellular carcinoma in cirrhosis: Is resection still the treatment of choice? *Hepatology* 47: 82–89.

27 Chen, M.S., Li, J.Q., Zheng, Y. et al. (2006). A prospective randomized trial comparing percutaneous local ablative therapy and partial hepatectomy for small hepatocellular carcinoma. *Ann. Surg.* 243: 321–328.

28 Huang, J., Yan, L., Cheng, Z. et al. (2010). A randomized trial comparing radiofrequency ablation and surgical resection for HCC conforming to the Milan criteria. *Ann. Surg.* 252: 903–912.

29 European Association for the Study of the Liver and European Organisation for Research and Treatment of Cancer (2012). EASL-EORTC Clinical Practice Guidelines: Management of hepatocellular carcinoma. *J. Hepatol.* 56: 908–943.

30 Beasley, R.P., Hwang, L.Y., Lin, C.C., and Chien, C.S. (1981). Hepatocellular carcinoma and hepatitis B virus: A prospective study of 22 707 men in Taiwan. *Lancet* 2: 1129–1133.

31 Tsukuma, H., Hiyama, T., Tanaka, S. et al. (1993). Risk factors for hepatocellular carcinoma among patients with chronic liver disease. *N. Engl. J. Med.* 328: 1797–1801.

32 Chen, C.J., Yang, H.I., Su, J. et al. (2006). Risk of hepatocellular carcinoma across a biological gradient of serum hepatitis B virus DNA level. *JAMA* 295: 65–73.

33 Lok, A.S., Seeff, L.B., Morgan, T.R. et al. (2009). Incidence of hepatocellular carcinoma and associated risk factors in hepatitis C-related advanced liver disease. *Gastroenterology* 136: 138–148.

34 Singal, A.G., Volk, M.L., Jensen, D. et al. (2010). A sustained viral response is associated with reduced liver-related morbidity and mortality in patients with hepatitis C virus. *Clin. Gastroenterol. Hepatol.* 8: 280–288.

35 Bolondi, L. (2003). Screening for hepatocellular carcinoma in cirrhosis. *J. Hepatol.* 39: 1076–1084.

36 Kim, C.K., Lim, J.H., Lee, W.J. (2001). Detection of hepatocellular carcinomas and dysplastic nodules in cirrhotic liver: Accuracy of ultrasonography in transplant patients. *J. Ultrasound Med.* 20: 99–104.

37 Singal, A., Volk, M.L., Waljee, A. et al. (2009). Meta-analysis: Surveillance with ultrasound for early-stage hepatocellular carcinoma in patients with cirrhosis. *Aliment. Pharmacol. Ther.* 30: 37–47.

38 Sato, T., Tateishi, R., Yoshida, H. et al. (2009). Ultrasound surveillance for early detection of hepatocellular carcinoma among patients with chronic hepatitis C. *Hepatol. Int.* 3: 544–550.

39 Singal, A.G., Pillai, A., and Tiro, J. (2014). Early detection, curative treatment, and survival rates for hepatocellular carcinoma surveillance in patients with cirrhosis: A meta-analysis. *PLoS Med.* 11: e1001624.

40 Sherman, M., Peltekian, K.M., and Lee, C. (1995). Screening for hepatocellular carcinoma in chronic carriers of hepatitis B virus: Incidence and prevalence of hepatocellular carcinoma in a North American urban population. *Hepatology* 22: 432–438.

41 Trevisani, F., D'Intino, P.E., Morselli-Labate, A.M. et al. (2001). Serum alpha-fetoprotein for diagnosis of hepatocellular carcinoma in patients with chronic liver disease: Influence of HBsAg and anti-HCV status. *J. Hepatol.* 34: 570–575.

42 Tong, M.J., Blatt, L.M., and Kao, V.W. (2001). Surveillance for hepatocellular carcinoma in patients with chronic viral hepatitis in the United States of America. *J. Gastroenterol. Hepatol.* 16: 553–559.

43 Bolondi, L., Sofia, S., Siringo, S. et al. (2001). Surveillance programme of cirrhotic patients for early diagnosis and treatment of hepatocellular carcinoma: A cost effectiveness analysis. *Gut* 48: 251–259.

44 Lok, A.S., Sterling, R.K., Everhart, J.E. et al. (2010). Des-gamma-carboxy prothrombin and alpha-fetoprotein as biomarkers for the early detection of hepatocellular carcinoma. *Gastroenterology* 138: 493–502.

45 Izuno, K., Fujiyama, S., Yamasaki, K. et al. (1995). Early detection of hepatocellular carcinoma associated with cirrhosis by combined assay of des-gamma-carboxy prothrombin and alpha-fetoprotein: A prospective study. *Hepatogastroenterology* 42: 387–393.

46 Zhang, B.H., Yang, B.H., and Tang, Z.Y. (2004). Randomized controlled trial of screening for hepatocellular carcinoma. *J. Cancer Res. Clin. Oncol.* 130: 417–422.

47 Chen, J.G., Parkin, D.M., Chen, Q.G. et al. (2003). Screening for liver cancer: Results of a randomised controlled trial in Qidong, China. *J. Med. Screen.* 10: 204–209.

48 Santi, V., Trevisani, F., Gramenzi, A. et al. (2010). Semiannual surveillance is superior to annual surveillance for the detection of early hepatocellular carcinoma and patient survival. *J. Hepatol.* 53: 291–297.

49 Chevret, S., Trinchet, J.C., Mathieu, D. et al. (1999). A new prognostic classification for predicting survival in patients with hepatocellular carcinoma. Groupe d'Etude et de Traitement du Carcinome Hepatocellulaire. *J. Hepatol.* 31: 133–141.

50 Mourad, A., Deuffic-Burban, S., Ganne-Carrie, N. et al. (2014). Hepatocellular carcinoma screening in patients with compensated hepatitis C virus (HCV)-related cirrhosis aware of their HCV status improves survival: A modeling approach. *Hepatology* 59: 1471–1481.

51 Cucchetti, A., Trevisani, F., Pecorelli, A. et al. (2014). Estimation of lead-time bias and its impact on the outcome of surveillance for the early diagnosis of hepatocellular carcinoma. *J. Hepatol.* 61: 333–341.

52 Sarasin, F.P., Giostra, E., and Hadengue, A. (1996). Cost-effectiveness of screening for detection of small hepatocellular carcinoma in western patients with Child-Pugh class A cirrhosis. *Am. J. Med.* 101: 422–434.

53 Andersson, K.L., Salomon, J.A., Goldie, S.J., and Chung, R.T. (2008). Cost effectiveness of alternative surveillance strategies for hepatocellular carcinoma in patients with cirrhosis. *Clin. Gastroenterol. Hepatol.* 6: 1418–1424.

CHAPTER 23

Ovarian cancer prevention and screening

Aleksandra Gentry-Maharaj, Michelle Griffin, and Usha Menon

Gynaecological Cancer Research Centre, UCL, London, UK

SUMMARY BOX

- Major efforts have been made to identify risk factors for ovarian cancer and to build risk-prediction models that combine epidemiological, genetic, and epigenetic factors in order to improve risk stratification.

- Future preventive strategies such as the oral contraceptive pill, aspirin, and opportunistic salpingectomy and screening strategies are likely to be based on individual risk estimates using such models.

- There is good evidence that multimodal screening using serum CA125 interpreted using ROCA with TVS as a second-line test has encouraging performance characteristics.

- Screening for ovarian cancer in the general population is currently not recommended. However, results of the UK Collaborative Trial of Ovarian Cancer Screening suggest a mortality reduction associated with multimodal screening of around 20%. If this is confirmed on further follow-up of two to three years, it is likely to have an impact on future recommendations.

- Women at high risk are advised to undergo risk-reducing salpingo-oophorectomy. For those opting not to undergo surgery, in the UK screening is currently not available on the NHS, but is advocated at six-monthly intervals in the USA.

- A drive to develop a new generation of screening tests based on tumour DNA and novel specimens such as cervical samples is under way.

Ovarian cancer (OC) is the most fatal of all gynaecological malignancies and accounts for around 4% of all cancers diagnosed in women. Worldwide, there are 239 000 new cases of OC each year, of whom 7270 are in the UK [1]. While 10-year age-standardized survival has increased in England from 18% during 1971–1972 to 35% during 2010–2011, two-thirds of women die within 10 years of diagnosis [2]. Most of the improvement in survival has occurred in early-stage

---

Cancer Prevention and Screening: Concepts, Principles and Controversies, First Edition.
Edited by Rosalind A. Eeles, Christine D. Berg, and Jeffrey S. Tobias.
© 2019 John Wiley & Sons, Inc. Published 2019 by John Wiley & Sons, Inc.

disease, highlighting the importance of diagnosing early-stage/low-volume disease. This has led to ongoing efforts to explore risk stratification, prevention, and screening, which form the focus of this chapter. Given that epithelial OC is a heterogeneous disease, it is unlikely that one strategy will be effective for all histological subtypes (high-grade serous, endometrioid, clear-cell, low-grade serous, mucinous). In addition, recent evidence on precursor lesions such as serous tubal intraepithelial carcinoma (STIC) in a proportion of high-grade serous cancers suggests the need to explore novel solutions beyond routine tests such as serum CA125 and transvaginal ultrasound.

Lifetime risk of ovarian cancer

The average woman's lifetime risk of ovarian cancer is 1.9% [3], but there are women at substantially higher (40–60%) and lower risk. It is increasingly possible to stratify women based on their genetic and epidemiological risk factors [3].

Risk factors

Age
There is a strong correlation with age, with 83% of cases occurring in women over 50 years. The incidence rates rise sharply from an age-standardized rate of 8.9 per 100 000 in women aged 35–39 to a peak of 69.2 per 100 000 in those aged 80–84 [4].

Family history
The strongest risk factor is a family history of breast and multiple ovarian cancers [5] or the Lynch syndrome cancers (bowel, endometrium, stomach, kidney, ovary, skin in multiple relatives) [6, 7]. Women with a single first-degree relative with ovarian cancer may have up to a threefold increased risk [8]. Genetic predisposition could be due to alterations in the following:

High-penetrance genes
These include mutations in the *BRCA1* and *BRCA2* genes, with average cumulative risk of epithelial OC by the age of 70 of 40–60% (*BRCA1*) and 11–27% (*BRCA2*) mutation carriers [9]. Emerging evidence suggests that *BRCA* germline mutations are present in 14% of women with invasive nonmucinous epithelial ovarian cancer, and 22% of those with high-grade serous epithelial ovarian cancer [10]. This has led to efforts to extend genetic testing for *BRCA* genes to all women with nonmucinous epithelial OC at the point of diagnosis. *BRCA* mutations occur at a rate of 1 in 300 to 1 in 500 in most populations [11], but significantly increase to 1 in 40 in the Ashkenazi Jewish population [11]. In the latter group, there is growing evidence that identification of individuals through family history alone misses over half of those with mutations in *BRCA1/2*

[12–15]. Using systematic testing in such populations with a high prevalence of mutations has recently been shown to be acceptable and cost-effective [16], and suggests that 3.6% of OCs could be prevented if population testing for *BRCA1/2* was available [17].

In Lynch syndrome, the lifetime risk of OC is lower and related to the specific mutations (approximately 2–15%) [18] in at least five different DNA mismatch repair genes [19], with the highest risk in *MLH1* and *MSH2* carriers.

Moderate-penetrance genes

Several susceptibility genes that confer more moderate penetrance risks of OC, such as *RAD51C* [20, 21], *RAD51D* [22], and *BRIP1* [23], have been described and may account for the excess familial risk in these women. The magnitude of risk associated with these alleles seems to be similar to those associated with *BRCA2* mutations. Most recent data suggest that *RAD51C* mutations are associated with a 6.8-fold increased risk of OC, *RAD51D* with a 10-fold increased risk [24], while *BRIP1* deleterious mutations carry a relative risk of OC of 11, increasing to 14 for high-grade serous OCs [25]. Some of these moderate-penetrance genes have been included in commercially available gene-testing panels for ovarian (OvaNEXT™) and breast and ovarian cancer (GeneDX™), without sufficient evidence to support their clinical significance. These multigene panels are constrained by the accuracy of prediction/definition of risk and clinical use [26].

Low-penetrance inherited genetic variants

Through the efforts of the Ovarian Cancer Association Consortium, a worldwide initiative currently consisting of 76 groups, 37 common low-risk (low-penetrance) loci have been identified [27–37], with the strongest association with the serous subtype. Subtype-specific single-nucleotide polymorphisms (SNPs) for the other histological subtypes have also been identified [38]. Individually, these loci confer an increase in relative risk of 1.2–1.4. Despite possible risk stratification based on these SNPs, the clinical implications are still not clear. Some of these loci have been shown to alter OC risk in mutation carriers, with four of these being associated with OC risk in *BRCA2* carriers and two in *BRCA1* carriers [39]. Despite the huge effort in identifying new disease susceptibility loci, the known genetic factors identified so far only account for less than half of the heritable risk for OC [8]. This indicates that other susceptibility alleles exist and that only a fraction of the risk variants have been identified. A major consortia-wide effort (Collaborative Oncological Gene-environment Study, COGS) has contributed to identifying some of the 37 loci included above [29]. However, risk stratification based on the emerging genetic factors will need to be carefully thought through [40].

Epidemiological factors

Established protective factors for OC include oral contraceptive pill (OCP) use, pregnancy, breast-feeding, and tubal ligation, thought to exert their effect through reduction of the number of ovulatory cycles in a woman, while nulliparity and infertility are associated with increased risk (Table 23.1). Of particular interest is

Table 23.1 Risk factors for ovarian cancer (OC).

Risk Factor	OR/RR	95% CI	Author	Year
Oral contraceptive pill (OCP)	0.73	0.66–0.81	Havrilesky et al. [85]	2013
OCP duration (>120 months)	0.43	0.37–0.51		
OCP age at first use (<20)	0.63	0.45–0.89		
OCP type (combined)	0.68	0.55–0.83	Faber et al. [86]	2013
OCP type (combined and progestin only)	0.5	0.28–0.87		
OCP type (progestin only)	0.97	0.45–2.14		
Tubal ligation	0.82	0.68–0.97	Rice et al. [41]	2013
Tubal ligation* (adjusted for age, OCP use, parity)	0.33	0.16–0.64	Hankinson et al. [87]	1993
Tubal ligation	0.87	0.78–0.98	Madsen et al. [44]	2015
Primary invasive epithelial ovarian cancer				
Serous	0.92	0.79–1.08		
Endometrioid	0.66	0.47–0.93		
Mucinous	1.25	0.94–1.67		
Clear cell	1.03	0.65–1.62		
Other	0.6	0.43–0.83		
Borderline	1.03	0.89–1.21		
Salpingectomy			Madsen et al. [44]	2015
Unilateral	0.9	0.72–1.12		
Bilateral	0.58	0.36–0.95		
Hysterectomy with unilateral oophorectomy	0.65	0.45–0.94	Rice et al. [41]	2013
Simple hysterectomy	1.09	0.83–1.42		
Age ≥45	0.64	0.40–1.02		
Underwent procedure within 10 years of questionnaire	0.65	0.38–1.13		
Overall (regardless of year of OC diagnosis)	0.81	0.72–0.92	Jordan et al. [43]	2013
Median year of OC diagnosis pre-2000	0.7	0.65–0.76		
Median year of OC diagnosis post-2000	1.18	1.06–1.31		

Continued

Table 23.1 Continued

Parity			Fortner et al. [88]	2015
Full-term pregnancy	0.73	0.58–0.92		
Borderline	1.12	0.59–2.13		
Type I invasive epithelial ovarian cancer	0.47	0.33–0.69		
Type II invasive epithelial ovarian cancer	0.81	0.61–1.06		
Parous	0.71	0.61–0.85	Yang et al. [89]	2012
Serous	0.83	0.65–1.06		
Endometrioid	0.49	0.30–0.80		
Mucinous	0.54	0.25–1.14		
Clear cell	0.28	0.13–0.62		
Other	0.76	0.56–1.04		
Breastfeeding			Fortner et al. [88]	2015
Borderline	1.02	0.54–1.93		
Type I	0.67	0.41–1.08		
Type II	0.85	0.64–1.13		
Infertility treatment			Jensen et al. [90]	2009
Gonadotrophins	0.83	0.50–1.37		
Clomifene	1.14	0.79–1.64		
Human chorionic gonadotrophin	0.89	0.62–1.29		
Gonadotrophin-releasing hormone	0.8	0.42–1.51		
Endometriosis			Pearce et al. [54]	2012
Low-grade serous	2.11	1.39–3.20		
Endometrioid	2.04	1.67–2.48		
Clear cell	3.05	2.43–3.84		
Obesity			Olsen et al. [46]	2013
Serous	0.98	0.94–1.02		
Low-grade serous	1.13	1.03–1.25		
Endometrioid	1.17	1.11–1.23		
Mucinous	1.19	1.06–1.32		
Borderline (serous)	1.24	1.18–1.30		

Continued

Table 23.1 Continued

Risk Factor	OR/RR	95% CI	Author	Year
Cigarette smoking			Faber et al. [47]	2013
Current				
Mucinous	1.13	1.03–1.65		
Borderline (mucinous)	1.83	1.39–2.41		
Former				
Borderline (serous)	1.3	1.12–1.50		
Hormone replacement therapy (HRT)	1.33	1.16–1.53	Yang et al. [89]	2012
Current users			Collaborative Group on Epidemiological Studies of Ovarian Cancer [48]	2015
<5 years duration	1.43	1.31–1.56		
≥5 years duration	1.41	1.34–1.49		
Past users (<5 years since last use)				
<5 years duration	1.17	0.97–1.38		
≥5 years duration	1.29	1.11–1.49		
Past users (≥5 years since last use)				
<5 years duration	0.94	0.88–1.02		
≥5 years duration	1.1	1.01–1.20		
Estradiol-only therapy (5 years or more)			Koskela-Niska et al. [49]	2013
Serous	1.45	1.20–1.75		
Mucinous	0.35	0.19–0.67		
Estradiol–progestin therapy (5 years or more)				
Sequential	1.35	1.20–1.63		
Sequential (endometrioid)	1.88	1.24–2.86		
Ever use			Fortner et al. [88]	2015
Borderline	0.62	0.33–1.03		
Type I	0.92	0.56–1.51		
Type II	1.12	0.85–1.48		

Continued

Table 23.1 Continued

Aspirin			Baandrup et al. [91]	2015
Low dose	0.94	0.85–1.05		
Low dose – long-term use (over 5 years)	0.77	0.55–1.08		
150 mg	0.82	0.68–0.99		
Statins	0.98	0.87–1.10	Baandrup et al. [53]	2015
Mucinous	0.63	0.39–1.00		

CI, confidence interval; OR, odds ratio; RR, risk ratio.

the reduction of OC risk associated with the OCP, with over 10 years' use associated with a 50% risk reduction. A stronger protective effect of the OCP has been found in women at high risk due to *BRCA1/2* mutations, and again the effect is proportional to duration of use.

Hysterectomy had for many years been thought to reduce the risk of OC. More recently, no evidence of an association between simple hysterectomy and ovarian cancer has been reported [41, 42] with an increased risk of OC with hysterectomy reported in women being diagnosed with OC after 2000 [43]. Although this temporal change is difficult to explain, it may possibly be due to a decrease in overall hysterectomy rates, move towards a vaginal rather than abdominal approach, decline in bilateral salpingo-oophorectomy performed at the same time, and increase in the age of those undergoing the procedure.

There is now observational population-based data that bilateral salpingectomy alone may be associated with a 42% (odds ratio [OR] 0.58; 95% confidence interval [CI] 0.36–0.95) decrease in ovarian cancer risk [44].

Lifestyle factors

A lot of work has been done to clarify the risk reduction of various lifestyle approaches, such as alcohol [45], obesity [46], cigarette smoking [47], and talc use. Some of these are subtype specific, such as endometriosis, cigarette smoking, and obesity, while others are 'general risk factors'. Use of talc in the genital area has consistently been shown to increase the risk of OC and therefore it is not recommended.

Drugs

Hormone replacement therapy

Data from the observational studies show an increased risk of OC with hormone replacement therapy (HRT) use. An individual participant meta-analysis of 52 epidemiological studies reported that women who use hormone therapy for five years from around age 50 have about one extra ovarian cancer per 1000 users [48]. Estradiol-only therapy (if used for five years or more) increases the risk of serous OC by 45%, but decreases the risk of mucinous OC by 65%, while estradiol–progestin therapy (five years or more), if used as a sequential regimen, increases the risk by 35% compared to the continuous regimen, which did not (Table 23.1) [49].

Aspirin
More recently, low-dose aspirin has been shown to be associated with a reduction of ovarian [50] and endometrial cancer [51] risk in the general population. There is emerging evidence of risk reduction of ovarian and endometrial cancers in high-risk women with Lynch syndrome as well [52].

Statins
Limited data indicate a decreased risk of ovarian cancer among those using statins. Recently, a large Danish nationwide study of 4103 cases and 58 706 controls reported a neutral association between ever using statins and OC risk (OR 0.98, 95% CI 0.87–1.10) [53].

Other risk factors
Women with endometriosis are at an increased risk of epithelial OC. An analysis of 13 ovarian cancer case-control studies from the Ovarian Cancer Association Consortium has shown that women who self-reported endometriosis were substantially more likely to develop clear-cell (OR 3.05, 95% CI 2.43–3.84), low-grade serous (OR 2.11, 95% CI 1.39–3.20), and invasive endometrioid ovarian cancers (OR 2.04, 95% CI 1.67–2.48) [54]. There was no association between endometriosis and risk of mucinous or high-grade serous invasive epithelial OC or borderline tumours of either subtype. Risk related to endometriosis was less pronounced in multiparous women compared to nulliparous, again suggesting the protective effect of parity.

Recent evidence indicates that endometriosis-associated OC shows favourable characteristics, including low-grade and early-stage disease. But it is unlikely that the presence of endometriosis affects disease progression after the onset of OC. Consequently, in those with a diagnosis of endometriosis, timely treatment may be advisable to reduce the OC risk.

Risk-prediction models

Significant efforts are under way to improve risk prediction. There are several predictive models that use family history to estimate mutation risk in *BRCA* genes and lifetime risk of OC, such as BRCAPRO, BODICEA, and Myriad II, as well as the Finnish, US National Cancer Institute, University of Pennsylvania, and Yale University models [55]. Although each model is unique based on the methods/ population used, their performances in identifying women who have a high probability of carrying a *BRCA1/2* mutation have similar discrimination ability, ranging from 71% (Yale) to 83% (BRCAPRO) [56]. Such models may prove as useful tools to assess cancer risk on a population basis in the future. Major efforts are now under way to further improve prediction using a combination of genetic and epidemiological factors. It is likely that in the future risks of a lower magnitude (<10% lifetime risk of OC) may instigate consultations between women and their gynaecologists [3].

Prevention

In the context of OC, all strategies available reduce risk but do not completely eliminate the possibility of a cancer arising in the future.

Risk-reducing surgery

Risk-reducing salpingo-oophorectomy (RRSO) reduces ovarian cancer risk in *BRCA* mutation carriers by 85% [57]. It is associated with a relatively low complication rate (3.9%; 95% CI 2.0–6.7%) [5]. RRSO is routinely recommended in high-risk women after completion of their families. While the standard recommendation is from the age of 35, it is important to individualize this, especially in women with *BRCA2* gene mutations. In Lynch syndrome women, the risk-reducing surgery includes hysterectomy. Removal of the ovaries leads to premature menopause, which is associated with increased morbidity and mortality, and hence RRSO is usually accompanied by use of HRT till the age of natural menopause [58]. Based on emerging evidence that most high-grade serous ovarian cancers originate in the fallopian tubes and involve the ovary secondarily [59], removal of the tubes alone has been put forward as an alternative risk-reducing strategy. McAlpine et al. [60] have already reported on the uptake, risk, and complications of opportunistic salpingectomy. This has been widely implemented in women undergoing pelvic surgery in Canada and endorsed by the Society of Gynecologic Oncology in the USA [61]. Gynaecologists surveyed in the UK have indicated that they would be willing to undertake bilateral salpingectomy at the time of hysterectomy (92%) or tubal ligation (65%) [62]. More recently, an approach based on bilateral salpingectomy with delayed oophorectomy in BRCA mutation carriers is being trialed in the United States [63]. Similar trial is to launch in the United Kingdom.

Aspirin

In the CAPP2 randomized controlled trial (RCT) of Lynch syndrome women, aspirin (600 mg a day for at least two years) reduced the risk of colorectal cancer (hazard ratio [HR] 0.63, 95% CI 0.35–1.13, p=0.12), with a similar effect on other noncolorectal Lynch syndrome cancers (HR 0.63, 95% CI 0.34–1.19, p=0.16) [52]. Hence it is increasingly applied (with some women using a 75 mg low-dose regime) to reduce the risk of ovarian and endometrial cancer in these women. The current trial (CaPP3) [64] due to report in 2020 is assessing the lowest dose (100, 300, and 600 mg per day) that confers such risk reduction in these women.

Oral contraceptive pill

Due to side effects, it is not currently recommended that women, especially those in their 40s, take OCP solely for OC risk reduction. That is, however, an added advantage, especially in those at high risk, who are considering using OCP for contraception or other medical indications.

Screening for ovarian cancer

Currently, there is no screening programme for ovarian cancer. In 2012, the US Preventative Task Force (USPSTF) reaffirmed its previous recommendation that screening should not be undertaken in the general population [65]. The National Institute for Health and Clinical Excellence (NICE) guidance in the UK advises that investigations should be carried out in women (especially if 50 years or over) only if reporting persistent or frequent symptoms (abdominal distension, early satiety, loss of appetite, pelvic or abdominal pain, or increased urinary urgency and/or frequency), particularly if more than 12 times per month [66]. However, recent evidence from the UK trial suggests that annual screening in the general population using a multimodal approach may be associated with a mortality benefit, which needs to be confirmed on further follow-up [67].

General population

In view of the improved survival in OC patients detected at an early stage, and the fact that a screening strategy based on CA125 and ultrasound demonstrated survival advantage in the screened women, large RCTs of OC screening were set up in the mid-1990s. The results of the ovarian arm of the Prostate, Lung, Colorectal and Ovarian (PLCO) Cancer Screening Trial, an RCT where 30 630 women aged 55–74 between 1993 and 2007 underwent screening using serum CA125 with a cut-off of ≥35 kU/l and transvaginal ultrasound (TVS) for four years, followed by CA125 alone for a further two years, showed no mortality benefit (mortality rate ratio 1.18, 95% CI 0.91–1.54) at a median follow-up of 12.4 years. Moreover, there was a high (15%) serious complication rate in women undergoing surgery for false-positive findings [68]. Updated data based on extended follow up at median of 14.7 years re-confirmed the lack of mortality benefit [69].

More encouraging data from the Kentucky single-arm ultrasound study of 37 293 women (a mean follow up of 5.8 years) found five-year survival rates in women with primary invasive epithelial cancer who were screened to be significantly higher (74.8% ± 6.6%) compared to unscreened nonstudy women (53.7% ± 2.3%) [70]. However, these rates are not comparable due to the 'lead-time effect' of screening and the likelihood of a significant healthy volunteer effect in those who participated in the screening study [71].

The largest RCT to date is the UK Collaborative Trial of Ovarian Cancer Screening (UKCTOCS), in which 202 638 women from the general population were randomized to no intervention (control) or annual screening using either transvaginal ultrasound (USS, n = 50 639) or serum CA125 interpreted using the 'Risk of Ovarian Cancer' algorithm (ROCA), with transvaginal ultrasound as a second-line test (multimodal screening, MMS, n = 50 640). Screening was completed at the end of 2011. On the prevalence screen, both MMS and USS strategies had encouraging sensitivity for primary invasive epithelial ovarian/tubal cancers (iEOC; 89.5% and 75%, respectively) [72]. During incidence screening in the MMS arm, sensitivity and specificity of the multimodal strategy for iEOC was 86%, with 4.8 women undergoing surgery/detected iEOC. The ROCA assigns risk of ovarian cancer based on age and CA125 profile. Interpreting the annual serum CA125 using the ROCA detected 86.5% (134/155) of iEOC diagnosed within one year of the screen, while an approach using fixed CA125 cut-off at the last annual screen of >35, >30, or >22U/mL would have identified 41.3%, 48.4%, and 66.5%, respectively. The area under the curve for ROCA (0.915) was significantly (p = 0.0027) higher than for a single threshold rule (0.869), with screening using ROCA doubling the number of screen-detected iEOCs compared to a fixed cut-off [73]. Independent validation of the UK findings of high specificity and positive predictive value of ROCA was reported from a single-arm US prospective study of 4051 low-risk postmenopausal women [74].

Mortality outcome data from UKCTOCS based on follow-up until 31 December 2014 suggests that screening using the multimodal strategy may result in a reduction in ovarian cancer mortality [67]. There was a significant stage shift of iEOC and primary peritoneal cancers in the MMS arm (36.1% Stage I/II) compared to control (23.9% Stage I/II). The reduction in ovarian and tubal cancer deaths (MMS 15%; USS 11%) over 14 years was not significant in the primary Cox analysis comparing either group to control. However, this overall estimate comprised a reduction of 8% in the first seven years of the trial and 23% in years 7–14 in the MMS group, and 2% and 21%, respectively, in the USS group. This delayed mortality effect of screening was similar to that seen in other screening trials, and was associated with a significant (p = 0.023) mortality reduction in the MMS versus control comparison, using the weighted log-rank analysis adopted by the PLCO trialists. A significant (p = 0.021) mortality reduction of 20% was also observed in the MMS group when the prevalent cases (women who had OC prior to the start of trial) were excluded from the analysis. The mortality reductions in the USS arm were not significant. With regard to harms, per 10 000 screens, 14 women in the MMS arm and 50 in the USS arm underwent trial surgery as a result of positive screen results and were then found to have only benign ovarian lesions or normal ovaries. The major surgical complication rate in the latter was low (3.1% MMS and 3.5% USS) and similar to those usually reported for such surgery. The initial cost-effectiveness analysis demonstrated that the MMS strategy falls within the NICE threshold [75]. Further follow up for four years is currently underway before firm conclusions on the efficacy and cost-effectiveness of screening can be reached.

High risk

Annual screening for OC is not recommended in high-risk women, as it is not effective in detecting early-stage disease [76]. A shorter screening interval of four months using serum CA125 interpreted by ROCA and transvaginal ultrasound was investigated in the UK Familial Ovarian Cancer Screening Study (UKFOCSS) Phase II. Such intensive screening will lead to women recalled for abnormal results experiencing transient cancer-specific distress, but there was no significant effect on general anxiety/depression or overall reassurance [77].

The results of Phase II demonstrate a significant stage shift in women diagnosed with invasive epithelial ovarian, tubal and peritoneal cancers within 1 year of last screen (63% Stage I-IIIA) compared with those diagnosed >1 year after screening ended (6% Stage I-IIIA; p=0.0004). Moreover, there were higher rates of zero residual disease after debulking (95% versus 72%; p=0.09) and lower rates of neoadjuvant chemotherapy (5% versus 44%; p=0.008) in those detected within a year of the last screen [78]. The performance of a similar strategy using ROCA has been evaluated prospectively in screening trials in women at high risk in the USA (Cancer Genetics Network, CGN, and Gynaecology Oncology Group, GOG) and reported similar stage shift [79].

There are currently differing views on whether screening should be offered to high-risk women. In the UK in the NHS there is no screening for OC in high-risk women, with risk management confined to RRSO and symptom awareness. However, in the USA, while the primary recommendation is risk-reducing surgery, the US National Comprehensive Cancer Network guidelines consider six-monthly screening using serum CA125 and TVS a reasonable approach for those who do not wish to undergo surgery.

Future directions

The goal is to develop a new generation of screening tests based on tumour DNA [80], in view of the recent emerging evidence that TP53 mutations could be detected in vaginal sections of 60% of patients with high-grade serous cancer, and novel specimens such as cervical samples [81]. More recently, a multi-analyte test (CancerSEEK) of eight biomarkers including CA125 and TP53 mutations exhibited a high sensitivity of 98% for ovarian cancer [82].

Symptom awareness

Symptoms for ovarian cancer, albeit nonspecific, are not 'silent', but may lead to earlier diagnosis with less tumour burden [83]. In the UK, NICE issued guidelines in 2011 stating that any women (especially those over 50) presenting to primary care with persistent abdominal distension/'bloating', feeling full and/or loss of appetite, pelvic/abdominal pain, increased urinary urgency and/or frequency, unexplained weight loss, fatigue, or changes in bowel habit should have a CA125 test followed by TVS. However, during the NHS campaign 'Be Clear on Cancer', the high prevalence (14% of those over 45 years presenting to primary care had frequent and/or severe symptoms) of these gynaecological cancer symptoms has become evident [84]. Use of public awareness campaigns is probably best aimed at those at high risk, as otherwise the burden in increase in consultation could be unmanageable.

Conclusion

There is a significant effort under way to identify epidemiological and genetic risk factors for ovarian cancer and improve on the current risk-prediction models so that prevention and screening can be tailored to the individual. In high-risk women, RRSO following completion of the family is recommended. There is an increasing trend to recommend low-dose aspirin to women with Lynch syndrome. There is good evidence that multimodal screening using serum CA125 interpreted using ROCA with TVS as a second-line test has the best performance characteristics to date. Recent data from UKCTOCS suggest that annual multimodal screening may be associated with a mortality benefit in the general population, with estimates of mortality reduction of around 20%. Further follow-up is required to confirm the effect size and the cost-effectiveness before any general population screening is considered. Recommendations for high-risk women who decide not to undergo RRSO are controversial. Whilst 4-monthly screening using ROCA demonstrated significant stage shift, screening is currently not available on the NHS in the UK, but is recommended six-monthly in the USA. In the meantime, major efforts are in progress to explore preventive strategies such as opportunistic bilateral salpingectomy in both the low- and high-risk populations, and to develop a new generation of screening tests based on tumour DNA and novel specimens such as cervical samples.

References

1 Cancer Research UK (2011). Ovarian cancer statistics. http://www.cancerresearchuk.org/health-professional/cancer-statistics/statistics-by-cancer-type/ovarian-cancer (accessed 14 March 2018).

2 Cancer Research UK (2011). Ovarian cancer survival statistics. http://www.cancerresearchuk.org/health-professional/cancer-statistics/statistics-by-cancer-type/ovarian-cancer/survival#heading-Two (accessed 14 March 2018).

3 Cancer Research UK (2011). Ovarian cancer statistics. http://www.cancerresearchuk.org/health-professional/cancer-statistics/statistics-by-cancer-type/ovarian-cancer#heading-Zero (accessed 14 March 2018).

4 Cancer Research UK (2011). Ovarian cancer incidence statistics. http://www.cancerresearchuk.org/health-professional/cancer-statistics/statistics-by-cancer-type/ovarian-cancer/incidence#heading-One (accessed 14 March 2018).

5 Manchanda, R., Abdelraheim, A., Johnson, M. et al. (2011). Outcome of risk-reducing salpingo-oophorectomy in BRCA carriers and women of unknown mutation status. *BJOG* 118 (7): 814–824.

6 Umar, A., Boland, C.R., Terdiman, J.P. et al. (2004). Revised Bethesda Guidelines for hereditary nonpolyposis colorectal cancer (Lynch syndrome) and microsatellite instability. *J. Natl Cancer Inst.* 96 (4): 261–268.

7 American College of Obstetricians and Gynecologists (2014). Lynch Syndrome. Society of Gynecologic Oncology: Practice Bulletin. https://www.sgo.org/wp-content/uploads/2012/09/2014-ACOG-bulletin.pdf (accessed 7 July 2015).

8 Jervis, S., Song, H., Lee, A. et al. (2014). Ovarian cancer familial relative risks by tumour subtypes and by known ovarian cancer genetic susceptibility variants. *J. Med. Genet.* 51 (2): 108–113.

9 Antoniou, A., Pharoah, P.D., Narod, S. et al. (2003). Average risks of breast and ovarian cancer associated with BRCA1 or BRCA2 mutations detected in case series unselected for family history: A combined analysis of 22 studies. *Am. J. Hum. Genet.* 72 (5): 1117–1130.

10 Alsop, K., Fereday, S., Meldrum, C. et al. (2012). BRCA mutation frequency and patterns of treatment response in BRCA mutation-positive women with ovarian cancer: A report from the Australian Ovarian Cancer Study Group. *J. Clin. Oncol.* 30 (21): 2654–2663.

11 Rosenthal, E., Moyes, K., Arnell, C. et al. (2015). Incidence of BRCA1 and BRCA2 non-founder mutations in patients of Ashkenazi Jewish ancestry. *Breast Cancer Res. Treat.* 149 (1): 223–227.

12 Manchanda, R., Loggenberg, K., Sanderson, S. et al. (2015). Population testing for cancer predisposing BRCA1/BRCA2 mutations in the Ashkenazi-Jewish community: A randomized controlled trial. *J. Natl Cancer Inst.* 107 (1): 379.

13 Metcalfe, K.A., Poll, A., Royer, R. et al. (2010). Screening for founder mutations in BRCA1 and BRCA2 in unselected Jewish women. *J. Clin. Oncol.* 28 (3): 387–391.

14 Gabai-Kapara, E., Lahad, A., Kaufman, B. et al. (2014). Population-based screening for breast and ovarian cancer risk due to BRCA1 and BRCA2. *Proc. Natl Acad. Sci. U. S. A.* 111 (39): 14205–14210.

15 King, M.C., Levy-Lahad, E., and Lahad, A. (2014). Population-based screening for BRCA1 and BRCA2: 2014 Lasker Award. *JAMA* 312 (11): 1091–1092.

16 Manchanda, R., Legood, R., Burnell, M. et al. (2015). Cost-effectiveness of population screening for BRCA mutations in Ashkenazi Jewish women compared with family history-based testing. *J. Natl Cancer Inst.* 107 (1): 380.

17 Finch, A., Bacopulos, S., Rosen, B. et al. (2014). Preventing ovarian cancer through genetic testing: A population-based study. *Clin. Genet.* 86 (5): 496–499.

18 Song, H., Cicek, M.S., Dicks, E. et al. (2014). The contribution of deleterious germline mutations in BRCA1, BRCA2 and the mismatch repair genes to ovarian cancer in the population. *Hum. Mol. Genet.* 23 (17): 4703–4709.

19 Bonadona, V., Bonaiti, B., Olschwang, S. et al. (2011). Cancer risks associated with germline mutations in MLH1, MSH2, and MSH6 genes in Lynch syndrome. *JAMA* 305 (22): 2304–2310.

20 Meindl, A., Hellebrand, H., Wiek, C. et al. (2010). Germline mutations in breast and ovarian cancer pedigrees establish RAD51C as a human cancer susceptibility gene. *Nature Genet.* 42 (5): 410–414.

21 Loveday, C., Turnbull, C., Ruark, E. et al. (2012). Germline RAD51C mutations confer susceptibility to ovarian cancer. *Nature Genet.* 44 (5): 475–476; author reply 6.

22 Loveday, C., Turnbull, C., Ramsay, E. et al. (2011). Germline mutations in RAD51D confer susceptibility to ovarian cancer. *Nature Genet.* 43 (9): 879–882.

23 Rafnar, T., Gudbjartsson, D.F., Sulem, P. et al. (2011). Mutations in BRIP1 confer high risk of ovarian cancer. *Nature Genet.* 43 (11): 1104–1107.

24 Song, H., Dicks, E., Ramus, S.J. et al. (2015). Contribution of germline mutations in the RAD51B, RAD51C and RAD51D genes to ovarian cancer in the population. *J. Clin. Oncol.* 33 (26): 2901–2907.

25 Ramus, S.J., Song, H., Dicks, E. et al. (2015). Germline mutations in the BRIP1, BARD1, PALB2 and NBN genes in women with ovarian cancer. *J. Natl Cancer Inst.* 107 (11): djv214.

26 Easton, D.F., Pharoah, P.D., Antoniou, A.C. et al. (2015). Gene-panel sequencing and the prediction of breast-cancer risk. *N. Engl. J. Med.* 372 (23): 2243–2257.

27 Song, H., Ramus, S.J., Tyrer, J. et al. (2009). A genome-wide association study identifies a new ovarian cancer susceptibility locus on 9p22.2. *Nature Genet.* 41 (9): 996–1000.

28 Goode, E.L., Chenevix-Trench, G., Song, H. et al. (2010). A genome-wide association study identifies susceptibility loci for ovarian cancer at 2q31 and 8q24. *Nature Genet.* 42 (10): 874–879.

29 Sakoda, L.C., Jorgenson, E., and Witte, J.S. (2013). Turning of COGS moves forward findings for hormonally mediated cancers. *Nature Genet.* 45 (4): 345–348.

30 Kuchenbaecker, K.B., Ramus, S.J., Tyrer, J. et al. (2015). Identification of six new susceptibility loci for invasive epithelial ovarian cancer. *Nature Genet.* 47 (2): 164–171.

31 Bolton, K.L., Tyrer, J., Song, H. et al. (2010). Common variants at 19p13 are associated with susceptibility to ovarian cancer. *Nature Genet.* 42 (10): 880–884.

32 Pharoah, P.D., Tsai, Y.Y., Ramus, S.J. et al. (2013). GWAS meta-analysis and replication identifies three new susceptibility loci for ovarian cancer. *Nature Genet.* 45 (4): 362–370.

33 Permuth-Wey, J., Lawrenson, K., Shen, H.C. et al. (2013). Identification and molecular characterization of a new ovarian cancer susceptibility locus at 17q21.31. *Nature Comm.* 4: 1627.

34 Shen, H., Fridley, B.L., Song, H. et al. (2013). Epigenetic analysis leads to identification of HNF1B as a subtype-specific susceptibility gene for ovarian cancer. *Nature Comm.* 4: 1628.

35 Couch, F.J., Wang, X., McGuffog, L. et al. (2013). Genome-wide association study in BRCA1 mutation carriers identifies novel loci associated with breast and ovarian cancer risk. *PLoS Genet.* 9 (3): e1003212.

36 Chen, K., Ma, H., Li, L. et al. (2014). Genome-wide association study identifies new susceptibility loci for epithelial ovarian cancer in Han Chinese women. *Nature Comm.* 5: 4682.

37 Phelan, C.M., Kuchenbaecker, K.B., Tyrer, J.P. et al. (2017). Identification of 12 new susceptibility loci for different histotypes of epithelial ovarian cancer. *Nature Genet.* 49 (5): 680–691.

38 Earp, M.A., Kelemen, L.E., Magliocco, A.M. et al. (2014). Genome-wide association study of subtype-specific epithelial ovarian cancer risk alleles using pooled DNA. *Human Genet.* 133 (5): 481–497.

39 Ramus, S.J., Antoniou, A.C., Kuchenbaecker, K.B. et al. (2012). Ovarian cancer susceptibility alleles and risk of ovarian cancer in BRCA1 and BRCA2 mutation carriers. *Human Mutat.* 33 (4): 690–702.

40 Hall, A.E., Chowdhury, S., Hallowell, N. et al. (2014). Implementing risk-stratified screening for common cancers: A review of potential ethical, legal and social issues. *J. Public Health.* 36 (2): 285–291.

41 Rice, M.S., Murphy, M.A., Vitonis, A.F. et al. (2013). Tubal ligation, hysterectomy and epithelial ovarian cancer in the New England Case-Control Study. *Int. J. Cancer* 133 (10): 2415–2421.

42 Wang, C., Liang, Z., Liu, X. et al. (2016). The Association between Endometriosis, Tubal Ligation, Hysterectomy and Epithelial Ovarian Cancer: Meta-Analyses. *Int. J. Environ. Res. Public Health.* 13 (11): 1138.

43 Jordan, S.J., Nagle, C.M., Coory, M.D. et al. (2013). Has the association between hysterectomy and ovarian cancer changed over time? A systematic review and meta-analysis. *Eur. J. Cancer* 49 (17): 3638–3647.

44 Madsen, C., Baandrup, L., Dehlendorff, C., and Kjaer, S.K. (2015). Tubal ligation and salpingectomy and the risk of epithelial ovarian cancer and borderline ovarian tumors: A nationwide case-control study. *Acta Obstet. Gynecol. Scand.* 94 (1): 86–94.

45 Kelemen, L.E., Bandera, E.V., Terry, K.L. et al. (2013). Recent alcohol consumption and risk of incident ovarian carcinoma: A pooled analysis of 5,342 cases and 10,358 controls from the Ovarian Cancer Association Consortium. *BMC Cancer* 13: 28.

46 Olsen, C.M., Nagle, C.M., Whiteman, D.C. et al. (2013). Obesity and risk of ovarian cancer subtypes: Evidence from the Ovarian Cancer Association Consortium. *Endocr. Relat. Cancer* 20 (2): 251–262.

47 Faber, M.T., Kjaer, S.K., Dehlendorff, C. et al. (2013). Cigarette smoking and risk of ovarian cancer: A pooled analysis of 21 case-control studies. *Cancer Causes Control* 24 (5): 989–1004.

48 Collaborative Group on Epidemiological Studies of Ovarian Cancer; Beral, V., Gaitskell, K., Hermon, C. et al. (2015). Menopausal hormone use and ovarian cancer risk: Individual participant meta-analysis of 52 epidemiological studies. *Lancet* 385 (9980): 1835–1842.

49 Koskela-Niska, V., Pukkala, E., Lyytinen, H. et al. (2013). Effect of various forms of post-menopausal hormone therapy on the risk of ovarian cancer: A population-based case control study from Finland. *Int. J. Cancer* 133 (7): 1680–1688.

50 Trabert, B., Ness, R.B., Lo-Ciganic, W.H. et al. (2014). Aspirin, nonaspirin nonsteroidal anti-inflammatory drug, and acetaminophen use and risk of invasive epithelial ovarian cancer: A pooled analysis in the Ovarian Cancer Association Consortium. *J. Natl Cancer Inst.* 106 (2): djt431.

51 Neill, A.S., Nagle, C.M., Protani, M.M. et al. (2013). Aspirin, nonsteroidal anti-inflammatory drugs, paracetamol and risk of endometrial cancer: A case-control study, systematic review and meta-analysis. *Int. J. Cancer* 132 (5): 1146–1155.

52 Burn, J., Gerdes, A.M., Macrae, F. et al. (2011). Long-term effect of aspirin on cancer risk in carriers of hereditary colorectal cancer: An analysis from the CAPP2 randomised controlled trial. *Lancet* 378 (9809): 2081–2087.

53 Baandrup, L., Dehlendorff, C., Friis, S. et al. (2015). Statin use and risk for ovarian cancer: A Danish nationwide case-control study. *Br. J. Cancer* 112 (1): 157–161.

54 Pearce, C.L., Templeman, C., Rossing, M.A. et al. (2012). Association between endometriosis and risk of histological subtypes of ovarian cancer: A pooled analysis of case-control studies. *Lancet Oncol.* 13 (4): 385–394.

55 Amir, E., Freedman, O.C., Seruga, B., and Evans, D.G. (2010). Assessing women at high risk of breast cancer: A review of risk assessment models. *J. Natl Cancer Inst.* 102 (10): 680–691.

56 Parmigiani, G., Chen, S., Iversen, E.S., Jr et al. (2007). Validity of models for predicting BRCA1 and BRCA2 mutations. *Ann. Intern. Med.* 147 (7): 441–450.

57 Marchetti, C., De Felice, F., Palaia, I. et al. (2014). Risk-reducing salpingo-oophorectomy: A meta-analysis on impact on ovarian cancer risk and all cause mortality in BRCA 1 and BRCA 2 mutation carriers. *BMC Women Health* 14: 150.

58 Parker, W.H., Feskanich, D., Broder, M.S. et al. (2013). Long-term mortality associated with oophorectomy compared with ovarian conservation in the nurses' health study. *Obstet. Gynecol.* 121 (4): 709–716.

59 Crum, C.P., Drapkin, R., Miron, A. et al. (2007). The distal fallopian tube: A new model for pelvic serous carcinogenesis. *Curr. Opin. Obstet. Gynecol.* 19 (1): 3–9.

60 McAlpine, J.N., Hanley, G.E., Woo, M.M. et al. (2014). Opportunistic salpingectomy: Uptake, risks, and complications of a regional initiative for ovarian cancer prevention. *Am. J. Obstet. Gynecol.* 210 (5): 471, e1–11.

61 Society of Gynecologic Oncology (2013). SGO Clinical Practice Statement: Salpingectomy for ovarian cancer prevention. https://www.sgo.org/clinical-practice/guidelines/sgo-clinical-practice-statement-salpingectomy-for-ovarian-cancer-prevention/ (accessed 22 July 2015).

62 Manchanda, R.C., Chandrasekaran, D., Saridogan, E. et al. (2015) Opportunistic bilateral salpingectomy (OBS) for prevention of ovarian cancer: Support for a clinical trial or routine care amongst UK clinicians. Newcastle: British Gynaecological Cancer Society.

63 Anderson M. (2017). Prophylactic salpingectomy with delayed oophorectomy, risk-reducing salpingo-oophorectomy, and ovarian cancer screening among BRCA mutation carriers: A proof-of-concept study (Study #2013-0340). [cited 23/07/2017]; Available from: https://www.mdanderson.org/patients-family/diagnosis-treatment/clinical-trials/clinical-trials-index/clinical-trials-detail.ID2013-0340.html.

64 CaPP3. CaPP3 Cancer Prevention Programme. (2017). Available from: http://www.capp3.org/.

65 Moyer, V.A.; Force USPST (2012). Screening for ovarian cancer: U.S. Preventive Services Task Force reaffirmation recommendation statement. *Ann. Intern. Med.* 157 (12): 900–904.

66 National Institute of Health and Clinical Excellence (2011). Ovarian cancer: Recognition and initial management. https://www.nice.org.uk/guidance/cg122 (accessed 14 July 2015).

67 Jacobs, I.J., Menon, U., Ryan, A. et al. (2016). Ovarian cancer screening and mortality in the UK Collaborative Trial of Ovarian Cancer Screening (UKCTOCS): A randomised controlled trial. *Lancet* 387 (10022): 945–956.

68 Buys, S.S., Partridge, E., Black, A. et al. (2011). Effect of screening on ovarian cancer mortality: The Prostate, Lung, Colorectal and Ovarian (PLCO) Cancer Screening Randomized Controlled Trial. *JAMA* 305 (22): 2295–2303.

69 Pinsky, P.F., Yu, F., Kramer, B.S. et al. (2016). Extended mortality results for ovarian cancer screening in the PLCO trial with median 15 years follow-up. *Gynecol. oncol.* 143 (2): 270–275.

70 van Nagell, J.R., Jr, DePriest, P.D., Ueland, F.R. et al. (2007). Ovarian cancer screening with annual transvaginal sonography: Findings of 25,000 women screened. *Cancer* 109 (9): 1887–1896.

71 Burnell, M., Gentry-Maharaj, A., Ryan, A. et al. (2011). Impact on mortality and cancer incidence rates of using random invitation from population registers for recruitment to trials. *Trials* 12: 61.

72 Menon, U., Gentry-Maharaj, A., Hallett, R. et al. (2009). Sensitivity and specificity of multimodal and ultrasound screening for ovarian cancer, and stage distribution of detected cancers: Results of the prevalence screen of the UK Collaborative Trial of Ovarian Cancer Screening (UKCTOCS). *Lancet Oncol.* 10 (4): 327–340.

73 Menon, U., Ryan, A., Kalsi, J. et al. (2015). Risk algorithm using serial biomarker measurements doubles the number of screen-detected cancers compared with a single-threshold rule in the United Kingdom Collaborative Trial of Ovarian Cancer Screening. *J. Clin. Oncol.* 33 (18): 2062–2071.

74 Lu, K.H., Skates, S., Hernandez, M.A. et al. (2013). A 2-stage ovarian cancer screening strategy using the Risk of Ovarian Cancer Algorithm (ROCA) identifies early-stage incident cancers and demonstrates high positive predictive value. *Cancer* 119 (19): 3454–3461.

75 Menon, U., McGuire, A.J., Raikou, M. et al. (2017). The cost-effectiveness of screening for ovarian cancer: results from the UK Collaborative Trial of Ovarian Cancer Screening (UKCTOCS). *Br. J. Cancer* 117 (5): 619–627.

76 Rosenthal, A.N., Fraser, L., Manchanda, R. et al. (2013). Results of annual screening in phase I of the United Kingdom familial ovarian cancer screening study highlight the need for strict adherence to screening schedule. *J. Clin. Oncol.* 31 (1): 49–57.

77 Brain, K.E., Lifford, K.J., Fraser, L. et al. (2012). Psychological outcomes of familial ovarian cancer screening: No evidence of long-term harm. *Gynecol. Oncol.* 127 (3): 556–563.

78 Rosenthal, A.N., Fraser, L.S.M., Philpott, S. et al. (2017). Evidence of stage shift in women diagnosed with ovarian cancer during phase II of the United Kingdom familial ovarian cancer screening study. Journal of clinical oncology: official journal of the American Society of Clinical Oncology 35 (13): 1411–1420.

79 Skates, S.J., Greene. M.H., Buys, S.S. et al. (2017). Early detection of ovarian cancer using the risk of ovarian cancer algorithm with frequent CA125 testing in women at increased familial risk – combined results from two screening trials. Clinical cancer research: an official journal of the American Association for Cancer Research. 23 (14): 3628–3637.

80 Erickson, B.K., Kinde, I., Dobbin, Z.C. et al. (2014). Detection of somatic TP53 mutations in tampons of patients with high-grade serous ovarian cancer. *Obstet. Gynecol.* 124 (5): 881–885.

81 Kinde, I., Bettegowda, C., Wang, Y. et al. (2013). Evaluation of DNA from the Papanicolaou test to detect ovarian and endometrial cancers. *Sci. Transl. Med.* 5 (167): 167ra4.

82 Cohen, J.D., Li, L., Wang, Y. et al. (2018). Detection and localization of surgically resectable cancers with a multi-analyte blood test. *Science* 359 (6378): 926–930.

83 Gilbert, L., Basso, O., Sampalis, J. et al. (2012). Assessment of symptomatic women for early diagnosis of ovarian cancer: Results from the prospective DOvE pilot project. *Lancet Oncol.* 13 (3): 285–291.

84 Cancer Research UK (2014). Ovarian cancer campaign: Be clear on cancer. http://www.cancerresearchuk.org/health-professional/early-diagnosis-activities/be-clear-on-cancer/ovarian-cancer-campaign (accessed 22 July 2015).

85 Havrilesky, L.J., Gierisch, J.M., Moorman, P.G. et al. (2013). Oral contraceptive use for the primary prevention of ovarian cancer. *Evid. Rep. Technol. Assess.* 2013 (212): 1–514.

86 Faber, M.T., Jensen, A., Frederiksen, K. et al. (2013). Oral contraceptive use and impact of cumulative intake of estrogen and progestin on risk of ovarian cancer. *Cancer Causes Control* 24 (12): 2197–2206.

87 Hankinson, S.E., Hunter, D.J., Colditz, G.A. et al. (1993). Tubal ligation, hysterectomy, and risk of ovarian cancer: A prospective study. *JAMA* 270 (23): 2813–2818.

88 Fortner, R.T., Ose, J., Merritt, M.A. et al. (2015). Reproductive and hormone-related risk factors for epithelial ovarian cancer by histologic pathways, invasiveness and histologic subtypes: Results from the EPIC cohort. *Int. J. Cancer* 137 (5): 1196–1208.

89 Yang, H.P., Trabert, B., Murphy, M.A. et al. (2012). Ovarian cancer risk factors by histologic subtypes in the NIH-AARP Diet and Health Study. *Int. J. Cancer* 131 (4): 938–948.

90 Jensen, A., Sharif, H., Frederiksen, K., and Kjaer, S.K. (2009). Use of fertility drugs and risk of ovarian cancer: Danish Population Based Cohort Study. *BMJ* 338: b249.

91 Baandrup, L., Kjaer, S.K., Olsen, J.H. et al. (2015). Low-dose aspirin use and the risk of ovarian cancer in Denmark. *Ann. Oncol.* 26 (4): 787–792.

CHAPTER 24

Screening for testicular cancer

Kevin Litchfield[1], Clare Turnbull[2], and Robert A. Huddart[3]

[1] Division of Genetics and Epidemiology, The Institute of Cancer Research; Translational Cancer Therapeutics Laboratory, The Francis Crick Institute, London, UK
[2] William Harvey Research Institute, Queen Mary University; Division of Genetics and Epidemiology, The Institute of Cancer Research; Department of Clinical Genetics, Guy's and St Thomas' NHS Foundation Trust, London, UK
[3] The Institute of Cancer Research, London, UK

SUMMARY BOX

- Carcinoma *in situ* (CIS) is a pre-invasive precursor state of testicular germ cell tumour (TGCT), which is clinically detectable postpuberty in men who would otherwise go on to develop TGCT.

- A set of genetic risk variants (single-nucleotide polymorphisms or SNPs) for TGCT has been identified, which offer much stronger stratification of genetic risk for TGCT than equivalent SNP sets for most common tumours.

- Screening tools available for TGCT include semen assay, SNP profiling, risk assessment based on clinical notes/family history, and testicular biopsy.

- Testicular biopsy is currently undertaken in many centres in men deemed at elevated risk of TGCT.

- No wide-scale programmes of TGCT screening are currently in place, largely due to the rare nature of TGCT, the effectiveness of current treatment, the high rates of survival, and the invasive nature of confirmatory testicular biopsy.

- The motivation for further developing TGCT screening programmes is threefold: preventing cancers in young men; reducing treatment-induced survivorship issues; and averting treatment resistance.

- Future scientific and technological developments may provide a rationale for a shift from the status quo and to offering screening for TGCT to more men.

Testicular germ cell tumour (TGCT) is the most common cancer affecting young men, with a mean age at diagnosis of 36 years [1, 2]. Germ cell tumours account for over 95% of all testicular cancers and are commonly divided into two main histological subtypes: seminomas, which resemble undifferentiated primary germ cells; and nonseminomas, which show differing degrees of differentiation. Over

---

Cancer Prevention and Screening: Concepts, Principles and Controversies, First Edition.
Edited by Rosalind A. Eeles, Christine D. Berg, and Jeffrey S. Tobias.
© 2019 John Wiley & Sons, Inc. Published 2019 by John Wiley & Sons, Inc.

18 000 new cases of TGCT are diagnosed annually in Europe, and incidence rates have increased rapidly in recent decades, approximately doubling over the last 40 years in Western European and North American populations [3]. Incidence of the disease varies considerably between ethnic groups, with the highest rates observed in Caucasians, where lifetime TGCT risk is 0.5%. There have been significant advances in the treatment of testicular cancer, owing to the exceptional sensitivity of malignant testicular germ cells to platinum-based chemotherapies. Today a cure is expected in over 95% of all patients, and in around 80% of patients presenting with metastatic disease [4, 5]. However, this is at the cost of considerable treatment-related survivorship issues, such as an increased risk of metabolic syndrome, infertility, and secondary cancer, experienced by men for many decades following diagnosis and treatment in their third or fourth decade [6–8]. In addition, there are limited options for patients who demonstrate platinum resistance, a group for whom the long-term survival rate is only 10–15% [9]. Studies in families have consistently demonstrated a strong familial relative risk, and twin and immigrant studies support a strong genetic basis to TGCT [10–12]. Negative results from linkage analysis along with recent successful findings from genome-wide association studies (GWAS) suggest that the genetic architecture of TGCT risk is highly polygenic. GWAS has so far identified 49 risk loci for TGCT [13–24], with individual SNPs carrying per allele odds ratios (OR) in excess of 2.5, among the highest reported in GWAS of any cancer type [25]. Collectively, the 19 risk SNPs explain over 30% of the excess familial risk of TGCT [26].

TGCT arises from a noninvasive precursor lesion, termed carcinoma in situ (CIS) [27]. Clinical and molecular observations demonstrate that oncogenesis is initiated during foetal development, when normal progenitor germ cells transform into CIS [28–30]. Subsequent proliferation of CIS cells occurs during puberty, likely secondary to hormonal influences [31, 32]. The incidence of CIS is equivalent to the lifetime risk of developing TGCT, which, combined with longitudinal studies, has led to wide acceptance that CIS invariably precedes and progresses to invasive TGCT. The strong genetics of TGCT, coupled with CIS acting as a robust biomarker, present in all those who will go on to develop invasive TGCT, offer an attractive schema for stratified disease screening. It is important to note, however, that while these factors offer a plausible theoretical model, no current large screening programmes for testicular cancer are in place [33, 34]. This is due to broader epidemiological and clinical factors, discussed in detail in what follows. In addition, we review in this chapter examples of ad hoc screening that are currently implemented and the tools used, as well as discussing the technological advancements which may lead to broader programmes.

Approaches to screening

Testicular self-examination

The majority of TGCTs present as a painless lump in the testis. Testicular self-examination (TSE) promotes regular self-examination to detect early changes in the testis. Diagnostic delay leads to patients presenting with more advanced disease [35]. It is hoped that this will lead to earlier presentation and a reduction in presentation of advanced disease, and thus improve survival. This approach has been widely promoted by men's charities, but robust evidence of its effectiveness is lacking. A number of charities (Cancer Research UK, Everyman, Orchid) promoted this approach in the UK, and its wider usage and increased awareness have been linked to shorter times of presentation, smaller tumours, and earlier stage at presentation [36]. The main criticism of this approach has been in increasing psychological distress and detection/presentation of men for medical care with incidental and benign testicular abnormalities. The US Preventive Services Task Force (USPSTF) recommended against TSE screening programmes based on the lack of evidence of effectiveness, presentation of false-positive findings, and good prognosis of treatment for more advanced disease [37]. Aberger et al. [38], however, have reported that the costs of screening may be offset by the excess cost of treating advanced disease. This excess cost was equivalent to 180–190 office visits with ultrasound examination, suggesting that promoting this 'free' screening test may not increase costs, and indeed may be cost saving. It seems reasonable to recommend this approach to patients at high risk of TGCT, due for example to personal or family history. It should be noted that this approach enables earlier cancer detection, not prevention.

Ultrasound screening

Ultrasound is commonly used to confirm the diagnosis of TGCT with a high degree of accuracy [39]. Ultrasound can detect impalpable lesions and thus detect TGCT at an earlier stage than clinical examination or TSE. There is, however, a significant false-positive rate, with difficulty in distinguishing between TGCT and benign stromal tumours and other testicular lesions. In some studies, as many as 25% of impalpable lesions detected by ultrasound had such a benign aetiology [40]. Routine ultrasound has been advocated for patients with ultrasound-detected testicular lesions such as microlithiasis that are considered to be a risk factor for developing TGCT, but its value has been questioned [41]. Currently there is no clear evidence that routine ultrasound screening improves outcomes or will be cost-effective.

Detection of CIS: Testicular biopsy

The presence of CIS can be ascertained in postpubertal males via testicular biopsy, with CIS taken as being a lesion highly or wholly predictive of future TGCT (see Figure 24.1). Testicular biopsy has an excellent diagnostic accuracy, with the current double-site biopsy procedure (as recommended in European guidelines) achieving sensitivity of 97.5% and overall accuracy of 99.8% in a large series of 2300 patients [42]. Following CIS detection, progression to invasive TGCT is observed in 50% of cases within five years, 70% of cases within seven years, and in almost all cases eventually [42]. On detection of CIS, typically orchidectomy would be performed. This therefore obviates waiting for the development of invasive disease, the potential requirement for chemotherapy or radiation treatment, and the risk of presentation with advanced and/or treatment-refractory disease.

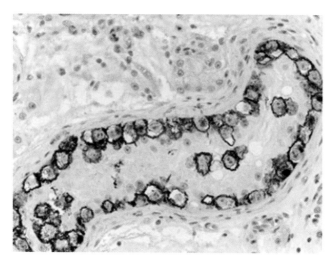

Figure 24.1 Histological section of testicular biopsy specimen: CIS cells are stained dark and are located at the basement membrane of the seminiferous tubule.

However, testicular biopsy is an invasive procedure, frequently conducted under general anaesthetic, and is associated with a surgical complication rate of 2.8% [42]. While the majority of surgical complications are superficial wound infections that can be managed conservatively, in a small minority of complications repeat surgery is required, and rarely loss of the biopsied testicle has been reported. Generally, testicular biopsy is considered a low-risk procedure assuming that the rules of good surgical care are followed. Nevertheless, testicular biopsy is invasive, costly, and time-consuming to the patient and health-care service, and therefore necessarily remains restricted to contexts in which there is a reasonably high detection rate.

Detection of CIS: Semen assay

Recently CIS has also been shown to be detectable by immunocytological techniques, based on identification of foetal germ cell markers in cells found in semen samples [43]. The technology underlying immunocytological detection is under ongoing development and trials of clinical implementation in high-risk groups of men have been undertaken [43]. However, this emerging technology could really transform screening for TGCT, as the assays are noninvasive and avoid unnecessary biopsy procedures. The current semen assays offer sensitivity of 67% and specificity of 98% [43]. While the high specificity means that false-positive results are rare, due to lower rates of sensitivity semen analysis will currently miss one in three cases of TGCT. However, it is anticipated that technical and technological developments in the assay will improve the sensitivity. If rates of 80–90% can be achieved, this technology offer a viable method to detect CIS and prevent invasive TGCT in broader population groups.

Identifying men at high risk

It is unlikely that population screening for TGCT will be viable due to disease frequency and prognosis (see later discussion). This raises the question of whether we can identify men with elevated risk that could be identified for future screening programmes.

Risk assessment based on medical history

Recognized risk factors for TGCT in the medical history include past history of germ cell tumour and history of undescended testis (UDT) [44]. The evidence supporting these as risk factors is strong. Several follow-up studies have demonstrated that TGCT in the ipsilateral testis confers a 12-fold elevated risk of disease in the contralateral testicle [45]. Based on these elevated risk factors, screening of the contralateral testis at the time of primary orchidectomy is routine practice in a number of centres in Germany and Denmark. However, this practice has been criticized and is not implemented in many other countries, such as the UK and USA [46]. The risk of TGCT in men with UDT has been widely studied, with a large meta-analysis of 20 case-control studies across 1976–2003 reporting a near fivefold elevation in TGCT risk [47].

Associations with other testicular abnormalities have also been variously reported, including microlithiasis, testicular dysgenesis, and infertility [44, 48, 49]. The rise in TGCT incidence has been accompanied by a comparable fall in global sperm counts, prompting the hypothesis that TGCT may be aetiologically linked to male reproductive abnormalities as a part of the so-called testicular dysgenesis syndrome. Genetic studies have found that shared risk factors, such as the chromosome Y GR/GR deletion, predispose to both sets of conditions [50]. A large meta-analysis shows that subfertile men have a 1.6-fold increased risk of TGCT. In a Danish study reviewing over 200 contralateral biopsy specimens in men after a first TGCT, evidence of testicular dysgenesis, such as CIS, undifferentiated sertoli cells, and microcalcifications, was observed in 25% of samples.

Overall, TGCT screening based on medical history varies widely, and the risk factors discussed are often used in combination. For example, the European Germ Cell Cancer Consensus Group recommends that contralateral screening should be offered to patients with history of cryptorchidism, age under 30 years, and a testicular volume <12 mL [46].

Risk assessment based on environmental risk factors

Due to the rapidly rising incidence of TGCT, intense focus has centred on environmental risk factors, with in utero exposures of particular focus on account of the likely prenatal initiation events for the disease. While an association between TGCT and certain perinatal factors, such as low birth weight (OR 1.28, 95% confidence interval [CI] 0.99–1.65), has been suggested, overall the data remain inconclusive [51]. In terms of postnatal exposures, weak associations with cannabis usage, sedentary lifestyle, certain occupations, and pesticide exposure have all been proposed for TGCT; again, findings have been inconsistent and often fail to replicate. For TGCT screening there are no current lifestyle factors that are considered sufficiently robust to be clinically utilized.

Risk assessment based on family history

Along with evaluation of past medical history, family history should also be taken into account in the risk estimation. Studies in families from multiple countries have consistently demonstrated an eightfold increased risk of TGCT for brothers of cases and a fourfold increased risk for father–son relationships [10]. Despite these high familial relative risks, due to the low absolute risk of TGCT, familial disease is relatively rare: approximately 2% of cases have an affected first-degree relative, while only 6% report any family history of TGCT [52]. Studies have reported that familial TGCT presents at a younger age than isolated TGCT [53], and interestingly a stronger association with microlithiasis when compared to sporadic cases has also been reported [54]. Examples of ovarian germ cell tumour have been recurrently reported in pedigrees along with TGCT, suggesting shared oncogenic pathways [55].

Elucidation of the genetic basis of familial TGCT was first approached through genome-wide linkage analysis. This was undertaken by the International Testicular Cancer Linkage Consortium (ITCLC), studying 237 pedigrees and 518 affected individuals. This analysis did not find any evidence of genetic linkage to specific loci beyond that predicted under the null hypothesis by chance [56, 57]. Conclusions from this study were that a single locus accounting for a sibling relative risk of greater than 4.0 is unlikely to exist, and instead TGCT susceptibility is likely to involve multiple genes. Furthermore, whole-exome sequencing has been recently undertaken in over 400 TGCT cases across more than 200 families, to search for rare high-penetrance mutations conferring susceptibility to TGCT. Large scale sequencing studies have excluded existence of a major high penetrance susceptibility gene for TGCT (Greene, Bishop, and Turnbull, personal communication) [58, 59]. Thus, there are no known Mendelian TGCT predisposition genes, akin to *BRCA1/BRCA2* for breast cancer, for which TGCT families can be tested and individuals can be deemed to be at 'high risk' or 'low risk'. Instead, the elevated risk in families appears likely to be driven by the combination of multiple common polygenic factors which segregate independently within the family. Accordingly, the influence of family history in risk estimation for an individual is typically estimated empirically from the data from the epidemiological family studies.

Risk assessment based on genetic profile

The high effect size of genetic markers identified through GWAS has raised the possibility of genetic risk profiling for TGCT. In fact, homozygote risk allele carriers for SNP rs995030 (*KITLG* locus) have a sevenfold increased TGCT risk compared to homozygote protective allele carriers, due to this one polymorphism alone. Polygenic risk scoring (PRS) models, considering the combined effect of all known SNPs on disease risk, have been presented for TGCT by a number of groups [14, 52]. The latest such model demonstrates that the top 1% of men with the highest genetic risk of TGCT carry a ninefold elevated disease risk compared to the population average. For comparison purposes, equivalent PRS models for ovarian, breast, and prostate cancer demonstrated that the top 1% of highest-risk genotypes have only a twofold, threefold, and fivefold increased risk, respectively [60]. This suggests that common TGCT SNPs demonstrate useful power in terms of risk discrimination. In addition, it may be possible to combine genetic and clinical risk factors, for example a US group has calculated that white males in the top 1% of genetic risk and with history of UDT would have a 50-fold elevation in risk [52], equating to a lifetime TGCT risk of 26%. However, this model assumes full independence of effects between genetic and nongenetic factors, an assumption not yet validated through observed clinical data. Complex modelling trained and tested on clinical datasets fully characterized for genotype and phenotype is required to correctly probe the nature of these interactions. While genetic risk models for TGCT have been evaluated as a theoretical exercise, to date to the best of our knowledge TGCT genetic risk profiling has not yet been implemented in the clinical setting.

Screening for testicular cancer: The challenges

Several challenges prevent large-scale programmes of screening for testicular cancer. First, it is essential to consider relative risks versus absolute risks. The absolute lifetime risk of TGCT in Caucasian males is 0.5%, comparatively low versus common cancers like breast and prostate cancer, affecting approximately 10–12% of women and men, respectively. This means that high relative risks only translate into modest absolute risks: for example, men with UDT have a fivefold elevated relative risk of TGCT, but only a 2.5% lifetime risk. Secondly, the high cure rate for TGCT means there is limited opportunity for any programme of screening to have a sizeable impact on disease mortality. Thirdly, the current clinically available follow-up test to screen for CIS is testicular biopsy, which is invasive, low throughput, and associated with a significant rate of surgical complications. This renders it challenging to justify applying this procedure to any large population group. Fourthly, any large-scale TGCT screening programme is unlikely to demonstrate savings in health-related expenditure. This is due to the low incidence of TGCT, meaning that very large numbers of disease-free men would need to be screened to identify a small number of cases. For these reasons, screening for testicular cancer is currently largely restricted to those with a past history of testicular cancer who have a significant risk of contralateral testicular cancer. Even in this population, it is debated as to whether all patients, selected patients with additional risk factors, or none should be screened [46].

Screening for testicular cancer: Future directions

It is possible that scientific and technological advances offer the potential to shift the current balance, to a position in which TGCT screening might offer a broader benefit and become viable. In particular, noninvasive semen assays to detect CIS, if they can be scaled to high-throughput tests with improved sensitivity, offer real transformative opportunities and avoidance of unnecessary biopsy. Secondly, identification of further genetic risk factors predisposing men to TGCT offers potential to stratify individuals into clinically actionable risk groups. Heritability analyses suggest that between 25% and 50% of TGCTs are caused by inherited genetic factors [61, 62], meaning that a large number of risk markers remain unidentified. As these risk markers are mapped, groups with lifetime TGCT risk of ≥10% may be conceivably identified.

Utilising these developments, it is possible to envisage an integrated multistage screening programme for TGCT, a theoretical example of which is presented in Figure 24.2. Such a model would work across three stages, the first of which

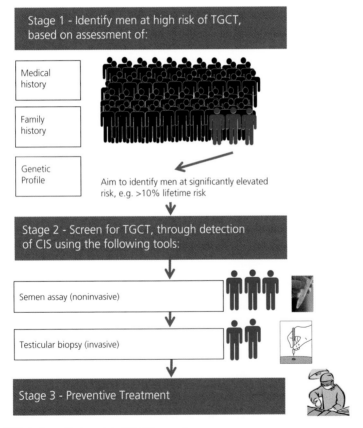

Figure 24.2 A theoretical model of TGCT screening.

would be identifying men at significantly elevated risk of TGCT, based on medical history, family history, and genetic risk profiling. Secondly, men at high risk could then go on to be screened for the presence/absence of CIS, using semen assay with or without testicular biopsy. Thirdly, men with confirmed CIS could then be eligible for preventive surgery, to eliminate the TGCT risk. Such an approach offers a number of benefits, for example overcoming the rare nature of TGCT by strict filtering to identify only those at high risk. Additionally, the integration of risk profiling with semen assay offers a noninvasive screening pathway with high specificity, reducing the number of unnecessary invasive negative biopsy procedures, while still identifying the majority of cases.

Conclusion

The pre-invasive biomarker CIS and high predictive value of the genetic risk profiling initially proffer TGCT as a clinical model that is likely to be amenable to screening. However, in consideration of population-based screening, with current technologies, these attributes are outweighed by broader epidemiological and clinical considerations. Targeted screening in individuals identified to be at elevated baseline risk, predominantly those with a contralateral tumour, are employed especially in Northern Europe, with evidence of clinical benefit. Future scientific and technological advances have the potential to alter the landscape, shifting the cost–benefit balance to enable broader TGCT screening. The motivation is clear for further developing methodologies, especially around semen analysis. Reducing the occurrence of invasive cancer arising in young men will contribute to reducing the burden of chemotherapy-related survivorship issues and to reducing mortality in the minority with a treatment-refractory disease state.

References

1 Bray, F., Ferlay, J., Devesa, S.S. et al. (2006). Interpreting the international trends in testicular seminoma and nonseminoma incidence. *Nature Clin. Pract. Urol.* 3 (10): 532–543.
2 Ruf, C.G., Isbarn, H., Wagner, W. et al. (2014). Changes in epidemiologic features of testicular germ cell cancer: Age at diagnosis and relative frequency of seminoma are constantly and significantly increasing. *Urol. Oncol.* 32 (1): 33, e1–6.
3 Le Cornet, C., Lortet-Tieulent, J., Forman, D. et al. (2014). Testicular cancer incidence to rise by 25% by 2025 in Europe? Model-based predictions in 40 countries using population-based registry data. *Eur. J. Cancer* 50 (4): 831–839.
4 Oldenburg, J., Fossa, S.D., Nuver, J. et al. (2013). Testicular seminoma and non-seminoma: ESMO Clinical Practice Guidelines for diagnosis, treatment and follow-up. *Ann. Oncol.* 24: 125–132.
5 Siegel, R., DeSantis, C., Virgo, K. et al. (2012). Cancer treatment and survivorship statistics, 2012. *CA Cancer J. Clin.* 62 (4): 220–241.

6 de Haas, E.C., Altena, R., Boezen, H.M. et al. (2013). Early development of the metabolic syndrome after chemotherapy for testicular cancer. *Ann. Oncol.* 24 (3): 749–755.

7 Bujan, L., Walschaerts, M., Moinard, N. et al. (2013). Impact of chemotherapy and radiotherapy for testicular germ cell tumors on spermatogenesis and sperm DNA: A multicenter prospective study from the CECOS network. *Fertil. Steril.* 100 (3): 673–680.

8 Rusner, C., Streller, B., Stegmaier, C. et al. (2014). Risk of second primary cancers after testicular cancer in East and West Germany: A focus on contralateral testicular cancers. *Asian J. Androl.* 16 (2): 285–289.

9 Nitzsche, B., Gloesenkamp, C., Schrader, M. et al. (2012). Anti-tumour activity of two novel compounds in cisplatin-resistant testicular germ cell cancer. *Br. J. Cancer* 107 (11): 1853–1863.

10 Hemminki, K., and Li, X. (2004). Familial risk in testicular cancer as a clue to a heritable and environmental aetiology. *Br. J. Cancer* 90 (9): 1765–1770.

11 Swerdlow, A.J., De Stavola, B.L., Swanwick, M.A., and Maconochie, N.E. (1997). Risks of breast and testicular cancers in young adult twins in England and Wales: Evidence on prenatal and genetic aetiology. *Lancet* 350 (9093): 1723–1728.

12 McGlynn, K.A., Devesa, S.S., Graubard, B.I., and Castle, P.E. (2005). Increasing incidence of testicular germ cell tumors among black men in the United States. *J. Clin. Oncol.* 23 (24): 5757–5761.

13 Rapley, E.A., Turnbull, C., Al Olama, A.A. et al. (2009). A genome-wide association study of testicular germ cell tumor. *Nature Genet.* 41 (7): 807–810.

14 Turnbull, C., and Rahman, N. (2011). Genome-wide association studies provide new insights into the genetic basis of testicular germ-cell tumour. *Int. J. Androl.* 34 (4, Part 2): e86–96; discussion e7.

15 Kanetsky, P.A., Mitra, N., Vardhanabhuti, S. et al. (2009). Common variation in KITLG and at 5q31.3 predisposes to testicular germ cell cancer. *Nature Genet.* 41 (7): 811–815.

16 Turnbull, C., Rapley, E.A., Seal, S. et al. (2010). Variants near DMRT1, TERT and ATF7IP are associated with testicular germ cell cancer. *Nature Genet.* 42 (7): 604–607.

17 Kanetsky, P.A., Mitra, N., Vardhanabhuti, S. et al. (2011). A second independent locus within DMRT1 is associated with testicular germ cell tumor susceptibility. *Hum. Mol. Genet.* 20 (15): 3109–3117.

18 Ruark, E., Seal, S., McDonald, H. et al. (2013). Identification of nine new susceptibility loci for testicular cancer, including variants near DAZL and PRDM14. *Nature Genet.* 45 (6): 686–689.

19 Schumacher, F.R., Wang, Z., Skotheim, R.I. et al. (2013). Testicular germ cell tumor susceptibility associated with the UCK2 locus on chromosome 1q23. *Hum. Mol. Genet.* 22 (13): 2748–2753.

20 Chung, C.C., Kanetsky, P.A., Wang, Z. et al. (2013). Meta-analysis identifies four new loci associated with testicular germ cell tumor. *Nature Genet.* 45 (6): 680–685.

21 Litchfield, K., Sultana, R., Renwick, A. et al. (2015). Multi-stage genome wide association study identifies new susceptibility locus for testicular germ cell tumour on chromosome 3q25. *Hum. Mol. Genet.* 24 (4): 1169–1176.

22 Wang, Z., McGlynn, K.A., Rajpert-De Meyts, E. et al. (2017). Meta-analysis of five genome-wide association studies identifies multiple new loci associated with testicular germ cell tumor. *Nat Genet.* 49 (7): 1141–1147.

23 Litchfield, K., Levy, M., Orlando, G. et al. (2017). Identification of 19 new risk loci and potential regulatory mechanisms influencing susceptibility to testicular germ cell tumor. *Nat Genet.* 49 (7): 1133–1140.

24 Litchfield, K., Holroyd, A., Lloyd, A. et al. (2015). Identification of four new susceptibility loci for testicular germ cell tumour. *Nat Commun.* 27 (6): 8690.

25 Chanock, S. (2009). High marks for GWAS. *Nature Genet.* 41 (7): 765–766.

26 Litchfield, K., Shipley, J., and Turnbull, C. (2015). Common variants identified in genome-wide association studies of testicular germ cell tumour: An update, biological insights and clinical application. *Andrology* 3 (1): 34–46.

27 Oosterhuis, J.W., and Looijenga, L.H. (2005). Testicular germ-cell tumours in a broader perspective. *Nature Rev. Cancer* 5 (3): 210–222.

28 Kristensen, D.M., Sonne, S.B., Ottesen, A.M. et al. (2008). Origin of pluripotent germ cell tumours: The role of microenvironment during embryonic development. *Mol. Cell. Endocrinol.* 288 (1–2): 111–118.

29 Skakkebaek, N.E., Berthelsen, J.G., Giwercman, A., and Muller, J. (1987). Carcinoma-in-situ of the testis: Possible origin from gonocytes and precursor of all types of germ cell tumours except spermatocytoma. *Int. J. Androl.* 10 (1): 19–28.

30 Rajpert-De Meyts, E. (2006). Developmental model for the pathogenesis of testicular carcinoma in situ: Genetic and environmental aspects. *Hum. Reprod Update* 12 (3): 303–323.

31 Horwich, A., Shipley, J., and Huddart, R. (2006). Testicular germ-cell cancer. *Lancet* 367 (9512): 754–765.

32 Rajpert-De Meyts, E., Bartkova, J., Samson, M. et al. (2003). The emerging phenotype of the testicular carcinoma in situ germ cell. *Apmis* 111 (1): 267–278; discussion 78–79.

33 Litchfield, K., Levy, M., Huddart, R.A. et al. (2016). The genomic landscape of testicular germ cell tumours: from susceptibility to treatment. *Nat Rev. Urol.* 13 (7): 409–419

34 Litchfield, K., Mitchell, J.S., Shipley, J. et al. (2016). Polygenic susceptibility to testicular cancer: implications for personalised health care. *Br. J. Cancer.* 114 (12): e22

35 Huyghe, E., Muller, A., Mieusset, R. et al. (2007). Impact of diagnostic delay in testis cancer: Results of a large population-based study. *Eur. Urol.* 52 (6): 1710–1716.

36 Powles, T.B., Bhardwa, J., Shamash, J. et al. (2005). The changing presentation of germ cell tumours of the testis between 1983 and 2002. *BJU Int.* 95 (9): 1197–1200.

37 Lin, K., and Sharangpani, R. (2010). Screening for testicular cancer: An evidence review for the U.S. Preventive Services Task Force. *Ann. Intern. Med.* 153 (6): 396–399.

38 Aberger, M., Wilson, B., Holzbeierlein, J.M. et al. (2014). Testicular self-examination and testicular cancer: A cost-utility analysis. *Cancer Med.* 3 (6): 1629–1634.

39 Wasnik, A.P., Maturen, K.E., Shah, S. et al. (2012). Scrotal pearls and pitfalls: Ultrasound findings of benign scrotal lesions. *Ultrasound Q.* 28 (4): 281–291.

40 Haas, G.P., Shumaker, B.P., and Cerny, J.C. (1986). The high incidence of benign testicular tumors. *J. Urol.* 136 (6): 1219–1220.

41 Tan, M.H., and Eng, C. (2011). Testicular microlithiasis: Recent advances in understanding and management. *Nature Rev. Urol.* 8 (3): 153–163.

42 Dieckmann, K.P., Kulejewski, M., Heinemann, V., and Loy, V. (2011). Testicular biopsy for early cancer detection: Objectives, technique and controversies. *Int. J. Androl.* 34 (4, Part 2): e7–e13.

43 Almstrup, K., Lippert, M., Mogensen, H.O. et al. (2011). Screening of subfertile men for testicular carcinoma in situ by an automated image analysis-based cytological test of the ejaculate. *Int. J. Androl.* 34 (4, Part 2): e21–e30; discussion e1.

44 Trabert, B., Zugna, D., Richiardi, L. et al. (2013). Congenital malformations and testicular germ cell tumors. *Int. J. Cancer* 133 (8): 1900–1904.

45 Fossa, S.D., Chen, J., Schonfeld, S.J. et al. (2005). Risk of contralateral testicular cancer: A population-based study of 29,515 U.S. men. *J. Natl Cancer Inst.* 97 (14): 1056–1066.

46 Beyer, J., Albers, P., Altena, R. et al. (2013). Maintaining success, reducing treatment burden, focusing on survivorship: Highlights from the third European Consensus Conference on Diagnosis and Treatment of Germ-cell Cancer. *Ann. Oncol.* 24 (4): 878–888.

47 Dieckmann, K.P., and Pichlmeier, U. (2004). Clinical epidemiology of testicular germ cell tumors. *World J. Urol.* 22 (1): 2–14.

48 Tan, I.B., Ang, K.K., Ching, B.C. et al. (2010). Testicular microlithiasis predicts concurrent testicular germ cell tumors and intratubular germ cell neoplasia of unclassified type in adults: A meta-analysis and systematic review. *Cancer* 116 (19): 4520–4532.

49 McGlynn, K.A., and Trabert, B. (2012). Adolescent and adult risk factors for testicular cancer. *Nature Rev. Urol.* 9 (6): 339–349.

50 Nathanson, K.L., Kanetsky, P.A., Hawes, R. et al. (2005). The Y deletion gr/gr and susceptibility to testicular germ cell tumor. *Am. J. Hum. Genet.* 77 (6): 1034–1043.

51 McGlynn, K.A., and Cook, M.B. (2009). Etiologic factors in testicular germ-cell tumors. *Fut. Oncol.* 5 (9): 1389–1402.

52 Greene, M.H., Mai, P.L., Loud, J.T. et al. (2015). Familial testicular germ cell tumors (FTGCT): Overview of a multidisciplinary etiologic study. *Andrology* 3 (1): 47–58.

53 Mai, P.L., Chen, B.E., Tucker, K. et al. (2009). Younger age-at-diagnosis for familial malignant testicular germ cell tumor. *Fam. Cancer* 8 (4): 451–456.

54 Coffey, J., Huddart, R.A., Elliott, F. et al. (2007). Testicular microlithiasis as a familial risk factor for testicular germ cell tumour. *Br. J. Cancer* 97 (12): 1701–1706.

55 Stettner, A.R., Hartenbach, E.M., Schink, J.C. et al. (1999). Familial ovarian germ cell cancer: Report and review. *Am. J. Med. Genet.* 84 (1): 43–46.

56 Crockford, G.P., Linger, R., Hockley, S. et al. (2006). Genome-wide linkage screen for testicular germ cell tumour susceptibility loci. *Hum. Mol. Genet.* 15 (3): 443–451.

57 Rapley, E.A., Crockford, G.P., Teare, D. et al. (2000). Localization to Xq27 of a susceptibility gene for testicular germ-cell tumours. *Nat. Genet.* 24 (2): 197–200.

58 Litchfield, K., Loveday, C., Levy, M. et al. (2018). Large-scale sequencing of testicular germ cell tumour (TGCT) cases excludes major TGCT predisposition gene. *Eur. Urol.* 73 (6): 828–831.

59 Litchfield, K., Levy, M., Dudakia, D. et al. (2016). Rare disruptive mutations in ciliary function genes contribute to testicular cancer susceptibility. *Nat Commun.* 20 (7): 13840.

60 Bahcall, O. (2013). Risk prediction and population screening for breast, ovarian and prostate cancers. *Nat. Genet.* http://www.nature.com/icogs/primer/risk-prediction-and-population-screening-for-breast-ovarian-and-prostate-cancers/ (accessed 3 January 2018).

61 Czene, K., Lichtenstein, P., and Hemminki, K. (2002). Environmental and heritable causes of cancer among 9.6 million individuals in the Swedish family-cancer database. *Int. J. Cancer* 99 (2): 260–266.

62 Litchfield, K., Thomsen, H., Mitchell, J.S. et al. (2015). Quantifying the heritability of testicular germ cell tumour using both population-based and genomic approaches. *Sci. Rep.* 5: 13889.

CHAPTER 25

Issues in paediatric cancers

David Malkin and Jonah Himelfarb

Division of Hematology/Oncology, Genetics and Genome Biology Program, The Hospital for Sick Children; Department of Pediatrics, University of Toronto, Ontario, Canada

---

SUMMARY BOX

- Paediatric cancers may have up to a 25% chance of being due to a genetic predisposition, and increasing availability of next-generation sequencing will result in identification of more genetic conditions over the coming years.

- There are rare instances of conditions with prevention options; some of these involve prophylactic surgery, e.g. familial adenomatous polyposis, multiple endocrine neoplasia.

- Testing of children for a genetic predisposition should only be offered if there is a management option or strong psychological implication.

- Children who survive childhood cancer have a 20% risk of a second malignancy, and screening for this needs to incorporate minimization of use of modalities that cause DNA damage.

"But I thought kids don't get cancer?"

The strongest risk factor for the development of cancer is advanced age. This is owing to the fact that cancer is typically the product of repeated damage to an individual's genetic and epigenetic make-up. These mutations ultimately culminate in deregulation of the cell cycle and aberrant cell division, leading to neoplastic transformation.

Acquired mutations usually develop through errors in cell division or exposure to environmental carcinogens, processes that are not thought to have sufficient time to accumulate in a child. As a result, the development of malignancies is relatively rare in children, occurring with an incidence of only 186.6 per 1 million in those aged 0–19 years compared with 4548 per 1 million in the general population [1].

However, when cancer does present in children, special considerations must be taken. The emotional repercussions of a diagnosis to a child and their family

---

Cancer Prevention and Screening: Concepts, Principles and Controversies, First Edition.
Edited by Rosalind A. Eeles, Christine D. Berg, and Jeffrey S. Tobias.
© 2019 John Wiley & Sons, Inc. Published 2019 by John Wiley & Sons, Inc.

are often devastating and require an additional degree of sensitivity. Children are also particularly vulnerable to both the psychological and physiological effects of screening and treatment. They have many decades, on completion of treatment, to manifest diverse and often devastating complications from the therapy received.

Children are also unique with respect to the types of cancer they develop. The most frequently diagnosed malignancies in young children are leukaemias (31%), tumours of the central nervous system (CNS; 21%), and lymphomas (10%) [1].

However, due to the relative infrequency of these cancers, there are currently no recommended formal cancer screening protocols for the healthy paediatric population. For targeted prevention or screening protocols to be implemented in a child, one must first prove that the child is at increased risk, most often by iden- tifying them with a cancer predisposition syndrome (CPS). CPSs impart an ele- vated susceptibility to the development of certain cancers due to inherited (or *de novo*) mutations in one of a wide spectrum of genes [2]. Historically, it had been suggested that fewer than 10% of cancers in children are attributable to underly- ing genetic factors. With the advent of next-generation sequencing (NGS) tech- nologies, the increased efforts to map greater portions of somatic and germline genomes of children with cancer, and the increased recognition by oncologists and primary care providers of the need to document and pay attention to tumour type and family cancer history, it has become apparent that an increasing fraction of paediatric cancers are associated with an underlying CPS [3]. Several recent studies, most notably including an extensive sequencing effort for 1120 paediatric cancer patients, confirmed the prevalence of germline mutations across a panel of known cancer genes to be 8.5%, likely an underestimate due to limitations within the study [4].

Herein, we discuss recognition and screening for CPSs, strategies for cancer prevention, as well as the late effects of treatment in these at-risk populations.

Prevention

Children are not generally perceived to be at high risk for cancer and the connec- tion to modifiable risk factors is less clear than for adult populations. Major risk factors associated with adult cancer, such as obesity, sun exposure, and lack of exercise, have not been shown to be linked with paediatric cancers [5]. As a result, most cancer prevention for paediatric patients has focused on simply avoid- ing possible carcinogens rather than active lifestyle modification. This begins *in utero* with maternal factors that can predispose a growing foetus to cancer. A nota- ble example was the maternal exposure to the teratogenic drug diethylstilbestrol (DES) from the 1940s to the 1970s. DES was the first orally active oestrogen, with marketers claiming it prevented spontaneous abortion and preterm delivery. It was later discovered that *in utero* exposure to DES caused gross morphological defects as well as an increased incidence of clear-cell adenocarcinoma of the cervix in daughters [6, 7].

Poor maternal diet has also been linked to increasing foetal risk of childhood cancer development. Studies show a child will be at greater risk if their mother had a lower intake of fruits and vegetables or consumed higher amounts of fried foods in the periconception period [8, 9]. Surprisingly, parental smoking has not been clearly linked to an elevated rate of cancer in children, although reports have varied. A recent meta-analysis of 17 studies showed that smoking during or before the pregnancy was not associated with a risk of brain tumours [10]. Another study found no correlation between maternal smoking and hepatoblastoma [11].

As children age, skin cancer becomes an increasing risk, with melanoma representing 7% of all cancers in those aged 15–19 years [12]; nearly 25% of lifetime ultraviolet radiation exposure occurs during childhood and is largely preventable [13]. Skin protection can be achieved by applying sunscreen, avoiding tanning beds, and implementing childhood education programmes.

Other common preventive measures include male circumcision to reduce penile cancer risk, and human papilloma virus (HPV) vaccination to prevent cervical cancer [14, 15].

For most children, these precautions reduce an already very low risk of developing cancer. For those with CPSs, however, little can be done to actively prevent progression to malignancy. If parents are identified as carrying a cancer-predisposing gene mutation or having a CPS, they can pass on the hereditary susceptibility to their children. This risk can be mitigated through the use of assisted reproductive technologies (ARTs). These include preimplantation genetic diagnosis (PGD) of embryos and prenatal diagnosis (PND) of the foetus. In PGD, embryos are analysed after fertilization to determine whether they harbour a deleterious disease-causing gene mutation. Once identified, at-risk embryos that can be selected out, whereas those that do not have mutations are selected for implantation. PND consists of sampling either chorionic villi or amniotic fluid from the conceptus and then performing genetic analysis. Depending on the results of the analysis, prospective parents are able to make choices regarding carrying the pregnancy to term. While PGD and PND are controversial under certain circumstances, they are largely viewed as acceptable for individuals at elevated risk of a serious foetal genetic disorder. Furthermore, a recent study showed that 72% of patients with a hereditary cancer syndrome feel that PGD should be offered [16]. When PND or PGD is considered, intensive prenatal and post-test genetic counselling are the standard of care. Multidisciplinary teams, including paediatric oncologists and genetic counsellors, work together to provide support during and after the decision-making process. Current recommendations are that the role of the paediatric oncologist should be to support a family's decision relating to PGD [17].

After delivery, preventive options are much more limited for a child with a CPS. In these children, neoplasms often develop at unpredictable times, with multiple organs at risk. This often makes definitive targeted interventions a challenge; however, prophylactic surgery is an option in certain syndromes. In multiple endocrine neoplasia type 2A (MEN2A), the risk of developing medullary thyroid carcinoma (MTC) is 100% and prophylactic thyroidectomy is usually recommended before the age of 5 [18, 19]. In multiple endocrine neoplasia type 2B (MEN2B), thyroidectomy is recommended even earlier, within the first year of life [19]. For Li-Fraumeni syndrome (LFS), the 'Toronto Protocol' encourages the consideration of risk-reducing bilateral mastectomy in female adult *TP53* mutation carriers [20]. In familial adenomatous polyposis (FAP), prophylactic colectomy has been able to greatly reduce death from colorectal cancer.

Although these examples of surgical interventions provide increased protection from certain cancers associated with the underlying CPS, they are only temporizing measures. MEN, LFS, and FAP can all cause malignancies in multiple organs. For many CPSs, the target organs preclude prophylactic surgery.

Screening

Cancer screening presents an opportunity to reduce morbidity and mortality by diagnosing malignancy at an earlier stage. Earlier in development, cancers are less likely to have invaded surrounding tissue or undergone metastasis. This results in a lower disease burden with fewer complications, and also reduces the risk of treatment sequelae. When the disease is localized, less aggressive techniques for management can be employed and systemic exposures can be avoided. Overall, early detection can often lead to positive health outcomes for paediatric cancer patients through altering the course of disease.

However, due to the low rates of cancer in children, the benefits conferred to healthy adults through regular screening cannot be extended to youths. It is important to note that screening is not without risks, including radiation exposure, reactions to contrast dyes, sedation, and anaesthesia [19]. Currently, it is neither cost-effective nor clinically responsible to screen the general paediatric population.

One notable attempt for paediatric cancer screening was performed during the 1990s for neuroblastoma. In the study, 425 816 children underwent urinalysis for detection of elevated levels of homovanillic acid (HVA) and vanillylmandelic acid (VMA), biomarkers of the disease. The authors concluded that while screening increased the detected incidence of neuroblastoma, it provided no reduction in morbidity or mortality [21].

The low prevalence of paediatric cancers makes the positive predictive value of many tests too low to be clinically useful. If the prevalence of a disease is 1% and a test has specificity and sensitivity of 95%, the probability of disease after a positive test result is still only 16% [22]. For a majority of patients this leads to unnecessary follow-up testing, which can result in undue patient anxiety, radiation exposure, and medical complications. A further concern is that some parents may not appreciate the significance of a false positive result. One study showed that 5% of parents who received a false-positive result on a newborn screen still believed their children may be at risk for disease [22, 23]. This effect can endure even after counseling. It is recommended that general screening not be performed unless the disease prevalence is at least 5%. At a prevalence of 5% and a test sensitivity and specificity of 95% the probability of disease after a positive result will be 50%.

For this reason, the first step to screening is identifying patients at higher risk by defining the characteristics of a CPS. Features associated with hereditary cancer syndromes have been well described and can be divided into family history factors and patient factors [17]. Based on similar criteria, a selection tool was recently developed to help identify patients that could benefit from genetic counselling [24]. The validation of this selection tool, or one like it, will aid detection of lesser-known CPSs and be crucial for the discovery of novel syndromes. It has been suggested that more than 1 in 4 children with cancer should undergo genetic evaluation [17]. If a CPS is suspected, a predisposition can be confirmed for many syndromes by genetic testing. It is important to note that absence of a positive genetic test does not preclude the diagnosis of a hereditary CPS.

Once a CPS has been recognized, a clinician/genetic counsellor should educate the family about the pattern of inheritance and the risk posed to other relatives. The presenting child, and others at risk, can begin to be monitored. For many syndromes established screening protocols exist, which have been shown to provide improved prognostic outcomes. Here we discuss a selection of significant cancer predisposition syndromes.

Li-Fraumeni syndrome

LFS is the prototypical CPS and is characterized by soft-tissue sarcomas, brain tumours, adrenocortical carcinomas, premenopausal breast cancer, leukaemia, and a myriad of other malignancies presenting at a young age [20]. Classic LFS is defined by fulfilling the following three criteria: a patient must (1) be diagnosed with sarcoma younger than 45 years of age; (2) have a first-degree relative who was diagnosed with cancer younger than 45 years; and (3) have a first- or second-degree relative who received a diagnosis of cancer younger than 45 or a sarcoma at any age [18]. Germline *TP53* mutations can be found in 70–83% of patients who meet these conditions [20]. The gene product p53 is a classic tumour suppressor and has diverse cellular functions, including DNA repair, initiation of apoptosis, and control of cell cycle. In mutation carriers, the risk of developing cancer throughout their life has been reported as up to 90%, with a 40% risk before the age of 20 [25]. The syndrome is inherited in an autosomal dominant pattern and is highly penetrant, leading to a large burden of disease within LFS families. An extensive screening protocol (Table 25.1) has been implemented, with promising results for LFS patients harboring the *TP53* germline mutation [20]. The protocol consists of biochemical screening in conjunction with regular whole-body magnetic resonance imaging (MRI) to monitor various at-risk tissues. The strategy has resulted in a three-year overall survival of 100% in the surveillance group, compared to only 21% in the nonsurveillance group (Figure 25.1) [20]. This screening strategy has proven to be an ideal example of the efficacy that regular, informed monitoring can have in extending life and reducing morbidity in patients with CPSs.

Table 25.1 Surveillance strategy for individuals with germline TP53 mutations*.

Children

Adrenocortical carcinoma
- Ultrasound of abdomen and pelvis every 3–4 months
- Complete urinalysis every 3–4 months
- Blood tests every 4 months: β-human chorionic gonadotropin, alpha-fetoprotein, 17-OH-progesterone, testosterone, dehydroepiandrosterone sulfate, androstenedione

Brain tumour
- Annual brain MRI

Soft tissue and bone sarcoma
- Annual rapid total body MRI

Leukaemia or lymphoma
- Blood test every 4 months: complete blood count, erythrocyte sedimentation rate, lactate dehydrogenase

Adults

Breast cancer
- Monthly breast self-examination starting at age 18 years
- Clinical breast examination twice a year, starting at age 20–25 years, or 5–10 years before the earliest known breast cancer in the family
- Annual mammography and breast MRI screening starting at age 20–25 years, or at earliest age of onset in the family
- Consider risk-reducing bilateral mastectomy

Brain tumour
- Annual brain MRI

Soft tissue and bone sarcoma
- Annual rapid total body MRI
- Ultrasound of abdomen and pelvis every 6 months

Colon cancer
- Colonoscopy every 2 years, beginning at age 40 years, or 10 years before the earliest known colon cancer in the family

Melanoma
- Annual dermatological examination

Leukaemia or lymphoma
- Complete blood count every 4 months
- Erythrocyte sedimentation rate, lactate dehydrogenase every 4 months

---

*In addition to regular assessment with family physician with close attention to any medical concerns or complaints.

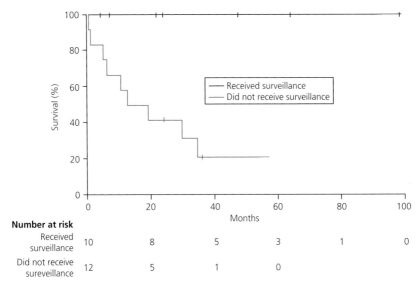

Figure 25.1 Surveillance in Li-Fraumeni syndrome demonstrates improvement in survival.

Retinoblastoma

Retinoblastoma is a malignant tumour of the developing retina caused by loss of expression of both copies of the *RB1* gene. Under normal circumstances, the protein coded by *RB1* binds to E2F proteins to regulate cell division. Gene mutations can occur sporadically in an autosomal dominant pattern of inheritance. In hereditary cases of retinoblastoma, a child inherits a mutated copy of the gene in their germline and somatic loss of the other copy will cause tumour formation. Patients with the hereditary disease have a 90% lifetime risk of developing retinoblastoma and represent 40% of all cases [26, 27]; 95% of diagnoses of retinoblastoma are made before the age of 5 years [28].

It is important to note that due to the high *de novo* germline mutation rate, the family history for retinoblastoma can often be negative [27]. All patients presenting with bilateral retinoblastoma, unilateral multifocal disease, or a positive family history should be suspected of carrying a germline mutation [28, 29]. Since 10–15% of patients with unilateral retinoblastoma can still harbour an inherited mutation, genetic testing is justified in any patient presenting with the disease [26, 29]. Children who carry a germline mutation are at high risk for retinoblastoma and require regular fundoscopy. An exact schedule for fundoscopy screening has not been agreed upon, but there is consensus that screening should be very frequent in early life and can be stopped around the age of 5 years. One proposed screening schedule risk-stratifies patients based on mutation status and family history. For children who harbour an *RB1* mutation or who have parents with bilateral retinoblastoma, the authors recommend a fundoscopic exam within the first eight days of birth, then every month up to 18 months of age, then gradually transitioning to every three months until 4 years of age. For children who have a sibling with bilateral retinoblastoma or a parent with a unilateral, unifocal tumour, the authors recommend fundoscopy within the first month after birth, every two months until 2 years of age, and then every six months until 4 years of age [29]. This surveillance strategy resulted in tumours detected at smaller size, and significantly reduced the number of patients requiring enucleation or external beam radiation for management [29].

Familial adenomatous polyposis

FAP is a highly penetrant, autosomal-dominant polyposis syndrome caused by mutation of the *APC* (adenomatous polyposis coli) gene in roughly 90% of cases [19, 30]. The APC protein acts as a tumour suppressor and monitors cell division. One of the ways APC controls the cell cycle is by triggering the degradation of beta-catenin, a signal transducer that goes to the nucleus and promotes proliferation [31]. The disease is characterized by the formation of hundreds to thousands of adenomatous colorectal polyps at a young age. In 8% of cases, patients present with a milder form of the disease, called attenuated FAP, and have later onset with fewer polyps [32]. The *APC* mutation can also result in numerous extracolonic manifestations, including hypertrophy of the retinal pigment epithelium, desmoid tumours, osteomas, epidermal cysts, and extracolonic malignancies [33].

A recent study of 163 patients with FAP found that the average age of diagnosis was 12.5 years old, with 69% found on colonoscopy and 25% found by genetic testing [33]. If these children do not receive appropriate care, there is nearly 100% progression to colorectal cancer (CRC) by age 35–40, with some progressing to malignancy in childhood [34]. In addition to mortality due to CRC, other leading causes of death in these patients are desmoid and duodenal tumors [35].

Current screening recommendations for carriers of the *APC* mutation consists of sigmoidoscopy every two years after the age of 10–12 years, with a transition to annual colonoscopies if adenomas are detected [36]. To detect upper gastrointestinal (GI) adenomas, esophagogastroduodenoscopy has been recommended starting at age 25–30, with the interval between exams being dependent on the severity of the disease [36]. To monitor the development of hepatoblastoma (*APC* mutant carriers have a 400-fold increased risk), routine abdominal ultrasound and measurements of serum alpha-fetoprotein have been recommended until age 5 [37]. In addition, patients should have annual physical examination with thyroid palpation [37]. One group has suggested a more intense screening schedule with endoscopy starting at age 7, or even earlier if a family member had an onset of symptoms at a younger age [33]. The potential for personalized screening schedules based on location of the inherited mutation within the *APC* gene has also been recognized. Mutations at certain amino acid residues are associated with development of CRC up to 10 years earlier, while other codons result in a mild phenotype [34].

For high-risk individuals who are not carriers of the *APC* mutation, screening protocols are less intensive and sigmoidoscopy can be discontinued after age 50 if there is no detection of adenomas [36].

Multiple endocrine neoplasia

MEN comprises a group of highly penetrant, autosomal-dominant syndromes that result in tumours of endocrine and nonendocrine organs. The two types, MEN1 and MEN2, are characterized by mutations in the *MEN1* tumour suppressor gene and the *RET* proto-oncogene, respectively [19]. MEN1 and MEN2 present differently, with a unique spectrum of tumours and affected tissues for each condition.

MEN1

MEN1 presents with pituitary adenomas, pancreatic islet tumours, and most commonly parathyroid adenomas. The disease can be clinically diagnosed when two of these three tumours are present [19]. Alternatively, the diagnosis can be made if there is one MEN1-related tumour and a positive family history, or with a molecular diagnosis alone [38]. The penetrance of MEN1 is close to 0% below the age of 5, 25% at age 15, and 95% at age 40 [18, 39]. Based on a systematic review of the literature, in 2012 a clinical practice guideline was developed for the screening of MEN1. Beginning at age 5, pituitary function is screened for with annual prolactin and IGF-1 levels, as well as an MRI every three years. Screening for insulinomas should also begin around age 5, with annual fasting glucose and insulin levels. At age 8, parathyroid testing is started with measurements of annual calcium and parathyroid hormone (PTH) levels. Before the age of 10, screening for other pancreatic malignancies begins through annual measurements of Chromogranin-A, pancreatic polypeptide, glucagon, and vasoactive intestinal peptide (VIP), as well as annual imaging with MRI, computed tomography (CT), or endoscopic ultrasound (EUS). At the same time, screening of the adrenal glands is started, with MRI or CT repeated alongside the pancreatic imaging. Conventionally, no biochemical testing has been performed for the adrenal glands unless there are symptoms or signs of a functioning tumour or if a tumour greater than 1 cm is identified on imaging. However, reevaluation of this practice suggests that biochemical surveillance may be an appropriate complement to imaging. After age 15, the thymic and bronchial carcinoid tumours are screened for by CT or MRI, repeating every one to two years. Finally, beginning at age 20, gastrin levels are measured (with or without gastric pH) for early detection of gastrinomas [38].

MEN2

MEN2 is further subdivided into MEN2A, MEN2B, and familial medullary thyroid carcinoma (MTC). MEN2A and MEN2B are both characterized by thyroid, parathyroid, and adrenal tumours, but MEN2B can present with numerous nonendocrine manifestations. For both MEN2A and MEN2B, MTC develops in nearly all patients and often at a very young age. In addition, each condition possesses roughly a 50% risk for development of pheochromocytoma. MEN2A accounts for 75% of all cases of MEN2 and is much less aggressive than MEN2B. In MEN2B, neoplasias develop 10 years earlier relative to MEN2A, with metastases from MTC occurring in children as young as 3 years old. Of note is that while 95% of patients with MEN2A have an affected parent, up to 90% of cases of MEN2B are the result of *de novo* mutations. MEN2B can be recognized clinically by a constellation of Hirschsprung's disease, oral lesions, 'tearless crying', and skeletal abnormalities [40]. Prophylactic thyroidectomy is performed before age 5 for MEN2A and within the first year of life for MEN2B, and then screening protocols are followed for pheochromocytoma. Beginning at age 5, patients with MEN2A undergo annual measurements of urinary catecholamines or plasma metanephrines, as well as MRI every three years. The pheochromocytoma screening protocol is identical for MEN2B, but begins at age 3. Screening for hyperparathyroidism starts at age 10 for both MEN2A and MEN2B and consists of an annual calcium profile [41].

Beckwith-Wiedemann syndrome

Beckwith-Wiedemann syndrome (BWS) is a congenital overgrowth condition, with affected children displaying macrosomia. Children exhibit various signs and symptoms, including macroglossia, hemihyperplasia, abdominal wall defects, and severe hypoglycaemia in the neonatal period. The condition is caused by aberrations in an imprinted locus that encodes insulin-like growth factor II (IGF2), CDKN1C, as well as other genes [19]. The exact mechanism for the defect varies, from hypomethylation of imprinting control region 2 (60% of cases), paternal uniparental disomy (20–25%), hypermethylation of imprinting control region 1 (10% of cases), and maternally inherited mutation of CDKN1C (5%) to chromosomal abnormalities of chr11p15 (<1%) [42]. The disease occurs sporadically in most cases with only around 15% of patients having a positive family history [43]. Most of those affected by BWS do not have serious complications due to the condition and enjoy a normal life expectancy. However, neoplasia will manifest in approximately 10% of patients, usually during childhood. Most commonly embryonal tumours will develop, including Wilms tumour (40–43% of cases) and hepatoblastoma (12–20% of cases) [19]. Tumour surveillance protocols consists of abdominal ultrasound examination every three months until the age of 8 [42]. Alpha-fetoprotein (AFP) level measurements are recommended every three months until the age of 4–6 years, although some studies have questioned the appropriateness of drawing blood for AFP screening for hepatoblastoma [42, 44]. In the future, dried blood spots may be an acceptable alternative for measuring and monitoring levels of AFP [44]. Lastly, the risk for neuroblastoma is small, but screening with quarterly urine catecholamine levels and annual chest X-ray can be appropriate [42]. Evidence suggests that BWS can be categorized into four molecular subtypes with unique phenotypic profiles. This will soon allow for risk stratification and individualized screening plans based on the unique molecular pathobiology of affected patients [44].

Von Hippel-Lindau disease

Von Hippel-Lindau (VHL) is a highly penetrant, autosomal-dominant syndrome caused by a germline mutation in the *VHL* tumour suppressor gene [45]. Under normal circumstances, *VHL* binds with other proteins, forming a complex to ubiquitinate and degrade hypoxia inducible factor (HIF). HIF is expressed in response to tissue hypoxia and results in angiogenesis, red blood cell production, and changes in cell cycle regulation. When *VHL* is mutated, HIF functions even in times of normoxia and results in a predisposition to both malignant and benign hypervascular tumours [45]. Characteristic tumours include CNS hemangioblastomas, retinal hemangiomas, and clear-cell renal cell carcinomas [46]. Other common tumours include pheochromocytomas, islet-cell tumours, and endolymphatic-sac tumours [19, 46]. Penetrance approaches 100% by age 60, with a mean age of presentation at roughly 26 years [46, 47]. Approximately 80% of patients inherit mutations, while the remaining 20% are due to *de novo* mutations [48]. The diagnosis can be made clinically if a patient presents with two or more CNS hemangioblastomas, or a solitary hemangioblastoma along with an additional characteristic lesion [19]. If a family history is present, the diagnosis can be made if there is presentation of a renal cell carcinoma, a pheochromocytoma, or a single CNS hemangioblastoma [19]. Screening recommendations for VHL involve regular investigations for retinal hemangioblastomas, pheochromocytomas, renal-cell carcinomas, pancreatic tumours, CNS hemangioblastomas, and endolymphatic-sac tumours (ELSTs). Retinal hemangioblastomas are screened for soon after birth with fundoscopy and repeated annually in at-risk children. Plasma metanephrines are measured starting at 2–5 years of age and are repeated annually to monitor possible development of pheochromocytomas. Work-up for renal-cell carcinoma begins around age 5–8 years with abdominal ultrasound or MRI performed annually. Work-up for pancreatic carcinoma is the same as renal cell, but imaging is not likely to be necessary prior to 20 years of age. However, because imaging of the pelvis and adrenal glands usually incorporates the pancreas, attention to pancreatic pathology can be part of the usual surveillance exam even at an early age. Screening recommendations for CNS hemangioblastomas are somewhat an area of contention, but most agree that gadolinium-enhanced MRI of the brain and spine should begin around age 11–15, with imaging repeated every one to two years. This imaging will also be able to visualize development of an ELST. ELSTs can be further monitored with regular audiological examinations [19, 49].

Hereditary pheochromocytomas and paragangliomas

Pheochromocytomas and paragangliomas (PHEO/PGL) are rare, benign tumours that occur at a combined annual incidence of approximately 3 per 1 million [50]. Although these tumours are commonly denoted as benign, they are capable of producing severe morbidity due to mass effect, secretion of catecholamines, malignant transformation, and metastatic spread [51]. Roughly 30% of PHEO/PGL are hereditary and attributable to autosomal-dominant germline mutations in tumour suppressor genes [50]. A majority (around 80%) of familial cases are caused by germline mutations in succinate dehydrogenase *(SDH)* genes [51]. *SDHA, SDHB, SDHC,* and *SDHD* encode proteins that assemble in the mitochondria to form the mitochondrial complex 2, a critical enzyme for cellular respiration [51]. When mutated, there is increased susceptibility to tumour development, with a lifetime penetrance approaching 70% [51]. In addition to PHEO/PGL, certain *SDH* gene mutations also predispose to the development of renal carcinomas as well as gastrointestinal stromal tumours (GISTs). Initiation of screening has been suggested in the second decade of life and includes annual physical examination, blood pressure measurement, and testing for urinary catecholamine elevation. Recommended imaging consists of biannual CT/MRI of the neck, skull base, thorax, abdomen, and pelvis [51]. To avoid excess radiation exposure, most groups now favor MRI over CT, reserving PET-CT to corroborate functional evidence of tumour development noted on MRI scans. A genotype–phenotype correlation has also been observed, with different *SDH* genes mutated with differences in penetrance, age of onset, type of primary, risk of multiple primaries, and rate of malignant transformation. The association between genotype and phenotype will allow for more personalized screening in the future. Currently it is already recommended that those with an *SDHB* mutation begin screening earlier, due to a younger age of onset and a striking propensity for metastatic spread of disease [51].

Nevoid basal cell carcinoma syndrome (Gorlin syndrome)

Gorlin syndrome is a rare, autosomal-dominant predisposition syndrome caused by a germline mutation in *PTCH1*. *PTCH1* is a cell surface protein that acts in the SHH signalling pathway, activating GLI transcription factors and promoting cell division [18]. Patients with Gorlin characteristically develop multiple basal-cell carcinomas, but also other manifestations of disease, including palmar/plantar pits, jaw cysts, calcification of the falx cerebri, and skeletal malformations [52]. The basal cell carcinomas can vary from several to thousands in number and can develop as young as 3 years old [18]. The diagnosis of Gorlin is made clinically based on physical examination and radiological imaging. Diagnostic criteria are separated into major and minor features. A diagnosis is made when there are presence of either two major criteria or one major and two minor criteria [52]. Children at risk for Gorlin should have a physical exam at birth, checking for palmar and plantar pitting as well as other minor features of the disease. Due to the propensity to develop basal-cell carcinoma, regular dermatological evaluation is imperative, especially during adolescence. It is also important to counsel patients to minimize ultraviolet exposure and avoid imaging using ionizing radiation whenever possible. Additionally, Gorlin is associated with cardiac fibromas and medulloblastomas. The former is monitored with periodic echocardiography and the latter is surveyed with annual MRI until the age of 7 [53].

Newly described syndromes

In recent years, new cancer predisposition syndromes have been identified and are still actively being characterized, including DICER1 syndrome and constitutional mismatch repair deficiency (CMMRD), also referred to as biallelic mismatch repair deficiency (bMMRD) syndrome. DICER1 syndrome is an autosomal-dominant CPS that was discovered due to its association with familial pleuropulmonary blastoma (PPB), a rare tumour of the lung parenchyma [54]. The syndrome is due to inheritance of a mutation in the *DICER1* gene, which encodes a RNase III endonuclease responsible for processing miRNAs and siRNAs [54]. These small RNAs allow for post-transcriptional regulation of gene expression and are responsible for key tasks, including regulation of organogenesis, cell cycle control, and oncogenesis [54]. In addition to PPB, children with DICER1 syndrome are at risk of developing cystic nephromas, cervical embryonal rhabdomyosarcoma, ovarian Sertoli–Leydig tumours, pituitary blastoma, pineoblastoma, and multinodular goitres [3].

CMMRD/bMMRD is a CPS wherein patients inherit mutations in the DNA mismatch repair genes (*MLH1*, *MSH2*, *MSH6*, and *PMS2*) from both parental lineages [55]. The vast majority of carriers of biallelic mismatch repair are the progeny of consanguineous parents. Under normal conditions, the role of the mismatch repair genes is to correct base substitution, insertions, and deletions, which occur naturally during DNA replication. Affected children are at risk of developing various cancers at a particularly young age. The most common cancers are haematological malignancies, brain tumours (glioblastoma, anaplastic astrocytoma, medulloblastoma), colorectal cancer, and Lynch syndrome–associated malignancies, although other tumours present as well. Physical findings including café-au-lait spots have also been associated with the disease [55]. Protocols have been suggested to identify patients who may be affected by CMMRD/bMMRD; screening regimens for affected patients have been developed and are currently being assessed [55].

Surveillance protocols for these two syndromes, and other recently described CPSs, are still currently in development, with no consensus having yet been reached. It is first necessary to identify all susceptible organs, and then investigations must be conducted to determine the screening modality and schedule that would be most appropriate.

Ethics of genetic testing

Testing for a CPS presents difficult ethical questions in paediatric patients. The largest challenge is that children are developing decision-making capacity throughout childhood. For capacity, a child must be able to understand information surrounding their diagnosis, critically reason, and express a set of values to apply. If a child cannot demonstrate capacity, parents may be used as substitute decision-makers. As a result, it is usually the decision of the parents if a young, at-risk child should undergo genetic testing. Screening asymptomatic children is generally only acceptable when the test result will change the medical care during childhood. Consistent with this, in 1994 the US Institute of Medicine concluded that 'childhood testing is not appropriate for … untreatable childhood diseases' [56]. Ethicists have argued this point, saying that even if a disease is 'untreatable' in childhood, families and children can still benefit from a predictive diagnosis. Once parents know their child is likely to develop disease, they can choose to live closer to tertiary care facilities, save money for future health-care expenditures, and prepare emotionally for the eventual onset of disease [57]. For parents, there is also a psychological aspect of testing, which is the ability to remove uncertainty about the future of their child [27, 57]. Studies have shown that 'not knowing' can be more stressful than either a positive or a negative result [58].

Nevertheless, there are many risks to screening. Making the decision to screen a presymptomatic patient can result in loss of autonomy for the child. When the child is older, they may have wished not to be tested or not to know, but these options are lost [27]. A positive test may change parents' attitudes and they could treat the child as ill before symptoms are developed [57]. Test results may strain relationships between siblings and can lead to survivor's guilt in an unaffected sibling [27]. Similarly, parents may feel responsible for passing on a gene to their children and become burdened with guilt [25].

Families should also understand that testing for a CPS in a previously undiagnosed family could have repercussions for all relatives. A positive result will affect the risk status of other family members and may prompt more testing.

Ultimately, population data regarding the risk/benefit of treatment are useful, but each family requires an individualized assessment [57]. This should be done through multiple sessions so families have time to make informed decisions and consider possible repercussions of genetic testing [27].

Screening: Future directions

Although patients with CPSs are a heterogeneous group, they are most often not treated as such. Tumours that patients develop vary with respect to age of onset, location, rate of growth, response to medical management, and numerous other prognostic factors. These differences are largely attributed to the unique genetic and epigenetic profile among the diverse patient population [18]. Despite this, screening protocols currently do not reflect this reality and are not tailored to address the variety of genetic modifiers. With the advent of next-generation sequencing (NGS) and the rapidly falling cost of inspecting genotypes, advancements in personalized medicine can be expected in the coming years.

NGS has allowed for the discovery of previously unidentified modifier genes within predisposition syndromes, which are already beginning to be used to risk-stratify patients. As these modifiers are characterized more thoroughly, surveillance protocols and treatments can be built around a patient's unique risks. The ability to shape clinical care has already been put into practice, with a recent study showing that 43% of cancer patients who were genetically profiled received clinically significant results [59]. Sequencing has also led to the discovery of CPSs that otherwise would not have been recognized. In one example, whole-exome sequencing was used to uncover the causative role of germline *MAX* mutations in three patients with pheochromocytoma [3]. It is important to identify these germline mutations, because in a subset of CPSs chemoprevention has been shown to be efficacious [3].

The interest in the role of germline mutations has spurred the CSER Tumor Working Group to develop recommendations whereby germline mutations can be identified from a somatic tissue biopsy [60]. This approach will aid in the detection of low-penetrance and low-expressivity phenotypes of CPSs. Improved knowledge of these syndromes will be an asset in informing future care and developing individualized cancer therapies.

Another important tool for tumour detection is circulating tumour DNA (ctDNA), which is released from cells following death by apoptosis or necrosis, and is then detectable in the bloodstream. The amount of ctDNA in the blood correlates with tumour staging and prognosis [61]. While ctDNA has not yet been introduced into regular clinical care, it shows promise to allow for early detection of tumour development. This form of liquid tumour biopsy will also allow for the identification of chemical susceptibility without invasive techniques. The advantages offered by this method of monitoring can help alleviate the burden of screening for children with a CPS.

It is evident that precision oncology is the next leap forward in cancer prevention, screening, and treatment. In the future, improved clinical acumen in conjunction with an appreciation for cancer genomics will culminate in a new standard of care.

Late effects of treatment

An important issue in paediatric cancer is the propensity to develop complications following treatment. Children often receive therapy during critical periods of development and maturation, and survivors of childhood cancer have a lifetime to develop morbidities secondary to the care they received. This issue is especially important given the rising population of patients surviving to adulthood due to improvements in treatment. In the USA, approximately 1 in 570 people aged 20–34 is a survivor of childhood cancer, and this fraction continues to rise [62]. Over 60% of these childhood cancer survivors will have at least one long-term side effect of treatment [63]. As mentioned earlier, the complications from treatment are best mitigated through prevention, screening, and early detection. This allows for disease management by local therapy and avoidance of systemic exposures.

By far the most common late effect of treatment is secondary neoplasms. Secondary malignancies mainly consist of solid tumours secondary to radiation, or acute leukaemia and myelodysplastic syndrome after chemotherapy [24]. At 25 years from diagnosis, there are more deaths due to secondary malignancy than deaths attributable to any other cause, including recurrence of the primary cancer

[64]. At 30 years from diagnosis, approximately 20% of survivors have developed a secondary malignancy [64]. Death from secondary neoplasia has been associated with young age of diagnosis, radiation, alkylating agents, anthracyclines, epipodophyllotoxins, family history of cancer, type of primary diagnosis, and female sex [63, 64]. Latency periods for these cancers can be extremely long; for example, radiation-induced thyroid cancer has a median latency of 20.8 years [63]. Special considerations must also be taken with childhood cancer survivors who have a CPS. This population has an increased susceptibility to secondary malignancy from radiation or other DNA-damaging agents. Closer monitoring is required and special efforts must be made to avoid inflicting DNA damage during screening or treatment.

Cardiovascular disease (CVD) and pulmonary disease are also common late effects from treatment. Mortality from CVD and pulmonary disease in survivors of childhood cancer is increased 7-fold and 8.8-fold, respectively [63, 64]. Cardiac complications that develop include valvular defects, arrhythmias, congestive heart failure, and myocardial infarction. Lung disease can range from subclinical to life threatening, and can result in lung fibrosis and reduction in exercise tolerance as early as six years after diagnosis [65].

Secondary neoplasia, CVD, and pulmonary disease are only a few complications from an extensive list of potential morbidities that can develop after treatment. Each medical intervention during the management of cancer is associated with unique risks and requires special screening protocols. To address this, the Children's Oncology Group (COG) has established comprehensive screening recommendations to monitor for the development of disease after treatment. It cites over 100 possible late effects and the associated causative agents, risk factors, and suggested screening protocols, and also provides additional resources for health counselling [66].

These recommendations highlight the need for long-term follow-up clinics and regular check-ups with primary care physicians. At the end of cancer treatment, patients should receive information regarding their risks and the screening required. Although risk of death from the primary cancer decreases with time after treatment, risk of death from late effects of treatment increases [64]. For this reason, it is imperative to remain vigilant for the development of possible treatment effects and to adhere to lifelong screening. As cure rates rise beyond 85% for paediatric cancer, increasing attention must be placed on the management of this vulnerable population of survivors.

Conclusion

Prevention for paediatric cancers is limited due to the rarity and unpredictability of cancer development in youth. For those truly at risk, children with predisposition syndromes, thorough screening protocols are being developed to reduce morbidity and mortality. As sequencing becomes more ubiquitous and bioinformatics analyses advance, these screening protocols will be individually tailored to better match the needs of each patient. Developments in technology and an improved understanding of childhood cancer pathogenesis are setting a foundation to anticipate and target childhood cancers.

After treatment, there is an ever-growing group of survivors who require ongoing support and continued monitoring for the development of complications. As screening and prevention improve, cancer will be managed at earlier stages and the long-term burden of disease will be reduced in this vulnerable population. Overall, paediatric cancer represents a unique and challenging area of oncology, with distinct considerations specific to the youths affected. Significant advancements have been made to the field in the preceding decades, with more exciting developments promising to revolutionize quality of life and patient care.

References

1 Ward, E., DeSantis, C., Robbins, A. et al. (2014). Childhood and adolescent cancer statistics, 2014. *CA Cancer J. Clin.* 64 (2): 83–103.

2 Garber, J.E., and Offit, K. (2005). Hereditary cancer predisposition syndromes. *J. Clin. Oncol.* 23 (2): 276–292.

3 Samuel, N., Villani, A., Fernandez, C.V., and Malkin, D. (2014). Management of familial cancer: Sequencing, surveillance and society. *Nature Rev. Clin. Oncol.* 11 (12): 723–731.

4 Zhang, J., Walsh, M.F., Wu, G. et al. (2015). Germline mutations in predisposition genes in pediatric cancer. *N. Engl. J. Med.* 373 (24): 2336–2346.

5 American Cancer Society (2016). Risk factors and causes of childhood cancer. https://www.cancer.org/cancer/cancer-in-children/risk-factors-and-causes.html (accessed 3 January 2018).

6 Mittendorf, R. (1995). Teratogen update: Carcinogenesis and teratogenesis associated with exposure to diethylstilbestrol (DES) in utero. *Teratology* 51 (6): 435–445.

7 Murakami, M., and Fukami, J.-I. (1983). The binding of steroid hormones and diethylstilbestrol to proteins of human cells in culture. *Arch. Toxicol.* 53 (3): 245–248.

8 Lombardi, C., Ganguly, A., Bunin, G.R. et al. (2015). Maternal diet during pregnancy and unilateral retinoblastoma. *Cancer Causes Control* 26 (3): 387–397.

9 Kleinjans, J., Botsivali, M., Kogevinas, M., and Merlo Domenico, F. (2015). Fetal exposure to dietary carcinogens and risk of childhood cancer: What the NewGeneris project tells us. *BMJ* 2015: h4501.

10 Huang, Y., Huang, J.,Lan, J. et al. (2014). A meta-analysis of parental smoking and the risk of childhood brain tumors. *PloS One* 9 (7): e102910.

11 Johnson, K.J., Williams, K.S., Ross, J.A. et al. (2013). Parental tobacco and alcohol use and risk of hepatoblastoma in offspring: A report from the Children's Oncology Group. *Cancer Epidemiol. Biomarkers Prevent.* 22 (10): 1837–1843.

12 Pappo, A.S. (2003). Melanoma in children and adolescents. *Eur. J. Cancer* 39 (18): 2651–2661.

13 Godar, D.E., Urbach, F., Gasparro, F.P., and van der Leun, J.C. (2003). UV doses of young adults. *Photochem. Photobiol.* 77 (4): 453–457.

14 Harper, D.M., Franco, E.L., Wheeler, C. et al. (2004). Efficacy of a bivalent L1 virus-like particle vaccine in prevention of infection with human papillomavirus types 16 and 18 in young women: A randomised controlled trial. *Lancet* 364 (9447): 1757–1765.

15 Larke, N.L., Thomas, S.L., dos Santos Silva, I., and Weiss, H.A. (2011). Male circumcision and penile cancer: A systematic review and meta-analysis. *Cancer Causes Control* 22 (8): 1097–1110.

16 Rich, T.A., Liu, M., Etzel, C.J. et al. (2014). Comparison of attitudes regarding preimplantation genetic diagnosis among patients with hereditary cancer syndromes. *Fam. Cancer* 13 (2): 291–299.

17 Schiffman, J.D., Geller, J.I., Mundt, E. et al. (2013). Update on pediatric cancer predisposition syndromes. *Pediatr. Blood Cancer* 60 (8): 1247–1252.

18 Schiffman, J.D. (2014). Predisposition to pediatric and hematologic cancers: A moving target. Alexandra, VA: American Society of Clinical Oncology.

19 Monsalve, J., Kapur, J, Malkin, D., and Babyn, P.S. (2011). Imaging of cancer predisposition syndromes in children. *Radiographics* 31 (1): 263–280.

20 Villani, A., Tabori, U., Schiffman, J. et al. (2011). Biochemical and imaging surveillance in germline TP53 mutation carriers with Li-Fraumeni syndrome: A prospective observational study. *Lancet Oncol.* 12 (6): 559–567.

21 Woods, W.G., Tuchman, M., Robison, L.L. et al. (1996). A population-based study of the usefulness of screening for neuroblastoma. *Lancet* 348: 1682–1687.

22 Obuchowski, N.A., Graham, R.J., Baker, M.E., and Powell, K.A. (2001). Ten criteria for effective screening: Their application to multislice CT screening for pulmonary and colorectal cancers. *Am. J. Roentgenol.* 176 (6): 1357–1362.

23 Tluczek, A., Mischler, E.H., Farrell, P.M. et al. (1992). Parents' knowledge of neonatal screening and response to false-positive cystic fibrosis testing. *Dev. Behav. Pediatr.* 13: 181–186.

24 Jongmans, M.C., Loeffen, J.L., Waanders, E. et al. (2016). Recognition of genetic predisposition in pediatric cancer patients: An easy-to-use selection tool. *Eur. J. Med. Genet.* 59 (3): 116–125.

25 Malkin, D. (2004). Predictive genetic testing for childhood cancer: Taking the road less traveled by. *J. Pediatr. Hematol. Oncol.* 26 (9): 546–548.

26 Field, M., Shanley, S., and Kirk, J. (2007). Inherited cancer susceptibility syndromes in paediatric practice. *J. Paediatr. Child Health* 43(4): 219–229.

27 Tischkowitz, M., and Rosser, E. (2004). Inherited cancer in children: Practical/ethical problems and challenges. *Eur. J. Cancer* 40 (16): 2459–2470.

28 Wong, J.R., Tucker, M.A., Kleinerman, R.A., and Devesa, S.S. (2014). Retinoblastoma incidence patterns in the US Surveillance, Epidemiology, and End Results program. *JAMA Ophthalmol.* 132 (4): 478–483.

29 Rothschild, P.R., Lévy, D., Savignoni, A. et al. (2011). Familial retinoblastoma: Fundus screening schedule impact and guideline proposal. A retrospective study. *Eye* 25 (12): 1555–1561.

30 Bodmer, W.F., Bailey, C.J., Bodmer, J. et al. (1987). Localization of the gene for familial adenomatous polyposis on chromosome 5. *Nature* 328: 614–616.

31 Aoki, K., and Taketo, M.M. (2007). Adenomatous polyposis coli (APC): A multi-functional tumor suppressor gene. *J. Cell Sci.* 120 (19): 3327–3335.

32 Knudsen, A.L., Bisgaard, M.L., and Bülow, S. (2003). Attenuated familial adenomatous polyposis (AFAP): A review of the literature. *Fam. Cancer* 2 (1): 43–55.

33 Kennedy, R.D., Potter, D.D., Moir, C.R., and El-Youssef, M. (2014). The natural history of familial adenomatous polyposis syndrome: A 24-year review of a single center experience in screening, diagnosis, and outcomes. *J. Pediatr. Surg.* 49 (1): 82–86.

34 Munck, A., Gargouri, L., Alberti, C. et al. (2011). Evaluation of guidelines for management of familial adenomatous polyposis in a multicenter pediatric cohort. *J. Pediatr. Gastroenterol. Nutr.* 53 (3): 296–302.

35 Belchetz, L.A., Berk, T., Bapat, B.V. et al. (1996). Changing causes of mortality in patients with familial adenomatous polyposis. *Dis. Colon Rectum* 39: 384–387.

36 Vasen, H.FA, Möslein, G., Alonso, A. et al. (2008). Guidelines for the clinical management of familial adenomatous polyposis (FAP). *Gut* 57 (5): 704–713.

37 D'Orazio, J.A. (2010). Inherited cancer syndromes in children and young adults. *J. Pediatr. Hematol. Oncol.* 32 (3): 195–228.

38 Thakker, R.V., Newey, P.J., Walls, G.V. et al. (2012). Clinical practice guidelines for multiple endocrine neoplasia type 1 (MEN1). *J. Clin. Endocrinol. Metab.* 97 (9): 2990–3011.

39 Trump, D., Farren, B., Wooding, C. et al. (1996). Clinical studies of multiple endocrine neoplasia type 1 (MEN1). *QJM* 89 (9): 653–670.

40 Giri, D., McKay, V., Weber, A., and Blair, J.C. (2015). Multiple endocrine neoplasia syndromes 1 and 2: Manifestations and management in childhood and adolescence. *Arch. Dis. Child.* 100 (10): 994–999.

41 Johnston, L.B., Chew, S.L., Lowe, D. et al. (2001). Investigating familial endocrine neoplasia syndromes in children. *Horm. Res. Paediatr.* 55 (Suppl. 1): 31–35.

42 Weksberg, R., Shuman, C., and Beckwith, J.B. (2010). Beckwith–Wiedemann syndrome. *Eur. J. Hum. Genet.* 18 (1): 8–14.

43 Elliott, M., and Maher, E.R. (1994). Beckwith-Wiedemann syndrome. *J. Med. Genet.* 31 (7): 560.

44 Mussa, A., and Ferrero, G.B. (2015). Screening hepatoblastoma in Beckwith-Wiedemann syndrome: A complex issue. *J. Pediatr. Hematol. Oncol.* 37 (8): 627.

45 Kim, J.J., Rini, B.I., and Hansel, D.E. (2010) Von Hippel Lindau syndrome. *Adv. Exp. Med. Biol.* 685: 228–249.

46 Poulsen, M.L., Budtz-Jørgensen, E., and Bisgaard, M.L. (2010). Surveillance in von Hippel-Lindau disease (vHL). *Clin. Genet.* 77(1): 49–59.

47 Maher, E.R., Yates, J.R., Harries, R. et al. (1990). Clinical features and natural history of von Hippel-Lindau disease. *Q. J. Med.* 77 (283): 1151.

48 Maher, E.R., Neumann, H.P.H., and Richard, S. (2011). von Hippel–Lindau disease: A clinical and scientific review. *Eur. J. Hum. Genet.* 19 (6): 617–623.

49 Teplick, A., Kowalski, M., Biegel, J.A., and Nichols, K.E. (2011). Educational paper. *Eur. J. Pediatr.* 170 (3): 285–294.

50 Gill, A.J. (2012). Succinate dehydrogenase (SDH) and mitochondrial driven neoplasia. *Pathology* 44 (4): 285–292.

51 Pasini, B., and Stratakis, C.A. (2009). SDH mutations in tumorigenesis and inherited endocrine tumours: Lesson from the phaeochromocytoma–paraganglioma syndromes. *J. Intern. Med.* 266 (1): 19–42.

52 Ponti, G., Pastorino, L., Pollio, A. et al. (2012). Ameloblastoma: A neglected criterion for nevoid basal cell carcinoma (Gorlin) syndrome. *Fam. Cancer* 11 (3): 411–418.

53 Kimonis, V.E., Goldstein, A.M., Pastakia, B. et al. (1997). Clinical manifestations in 105 persons with nevoid basal cell carcinoma syndrome. *Am. J. Med. Genet.* 69 (3): 299–308.

54 Hill, D.A., Ivanovich, J., Priest, J.R. et al. (2009). DICER1 mutations in familial pleuropulmonary blastoma. *Science* 325 (5943): 965–965.

55 Bakry, D., Aronson, M., Durno, C. et al. (2014). Genetic and clinical determinants of constitutional mismatch repair deficiency syndrome: Report from the constitutional mismatch repair deficiency consortium. *Eur. J. Cancer* 50 (5): 987–996.

56 Institute of Medicine (1994). Assessing genetic risks: Implications for health and social policy. Washington, DC: National Academy Press.

57 Ross, L.F. (2002). Predictive genetic testing for conditions that present in childhood. *Kennedy Inst. Ethics J.* 12 (3): 225–244.

58 Broadstock, M., Michie, S., and Marteau, T. (2000). Psychological consequences of predictive genetic testing: A systematic review. *Eur. J. Hum. Genet.* 8: 731–738.

59 Harris, M.H., DuBois, S.G., Glade Bender, J.L. et al. (2016). Multicenter feasibility study of tumor molecular profiling to inform therapeutic decisions in advanced pediatric solid tumors: The Individualized Cancer Therapy (iCat) Study. *JAMA Oncol.* Jan. 28

60 Raymond, V.M., Gray, S.W., Roychowdhury, S. et al. (2016). Germline findings in tumor-only sequencing: Points to consider for clinicians and laboratories. *J. Natl Cancer Inst.* 108 (4): djv351.

61 Diaz, L.A., and Bardelli, A. (2014). Liquid biopsies: Genotyping circulating tumor DNA. *J. Clin. Oncol.* 32 (6): 579–586.

62 Hewitt, M.W.S., and Simone, J.V. (2003). *Childhood Cancer Survivorship: Improving Care and Quality of Life*. Washington, DC: National Academies Press.

63 Kopp, L.M., Gupta, P., Pelayo-Katsanis, L. et al. (2012). Late effects in adult survivors of pediatric cancer: A guide for the primary care physician. *Am. J. Med.* 125 (7): 636–641.

64 Record, E.O., and Meacham, L.R. (2015). Survivor care for pediatric cancer survivors: A continuously evolving discipline. *Curr. Opin. Oncol.* 27 (4): 291–296.

65 Huang, T.-T., Hudson, M.M., Stokes, D.C. et al. (2011). Pulmonary outcomes in survivors of childhood cancer: A systematic review. *CHEST* 140 (4): 881–901.

66 Children's Oncology Group (2013). Long-term follow-up guidelines for survivors of childhood, adolescent, and young adult cancers, Version 4.0. www.survivorshipguidelines.org (accessed 3 January 2018).

CHAPTER 26

Obesity and dietary approaches to cancer prevention

Andrew G. Renehan

Division of Cancer Sciences, School of Medical Sciences, University of Manchester; Manchester Cancer Research Centre and NIHR Manchester Biomedical Research Centre; Colorectal and Peritoneal Oncology Centre, The Christie NHS Foundation Trust, Manchester, UK

SUMMARY BOX

- Dietary influences on cancer risk are considered in three broad exposure categories: global excess caloric intake (eventually manifesting as overweight and obesity); macronutrients; and micronutrients. For each exposure, this chapter refers to a World Cancer Research Fund report, which arrives at judgements of 'convincing', 'probably', and 'limited', taking into account several a priori criteria.

- There is convincing and probable evidence that excess body weight, commonly expressed as body mass index (BMI), is associated with increased risk of more than 10 different adult cancer types.

- There is convincing evidence that red meat and processed meat are causes of colorectal cancer; and that foods containing dietary fibre, nonstarchy vegetables, and fruit probably protect against several gastrointestinal cancers.

- There is convincing and probable evidence that alcoholic drinks are a cause of cancers of the gastrointestinal tract, breast, and liver.

- There is limited evidence that micronutrients protect against cancer; there is convincing evidence that high-dose beta-carotene supplements are a cause of lung cancer in tobacco smokers.

- Cancer prevention through weight control and dietary modification is mainly via public awareness (though the promotion of a healthy diet is poorly defined) and legislation in selected cases. The multidimensionality of these approaches is encapsulated in the Manchester Cancer Prevention strategy grid.

Cancer Prevention and Screening: Concepts, Principles and Controversies, First Edition.
Edited by Rosalind A. Eeles, Christine D. Berg, and Jeffrey S. Tobias.
© 2019 John Wiley & Sons, Inc. Published 2019 by John Wiley & Sons, Inc.

For the purpose of this chapter, dietary influences on cancer risk are considered in three broad exposure categories: global excess caloric intake (eventually manifesting as overweight and obesity); macronutrients; and micronutrients. Precise quantification of exposure–disease risk underpins approaches to cancer prevention in this field. Over the past decade, a large volume of epidemiological and mechanistic studies have established and clarified these exposure–cancer risks. The 2007 World Cancer Research Fund (WCRF) [1], and its Continuous Update Project (CUP) [2], has been a central informative source for this subject, and forms a key part of this chapter. For each exposure, the WCRF arrives at a judgement of 'convincing', 'probable', or 'limited', taking into account several a priori criteria supporting (or not) causality, the susceptibility of data to confounding, and bias.

Smoking and physical inactivity are important risk factors for several cancer types, where diet and excess body weight also modify risk. These risk factors are beyond the scope of this chapter, as they are covered elsewhere in this book. Nonetheless, it is important to note that these multiple risk factors often interact and modify effect sizes of associations – for example, smoking and body mass index (BMI) [3] and smoking and diet [4] – on incident cancer risk, such that the risk factors discussed in this chapter should not be considered in isolation.

Assessment of the evidence

WCRF criteria for grading evidence
Table 26.1 lists the criteria agreed by the WCRF Panel that were necessary to support the judgements made regarding exposure–cancer associations. The grades are 'convincing', 'probable', 'limited–suggestive', 'limited–no conclusion', and 'substantial effect on risk unlikely'. The WCRF report [1] notes that 'in addition, interpretation of epidemiological evidence on any and all aspects of foods and drinks, body composition, and associated factors, with the risk of cancer, is never simple. General considerations include … methodological issues …, which need to be taken into account when evidence is assembled and assessed.'

Energy adjustment and dietary patterns
The first basic principle when evaluating the effect of a specific dietary factor on disease risk (here, cancer) is that the diets should be isocaloric (i.e. total energy intake is the same in both groups). This applies to animal experiments, and whenever possible (usually through adjustment) for human studies. Calorie intake and weight control are intrinsically related. Without taking caloric intake into account, if risk differences emerge attributed to the effects of the specific dietary factor of interest, the effects might simply reflect the influence of weight differences. Furthermore, differences in weight per se might have different physiological effects, independent of the dietary factors under investigation.

Table 26.1 WCRF judgement criteria.

Convincing	The following criteria are generally required: • Evidence from more than one study type. • Evidence from at least two independent cohort studies. • Absence of unexplained heterogeneity. • Good-quality studies to exclude with confidence the possibility that the observed association results from confounding or bias. • Presence of a plausible biological gradient ('dose response') in the association. • Strong and plausible experimental evidence, either from human studies or relevant animal models.
Probable	The following criteria are generally required: • Evidence from at least two independent cohort studies, or at least five case-control studies. • No substantial unexplained heterogeneity between or within study types in the presence or absence of an association, or direction of effect. • Good-quality studies to exclude with confidence the possibility that the observed association results from confounding or bias. • Evidence for biological plausibility.
Limited – suggestive evidence	These criteria are for evidence that is too limited to permit a probable or convincing causal judgement, but where there is evidence suggestive of a direction of effect. The evidence may have methodological flaws, or be limited in amount, but shows a generally consistent direction of effect. This almost always does not justify recommendations designed to reduce the incidence of cancer. The following criteria are generally required: • Evidence from at least two independent cohort studies or at least five case-control studies. • The direction of effect is generally consistent though some unexplained heterogeneity may be present. • Evidence for biological plausibility.
Limited – no conclusion	Evidence is so limited that no firm conclusion can be made. This category represents an entry level, and is intended to allow any exposure for which there are sufficient data to warrant Panel consideration, but where insufficient evidence exists to permit a more definitive grading. This does not necessarily mean a limited quantity of evidence. A body of evidence for a particular exposure might be graded 'limited – no conclusion' for a number of reasons. The evidence might be limited by the amount of evidence in terms of the number of studies available, by inconsistency of direction of effect, by poor quality of studies (for example, lack of adjustment for known confounders), or by any combination of these factors.
Substantial effect on risk unlikely	Evidence is strong enough to support a judgement that a particular food, nutrition, or physical activity exposure is unlikely to have a substantial causal relation to a cancer outcome. The evidence should be robust enough to be unlikely to be modified in the foreseeable future as new evidence accumulates.

Source: World Cancer Research Fund 2007 [1].

Secondly, most studies on diet and cancer risk have been undertaken in high-income countries. Thus, results from these studies might not necessarily be generalizable to other countries and populations. Furthermore, important dietary constituents in some foods consumed outside high-income countries might not have been evaluated.

Thirdly, as an additional dimension to the above (that most studies have been undertaken in high-income countries), the ranges and distributions that define (in statistical terms, parameterize) food and drink distributions may not apply to other countries. If distributions are wide, findings from studies may overemphasize the significance (or insignificance) of foods and drinks commonly consumed in high-income countries, but not applicable to middle- and low-income countries.

Finally, many studies on the diet–cancer link, in the past, frequently failed to take account of the effects of methods of food and drink production, preservation, processing, and preparation (including cooking). Historically, studies were inclined to underestimate the significance of foods and drinks where these were combined in dishes or meals. Again, these processes may vary between countries.

Measurement errors

The study of nutritional epidemiology is noted for difficulties in measuring and precisely quantifying dietary factor consumption. In general terms, it is easier to measure food intakes than intakes of dietary constituents of foods: 'This can lead to an undue degree of importance being given to studies of aspects of food and nutrition that happen to be more easily measured' [1]. Furthermore, for some dietary constituents there are no generally agreed definitions. For example, it is increasingly appreciated that there are different types of 'dietary fibre', each with different biological effects.

One of the greatest challenges in nutritional epidemiology is quantifying dietary exposure over time. A commonly used tool is the food-frequency questionnaire (FFQ), but this may be too crude to elicit modest (but important) dietary–cancer associations. This was illustrated in a seminal paper from Bingham and colleagues [5], who noted that cohort studies using the FFQ failed to show a relation between fat intake and breast cancer risk (speculating that the FFQ methods were prone to measurement error), but that a positive association was noted when a detailed seven-day food diary was used. However, the latter approach is resource heavy, restricting studies to modest sample sizes.

Study design, confounding, and biases

Almost all studies that contribute to the evidence presented here are observational. These study designs are inevitably susceptible to confounding and biases. The STROBE (Strengthening the Reporting of Observational Studies in Epidemiology) reporting guidance includes three main design categories: cohort, case-control, and cross-sectional [6]. There are many investigators who believe that there is a hierarchical structure to the relative merits of these different design types – for example, recall bias in case-control studies and the lack of direct assessment of disease risk in cross-sectional data are major limitations, but this dictum remains a matter of opinion. A small number of randomized controlled trials contribute to the evidence in this chapter, but these are invariably interventions of specific micronutrients. The WCRF report [1] notes that these trials often 'test the effects of dietary constituents as opposed to whole diets' and 'could lead to over-emphasis of the importance of isolated constituents which, within the context of food and diets, may have other effects'.

The STROBE reporting guidance states that 'confounding literally means confusion of effects' [6]. A confounder is a factor associated with both the outcome (in this case, cancer) and the exposure being studied, but is not an effect of the exposure. It is never possible for observational studies to eliminate completely the possibility that an evident effect of a constituent, or aspect of a food or drink, is at least in part caused by another factor. This is a common scenario in nutritional epidemiology, and obesity and cancer epidemiology.

On the other hand, a 'bias is a systematic deviation of a study's result from a true value' [6]. The STROBE reporting guidance makes a clear statement that 'bias and confounding are not synonymous' [6], and that biases arise either from false information (i.e. information bias) or subject selection (i.e. selection bias). Studies reliant on self-reporting of dietary intake are prone to bias. Notably, study participants tend to over-report consumption of foods that they believe to be healthy, and under-report foods that they believe to be unhealthy. Under-reporting of energy intake has been shown to be associated with factors such as age, overweight and obesity, and perceived body size [1].

It is worth briefly discussing *dose response*, a term borrowed from pharmacology, which can be applied in epidemiological studies of an exposure (including food and nutrition) and cancer risk. If a study observes a graded response, or a *biological gradient*, this might support the notion of biological plausibility, in that higher exposure leads to increased, or to reduced, risk. However, dose–response relationships are not straightforward, and commonly are nonlinear. This is well illustrated, for example, in the relationships between BMI and cancer outcome (the author has elsewhere described at least four common nonlinear relationships [7]).

Effect modification (or interaction) occurs when a measure of effect for an exposure changes over levels of another variable (the modifier) [6]. There are several examples of effect modifiers on the relation between excess weight (commonly expressed as elevated BMI) and cancer risk [8]. These include cigarette smoking, hormonal replacement therapy (HRT), and viral drivers of cancer, such as viral hepatitis and liver cancer. These will be illustrated in detail in the next sections. Effect modifiers are generally other cancer risk factors, and an effect modifier can also be a confounder. Smoking is an example, as ever smokers tend to have lower mean BMI levels compared with never smokers [9].

Excess body weight (elevated body mass index) and cancer risk

List of obesity-related cancers

In 2007, the WCRF [1] reported that there was 'convincing' evidence that body fatness, generally measured by calculating BMI (kg/m^2), was associated with an increased risk of oesophageal adenocarcinoma, and cancers of the pancreas, colorectum, postmenopausal breast, endometrium, and kidney, and evidence of 'probable' association with increased risk of gall-bladder cancer. Simultaneously, the present author led an overview systematic review and dose–response meta-analysis of prospective observational studies (221 datasets including 281 137 incident cancer diagnoses), published in 2008, quantifying cancer risk among 20 cancer types, expressed as risk per increase of $5\,kg/m^2$ [10]. By using a standardized approach across a large number of cancer types, that analysis demonstrated that associations are (1) sex specific (for example, a stronger association for men versus women for colon cancer); (2) site specific (for example, a stronger association for colon versus rectal cancer); (3) histology specific (for example, an association exists for oesophageal adenocarcinoma but not squamous cell carcinoma, SCC); (4) broadly consistent across geographical populations; and (5) present for BMI–cancer for a wider range of malignancies not previously thought to be linked with obesity [8].

Since the above two reports in 2007/2008, the most comprehensive updated evaluations of the associations between measures of body fatness and cancer risk have been undertaken through the WCRF CUP, which now links excess weight or body fatness to 11 cancers [2]. In 2016, an expert working group of 21 scientists from eight countries (including the present author) gathered, under the auspices of the International Agency for Research on Cancer (IARC) [11], to specifically evaluate the preventive effects of avoidance of excess body fatness on cancer risk. This group extended the list of obesity-related cancer, for which *sufficient* evidence exists, to 13 malignancies, as follows: cancers of the colon and rectum, oesophagus (adenocarcinoma), kidney (renal cell), breast (postmenopausal), endometrium, gastric cardia, liver, gall-bladder, pancreas, ovary, thyroid, multiple myeloma, and meningioma. A summary of the updated list of obesity-related cancers by gender is shown in Table 26.2 [10–16].

For the majority of these cancers, there are plausible biological mechanisms to explain these links. These candidates are three hormonal (systemic) systems, namely circulating sex hormones; the insulin and the insulin-like growth factor (IGF) system; and circulating adipokines and subclinical systemic inflammation [8]. In addition, the local peri-tumour adipose micro-environment or local ectopic fat is likely to be important [8, 17].

Other anthropometric measures, such as waist circumference (WC), and cancer risk have been evaluated. There are fewer studies, but the list of cancers associated with WC is similar to that for BMI [18]. Where comparative analyses are standardized, the magnitude of effect by WC is similar to that for BMI and cancer risk [19].

Table 26.2 Sex-specific risk estimates for increase in body mass index (BMI) by cancer types and gender (where data available).

Site	No. of studies (reference)	Summary estimates per 5 kg/m² (95% confidence intervals)	
		Men	**Women**
Oesophageal adenocarcinoma	5 cohorts [10]	1.52 (1.33–1.74)	1.51 (1.31–1.74)
Gastric cardia	IARC [11]	Highest vs lowest: 1.8 (1.3–2.5)	
Colorectal	29 cohorts [10]		
Colon		1.24 (1.20–1.28)	1.09 (1.05–1.13)
Rectum		1.09 (1.06–1.12)	1.02 (1.00–1.05)
Liver	14 pooled cohorts [12]	1.19 (1.09–1.29)	1.12 (1.03–1.22)
Gallbladder	4 cohorts [10]	1.09 (0.99–1.21)	1.59 (1.02–2.47)
Pancreatic	23 cohorts [14]	1.13 (1.04–1.22)	1.10 (1.04–1.16)
Kidney: renal cell	12 cohorts [10]	1.24 (1.15–1.34)	1.34 (1.25–1.43)
Meningioma	IARC [11]	Highest vs lowest: 1.5 (1.3–1.8)	
Thyroid	22 pooled cohorts [13]	1.06 (1.02–1.10)	
Multiple myeloma	IARC [11]	Highest vs lowest: 1.5 (1.2–2.0)	
Breast	34 cohorts [10]		
Postmenopausal breast			1.12 (1.08–1.16)
Premenopausal breast			0.92 (0.88–0.97)
Endometrial	19 cohorts [10]		1.59 (1.50–1.68)
Ovarian	34 cohorts [15]		1.06 (1.00–1.12)
Advanced prostate*	23 cohorts [16]	1.08 (1.04–1.12)	

*Prostate cancer is not on the IARC list, but is included here as it is on the WCRF list. Advanced prostate cancer is defined differently across studies, but including AJCC stages 3 and 4; metastatic cancer; Whitmore/Jewett stages C and D; high grade; and Gleason grade ≥7.

Effect modification of the BMI–cancer association

Over the past five years, it has become clear that in addition to the common effect modifiers such as age and sex, there are other effect modifiers of the BMI–cancer associations listed. Two clear examples are smoking status [20] and HRT [8, 21]. For example, studies show a higher risk of pancreatic cancer due to elevated BMI among never and ex-smokers as compared with current smokers with an equivalent elevated BMI [14]. Meta-analyses generally show inverse associations between BMI and smoking-related cancers, such as lung cancer and oesophageal squamous cell carcinoma. When these analyses are stratified by smoking status, null associations are generally observed in the never smoker strata. In the example of HRT use, meta-analyses of prospective studies evaluating the associations between BMI and subsequent risk of postmenopausal breast, endometrial, and ovarian cancers, stratified by HRT use, demonstrate that per incremental increase of 5 kg/m^2, there are increased risks of 18%, 90%, and 10%, respectively, in never HRT users. Among ever HRT users, there are no associations between BMI and postmenopausal breast and ovarian cancers, and an attenuated association (from 90% to 18% increase per 5 kg/m^2) for endometrial cancer [8].

A further effect modifier might be positivity for the presence of a viral oncogene. In a recently reported pooled analysis of 14 US-based prospective studies, Campbell and colleagues [12] (including the present author) confirmed an expected association between BMI and incident liver cancer, additionally showing a stronger association for men compared with women (Figure 26.1). The study also had the opportunity to explore the BMI–cancer association in a nested case-control analysis in individuals with measured serology for hepatitis B and C (HBV/HCV). In the presence of positive HBV/HCV serology, the BMI–liver cancer association was null; but there was a positive association where HBV/HCV serology was negative ($P_{interaction} = 0.04$) (Figure 26.1).

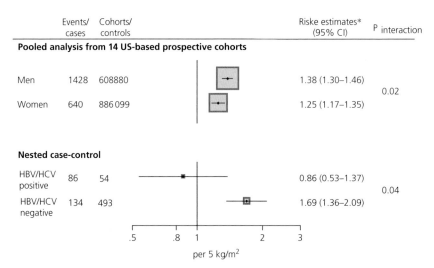

Figure 26.1 Summary plots of risk estimates for the associations of body mass index (BMI) and incident liver cancer, by gender and by hepatitis serology status (the latter in a nested case-control study). The horizontal lines represent risk confidence intervals. Size of box is proportionate to number of participants per category; proportionality is retained across the categories for illustrative reasons.
HBV, hepatitis B virus; HCV, hepatitis C virus.
* Risk estimates were hazard ratios for pooled analysis and odds ratios for nested case-control.
Constructed *de novo* using data directly supplied by Dr Peter Campbell [12].

It is tempting to speculate on the implications of these effect modification observations as follows. If there is a strong oncogenic driver (such as smoking, HRT, or a viral oncogene), the BMI–cancer association is significantly attenuated or 'drowned out'. This might have implications for prevention recommendations.

Population-attributable risk

As body weight is modifiable, there is a potential for cancer prevention. Calculation of attributable risk (often expressed as population-attributable fraction, PAF) offers an estimate of the burden of excess cancers attributable to elevated BMI in populations, and thus an approximation of avoidable cases and the potential for prevention. A research team, led from IARC (and including the present author), estimated that the PAF worldwide attributed to elevated BMI is 3.6%, or nearly half a million new cancer cases in adults [22]. PAFs are higher in women compared with men (5.4% versus 1.9%).

The methodologies used in these analyses were similar to those used in the Global Burden of Disease Project, in turn allowing ranking with analyses of attribution from other cancer risk factors using equivalent methodologies. Thus, at a global level, excess body weight is the third commonest attributable risk factor for cancer, after smoking (PAF 21%) [23] and infection (PAF 16%) [24]. In the UK, excess weight ranks as the second commonest risk factor, with a PAF of 5.5%, after smoking with a PAF of 19% [23, 24]. Thus, obesity is now a major public health issue not just for cardiovascular disease and diabetes risk, but also for cancer prevention.

Macronutrients and cancer risk

There are volumes of evidence and studies in this field, and a comprehensive overview is beyond the scope of this chapter. Instead, summary key findings are listed next, tabulated in Table 26.3. Several findings are cited directly from the 2007 WCRF report [1], with additional key updates as appropriate.

Meat consumption

Meat is an energy-dense macronutrient. Red meat may be high in animal fats, and fats may independently contribute to cancer risk. Subpopulations with high meat consumption also have elevated BMI values [25], a potential confounder. The 2007 WRCF report [1] concluded that there is convincing evidence that red meat and processed meat are causes of colorectal cancer:

> There is limited evidence suggesting that red meat is a cause of cancers of the oesophagus, lung, pancreas and endometrium; that processed meat is a cause of cancers of the oesophagus, lung, stomach and prostate; and that foods containing iron are a cause of colorectal cancer. There is also limited evidence that animal foods that are grilled (broiled), barbecued (charbroiled), or smoked, are a cause of stomach cancer.

These conclusions have been subject to ongoing quantification and interpretation over the past decade. In 2015, an IARC monograph working group evaluated the

Table 26.3 WCRF summary judgements on key foods as factors that modify risk of cancer.

	Meat consumption		Cereals/fibres		Vegetables and fruit		Milk/dairy products/ sugars		Fats and oils	
	Exposure	Cancer site	Exposure	Cancer site	Exposure	Cancer site	Exposure	Cancer site	Exposure	Cancer site
DECREASES RISK										
Convincing			Foods containing dietary fibres	Colorectum	Nonstarchy vegetables	Mouth, pharynx, larynx, oesophagus, stomach	Milk	Colorectum		
Probable					Allium vegetables	Stomach				
					Garlic	Colorectum				
					Fruits	Mouth, pharynx, larynx, lung, oesophagus, stomach				

Food / factor	Cancer site
Limited – suggestive/ no conclusion*	
Fish	Colorectum, liver[2]
Foods containing dietary fibres	Oesophagus
Nonstarchy vegetables	Nasopharynx, lung, colorectum, ovary, endometrium
Milk	Bladder
Soya, soya products	Pre- and postmenopausal breast[4]
Carrots	Cervix
Fruits	Nasopharynx, pancreas, liver, colorectum, stomach[1]
Pulses (legumes)	Stomach, prostate

Increases risk

Food / factor	Cancer site
Convincing	
Red meat	Colorectum
Processed meat	Colorectum
Processed meat	Stomach (noncardia)[1]
Aflatoxins	Liver
Diets high in calcium	Prostate
Probable	
Foods preserved by salting	Stomach[1]
Cantonese-style salted fish	Nasopharynx

Continued

Table 26.3 Continued

	Meat consumption		Cereals/fibres		Vegetables and fruit		Milk/dairy products/ sugars		Fats and oils	
	Exposure	Cancer site	Exposure	Cancer site	Exposure	Cancer site	Exposure	Cancer site	Exposure	Cancer site
Limited – suggestive/ no conclusion*	Red meat	Oesophagus, lung, pancreas, endometrium			Chilli	Stomach	Milk and dairy products	Prostate	Total fat	Lung, postmenopausal breast
	Processed meat	Oesophagus, lung, stomach, prostate					Cheese	Colorectum	Foods containing animal fats	Colorectum
	Smoked foods	Stomach					Foods containing sugars†	Colorectum[3]	Butter	Lung
									Foods containing saturated fatty acids	Pancreas[5]

Source: All entries are taken from the 2007 WCRF report [1], unless otherwise stated.

*The WCRF report had two limited evidence categories: suggestive and no conclusion. For simplicity of presentation, these have been combined here. An exhaustive list is not included.

†'Sugars' here means all 'nonmilk extrinsic' sugars, including refined and other added sugars, honey, and as contained in fruit juices and syrups. It does not include sugars naturally present in whole foods, such as fruit, and does not include lactose, as contained in animal or human milks.

[1] Added in the WCRF Stomach Cancer CUP 2016 [2]. [2] Added in the WCRF Liver Cancer CUP 2015 [2]. [3] Added in the WCRF Colorectal Cancer CUP 2011 [2]. [4] Added in the WCRF Breast Cancer CUP 2010 [2]. [5] Added in the WCRF Pancreas CUP 2012 [2].

carcinogenicity of the consumption of red meat and processed meat [26]. It defined red meat as 'unprocessed mammalian muscle meat – for example, beef, veal, pork, lamb, mutton, horse, or goat meat – including minced or frozen meat' and processed meat as 'meat that has been transformed through salting, curing, fermentation, smoking, or other processes to enhance flavour or improve preservation'. The working group pointed out that that there are many potentially important 'healthy' constituents in meat, including high biological value proteins and micronutrients such as B vitamins, iron (both free iron and haem iron), and zinc. However, biological concerns of carcinogenicity arise: first, through meat processing, such as curing and smoking, which can result in the formation of carcinogenic chemicals, including N-nitroso-compounds (NOCs) and polycyclic aromatic hydrocarbons (PAHs); and secondly, through cooking, which may produce known or suspected carcinogens, such as heterocyclic aromatic amines (HAAs) and PAHs.

The IARC monograph quantified colorectal cancer risk, citing a meta-analysis of 10 cohort studies [27] that reported a statistically significant dose–response relationship, with a 17% increased risk per 100 g per day of red meat and an 18% increase per 50 g per day of processed meat. The IARC monograph [26] examined 15 other types of cancer, and reported positive associations between consumption of red meat and cancers of the pancreas and the prostate (mainly advanced prostate cancer), and between consumption of processed meat and cancer of the stomach.

There remains a considerable amount of controversy around the exact extent of the association between meat (food) per se, and whether or not other constituents are the contributing influences. Some researchers claim that the cancer risk estimates associated with meat consumption are inflated [28]. There is an 'industry' of meta-analyses on this topic: for example, one arguing that after taking account of various methodological considerations, associations are weak [29]; another claiming that the type of meat product matters, and that, for example, there may be no association between pork consumption and colorectal cancer risk [30]. These inconsistencies make it difficult to give clear and consistent recommendations.

Vegetables, fruits, pulses (legumes), nuts, seeds, herbs, and spices

Fruits and nonstarchy vegetables are generally low energy-dense foods. The 2007 WRCF report [1] summarized that non-starchy vegetables are probably protective against cancers of the mouth, pharynx, larynx, oesophagus, and stomach: 'There is limited evidence suggesting that these macro-nutrients protect against cancers of the nasopharynx, lung, colorectum, ovary, and endometrium.' Additionally, 'allium vegetables probably protect against stomach cancer. Garlic (an allium vegetable) probably protects against colorectal cancer. There is limited evidence suggesting that carrots protect against cervical cancer; and that pulses (legumes), including soya and soya products, protect against stomach and prostate cancers.'

In general, fruits probably protect against cancers of the mouth, pharynx, and larynx, oesophagus, lung, and stomach. There is limited evidence suggesting that fruits also protect against cancers of the nasopharynx, pancreas, liver, and colorectum. There is limited evidence suggesting that chilli is a cause of stomach cancer.

Cereals (grains), roots, tubers, and plantains

Foods containing dietary fibre probably protect against colorectal cancer; and there is limited evidence suggesting that such foods protect against oesophageal cancer. Dietary fibre is found in plant foods such as vegetables, fruits, and pulses (legumes), as well as in cereals, roots, tubers, and plantains. All these foods are highest in dietary fibre when in whole or minimally processed form. Foods high in dietary fibre may have a protective effect because of being bulky and relatively low in energy density. [1]

The WRCF report [1] concluded that 'the evidence that foods contaminated with aflatoxins are a cause of liver cancer is convincing. Cereals (grains) and peanuts are the foods most commonly infested by these fungal toxins. Contamination is most widespread in countries with hot, damp climates and poor storage facilities.'

Fish consumption

The finding of the WRCF Report was that 'There is limited evidence suggesting that fish protect against colorectal cancer. Cantonese-style salted fish is probably a cause of nasopharyngeal cancer' [1].

Milk and dairy products

The conclusion of the WRCF report [1] was that 'milk probably protects against colorectal cancer; but limited evidence suggesting that milk protects against bladder cancer. There is limited evidence suggesting that cheese is a cause of colorectal cancer.'

It added that 'There is limited evidence suggesting that high consumption of milk and dairy products is a cause of prostate cancer" [1]. Milk is high in calcium, and there is evidence that diets high in calcium are a probable cause of prostate cancer.

Fats and oils

The WRCF report [1] found that 'there is limited evidence suggesting that total fat is a cause of lung cancer, and of postmenopausal breast cancer; that animal fat is a cause of colorectal cancer; and that consumption of butter is a cause of lung cancer'. The earlier reference in the comments on measurement error illustrated the challenges of accurately capturing dietary fat exposure using dietary questionnaires [5], and how the type of questionnaire used (FFQ versus detailed seven-day food diary) influences whether or not associations might be noted.

Salt and sugars

The conclusion of the WRCF report was that 'Salt is a probable cause of stomach cancer. Salt-preserved foods are also a probable cause of stomach cancer. There is limited evidence suggesting that sugars are a cause of colorectal cancer' [1].

Alcohol and other drinks

Alcoholic drinks

The WRCF report [1] concluded that 'the evidence that alcoholic drinks are a cause of cancers of the mouth, pharynx, and larynx, oesophagus, colorectum (men), and breast is convincing. Alcoholic drinks are probably a cause of liver cancer, and of colorectal cancer in women. It is unlikely that alcoholic drinks have a substantial adverse effect on the risk of kidney cancer.'

Since the 2007 WCRF report, there has been a considerable literature further defining the relationship between alcohol consumption and breast cancer risk. Large-scale analyses suggest that the alcohol–breast associations are not present for all breast cancer subtypes [31], and there is some evidence that alcohol use may be more strongly associated with risk of hormone-sensitive breast cancers compared with hormone-insensitive subtypes, suggesting distinct aetiological pathways for these two breast cancer subtypes [32]. It is also worth noting that the magnitude of association between alcohol and breast cancer risk is substantial – for example, hazard ratios for women consuming seven or more drinks per week versus never drinkers are of the order of twofold differences [31].

Coffee

The updated reports from the WCRF noted that there is evidence that coffee probably decreases the risk of endometrial [33] and liver [34] cancers; while that on pancreatic cancer noted that there was evidence that a substantial effect on risk was unlikely for coffee and pancreatic cancer [35].

Micronutrients and cancer risk

The 2007 WRCF report [1] summarized that 'foods containing *selenium* probably protect against prostate cancer; and there is limited evidence suggesting that these foods protect against stomach and colorectal cancers. There is limited evidence suggesting that foods containing *pyridoxine* protect against oesophageal and prostate cancers; and that foods containing *vitamin E* protect against oesophageal and prostate cancers.'

Macronutrients, such as vegetables, fruits, and pulses (legumes), and nuts and seeds, are rich in certain micronutrients that in themselves might influence cancer risk. Thus:

foods containing *folate* probably protect against pancreatic cancer, and there is limited evidence suggesting that these foods also protect against oesophageal and colorectal cancers. Foods containing *carotenoids* probably protect against cancers of the mouth, pharynx, and larynx, and lung cancer. Foods containing the carotenoid *beta-carotene* probably protect against oesophageal cancer; and foods containing *lycopene* probably protect against prostate cancer. *Calcium* probably protects against colorectal cancer. Foods containing *vitamin C* probably protect against oesophageal cancer.

> There is limited evidence suggesting that foods containing *quercetin* protect against lung cancer. There is also limited evidence suggesting that *alpha-tocopherol* protects against prostate cancer. [1]

It is important to note that many cancer protective effects from these micronutrients relate to specified doses.

The report also noted that 'The evidence that high-dose *beta-carotene supplements* are a cause of lung cancer in tobacco smokers is convincing. There is limited evidence suggesting that *high-dose retinol* supplements are a cause of lung cancer in tobacco smokers' [1]. This is the one research area where there are supporting data from randomized controlled trials (for example, the ATBC study, the CARET study, the Antioxidant Polyp Prevention trial), and demonstrates an example where trials reveal contrasting findings to those findings noted in epidemiological studies (reviewed elsewhere [36]).

It is unlikely that beta-carotene has a substantial effect on the risk of either prostate cancer or nonmelanoma skin cancer. There is limited evidence suggesting that retinol, at specific doses, protects against squamous cell carcinoma of the skin. There is also limited evidence suggesting that selenium supplements are a cause of skin cancer.

Controversy remains whether or not vitamin D protects against colorectal cancer. Various approaches have been employed to estimate vitamin D status in populations, including direct measures of circulating 25(OH)vitamin levels, and surrogates or alternative determinants of vitamin D (for example, region of residence, sun exposure estimates). While there is consistency of associations across geographical populations, confounding factors cannot be entirely excluded [37]. The updated WCRF report on colorectal cancer concluded that evidence was limited but suggestive on this question [38].

Dietary patterns

The 2007 WCRF reported noted that 'existing studies of specific dietary patterns use different definitions and that the evidence of their effect is unclear'. It concluded that no judgements can be made on any possible relationship between dietary patterns and the risk of cancer [1].

There is evidence from observational studies that adherence to a Mediterranean diet is associated with reduced cancer risk, but confounding cannot be excluded. Recently published trial evidence now supports this hypothesis. The PREDIMED study was a 1:1:1 randomized, single-blind, controlled-field dietary trial conducted at primary care level in Spain. Breast cancer incidence was a prespecified secondary outcome. The study was the first trial to show a beneficial effect of an immediate-term (median 4.8 years follow-up) Mediterranean diet supplemented with extra-virgin olive oil in the primary prevention of breast cancer. However, the authors acknowledged that their findings are 'based on few incident cases and, therefore, need to be confirmed in longer-term and larger studies' [39].

Cancer prevention through weight control and dietary modification

The Manchester Cancer Prevention strategy grid

Against the large volume of evidence laid out in this chapter on diet, obesity, and cancer risk, there is a need to channel this information through pathways to cancer prevention. In practice, in a social and health-care system such as that in the UK, the main strategies for weight control and dietary modification are through public awareness and legislation in selected cases. The former requires the promotion of a *healthy diet* – though this is poorly defined.

There are additional dimensions to cancer prevention, including type of prevention (primary, secondary, and tertiary); level of intervention (population, patient – namely, high-risk individuals, and personalized prevention at an individual level); and type of intervention. To address these multidimensional relationships, this chapter introduces the Manchester Cancer Prevention strategy grid (Table 26.4). This grid goes beyond cancer prevention through weight control and dietary interventions, to include other strategies such as screening, lifestyle interventions, vaccinations, chemoprevention, and prophylactic surgical interventions. There is a wealth of evidence that several prevention strategies are effective (for example bowel cancer screening; chemoprevention in women at high-risk of developing breast cancer) but at a real-world level, these strategies have been under-realized. Currently, there is a need for more integrated approaches – the grid offers this framework.

WCRF recommendations

As a follow-on to the 2007 report, in 2009 the WCRF published a policy and action document on cancer prevention: 'Food, Nutrition and Physical Activity' at a global level [40]. It developed an eight-point recommendation list, detailed in Table 26.5. The report estimated that about a third of the 13 most common cancers in the UK could be prevented through improved diet and body weight control.

There is currently an increasing focus on tackling the 'obesity' epidemic. Thus, for example, a recent report jointly from Cancer Research UK and the UK Health Forum [41] estimated that 72% of UK adults will be overweight or obese by 2035. The obesity uplift is predicted to increase the number of new cancer cases over 20 years by 670 000 along with other chronic diseases. It is estimated that 1% annual reduction from the predicted trend could avoid around 64 200 cancer cases over the next 20 years, with a potential economic saving of £2.5 billion.

Legislation

Further avenues to cancer prevention are through legislation. An example of this is the 'sugar tax' in England. In 2016, the UK government announced a new taxation system for sugary drinks. In addition to combating the growing proportion of

Table 26.4 Manchester Cancer Prevention strategy grid (3 × 3 × 3).

Levels (x3)	3 x 3	Tier	Illustrative examples
Population	Prevalence (reducing risk factors)	Primary	Meat consumption reduction at population level; population-level weight control and increased physical activity.
		Secondary	Weight-reduction interventions in populations with colorectal polyps/ endometrial hyperplasia.
		Tertiary	Lifestyle and smoking cessation interventions among cancer survivors.
	Political and cultural changes	Primary	Legislation, e.g. smoking ban; fortification of foodstuffs.
		Secondary	Population-level awareness of cancer-related symptoms leading to earlier-stage diagnosis.
		Tertiary	Regulation/monitoring of radiation doses received by cancer survivors and prevention of second primary cancers.
	Public health strategies	Primary	HPV vaccination against cervical cancer; some cancer screening programmes, e.g. colonoscopy and colorectal cancer.
		Secondary	Cancer screening programmes, e.g. breast cancer screening.
		Tertiary	Cancer surveillance programmes among chronic patients, e.g. anal cancer among male homosexuals and HIV-positive patients.
Patient	Gene penetrance and genetic risk assessment	Primary	Identification of high-penetrance inheritable cancer syndromes.
		Secondary	Identification of low-penetrance genetic predisposition followed by enhanced cancer screening.
		Tertiary	Identification of allelic polymorphisms that determine tamoxifen efficiency.
	Prophylaxis	Primary	Thyroidectomy among children with MEN type 1 syndrome; hysterectomy in women with Lynch syndrome; procto-colectomy in FAP family members; bilateral mastectomy in *BRCA* carriers.
		Secondary	Bilateral oophorectomy to reduce ovarian metastases among patients with rectal cancer.
		Tertiary	Total colectomy in patients with two or more synchronous nonhereditary colorectal cancers.

Continued

Table 26.4 Continued

	Chemo-prevention	Primary	Aspirin use over age 50 years and the prevention of colorectal cancer.
		Secondary	Nonchemotherapy agents (e.g. tamoxifen) and the reduction of cancer recurrence.
		Tertiary	Aromatase inhibitor use in breast cancer survivors to reduce risk of contra-lateral breast cancer.
Personalized	**Profiling individual risk**	Currently research only	The research target here is combining lifestyle and genetic information to maximize risk stratification.
	Prescription		The research target is personalized cancer risk reduction. For example, weight control and cancer prevention is likely to vary by gender.
	Time period and adherence		The research target here is around timing (when in adulthood) of cancer prevention intervention. For example, early-life adiposity might be inversely while later-life adiposity is positively associated with postmenopausal breast cancer.

FAP, familial adenomatous polyposis; HPV, human papilloma virus; MEN, multiple endocrine neoplasia syndrome.
Primary prevention: preventing the disease developing through tackling the social and behavioural determinants at a public health level.
Secondary prevention: early detection of the disease at a presymptomatic stage, e.g. cost-effective population screening programmes.
Tertiary prevention: cost-effective management of disease, reducing the impact of the disease post-diagnosis.

obesity in the UK, especially among children, this initiative will have a large impact on various chronic diseases in adults, such as diabetes and cardiovascular disease, as well as cancer. The consumption of sugary drinks has been increasing worldwide, and its relation to the obesity epidemic has been established [42]. Opposition from industry has, as expected, been strong, keeping implementation of such a tax at bay for most nations globally. Outside of Europe, Chile and Mexico have implemented similar sugar taxes, and preliminary results show positive impacts of taxation in reducing sugar sales. Although the health impacts remain to be assessed (including those on cancer), these initiatives are ground-breaking, with opportunities to prevent future cancers in hundreds of thousands of people worldwide.

Table 26.5 WCRF recommendations on weight, physical activity, and diet to reduce cancer risk.

Weight	Keep your weight as low as you can within the healthy range
Physical activity	Be physically active for at least 30 minutes every day, and sit less
High-calorie foods and drinks	Limit high-calorie foods and avoid sugary drinks
Fruit and vegetables	Eat a wide variety of whole grains, vegetables, fruits, and pulses such as beans
Red meat	Eat no more than 500 g (cooked weight) a week of red meat and eat little, if any, processed meat
Alcohol	If you do drink, limit alcoholic drinks to two for men and one for women a day
Salt	Limit your salt intake to less than 6 g (2.4 g sodium) a day by adding less salt and eating less food processed with salt
Supplements	Eat a healthy diet rather than relying on supplements to protect against cancer

Source: World Cancer Research Fund 2009 [40].

References

1 World Cancer Research Fund (2007). Food, nutrition, physical activity, and the prevention of cancer: A Global Perspective, 2e. Washington, CD: American Institute for Cancer Research.

2 World Cancer Research Fund (n.d.). Continuous Update Project findings and reports. http://www.wcrf.org/int/research-we-fund/continuous-update-project-findings-reports (accessed 26 October 2016).

3 Renehan, A.G., Leitzmann, M.F., and Zwahlen, M. (2012). Re: body mass index and risk of lung cancer among never, former, and current smokers. *J. Natl Cancer Inst.* 104 (21): 1680–1681; author reply 1.

4 Menvielle, G., Boshuizen, H., Kunst, A.E. et al. (2009). The role of smoking and diet in explaining educational inequalities in lung cancer incidence. *J. Natl Cancer Inst.* 101 (5): 321–330.

5 Bingham, S.A., Luben, R., Welch, A. et al. (2003). Are imprecise methods obscuring a relation between fat and breast cancer? *Lancet* 362 (9379): 212–214.

6 Vandenbroucke, J.P., von Elm, E., Altman, D.G. et al. (2007). Strengthening the Reporting of Observational Studies in Epidemiology (STROBE): Explanation and elaboration. *Ann. Intern. Med.* 147 (8): W163–W194.

7 Renehan, A.G., Harvie, M., Cutress, R.I. et al. (2016). How to manage the obese patient with cancer. *J. Clin. Oncol.* 34 (35): 4284–4294.

8 Renehan, A.G., Zwahlen, M., and Egger, M. (2015). Adiposity and cancer risk: New mechanistic insights from epidemiology. *Nat. Rev. Cancer* 15 (8): 484–498.

9 Akbartabartoori, M., Lean, M.E., and Hankey, C.R. (2005). Relationships between cigarette smoking, body size and body shape. *Int. J. Obes.* 29 (2): 236–243.

10 Renehan, A., Tyson, M., Egger, M. et al. (2008). Body mass index and incidence of cancer: A systematic review and meta-analysis of prospective observational studies. *Lancet* 371 (9612): 569–578.

11 Lauby-Secretan, B., Scoccianti, C., Loomis, D. K. et al. (2016). Body fatness and cancer: Viewpoint of the IARC Working Group. *N. Engl. J. Med.* 375 (8): 794–798.

12 Campbell, P.T., Newton, C.C., Freedman, N.D. et al. (2016). Body mass index, waist circumference, diabetes, and risk of liver cancer for U.S. Adults. *Cancer Res.* 76 (20): 6076–6083.

13 Kitahara, C.M., McCullough, M.L., Franceschi, S. et al. (2016). Anthropometric factors and thyroid cancer risk by histological subtype: Pooled analysis of 22 prospective studies. *Thyroid* 26 (2): 306–318.

14 Aune, D., Greenwood, D.C., Chan, D.S. et al. (2012). Body mass index, abdominal fatness and pancreatic cancer risk: A systematic review and non-linear dose-response meta-analysis of prospective studies. *Ann. Oncol.* 23 (4): 843–852.

15 World Cancer Research Fund (2014). Continuous Update Project report: Food, nutrition, physical activity, and the prevention of ovarian cancer. London: World Cancer Research Fund and American Institute for Cancer Research.

16 World Cancer Research Fund International (2014). Continuous Update Project report: Diet, nutrition, physical activity, and prostate cancer. London: World Cancer Research Fund.

17 Park, J., Morley, T.S., Kim, M. et al. (2014). Obesity and cancer: Mechanisms underlying tumour progression and recurrence. *Nat. Rev. Endocrinol.* 10 (8): 455–465.

18 Keum, N., Greenwood, D.C., Lee, D.H. et al. (2015). Adult weight gain and adiposity-related cancers: A dose-response meta-analysis of prospective observational studies. *J. Natl Cancer Inst.* 107 (3): pii: djv088.

19 Keimling, M., Renehan, A.G., Behrens, G. et al. (2013). Comparison of associations of body mass index, abdominal adiposity, and risk of colorectal cancer in a large prospective cohort study. *Cancer Epidemiol Biomarkers Prevent.* 22 (8): 1383–1394.

20 Song, M., and Giovannucci, E. (2016). Estimating the influence of obesity on cancer risk: Stratification by smoking is critical. *J. Clin. Oncol.* 34 (27): 3237–3239.

21 Renehan, A.G., Soerjomataram, I., and Leitzmann, M.F. (2010). Interpreting the epidemiological evidence linking obesity and cancer: A framework for population-attributable risk estimations in Europe. *Eur. J. Cancer* 46 (14): 2581–2592.

22 Arnold, M., Pandeya, N., Byrnes, G. et al. (2015). Global burden of cancer attributable to high body-mass index in 2012: A population-based study. *Lancet Oncol.* 16 (1): 36–46.

23 Ezzati, M., Henley, S.J., Lopez, A.D., and Thun, M.J. (2005). Role of smoking in global and regional cancer epidemiology: Current patterns and data needs. *Int. J. Cancer* 116 (6): 963–971.

24 de Martel, C., Ferlay, J., Franceschi, S. et al. (2012). Global burden of cancers attributable to infections in 2008: A review and synthetic analysis. *Lancet Oncol.* 13 (6): 607–615.

25 Renehan, A.G., Flood, A., Adams, K.F. et al. (2012). Body mass index at different adult ages, weight change, and colorectal cancer risk in the National Institutes of Health-AARP Cohort. *Am. J. Epidemiol.* 176 (12): 1130–1140.

26 Bouvard, V., Loomis, D., Guyton, K.Z. et al. (2015). Carcinogenicity of consumption of red and processed meat. *Lancet Oncol.* 16 (16): 1599–1600.

27 Chan, D.S., Lau, R., Aune, D. et al. (2011). Red and processed meat and colorectal cancer incidence: Meta-analysis of prospective studies. *PLoS One* 6 (6): e20456.

28 Gallus, S., and Bosetti, C. (2016). Meat consumption is not tobacco smoking. *Int. J. Cancer* 138 (10): 2539–2540.

29 Alexander, D.D., Weed, D.L., Miller, P.E., and Mohamed, M.A. (2015). Red meat and colorectal cancer: A quantitative update on the state of the epidemiologic science. *J. Am. Coll. Nutr.* 34 (6): 521–543.

30 Carr, P.R., Walter, V., Brenner, H., and Hoffmeister, M. (2016). Meat subtypes and their association with colorectal cancer: Systematic review and meta-analysis. *Int. J. Cancer* 138 (2): 293–302.

31 Falk, R.T., Maas, P., Schairer, C. et al. (2014). Alcohol and risk of breast cancer in postmenopausal women: An analysis of etiological heterogeneity by multiple tumor characteristics. *Am. J. Epidemiol.* 180 (7): 705–717.

32 Li, C.I., Chlebowski, R.T., Freiberg, M. et al. (2010). Alcohol consumption and risk of postmenopausal breast cancer by subtype: The Women's Health Initiative observational study. *J. Natl Cancer Inst.* 102 (18): 1422–1431.

33 World Cancer Research Fund (2013). Continuous Update Project report: Food, nutrition, physical activity, and the prevention of endometrial cancer. London: World Cancer Research Fund and American Institute for Cancer Research.

34 World Cancer Research Fund (2015). Continuous Update Project report: Diet, nutrition, physical activity, and liver cancer. London: World Cancer Research Fund and American Institute for Cancer Research.

35 World Cancer Research Fund (2012). Continuous Update Project report: Food, nutrition, physical activity, and the prevention of pancreatic cancer. London: World Cancer Research Fund and American Institute for Cancer Research.

36 Goralczyk, R. (2009). Beta-carotene and lung cancer in smokers: Review of hypotheses and status of research. *Nutr. Cancer* 61 (6): 767–774.

37 Giovannucci, E. (2010). Epidemiology of vitamin D and colorectal cancer: Casual or causal link? *J. Steroid Biochem. Mol. Biol.* 121 (1–2): 349–354.

38 World Cancer Research Fund (2010). Continuous Update Project report: Food, nutrition, physical activity, and the prevention of colorectal cancer. London: World Cancer Research Fund and American Institute for Cancer Research.

39 Toledo, E., Salas-Salvado, J., Donat-Vargas, C. et al. (2015). Mediterranean diet and invasive breast cancer risk among women at high cardiovascular risk in the PREDIMED trial: A randomized clinical trial. *JAMA Intern. Med.* 175 (11): 1752–1760.

40 World Cancer Research Fund (2009). Policy and action for cancer prevention. Food, nutrition and physical activity: A global perspective. Washington, DC: American Institute for Cancer Research.

41 Cancer Research UK (2016). Tipping the scales: Why preventing obesity makes economic sense. London: Cancer Research UK, UK Health Forum.

42 Imamura, F., O'Connor, L., Ye, Z. et al. (2015). Consumption of sugar sweetened beverages, artificially sweetened beverages, and fruit juice and incidence of type 2 diabetes: Systematic review, meta-analysis, and estimation of population attributable fraction. *BMJ* 351: h3576.

CHAPTER 27

Risk profiling for cancer prevention and screening – lessons for the future

Rosalind A. Eeles[1], Paul Pharoah[2], Alison Hall[3], Susmita Chowdhury[4], and Hilary Burton[3]

[1] The Institute of Cancer Research, The Royal Marsden NHS Foundation Trust, London, UK
[2] Centre for Cancer Genetic Epidemiology, University of Cambridge, Cambridge, UK
[3] PHG Foundation, Cambridge, UK
[4] West Suffolk NHS Foundation Trust; PHG Foundation, Cambridge, UK

SUMMARY BOX

Genetic predisposition to cancer: The models

- Genetic predisposition to cancer incorporates both common and rarer genetic variants, which have low and higher relative risks of cancer, respectively.

- Large consortia have been very effective in finding the lower-risk common variants, which are important for stratifying populations in order to target screening to population strata.

- Risk profiling models predict that population stratification should improve the efficiency of population screening and reduce overdiagnosis.

- Rarer, higher-risk mutations have implications for cascade testing of family members.

- Targeted screening studies incorporating genetic profiling in the coming years will have implications for public health implementation of mass genetic analysis, and this will require wider ethico-legal and social consideration.

- Risk profiling will also enable targeted prevention: primary or secondary.

- Education of health-care professionals and the public will be essential in the implementation.

Genetic predisposition to cancer: The models

Evidence that there is a genetic predisposition to common and rare cancers comes from several sources. There is epidemiological evidence of an increased relative risk at all common cancer sites to relatives of cases [1]. This risk rises as the age of

---

Cancer Prevention and Screening: Concepts, Principles and Controversies, First Edition.
Edited by Rosalind A. Eeles, Christine D. Berg, and Jeffrey S. Tobias.

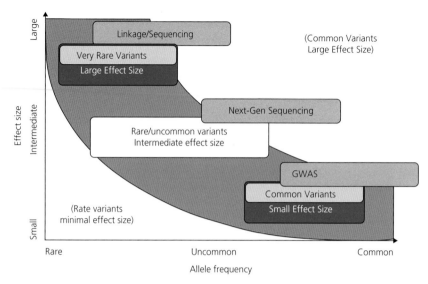

Figure 27.1 Finding the full spectrum of genetic variants in complex disease.GWAS, genome-wide association study.

the proband case decreases and as the number of cases in a family increases. In many common cancers, this rise in relative risk as these variables alter is too large to be due solely to a shared environment [2]. Manolio has proposed a model of genetic predisposition where some genetic variants are common (present in >5%) in the population, but each variant individually increases relative risk (RR) by only a small amount (often a RR of 1.2 or less); however, as such variants are common, often individuals harbour more than one variant and the risk from each is log additive or multiplicative. This can lead to cumulative, large relative risks at the extremes of the population distribution.

Other genetic variants are much rarer (<<1% of the population) and confer a larger RR (often over threefold). There is now evidence also of variants of intermediate frequency and intermediate RR [3] in many of the common cancers (1–5%). This is illustrated in Figure 27.1, together with the techniques used to find these variants [4].

Distribution of genetic risk in a population

The distribution of genetic risk to common cancers in the general population is similar to that for height. The distribution of absolute height values ranges from the extremes of very tall to very short compared with the average, with most individuals' values falling in the middle of the distribution; that is, a normal distribution. It is the same for the distribution of absolute risk of a common cancer in the general population. The cases of cancer have a risk distribution which is shifted to the right of this general population risk curve [5]. To date there are thousands of common genetic variants throughout the genome, which are described in the GWAS catalogue [6]. Most of these are noncoding and the mechanism by which they increase cancer risk is thought to be due to regulation of gene expression. Mapping of these variants on the regulatory parts of the genome has shown that they are preferentially sited in regulatory regions [7].

Rare cancers do not follow this pattern, as the genetic predisposition is rare and confers a high risk to those who harbour the genetic mutation.

Identification of those at risk of cancer due to a genetic predisposition

Those individuals with rarer genetic mutations have genetic variants which confer higher absolute risk to the person carrying the variant, and therefore if it has been inherited it is likely to have caused cancer in other family members. Consideration needs to be given regarding cascade testing of other family members. Furthermore, higher-risk variants are more likely to cause cancer earlier and on multiple occasions (see Table 27.1).

The probability that a germline genetic variant will cause the development of a cancer is called the penetrance. For most germline genetic variations, the penetrance is less than 100% (incomplete penetrance); for some conditions it nearly approaches this value (e.g. familial adenomatous polyposis with 100% penetrance for colorectal cancer by age 35; Li-Fraumeni syndrome with 90% penetrance in women by age 60). The penetrance for specific genetic mutations can be complicated by the context (for example, there are variable penetrance figures for different strengths of family history, which may be due to modifier genes altering the effect of the mutation [8]; and studies of gene–environment interactions have shown that some mutations are altered by the environment, for example the risk of cancer in *TP53* mutation carriers is increased by smoking).

Table 27.1 Features of genetic variation conferring cancer risk.

Variant Frequency	Lifetime Relative Risk of Cancer from the Variant	Features
Rare	≥Threefold	Younger onset of cancer than general population Multiple tumours Strong family history (multiple cases; clear lineage)
Common	≤Twofold	Cancers may occur at younger age but not always Less likely to have a strong family history No clear lineage

Technical aspects

The development of next-generation sequencing technologies and the mapping of genetic variation across the genome (the HapMap project of common human genetic variation and the Human Genome Project for sequencing of the human genome) have created a reference set of genetic variation. This was undertaken in several populations across the globe, and is used to compare the results of genetic analysis in test research sample sets or clinical samples to determine if the variants found are benign normal human variation or likely to be disease-associated variants. Studies to identify common genetic variation involve case-control analyses of large sample sets genotyped using gene chips containing thousands of single-nucleotide changes across the genome – so-called genome-wide association studies (usually over thousands of samples as the per allele odds ratio is low, as already noted) – and as the number of data points is large, the p value for genome-wide significance is stringent at $<p\ 5\times10^{-8}$ to minimize false discovery rates. The identification of intermediate/rarer germline genetic variation is now undertaken using next-generation sequencing and comparing the frequency of mutations in samples from cancer cases and population controls (Figure 27.1). Formerly linkage was used, which is the co-inheritance of segments of the genome with the disease phenotype. Since the advance of next-generation sequencing, linkage is now rarely used. The dilemma in efforts to identify such variants is that these can be present at low frequency in the normal population and not all may be disease causing. Tools are used to determine if such variation is more likely to be pathogenic: (1) pathogenic mutations are more often (but not always) disruptive to the reading of the genetic code, such as insertions, deletions, or nonsense mutations; (2) they are more likely to be in conserved regions of the genome (conserved across species); (3) computer models such as predictive programs which predict protein structure can model the effect of the genetic mutation on protein product crystal structure; and (4) functional assays on the *in vitro* and *in vivo* effects of the mutation can be used to predict downstream effects.

The classification of variants is one of the major challenges in genomics at present. This is crucial to determine which variants are clinically actionable, and therefore are important for targeting screening and management for higher-risk individuals and testing of relatives.

Plon et al. [9] have published an algorithm for classification of variants from Classes 1 to 5, with 5 being pathogenic (see Table 27.2). Class 4 has a 95–99% probability of pathogenicity. Classes 4 and 5 are reported and used in clinical decision-making (with clear counselling advice that Class 4 is not 100% certainty of pathogenicity) and, depending on the mode of inheritance, in some cases it may be appropriate to proactively identify other family members who might be at risk of disease, and would benefit from genetic testing to clarify whether they carry the genetic variant in question.

Table 27.2 Proposed classification system for sequence variants identified by genetic testing.

Class	Label of Classification	Probability of Pathogenicity
5	Pathogenic	1.00
4	Likely pathogenic	0.95–0.99
3	Uncertain	0.05–0.949
2	Likely not pathogenic	0.001–0.049
1	Not pathogenic	<0.001

Class 3 variants are not reported by all laboratories, and to date most variants turn out to be nonpathogenic on further research. Since Class 3 variants are in the intermediate zone between nonpathogenic and probably pathogenic, these are the most likely to alter over time with further research (research on segregation with disease and functional assays), so many laboratories keep them under review. However, not all laboratories do undertake regular review of Class 3 and 4 variants, and when tests are ordered the geneticist has to be cognizant of this so that they know if they need to review the results over time.

Risk profiling models and stratification effects on the screening paradigm

Common genetic variation is predicted to be most useful for stratifying populations into risk groups, whereas rarer variation is more relevant to individual risk currently. Numerous GWAS have yielded thousands of variants across the genome associated with increased disease risk, and typing of these can be used to divide the population into sectors of risk [5]. Figure 27.2 shows the risk distribution of a population typed for common variants, and demonstrates how the normal distribution of risk is moved to the right in cases versus controls in prostate cancer [10].

Pharoah [5] has modelled the population risk distribution for breast cancer and, assuming all the susceptibility genes were identified, the population in the half of the risk distribution at highest risk would account for 88% of all affected individuals.

Studies of targeted screening in populations profiled for common variants are starting to be reported; for example, in breast cancer, Evans et al. [11] have undertaken a study, PROCAS, to demonstrate whether SNP profiling (genotyping of the single-nucleotide polymorphisms [SNPs] and subsequent calculation of the polygenic risk score) in women would enable targeted mammography to find more cancers in the higher-risk strata. Studies are also under way in prostate cancer

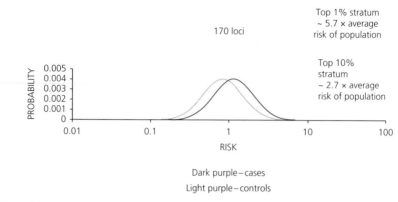

Figure 27.2 Prostate cancer risk prediction.

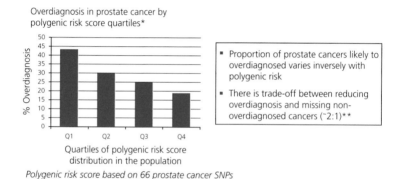

Figure 27.3 Polygenic risk and overdiagnosis: Prostate cancer.* Pashayan 2015 [13].
** Pashayan 2015 [14]. Source: Pashayan et al_https://www.ncbi.nlm.nih.gov/pmc/articles/
PMC4430305/-CC BY 3.0.

following feasibility studies in men with a family history of the disease [12].
Pashayan et al. [13, 14] have reported that the use of SNP profiling in a population should reduce the risk of overdiagnosis, and that this is particularly so in the
lower-risk quartile (Figure 27.3).

This group has also modelled the health economics of SNP profiling a population in order to target screening to those in the highest-risk strata versus using
merely an aged-based approach, and has shown that the former has a greater
efficacy at reducing overdiagnosis and therefore should be more beneficial on a
health economic assessment [15].

While rarer germline genetic variants are important for individuals and their
blood relatives as they confer high relative risks, for population screening these
rare variants have less impact, as they are rarer than common variants. The

exception is a population with a higher mutation frequency due to founder mutations. For example, a study in London of the Ashkenazim with four Ashkenazi grandparents who were tested for the founder mutations in the *BRCA1* and *BRCA2* genes showed that 2.5% had a mutation which is 10 times more frequent than in non-Ashkenazim from the same country [16]. Carriers of rarer genetic mutations have a level of cancer risk that warrants more intensive screening, which is often outside of the population screening age groups; for example, breast screening using a more sensitive technology (magnetic resonance imaging, MRI) from the age of 30 years as opposed to population screening using only mammography from age 47 (see Chapter 11).

As next-generation sequencing becomes more widespread, testing for rarer variants will progress from single gene sequencing to multiple genes (panel testing, which is starting to be undertaken, particularly in private health-care systems) to whole exome to whole genome. At present many health-care providers, particularly in public systems, are only offering single-gene sequencing. Multiple commercial platforms are now providing gene panels for particular diseases, for instance multiple cancer gene panels. The dilemma with such tests is that for some of the genes in the panel there is controversy about the precise penetrance estimates that should be quoted, and therefore the particular screening that should be offered (e.g. mutations in *PALB2, ATM*), and the high rate of variants of uncertain significance (Class 3 variants – see earlier discussion). Initiatives such as The 100,000 Genomes Project delivered by Genomics England, which aims to sequence 100 000 whole genomes, and the International Cancer Genome Consortium (tumour sequencing of whole genomes of various cancers worldwide with corresponding germline sequences), which are presently research initiatives, are likely to be brought into the clinical care pathway in the future; indeed, plans for integration of whole-genome sequencing within the NHS are already under way [17].

One development which requires much more evaluation is the extent to which those undergoing genomic sequencing for clinical reasons should also be offered the opportunity to have 'additional findings' actively sought and returned to them. As part of The 100,000 Genomes Project, this is currently being done on a research basis, and the findings being looked for include the rare high-penetrance variants in the *BRCA1* and *BRCA2* genes, which confer a high likelihood of developing breast cancer in affected individuals. Another consideration is how to manage the increasing volume of variants of uncertain significance which are likely to be generated. The question of how variants of uncertain significance should be dealt with in the face of an evolving evidence base is not trivial, since this will become increasingly burdensome as more DNA is sequenced. In the future, a significant amount of data will need to be reanalysed given that mutation-calling computer programs are imperfect, particularly those which call insertions and deletions, which is the majority of the Class 4 and 5 mutations.

Prevention

The use of risk profiling can target prevention, both primary, which is the administration of preventive surgery or medication to prevent a cancer occurring, and secondary prevention, which is screening to detect cancer earlier. The previous chapters outline the primary and secondary prevention strategies in each cancer site.

Ethical, legal, and social aspects

The addition of a range of modifiers including lifestyle and environmental factors to genetic profiling using susceptibility variants could allow the stratification of the population according to risk and, it is postulated, could be used in population cancer prevention programmes.

Conceptually, risk-stratified screening brings another dimension to Geoffrey Rose's approaches to prevention [18]. In his classic paper he highlighted two contrasting approaches. The first was a high-risk approach, which aimed to segregate 'a minority with special problems [at high risk of developing disease] from a majority who are regarded as normal and not needing attention'. This requires some means by which such high-risk individuals may be identified and the application of an intensive intervention such as prophylactic drug treatment to this group. Rose warned that the high-risk interventions would, at the very least, cause inconvenience and anxiety to individuals, and may even harm them. His second, contrasting approach aimed to shift the whole population risk through some generalized intervention, such as an overall change in diet. Both primary and secondary prevention in which an undifferentiated offer is made to the whole population may come into the second category.

The further dimension added by systematic stratification based on risk profiling is that following risk assessment offered to the whole population, individuals would be assigned to different strata or risk groups, each with their own package of care. Thus those at lower risk would receive minimal or no intervention, while those at higher risk might receive a more intensive, or potentially harmful or costly intervention. This is balanced against the greater potential benefit derived from using the intervention in this higher-risk group. There might be various gradations for strata in between low and high risk. The theoretical advantage of such an approach at a population level would be increased effectiveness, while minimizing harm and increasing cost-effectiveness.

Screening programmes characteristically involve the unsolicited offer of a screening test to large populations that are relatively undifferentiated, except for major features such as age or sex. In most countries of the developed world, the introduction of new programmes or the modification of existing ones is guided by systems of decision-making usually based on the original Wilson and Jungner screening criteria [19]. These establish a framework for judging the utility of an intervention based on the importance of the condition, the performance of the proposed screening test, the effectiveness of the intervention, and aspects related to the programme as a whole. Critical to such judgements are considerations of the practicality of implementing such a programme and its acceptability to patients and professionals. The PHG Foundation used results from consortia studies of common genetic variants (the COGS studies) associated with breast and prostate cancers to model risk-stratified prevention for these cancers [20]. Their report showed from focus group discussions [21] that such strategies would require consideration of the use and storage of genetic information, development of accurate risk assessment tools, new protocols for consent, and programmes of professional education and public engagement [22, 23].

The introduction of some form of risk assessment and stratification as a preliminary to the offer of the screening intervention *per se* is considered in what follows in the context of breast cancer screening programmes, using evidence derived from analysis of potential models for implementation. In particular, a number of ethical, legal, and social (ELS) issues would need to be considered before deciding to modify current programmes. As a preliminary, it is noted that the evidence for the benefit of mammography in breast cancer detection for the general population is controversial [24], and that 'all measures for primary prevention' should be considered first as ways of reducing breast cancer morbidity and mortality; for breast cancer this would include advice about alcohol intake, exercise, and avoidance of obesity.

As shown earlier in this chapter, when specifically applied to breast screening, modelling showed that stratified screening programmes based on age and genetic risk had the potential to improve the efficiency and benefit–harm ratio of a mammography screening programme. Such a stratified approach to prevention, while attractive, is more complex to implement than existing age-based programmes, and brings with it a new set of ELS dimensions, particularly when involving genetic biomarkers. At the very least it involves a two-step approach: administration of the risk assessment tool, followed by the offer and provision of the appropriate preventive intervention.

The ELS issues that arise depend to some extent on how the risk stratification is implemented. For stratification based on genomic susceptibility, all models require a DNA sample to be taken and analysed, relevant data to be obtained and interpreted so that the individual can be assigned to a risk stratum, and then the offer and provision of the indicated level and type of intervention. For example, stratified approaches might mean that women at higher risk commence screening at an earlier age, have more frequent mammography or a different modality of testing such as MRI, and continue to an older age [21, 22, 25].

An important variable that will underpin consideration of ELS issues is the breadth of genetic sampling and the subsequent management of the resulting samples and data. A possible model would be a 'targeted, disposable' model, where genotyping is performed using limited variants for a single disease, promptly analysed, and then routinely destroyed, retaining only the risk score. An alternative model would involve wider genetic testing (possibly even whole-genome testing), potentially providing information on risk for a whole range of conditions in addition to breast cancer. In this model, genotypic and phenotypic data may be retained for subsequent analysis for different purposes over an individual's lifetime. Such purposes may relate to the individual and to the wider population. The data could include information relevant to personal health or treatment of disease, or they could be stored in a database that may be used for health service or research purposes: for example, understanding genotype–phenotype interaction, disease epidemiology and natural history, or response to preventive or treatment interventions [25].

In the following discussion of ELS issues, those that are contingent on the particular model will be highlighted. Ethical challenges arising from breast screening programmes that incorporate some form of genetic testing include, among other things, data security; respect for autonomy and obtaining meaningful consent; minimizing harm and optimizing benefit; and the principle of justice, ensuring that practice is fair, equitable, and appropriate [25].

Privacy, data security, and storage

The issues relating to the use of genomic data differ significantly between the two models described earlier. In the 'targeted, disposable' model, such issues are relatively modest, being similar to the processing of other predictive health information. If genetic variant data are destroyed, then foreseeable harms (namely that an individual's privacy may be breached if identifiable genetic information is disclosed, particularly if it is linked to personal or health data such as disease or lifestyle) would be much decreased, although care would have to be taken to protect against disclosure of the risk score, which could be potentially stigmatizing. However, in the second 'wider testing and storage model', a much larger range of issues would arise, including identifying the individual from whom the data have come, but would expand to include data security and potential access by third parties. As well as the need to have systems to safeguard data security, it will be necessary also to carefully control such aspects as duration of storage and samples and/or identifiable data, and to closely monitor arrangements for access by legitimate third parties, including other health services, insurers or employers, family members, and wider research use, whether academic or commercial.

Autonomy and consent

Individuals offered risk-stratified screening should understand what is proposed and the potential consequences, both pros and cons. Processes for seeking consent should reflect the breadth of testing that will be undertaken; the target condition for screening; the potential for unrelated or incidental findings; and any implications of risk assessment results for employment or insurance. In the 'targeted disposable' model, the potential consequences of testing are relatively circumspect and immediate, therefore simpler to communicate and understand, and so will have fewer (but still important) ethical implications. In the 'wider testing and storage' scenario, there are many more implications that individuals need to understand before they can give consent. For example, what the potential is for subsequent recontact over findings that may or may not be related to the initial question of breast cancer risk; how predictive information might be fed back and whether this might affect family members; how data might be used for secondary purposes, for example by researchers or other third parties; and whether there is potential for discrimination or stigmatization, for example by insurers charging higher premiums for those at higher risk. At present in the UK a voluntary concordat and moratorium [26] prevents insurers who are members of the Association of British Insurers from requesting predictive genetic tests or disclosure of results of existing tests in presymptomatic individuals; this seems likely to cover genomic tests generated for risk stratification. However, this is a voluntary arrangement and is currently under review.

Minimizing harm and optimizing benefit from risk information

With a two-step approach of risk assessment followed by intervention, it is most likely that the individual will be informed of their risk or risk group and advised about the most appropriate preventive intervention. A number of social factors come into play at this point, when the individual needs to react to their risk information and take appropriate and informed action.

For breast cancer, this stage requires that people understand their personal risk, receive and understand information about screening options available and those that might be most suitable for their level of risk, and decide, with appropriate advice, whether or not to take up the screening offered. Important aspects to understand include risk perception: their concept of risk and the accuracy with which they perceive it; their psychological reaction to personal risk information; and their response in terms of health-seeking behaviour, which may be a change in lifestyle or acceptance of the offer of mammography. To date there is no empirical evidence on these aspects for genetically stratified breast screening, but some inferences can be made from studies of other circumstances. For example, in diabetes prevention, communication of genetic risk based either on genotype or on phenotype did not motivate changes in behaviour, such as increase in physical activity or improvements in self-reported diet or weight. On the other hand, it was reassuring that such information did not cause anxiety or worry in the participants [26].

To aid people in the understanding of their own personal risk, it seems clear that good communication tools will be required in a variety of formats (verbal, written, computer based). For risk assessment, there will need to be underlying health literacy and it will be important that genomic concepts are grasped, at least at a very basic level [22, 23]. There is some general concern that communication of genetic risk information may lower perceived control over the preventability and treatability of disease or may precipitate feelings of fatalism; or, conversely, that feedback of normal or a low risk of disease may lead to false reassurance, which may discourage behaviour change and possibly lead to people ignoring early symptoms of disease. A systematic meta-analysis in 2011 using the limited evidence available concluded that there was no impact of personalized genomic information on perceived control in either the short or longer term, or on the perceived effectiveness of behaviour interventions [27].

With regard to the subsequent uptake of the recommended screening programme, there is no empirical evidence about the impact of knowledge of risk arising from common genetic variants. A Cochrane systematic review of personalized risk communication in screening (not including genetic information) showed that this did increase informed choice, but not necessarily the uptake of screening [28]. However, there is some evidence in the case of breast cancer that receiving evidence about personal risk, derived from models that include age, family history, and standard phenotypic risk factors, increased the uptake of screening in women assessed as being at high risk of the disease [29].

Justice, equity, and appropriateness

Genetically stratified screening also raises wider issues of justice, equity, and appropriateness. Particularly where large-scale national screening programmes are involved, there needs to be transparency about the criteria by which particular screening policies are adopted and implemented which take demonstrable account of these three factors. Some potentially problematic areas include the need to be inclusive of population subgroups, the need for cultural sensitivity, and the need to manage individuals at low risk, especially those who may have been eligible for screening under a stratification programme based on age, but who are ineligible based on a risk-based assessment.

Various subpopulations may be disadvantaged by a genetic risk–stratified approach. Those from ethnic backgrounds other than white Caucasian may be effectively excluded from risk assessment because relevant variants in their population were not included in the original research on which the subsequent risk estimates were based. Others with less health or genetic literacy, possibly associated with low socio-economic status or educational background, may find the programme less accessible because of the complexity of decision-making required. It is therefore important to identify how such groups might be supported to participate, possibly through the provision of culturally or educationally appropriate materials or through targeted forms of engagement.

Finally, there are important concerns about how the programme would continue to engage with low-risk individuals, particularly those whose initial risk assessment may have led to advice not to undergo mammographic screening. This group remains at risk of disease, and should be encouraged to understand how adopting healthy lifestyle approaches might minimize this risk, as well as the potential benefits involved. Even more problematic will be how the programme deals with the inevitability of such low-risk women subsequently developing cancer. In order not to undermine the wider trust in these services, it will be vital that effective communication strategies are in place for all programme participants, explaining that for women judged to be at low risk, the potential harms due to false positives and unnecessary investigation actually outweigh the potential benefits for breast cancer detection and prevention.

Conclusion

Genetic predisposition to cancer involves both common and rarer genetic variants, which have low and higher relative risks of cancer, respectively. Large consortia have been very effective in finding the lower-risk common variants, which are important for stratifying populations in order to target screening to population strata. Risk profiling models predict that population stratification should improve the efficiency of population screening and reduce overdiagnosis. Rarer, higher-risk mutations have implications for cascade testing of family members. Targeted screening studies incorporating genetic profiling in the coming years will have implications for public health implementation of mass genetic analysis, and this will require wider ethico-legal and social considerations.

The ability to use genetic variants to stratify individuals according to cancer risk can provide an opportunity for cancer prevention in which preventive interventions are offered according to risk. This may increase the efficiency of interventions offered. A case study is presented for stratified breast cancer screening where it is shown that the ethical dimensions of this depend on how the risk data are used and potentially stored. Issues include privacy, data security and storage, how to promote autonomy and consent and the broad areas of justice, equity and appropriateness. This case study is based on theoretical modeling but will provide a framework for the issues that should be considered if stratified cancer screening is to be implemented.

Education of health-care professionals and the public will be essential in this implementation.

References

1 Goldgar, D.E., Easton, D.F., Cannon-Albright, L.A., and Skolnick, M.H. (1994). Systematic population-based assessment of cancer risk in first-degree relatives of cancer probands. *J. Natl Cancer Inst.* 86 (21): 1600–1608.

2 Carter, B.S., Beaty, T.H., Steinberg, G.D. et al. (1992). Mendelian inheritance of familial prostate cancer. *Proc. Natl Acad. Sci. U. S. A.* 89 (8): 3367–3371.

3 Turnbull, C., and Rahman, N. (2008). Genetic predisposition to breast cancer: Past, present, and future. *Annu. Rev. Genomics Hum. Genet.* 9: 321–345.

4 Hindorff, L.A., Gillanders, E.M., and Manolio, T.A. (2011). Genetic architecture of cancer and other complex diseases: Lessons learned and future directions. *Carcinogenesis* 32 (7): 945–954.

5 Pharoah, P.D., Antoniou, A., Bobrow, M. (2002). Polygenic susceptibility to breast cancer and implications for prevention. *Nature Genet.* 31 (1): 33–36.

6 National Human Genome Research Institute (2018). GWAS Catalog: The NHGRI-EBI Catalog of published genome-wide association studies. http://www.ebi.ac.uk/gwas/ (accessed 3 January 2018).

7 Han, Y., Hazelett, D.J., Wiklund, F. et al. (2015). Integration of multiethnic fine-mapping and genomic annotation to prioritize candidate functional SNPs at prostate cancer suscepti-bility regions. *Hum Mol. Genet.* 24 (19): 5603–5618.

8 Lecarpentier, J., Silvestri, V., Kuchenbaecker, K.B. et al. (2017). Prediction of breast and prostate cancer risks in male BRCA1 and BRCA2 mutation carriers using polygenic risk scores. *J. Clin. Oncol.* 35 (20): 2240–2250.

9 Plon, S.E., Eccles, D.M., Easton, D. et al. (2008). Sequence variant classification and report-ing: Recommendations for improving the interpretation of cancer susceptibility genetic test results. *Hum. Mutat.* 29 (11): 1282–1291.

10 Schumacher, F., Al Olama, A.A., Berndt, S.I. et al. (2018). Association analyses of more than 140,000 men identify 63 new prostate cancer susceptibility loci. *Nat Genet.* doi: 10.1038/s41588-018-0142-8. [Epub ahead of print].

11 Evans, D. Gareth, A.S., Stavrinos, P. et al. (2016). Improvement in risk prediction, early detection and prevention of breast cancer in the NHS Breast Screening Programme and family history clinics: A dual cohort study. *Programme Grants Appl. Res.* 4 (11).

12 Castro, E., Mikropoulos, C., Bancroft, E.K. et al. (2016). The PROFILE feasibility study: Targeted screening of men with a family history of prostate cancer. *Oncologist* 21 (6): 716–722.

13 Pashayan, N., Duffy, S.W., Neal, D.E. et al. (2015). Implications of polygenic risk-stratified screening for prostate cancer on overdiagnosis. *Genet. Med.* 17 (10): 789–795.

14 Pashayan, N., Pharoah, P.D., Schleutker, J. et al. (2015). Reducing overdiagnosis by polygenic risk-stratified screening: Findings from the Finnish section of the ERSPC. *Br. J. Cancer* 113 (7): 1086–1093.

15 Pashayan, N., and Pharoah, P. (2012). Population-based screening in the era of genomics. *Pers. Med.* 9 (4): 451–455.

16 Manchanda, R., Loggenberg, K., Sanderson, S. et al. (2015). Population testing for cancer predisposing BRCA1/BRCA2 mutations in the Ashkenazi-Jewish community: A randomized controlled trial. *J. Natl Cancer Inst.* 107 (1): 379.

17 Genomics England (n.d.) What can participants find out? https://www.genomicsengland.co.uk/taking-part/results/ (accessed 3 January 2018).

18 Burton, H., Sagoo, G.S., Pharoah, P., and Zimmern, R.L. (2012). Time to revisit Geoffrey Rose: Strategies for prevention in the genomic era? *Ital. J. Public Health* 9(4).

19 Wilson, J.M.G., and Jungner, G. (1968) Principles and practice of screening for disease. *Public Health Papers*. Geneva: World Health Organization.

20 Pashayan, N., Hall, A., Chowdhury, S. et al. (2013). Public health genomics and personalized prevention: Lessons from the COGS project. *J. Intern. Med.* 274 (5): 451–456.

21 Chowdhury, S., Dent, T., Pashayan, N. et al. (2013). Incorporating genomics into breast and prostate cancer screening: Assessing the implications. *Genet. Med.* 15 (6): 423–432.

22 Burton, H., Chowdhury, S., Dent, T. et al. (2013). Public health implications from COGS and potential for risk stratification and screening. *Nature Genet.* 45 (4): 349–351.

23 Chowdhury, S., Henneman, L., Dent, T. et al. (2015). Do health professionals need additional competencies for stratified cancer prevention based on genetic risk profiling? *J. Pers. Med.* 5 (2): 191–212.

24 Independent UKPoBCS (2012). The benefits and harms of breast cancer screening: An independent review. *Lancet* 380 (9855): 1778–1786.

25 Hall, A.E., Chowdhury, S., Hallowell, N. et al. (2014). Implementing risk-stratified screening for common cancers: A review of potential ethical, legal and social issues. *J. Public Health* 36 (2): 285–291.

26 Godino, J.G., van Sluijs, E.M., Marteau, T.M. et al. (2016). Lifestyle advice combined with personalized estimates of genetic or phenotypic risk of type 2 diabetes, and objectively measured physical activity: A randomized controlled trial. *PLoS Med.* 13 (11): e1002185.

27 Collins, R.E., Wright, A.J., and Marteau, T.M. (2011). Impact of communicating personalized genetic risk information on perceived control over the risk: A systematic review. *Genet. Med.* 13 (4): 273–277.

28 Edwards, A.G., Naik, G., Ahmed, H. et al. (2013). Personalised risk communication for informed decision making about taking screening tests. *Cochrane Database Syst. Rev.* 2 (Art. No.: CD001865). doi: 10.1002/14651858.CD001865.pub3.

29 Evans, D.G., Donnelly, L.S., Harkness, E.F. et al. (2016). Breast cancer risk feedback to women in the UK NHS breast screening population. *Br. J. Cancer* 114 (9): 1045–1052.

CHAPTER 28

Cancer prevention and screening: Advances to carry forward

Christine D. Berg[1], Rosalind A. Eeles[2], and Jeffrey S. Tobias[3]

[1] Division of Cancer Epidemiology and Genetics, National Cancer Institute, National Institutes of Health, Maryland, USA
[2] The Institute of Cancer Research, The Royal Marsden NHS Foundation Trust, London, UK
[3] Department of Oncology, University College London; University College Hospital Foundation Trust, London, UK

The global burden of cancer is increasing as other causes of death such as infectious diseases are brought under control. Additionally, as many countries become Westernized, such as with the adoption of cigarette smoking and dietary patterns, cancer incidence increases [1]. Importantly, international differences in cancer incidence have led to an understanding of the variable environmental and genetic causes of malignancy. As the aetiology of cancer has been better understood, methods targeted at prevention have improved. The prevention of malignancy is preferable to either early detection or effective treatment, both of which have drawbacks. Early detection has led to declines in cancer mortality for the diseases for which effective approaches have been developed and implemented. Cancer screening modalities have built on the success of the Papanicolaou cytological screening for cervical cancer. The technology of diagnostic imaging modalities and image recognition has improved accuracy, lowered or eliminated radiation exposure, and made many devices more affordable. As an indication of success of cancer detection and improved treatment modalities, the burden of second cancer in survivors, particularly of those with paediatric malignancies, is an increasing problem for which approaches are being developed. An overview of the advances made and the successes achieved in cancer prevention and screening is a useful coda to this book. Details of these advances and their impacts have been chronicled excellently and extensively by our authors and can be found in their specific chapters.

Different health systems approach cancer control differently, but certain policies that can improve results can be brought to bear [2]. Registries to document the nature and magnitude of the cancer burden in the specific region are needed and should be of high quality. This allows the government or health-care system to focus resources and to evaluate progress, or lack thereof. High-quality treatment

Cancer Prevention and Screening: Concepts, Principles and Controversies, First Edition.
Edited by Rosalind A. Eeles, Christine D. Berg, and Jeffrey S. Tobias.
© 2019 John Wiley & Sons, Inc. Published 2019 by John Wiley & Sons, Inc.

that is accessible to the population is also critical. Screening without referral networks for diagnosis and treatment is not useful. Inequality of access based on economic constraints and cultural barriers can be significant impediments to population-based approaches.

Tobacco control has had great success, but more needs to be done. The discoveries of the viral aetiology of several malignancies, cervical, oropharyngeal, and hepatocellular cancer being the prime examples, have led to the development of successful vaccines. Vaccine programmes have varied by country. For example, Australia has a widely adopted human papilloma virus (HPV) vaccination programme, which has led to some evidence of herd immunity [3]. Anal cancer, while rare, is more prevalent in certain demographic groups, such as men who have sex with men. Screening of this group with cytology and digital examination may prove to be efficacious and vaccination strategies should also help. The discovery of the role of *Helicobacter pylori* in the pathogenesis of gastric cancer was a major advance, and a straightforward antibiotic regimen can eliminate colonization with the pathogen. However, in many Western countries stomach cancer incidence had fallen even prior to this discovery. The cause of this decline is presumed to be food refrigeration, but it has not been definitively elucidated. Unfortunately, an uptick in carcinoma of the gastric fundus has been noted in younger cohorts in the USA [4].

Exposure to carcinogens can also occur through environmental means such as airborne pollution, for example ozone, and particulates, which can increase the risk of lung cancer. The Boston-based Health Effects Institute, and the Institute of Health Metrics and Evaluation based at the University of Washington, released a report detailing environmental deaths around the world due to pollution [5]. The estimate is that for 2015 more than 4.2 million people died prematurely. Coal burning, home heating, and exhaust from vehicular traffic are major culprits. Renewable energy sources and a transition to electric vehicles should help lower the disease burden. This will be a major undertaking spanning decades. It should also have an ameliorative effect on the progress of climate change as a side benefit to decreasing cancer incidence and other adverse health outcomes. Occupational exposures are also associated with a variety of cancers. Well-known examples include mesothelioma from asbestos and lung cancer from diesel exhaust. In countries with well-developed occupational health and safety programmes these problems are on the decline; however, continued vigilance is warranted, as regulations can be unwound [6].

A spreading problem is the obesity epidemic. While it is well known to be associated with diabetes and cardiovascular disease, there are also links to many cancers. The enlarging list includes endometrial, breast, kidney, liver, gall-bladder, pancreas, ovary, thyroid, multiple myeloma, meningioma, and colorectal. The UK has the dubious distinction of now having the highest rate in the world for adenocarcinomas of the lower oesophagus, thought to be related to increased reflux from abdominal obesity [7]. Effective public health approaches to obesity are sought, for instance improvement in the built environment to encourage exercise, such as bicycle paths for commuting.

Chemoprevention is an additional approach. Both oestrogenic and androgenic modifiers have been shown to lower the risk of their respective sex-linked cancers. Neither, though, has found widespread acceptance. Tamoxifen for breast cancer prevention is associated with an increased risk of venous thromboembolism and endometrial cancer. Five-alpha reductase inhibitors have been studied for prostate cancer prevention, but may be associated with an increase in the risk of high-grade disease [8].

Cervical cancer screening commenced at the time of the development of the Papanicolaou smear. Early pre-invasive lesions can be detected and successfully treated with procedures targeting the cervical *os*, so not only has the mortality declined, the incidence has declined as well. This is even amid a sexual revolution which has changed practices in many locales. However, trends in sub-Saharan African countries for which there are reliable data show a different picture [9].

Colorectal cancer is another malignancy for which the screening modalities, such as sigmoidoscopy and colonoscopy, can remove premalignant adenomas and have led to a decline in the incidence of the disease. Uptake of colorectal cancer screening in the population is uneven. Colonoscopy is preceded by an unpleasant bowel cleansing preparation. Some programmes that embrace noninvasive stool testing, such as FIT or FIT accompanied by stool DNA testing, have more acceptance in some populations. Also for countries without the capacity for colonoscopy screening of the population, these noninvasive tests can be implemented in a widespread fashion and the sensitivity targeted to the availability of follow-up procedures [10].

A very controversial screening test, the prostate specific antigen blood test, has been shown to have a benefit in decreasing prostate cancer mortality, with the downside of an increase in the detection of low-grade malignancies which may be so indolent as to not influence life expectancy (overdiagnosis). Also, false positives are a problem leading to invasive biopsies, which can be associated with an increased risk of infection. The European Randomized Study of Prostate Cancer (ERSPC) showed a 20% decline in mortality with every four-year screening compared to no screening. A similar study, the Prostate, Lung, Colorectal and Ovarian Cancer Screening Trial (PLCO) in the USA, had a very high level of contamination in the control group. This eliminated the ability to determine whether there would be a benefit from screening. In the USA the advent of prostate-specific antigen (PSA) screening, which had extensive uptake, was associated with a subsequent decline in men presenting with advanced/metastatic prostate cancer. The US Preventive Services Task Force (USPSTF) recommended against screening in the elderly with limited life expectancies, and then later expanded to advising against routine screening, although physicians were informed that they could discuss the controversies with their patients and informed decisions could be made on an individual basis, particularly in those with family histories of the disease or those of African American ancestry, who are at higher risk. Recently, the USPSTF 'D' Recommendation has been revised to a 'C' in its draft statement, which more reflects the role for informed-decision making [11]. The controversies in this common cancer are discussed further in Chapter 13.

Breast cancer screening has been subject to more randomized clinical trials (RCTs) with a total of more participants than any other screening test. Screening with mammography has been definitively proven to lower breast cancer mortality in women between 40 and 70 in Western developed countries. Many countries have breast cancer screening programmes. Some of these programmes are run by government health systems and others, such as in the USA, are through insurance-based mechanisms. Breast cancer mortality has fallen in many Western countries. The available evidence suggests that this is a result of a combination of treatment and screening. The focus now is balancing benefits and harms [12]. This can be accomplished by less frequent screening; for example, in those with less-dense breasts. Also, more sensitive techniques such as breast tomosynthesis can be employed in those with denser breasts. Magnetic resonance imaging (MRI) is more sensitive, but has a higher rate of false positives and is more expensive, so is reserved usually for the highest-risk subset.

Ovarian cancer screening is also a subject of intense research. The long-awaited UK Collaborative Trial of Ovarian Cancer Screening (UKCTOCS) study shows promise with a multimodal approach. In one arm of the study, the 'Risk of Ovarian Cancer' algorithm (ROCA) is employed: a woman's own CA-125 serves as a baseline and is measured annually, and with certain levels or changes ovarian ultrasound is added. This arm was the multimodal screening (MMS). Another arm was transvaginal ultrasound (USS) annually. There were 50% of the women in the control, no-screening group. This very well-done, large study (202 638 women) shows an encouraging decline, albeit small, in ovarian cancer mortality at 14 years (MMS 15%; USS 11%) [13]. There was a significant stage shift in the MMS arm compared to control. Risk-reducing salpingo-oophorectomy is highly effective in those at high risk: for example, those with *BRCA1* and *BRCA2* mutations were found in a cohort study to have a 77% decrease in all-cause mortality by age 70 [14]. Screening is highly unlikely to develop to the point where mortality reduction of that scale can be achieved in the high-risk population.

A problem with many screening strategies is overdiagnosis. This refers to finding indolent cancers that individuals may die with but not from. The frequency of this problem cannot be determined outside the context of an RCT. Long follow-up of these RCTs is also required after the screening stops, to allow catch-up of the clinically important cancers in the control group. With the advent of widespread computerized tomographic (CT) testing in many countries, because of the enhanced diagnostic potential of these imaging tests an example of a cancer found with increasing frequency is thyroid cancer. A new report on trends in thyroid cancer incidence and mortality rates used data from the Surveillance, Epidemiology, and End Results-9 (SEER-9) cancer registry programme. There was evidence for both overdiagnosis and an increase in incidence and mortality in the more aggressive cancers [15]. The reason for this increase is unknown. There is a rationale for revision of the terminology referring to low-grade papillary carcinoma and no longer considering it a malignancy, given the outstanding prognosis [16].

The most notable success has come with effective tobacco control policies in developed countries such as the USA. The landmark World Health Organization (WHO) Framework on Tobacco Control can be used as a model globally to further lower the burden from smoking-related diseases [17]. The list of smoking-related cancers continues to grow. In the USA, lung cancer in males has been falling and lung cancer in females has begun to decline. An emerging issue is that as the population of former smokers age, they remain at risk of lung cancer, and a growing fraction of lung cancers occur in the former-smoking population. This further emphasizes the need for effective public health measures to ensure that younger generations never start smoking. However, the current epidemic will be with us for some time.

Electronic cigarettes emerged onto the market with great fanfare. There are mixed opinions as to their benefits and harms. Considering them as an interim strategy for coming off a nicotine addiction has intuitive appeal. One of the habits of smoking, having something in your hand that you can bring to your mouth rather than a cookie, is satisfied with e-cigarettes. Nevertheless, there is still a need for subsequent cessation. Since e-cigarettes have not been on the market very long, there are little data on their harms. There are concerns regarding inhalation of the solvent and the potential for pulmonary and liver damage with intense use or long-term use. Again, there is intuitive appeal to strong discouragement of the young from taking up the habit, as continual exposure could well turn out to be detrimental in ways not predicted.

The President of Uruguay has instituted a very successful tobacco control programme since he assumed office. His background as a physician had made him very aware of the dreadful toll of tobacco products. The programme is multipronged and a part includes new warning labels on cigarettes and other tobacco products, and limitations on tobacco-product advertising. Tobacco company Philip Morris chose to sue Uruguay as violating a free-trade agreement between Switzerland and Uruguay. Uruguay won in a global court. The health of a country's public was deemed important, and the measures Uruguay took to improve it were deemed to over-ride free-trade concerns [18]. This achievement sends a strong message to other governments implementing aspects of tobacco control and the WHO Framework. Also, environmental and occupational hazards can contribute to premature deaths, including cancers, and countries may be able to utilize the same logic as tobacco control to regulate these hazards as well without running foul of trading partner concerns.

Even with effective tobacco control, lung cancer will remain a scourge in former smokers for many decades. Targeted treatments and immunotherapies have made inroads on mortality rates. Screening for lung cancer has finally, after decades of studies, been definitively shown to reduce lung cancer mortality. The US National Cancer Institute funded a National Lung Screening Trial which showed a 20% decrease in lung cancer mortality in a high-risk population after three annual low-dose CT scans. CT screening in these high-risk groups is now reimbursed in the USA by many insurance companies and Medicare [19].

Many European countries are awaiting the findings of the Dutch–Belgian randomized lung cancer screening trial, Nederlands-Leuvens Longkanker Screenings Onderzoek (NELSON), prior to making decisions about screening [20]. Improved risk stratification and perhaps other markers of early detection could make the process more efficient. Currently, screening programmes are technically challenging to set up and administer. Countries with more limited public health resources may choose to focus on tobacco control efforts until the screening process becomes less costly.

Tobacco chewing is very prevalent in many societies and leads to oral cancers being the sixth most common malignancy in the world. Other aetiological factors include alcohol, areca nut, and HPV. Tobacco control initiatives do target these other forms of tobacco. HPV-related oropharyngeal malignancy has emerged as a growing problem, thought to be related to changes in sexual practice. As HPV16 is the strain that is the causative factor for HPV-related oropharyngeal malignancy, it is thought that widespread vaccination, being undertaken primarily for cervical cancer prevention and wart prevention, may lower the incidence of this cancer as well, but of course trends in the incidence of the disease need to be carefully followed [21]. A variety of oral potentially malignant lesions (OPML) like leukoplakia, erythroplakia, and submucosal fibrosis may precede oral cancers. This has led to research on a variety of approaches for early detection, none of which have proven useful to date.

The genetics and genomic revolutions have led to a better understanding of the hereditary cancer syndromes and to the better stratification of cancer risk assessment in the population. The discovery of the *BRCA1* and *BRCA2* genes, which confer high lifetime risks of breast and ovarian cancer, has resulted in testing recommendations for families at high risk and calls for screening in certain high-risk populations, such as the Ashkenazim [22]. Prophylactic surgery with risk-reducing salpingo-oophorectomy and bilateral mastectomies has proved efficacious. In fact, cohort data suggest that oophorectomy is associated with a lowering of overall mortality [14]. Colorectal cancer is also increased in hereditary cancer syndromes such as Lynch and hereditary polyposis. Genetic testing of probands and then family members who may be gene carriers is recommended. More frequent colonoscopy is advocated. Total colectomy may be warranted in individuals with a disease such as ulcerative colitis.

As next-generation sequencing has emerged, genetic polymorphisms associated with increased risk of malignancy have been delineated [23]. These are most frequently single-nucleotide polymorphisms (SNPs). However, copy number variation, epigenetic mechanisms, may also be found to confer hereditary risks. Polygenic risk scores (PRS) have been developed as the number of SNPs discovered has increased. These PRS distribute in a Gaussian normal distribution, with those individuals with few disease-associated SNPs having low risk and those with numerous SNPs having high risk. It is unclear if either of these two groups could benefit from different screening frequencies, respectively fewer or more with more sensitive tests such as MRI for breast cancer.

As the fields of cancer prevention, early detection, and genetic evaluation become more complex, communication to health-care providers and the public is critical [24]. The proliferation of research and the increase in the rapidity of dissemination of findings due to electronic media add to the challenge. The lack, for the most part in many regions, of a well-educated populace with literacy and numeracy skills adequate to understand some of the inherent complexities increases the obstacles. Budget constraints and other governmental priorities need to be considered as well.

The future should be even more exciting than the current advances we could cover in this book. The challenges are clear, but the opportunities are enormous.

References

1 Global Burden of Disease 2013 Mortality and Causes of Death Collaborators (2015). Global, regional and national age-sex specific all-cause and cause-specific mortality for 240 causes of death, 1990–2013: A systematic analysis for the Global Burden of Disease Study 2013. *Lancet* 385: 117–171.

2 World Health Organization (2002). *National cancer control programmes: Policies and managerial guidelines.* Geneva: WHO.

3 Garland, S.M. (2014). The Australian experience with the human papillomavirus vaccine. *Clin. Ther.* 36: 17–23.

4 Anderson, W.F., Camargo, M.C., Fraumeni, J.F., Jr et al. (2010). Age-specific trends in incidence of noncardia gastric cancer in US adults. *JAMA* 303: 1723–1728.

5 Health Effects Institute (2017). *State of global air 2017: Special report.* Boston, MA: Health Effects Institute.

6 Fingerhut, M., Nelson, D.I., Driscoll, T. et al. (2006). The contribution of occupational risks to the global burden of disease: Summary and next steps. *Med. Lav.* 97: 313–321.

7 Arnold, M., Soerjomataram, I., Ferlay, J. et al. (2015). Global incidence of oesophageal cancer by histological subtype in 2012. *Gut* 64: 381–387.

8 Lazzeroni, M., and DeCensi, A. (2016). Alternate dosing schedules for cancer chemopreventive agents. *Semin. Oncol.* 43: 116–122.

9 Vaccarella, S., Laversanne, M., Ferlay, J. et al. (2017). Cervical cancer in Africa, Latin America and the Caribbean, and Asia: Regional inequalities and changing trends. *Int. J. Cancer* 141 (10): 1997–2001.

10 Alberti, L.R., Garcia, D.P., Coelho, D.L. et al. (2015). How to improve colon cancer screening rates. *World J. Gastrointest. Oncol.* 15: 484–491.

11 U.S. Preventive Services Task Force (2017). Draft recommendation statement: Prostate cancer screening. https://www.uspreventiveservicestaskforce.org/Page/Document/RecommendationStatementDraft/prostate-cancer-screening1 (accessed 24 July 2017).

12 U.S. Preventive Services Task Force (2016). Breast cancer: Screening. https://www.uspreventiveservicestaskforce.org/Page/Document/UpdateSummaryFinal/breast-cancer-screening1 (accessed 24 July 2017).

13 Jacobs, I.J., Menon, U., Ryan, A. et al. (2016). Ovarian cancer screening and mortality in the UK Collaborative Trial of Ovarian Cancer Screening (UKCTOCS): A randomised controlled trial. *Lancet* 387: 945–956. Erratum in *Lancet* (2016) 387: 944.

14 Finch, A.P., Lubinski, J., Møller, P. et al. (2017). Impact of oophorectomy on cancer incidence and mortality in women with a BRCA1 or BRCA2 mutation. *JAMA* 317: 1338–1348.

15 Lim, H., Devesa, S.S., Sosa, J.A. et al. (2017). Trends in thyroid cancer incidence and mortality in the United States, 1974–2013. *JAMA* 317: 1338–1348.

16 Nikiforov, Y.E., Seethala, R.R., Tallini, G. et al. (2016). Nomenclature revision for encapsulated follicular variant of papillary thyroid carcinoma: A paradigm shift to reduce overtreatment of indolent tumors. *JAMA Oncol.* 2: 1023–1029.

17 World Health Organization (2005). WHO Framework Convention on Tobacco Control. http://www.who.int/fctc/cop/about/en/ (accessed 24 July 2017).

18 Wikipedia (2017). Philip Morris v. Uruguay. https://en.wikipedia.org/wiki/Philip_Morris_v._Uruguay (accessed 24 July 2017).

19 Tanoue, L.T., Tanner, N.T., Gould, M.K. et al. (2015). Lung cancer screening. *Am. J. Respir. Crit. Care Med.* 191: 19–33.

20 Veronesi, G. (2015). Lung cancer screening: The European perspective. *Thorac. Surg. Clin.* 25: 161–174.

21 Guo, T., Eisele, D.W., and Fakhry, C. (2016). The potential impact of prophylactic human papillomavirus vaccination on oropharyngeal cancer. *Cancer* 122: 2313–2323.

22 Gabai-Kapara, E., Lahad, A., Kaufman, B. et al. (2014). Population-based screening for breast and ovarian cancer risk due to BRCA1 and BRCA2. *Proc. Natl Acad. Sci. U. S. A.* 111: 14205–14210.

23 Chatterjee, N., Shi, J., García-Closas, M. (2016). Developing and evaluating polygenic risk prediction models for stratified disease prevention. *Nat. Rev. Genet.* 17: 392–406.

24 Kissane, D.W., Bultz, B.D., Butow, P.N. et al., ed. (2017). *Oxford Textbook of Communication in Oncology and Palliative Care*, 2e. Oxford: Oxford University Press.

Index

Note: Page numbers in *italic* denote figures, those in **bold** denote tables.

Cancer Prevention and Screening: Concepts, Principles and Controversies, First Edition.
Edited by Rosalind A. Eeles, Christine D. Berg, and Jeffrey S. Tobias.
© 2019 John Wiley & Sons, Inc. Published 2019 by John Wiley & Sons, Inc.

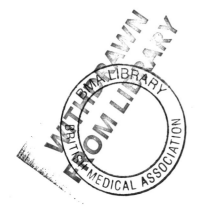